Handbook of Pediatric Surgery

Handbook of Pediatric Surgery

Editor: Aden Breland

AMERICAN
MEDICAL PUBLISHERS
www.americanmedicalpublishers.com

AMERICAN
MEDICAL PUBLISHERS
www.americanmedicalpublishers.com

Cataloging-in-Publication Data

Handbook of pediatric surgery / edited by Aden Breland.
p. cm.
Includes bibliographical references and index.
ISBN 979-8-88740-157-7
1. Children--Surgery. 2. Infants--Surgery. 3. Surgery, Operative.
4. Children--Diseases--Treatment. I. Breland, Aden.
RD137 .H36 2023
617.98--dc23

American Medical Publishers,
41 Flatbush Avenue,
1st Floor, New York,
NY 11217, USA

ISBN 979-8-88740-157-7 (Hardback)

Contents

Preface

The purpose of the book is to provide a glimpse into the dynamics and to present opinions and studies of some of the scientists engaged in the development of new ideas in the field from very different standpoints. This book will prove useful to students and researchers owing to its high content quality.

Pediatric surgery is a surgical subspecialty that deals with the surgery of fetuses, infants, children, adolescents, and young adults. It is used for the treatment of several pediatric diseases, including congenital malformations, abdominal wall defects, pectus excavatum and separation of conjoined twins. It also focuses on childhood tumors such as neuroblastoma, Wilms' tumor, rhabdomyosarcoma, liver tumors, teratomas and kidney tumor. There are mainly two sub categories that fall under pediatric surgery, namely, neonatal surgery and fetal surgery. Neonatal surgery involves the medical care of newborn infants, particularly who have illness or were born premature. Fetal surgery is a type of pediatric surgery that is used for the treatment of birth defects in fetuses. This book provides significant information of this discipline to help develop a good understanding of pediatric surgery. A number of latest researches have been included to keep the readers up-to-date with the global concepts in this branch of surgery. The book is an essential guide for both medical professionals and students.

At the end, I would like to appreciate all the efforts made by the authors in completing their chapters professionally. I express my deepest gratitude to all of them for contributing to this book by sharing their valuable works. A special thanks to my family and friends for their constant support in this journey.

Editor

1

Robotic Assisted Surgery in Pediatric Urology: Current Status and Future Directions

*Catherine J. Chen and Craig A. Peters**

Pediatric Urology, Children's Health System Texas, University of Texas Southwestern, Dallas, TX, United States

***Correspondence:**
Craig A. Peters
craig.peters@utsouthwestern.edu

The evolution of robotic surgical technology and its application in Pediatric Urology have been rapid and essentially successful. Further development remains limited in three key areas: procedural inefficiencies, cost and integration of surgical and clinical information. By addressing these challenges through technology and novel surgical paradigms, the real potential of surgical robotics in pediatric, as well as adult applications, may ultimately be realized. With this evolution, a continued focus on patient-centered outcomes will be essential to provide optimal guidance to technical innovations.

Keywords: robotic surgery, pyeloplasty, ureteral reimplantation, pediatric, minimally invasive surgery

BACKGROUND

Robot assisted surgical systems have revolutionized minimally invasive surgery, providing many advancements, including three-dimensional visualization, elimination of surgeon tremor, wristed instruments, and improved surgeon ergonomics. Since the first Intuitive Surgical da Vinci® surgical system was approved by the Food and Drug Administration in 2000, robot assisted surgery has been embraced by surgeons worldwide. As of September 30, 2017, 4,271 da Vinci® units have been installed, with 65% of these units installed in the United States, 17% in Europe, 15% in Asia, and 3% in the rest of the world (1).

The initial application of robot assisted surgery in the field of urology began with adult robot assisted prostatectomies and was soon applied to the pediatric population with robot assisted pyeloplasties (2). In pediatric urology, robot assisted surgery has subsequently been reported for ureteral reimplant, ureteroureterostomy, appendicovesicostomy creation, bladder neck reconstruction, and augmentation ileocystoplasty (3–8). In addition, robot assisted procedures have been reported in infants and as well as with 5 mm robotic instruments (9, 10).

Over the past 20 years, there has been continued improvement in robot assisted surgical systems with Intuitive Surgical releasing several upgrades and several other companies developing competing robotic platforms (11). As with all technological advances in medicine, patient-centered outcomes must be critically assessed and limitations identified so that technology can be continuously improved. Current limitations in robot assisted surgery can be distilled into three major categories: procedural inefficiencies, cost, and integration of surgical information.

PATIENT-CENTERED OUTCOMES

As the most common robot assisted surgery performed in children, robot assisted pyeloplasty has a more robust literature compared to that of other procedures; however, published studies are case series and not randomized controlled trials (12). Furthermore, these different studies used different criteria of outcomes such as resolution of pain, decrease in hydronephrosis on ultrasound, improved MAG3 lasix scans, duration of surgical procedure, duration of hospitalization, or use of postoperative pain medications, making meta-analysis difficult.

While the number of robot assisted ureteral reimplants is increasing in the United States, the literature demonstrates mixed results, with some groups reporting similar reflux resolution rates and other groups reporting inferior resolution rates compared to known open reimplant reflux resolution rates (3, 13–16). The variation of outcomes likely is secondary to variation in surgical technique, grades of reflux, and criteria used to evaluate resolution.

In order to truly assess patient outcomes, such as disease resolution, pain, and recovery, as well as compare results to that of open procedures, it is paramount for future research to clearly delineate all potential factors that can affect outcomes in order to accurately evaluate the efficacy of robot assisted pediatric urological surgery. As research consortia develop, it is critical for study protocols to be clearly defined so that data from different institutions can be combined. Current limitations in the literature center on the lack of consistency in terms of preoperative pathology grading as well as postoperative follow-up and definition of resolution.

In addition to disease resolution, there has been a small focus on scar location and robotic trocar placement to minimize visible scars. In many open procedures in pediatric urology, the incision site can often be placed in a location that can be easily hidden. The hidden incision endoscopic surgery (HIDES) trocar placement allows for the incision site of the trocar to be placed in a similar easily to conceal location on the abdomen while skiving in the subcutaneous fat and entering through the fascia at a higher more optimal location for robotic assisted surgery (17). In a recent survey of the general population regarding incision location for pediatric urologic surgery, many preferred incisions that could be covered by undergarments; however, this study fails to address that surgical incisions especially in children tend to heal well and fade over time (18). We have noticed in our patients who underwent laparoscopic surgery, that their port site incision scars are barely noticeable at follow-up appointments. While outcomes have been shown to be similar with the HIDES trocar placement, we recommend for surgeons especially at the beginning of their learning curve to use trocar placement locations that decrease the level of procedural difficulty (19).

LIMITATIONS: PROCEDURAL INEFFICIENCIES

A major roadblock in the implementation of robot assisted surgery to a wider spectrum of pediatric reconstructive urologic procedures centers on procedural inefficiencies. After demonstration of feasibility, any robot assisted surgical procedure is subsequently compared to the same procedure performed in an open fashion. While robot assisted pyeloplasties and less so, robot assisted ureteral reimplants have been well-integrated into the pediatric urology practice, other applications of robot assisted surgery fail to be adapted into routine practice mainly due to the extended time required to complete the procedure with robot assistance compared to the traditional open approach. This extended time can be attributed to procedural inefficiencies with robotic technology.

A key difference between open and robot assisted surgery is that in open surgery, the surgical assistant, either a trainee or a surgical first assist, actively facilitates the procedure, to allow the surgeon to perform the operation. This facilitation can range from staying still, retracting and stabilizing tissue, to active movement such as suture management, cutting, and suctioning. The key to this type of facilitation is that it is dynamic and involves an additional person working in tandem with the primary surgeon.

Our current use of the robot limits the use of an assistant and eliminates the ability for **dynamic facilitation**. While the use of the robotic fourth arm provides some facilitation in retraction, it is a static assist. If any changes need to be made, the surgeon must pause what they are currently doing to move the fourth arm, decreasing surgical efficiency.

In adult urology, the placement of additional laparoscopic ports allows for an active bedside assistant which has allowed for improved outcomes in complex procedures such as robot assisted partial nephrectomies. However, the reluctance to place additional ports due to cosmetic considerations in the pediatric population eliminates the role of a dynamic surgical facilitator. In an attempt to circumvent this limitation, many surgeons will use a hitch stitch to act as a retractor. While this technique is sufficient in simpler reconstructive procedures, the hitch stitch is static with limited ability to change positioning once it is placed.

One of the challenges of robot assisted surgical procedures is the inefficiency of suturing. Given the amount of limited working space, significant time can be spent pulling suture through as well as making sure that the suture does not tangle. While the impact is minimal in procedures with limited suturing, it can increase the surgical time significantly in cases that require large amounts of sewing, such as in robot assisted bladder augmentations.

Currently, robot assisted bladder augmentation has yet to be incorporated into routine practice due to the significant operative time needed to sew the bowel patch onto the bladder. When this procedure is performed in an open fashion, the dynamic facilitator assists the surgeon by ensuring the bowel segments are lined up to enable efficient throws as well as managing the suture and cinching down each throw so that the surgeon can focus on loading the needle and throwing the next stitch. The use of a dynamic surgical facilitator could potentially decrease operative time for this procedure robotically. Megaureter tapering is another procedure that requires increased suturing length as well as increased complexity.

There are many different approaches to improve sewing inefficiencies in robot assisted bladder augmentations. From a procedural approach, an immediate solution would be to place additional laparoscopic ports and have a bedside dynamic facilitator to assist with suture management. This does require a very skilled assistant who is completely familiar with the procedure. From a technological standpoint, development of a multi-arm surgical platform that allows for two surgeons to be operating robotically at the same time would enable robotic technology to incorporate dynamic facilitation. Currently, the

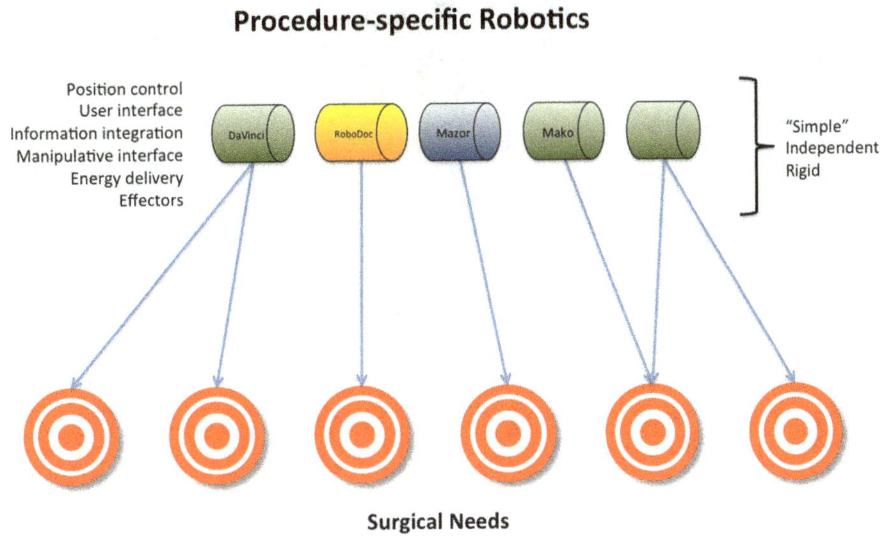

FIGURE 1 | Procedure-specific robotics.

operator sitting on the second console in a dual console system is only able to make changes in camera position while the primary surgeon console retains control over the working arms. The surgical assistant's role is significantly minimized and the assistant is often times more a spectator than a dynamic facilitator. Another technological solution might be development of a tool that could facilitate sewing and suture management.

Currently, there are two types of robotic instruments available: 5 and 8 mm instruments. In addition to the size difference, there are differences in the design of the instrument. While the 5 mm instruments are smaller, they have a different type of articulation mechanism, necessitating a larger radius of curve in order to make the similar movements compared to 8 mm instruments. This makes them suboptimal in smaller spaces such as in pediatric cases. Also, there are limited instrument options in the 5 mm size and the mechanical motion is less precise. The development of robotic instruments designed specifically for pediatric robot assisted surgery and small working spaces would be distinctly helpful. While there are studies demonstrating feasibility of 5 mm instruments in pediatric cases, many surgeons do not notice a significant difference in skin incision size and thus, use the 8 mm instruments because of more instrument options as well as increase ease of movement (10, 20). Although the first impression might be that such instruments would represent a small market, it is likely that they would find significant application in the evolving areas of adult oncological practice and reconstruction, such as trans-oral robotic procedures or endocrine surgery.

LIMITATIONS: COST

With healthcare costs increasing, we must evaluate the cost of surgical advancement. It is well-established that a robot assisted procedure costs more than its equivalent open procedure (12, 21). The majority of this is due to the high cost to purchase and maintain a robotic system and its disposable supplies. While the number of robot assisted cases are increasing, we are far from offsetting the significant cost of the robot platform.

With the da Vinci® system being the sole FDA-approved robot platform for urological surgery, it has had a monopoly on the market. There are also other robotic platforms that have been approved by the FDA; however, they are specialty and procedure specific and cannot be generally applied. The Flex® Robotic System is used and developed for transoral surgery and the Senhance™ Surgical Robotic System is designed for colorectal, transabdominal, and transthoracic procedures (11, 22–24). The inability to apply these robotic systems across specialties only increases the overall cost of healthcare. The ideal robot platform would be universal for all surgical and procedural specialties.

A potential solution to these challenges that push costs upward might be the development of robust modular robotic surgical systems. All current robotic systems involve two basic elements: positional control and end effectors (**Figure 1**). A modular robotic surgical system would integrate positional control with end-effectors that are designed to interact with specific anatomy, eliminating the need for procedure specific surgical systems (**Figure 2**). Such a design would be more cost-effective than the current designs that are limited to specific anatomy sites and procedures.

Furthermore, potentially lower value technological research and development also contributes to increased costs. While some have focused on haptics, ultimately, it is not the absence of haptics that is contributing to the ultimate problem of complex reconstructive cases taking significantly more time when performed with robot assistance compared to open surgery. There are many surrogates, such has visual cues of the tissue, that provide the same feedback to the surgeon.

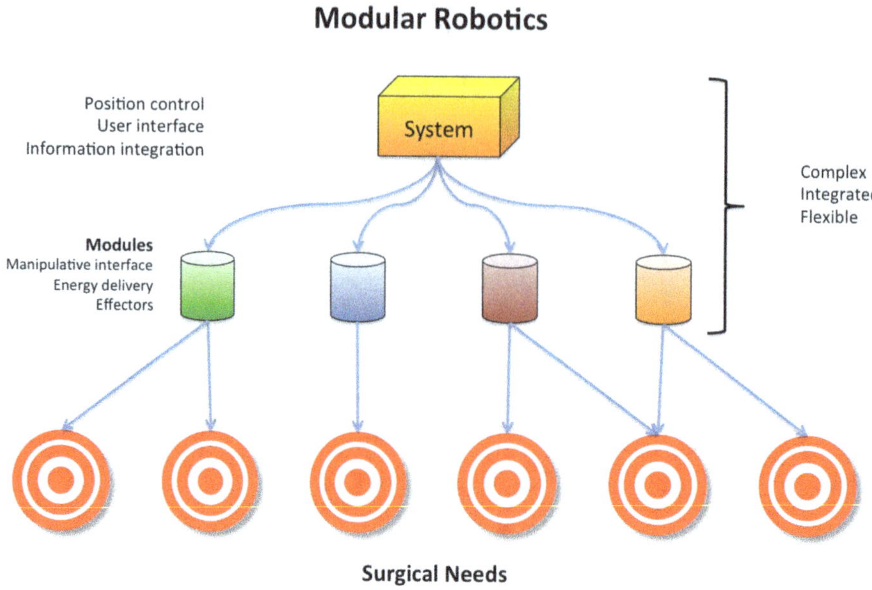

FIGURE 2 | Modular robotics.

Thus, it is crucial for surgeons to work with scientists and engineers to guide robotic advances. It is key for surgeons to step back and critically assess the barriers that we are encountering in procedures in order to better guide robotic research and development.

LIMITATIONS: INTEGRATION OF SURGICAL INFORMATION

Currently, the majority of surgeons use the robot as a surgical tool; however, there are adjunctive features that enhance the surgeon's ability to make surgical decisions, including Firefly™ and intraoperative ultrasound. The Firefly™ technology uses fluorescent aided imaging to help the surgeon identify vascular perfusion, which can help identify healthy tissue as well as normal vs. malignant tissue. The intraoperative ultrasound feature allows the surgeon to identify difficult to visualize structures. These technologies represent the simplest forms of informational integration in robotic surgery.

There is significant potential for the robot platform to become an information integration system, where digital imaging such as CT or MRI scans can be superimposed on the surgical field to allow for more precise surgical planning and mapping, as well as aid in difficult dissections. This allows the procedure to be personalized to the individual and the individual's pathology, and provides a more robust "view" of the surgical field. Even further informational integration may be feasible as well, with the fusion of anatomic and instrument positional data to facilitate surgical navigation. Autonomous or semi-autonomous actions of the robot have been explored and may further permit more efficient and effective interventions (25).

CONCLUSION

While robot assisted surgery has greatly improved minimally invasive surgery, we are far from perfecting this technology. Going forward, teamwork is key. Given the small procedural numbers at single pediatric institutions, the application of research consortia can help identify specific needs for surgical techniques to optimize outcomes. It is also critical to have open communication between physicians and engineers to develop new technology that will truly increase the applicability of robot assisted surgical technology.

AUTHOR CONTRIBUTIONS

CC researched and wrote the review. CP conceived the theme and key elements, reviewed, and edited the article.

REFERENCES

1. FAQ. Available online at: https://isrg.gcs-web.com/investor-faqs
2. Atug F, Woods M, Burgess SV, Castle EP, Thomas R. Robotic assisted laparoscopic pyeloplasty in children. *J Urol.* (2005) 174(4 Pt 1):1440–2. doi: 10.1097/01.ju.0000173131.64558.c9
3. Akhavan A, Avery D, Lendvay TS. Robot-assisted extravesical ureteral reimplantation: outcomes and conclusions from 78 ureters. *J Pediatr Urol.* (2014) 10:864–8. doi: 10.1016/j.jpurol.2014.01.028
4. Biles MJ, Finkelstein JB, Silva MV, Lambert SM, Casale P. Innovation in robotics and pediatric urology: robotic ureteroureterostomy for

duplex systems with ureteral ectopia. *J Endourol.* (2016) 30:1041–8. doi: 10.1089/end.2015.0645

5. Gundeti MS, Eng MK, Reynolds WS, Zagaja GP. Pediatric robotic-assisted laparoscopic augmentation ileocystoplasty and Mitrofanoff appendicovesicostomy: complete intracorporeal–initial case report. *Urology.* (2008) 72:1144–7; discussion: 1147. doi: 10.1016/j.urology.2008.06.070
6. Gundeti MS, Petravick ME, Pariser JJ, Pearce SM, Anderson BB, Grimsby GM, et al. A multi-institutional study of perioperative and functional outcomes for pediatric robotic-assisted laparoscopic Mitrofanoff appendicovesicostomy. *J Pediatr Urol.* (2016) 12:386.e1–e5. doi: 10.1016/j.jpurol.2016.05.031
7. Nguyen HT, Passerotti CC, Penna FJ, Retik AB, Peters CA. Robotic assisted laparoscopic Mitrofanoff appendicovesicostomy: preliminary experience in a pediatric population. *J Urol.* (2009) 182:1528–34. doi: 10.1016/j.juro.2009.06.055
8. Bagrodia A, Gargollo P. Robot-assisted bladder neck reconstruction, bladder neck sling, and appendicovesicostomy in children: description of technique and initial results. *J Endourol.* (2011) 25:1299–305. doi: 10.1089/end.2011.0031
9. Avery DI, Herbst KW, Lendvay TS, Noh PH, Dangle P, Gundeti MS, et al. Robot-assisted laparoscopic pyeloplasty: multi-institutional experience in infants. *J Pediatr Urol.* (2015) 11:139.e1–5. doi: 10.1016/j.jpurol.2014.11.025
10. Paradise HJ, Huang GO, Elizondo Sáenz RA, Baek M, Koh CJ. Robot-assisted laparoscopic pyeloplasty in infants using 5-mm instruments. *J Pediatr Urol.* (2017) 13:221–2. doi: 10.1016/j.jpurol.2016.12.011
11. Sheth KR, Van Batavia JP, Bowen DK, Koh CJ, Srinivasan AK. Minimally invasive surgery in pediatric urology: adaptations and new frontiers. *Urol Clin North Am.* (2018) 45:611–21. doi: 10.1016/j.ucl.2018.06.008
12. Mahida JB, Cooper JN, Herz D, Diefenbach KA, Deans KJ, Minneci PC, et al. Utilization and costs associated with robotic surgery in children. *J Surg Res.* (2015) 199:169–76. doi: 10.1016/j.jss.2015.04.087
13. Arlen AM, Broderick KM, Travers C, Smith EA, Elmore JM, Kirsch AJ. Outcomes of complex robot-assisted extravesical ureteral reimplantation in the pediatric population. *J Pediatr Urol.* (2016) 12:169.e1–6. doi: 10.1016/j.jpurol.2015.11.007
14. Timberlake MD, Peters CA. Current status of robotic-assisted surgery for the treatment of vesicoureteral reflux in children. *Curr Opin Urol.* (2017) 27:20–6. doi: 10.1097/MOU.0000000000000357
15. Grimsby GM, Dwyer ME, Jacobs MA, Ost MC, Schneck FX, Cannon GM, et al. Multi-institutional review of outcomes of robot-assisted laparoscopic extravesical ureteral reimplantation. *J Urol.* (2015) 193(5 Suppl.):1791–5. doi: 10.1016/j.juro.2014.07.128
16. Bowen DK, Faasse MA, Liu DB, Gong EM, Lindgren BW, Johnson EK. Use of Pediatric Open, Laparoscopic and Robot-Assisted Laparoscopic Ureteral Reimplantation in the United States: 2000 to 2012. *J Urol.* (2016) 196:207–12. doi: 10.1016/j.juro.2016.02.065
17. Gargollo PC. Hidden incision endoscopic surgery: description of technique, parental satisfaction and applications. *J Urol.* (2011) 185:1425–31. doi: 10.1016/j.juro.2010.11.054
18. Garcia-Roig ML, Travers C, McCracken C, Cerwinka W, Kirsch JM, Kirsch AJ. Surgical scar location preference for pediatric kidney and pelvic surgery: a crowdsourced survey. *J Urol.* (2017) 197(3 Pt 2):911–9. doi: 10.1016/j.juro.2016.11.033
19. Hong YH, DeFoor WR, Reddy PP, Schulte M, Minevich EA, VanderBrink BA, et al. Hidden incision endoscopic surgery (HIdES) trocar placement for pediatric robotic pyeloplasty: comparison to traditional port placement. *J Robot Surg.* (2018) 12:43–7. doi: 10.1007/s11701-017-0684-2
20. Baek M, Silay MS, Au JK, Huang GO, Elizondo RA, Puttmann KT, et al. Does the use of 5 mm instruments affect the outcomes of robot-assisted laparoscopic pyeloplasty in smaller working spaces? A comparative analysis of infants and older children. *J Pediatr Urol.* (2018) 14:537.e1–6. doi: 10.1016/j.jpurol.2018.06.010
21. Behan JW, Kim SS, Dorey F, De Filippo RE, Chang AY, Hardy BE, et al. Human capital gains associated with robotic assisted laparoscopic pyeloplasty in children compared to open pyeloplasty. *J Urol.* (2011) 186(4 Suppl):1663–7. doi: 10.1016/j.juro.2011.04.019
22. U.S. Food & Drug Administration. *FDA Clears New Robotically-Assisted Surgical Device for Adult Patients.* (2017). Available online at: http://news.doximity.com/entries/9699292?authenticated=false
23. Medrobotics. *Medrobotics® Corporation Receives FDA Clearance for Flex® Robotic System for Scarfree® Colorectal Procedures.* (2017).
24. Medrobotics. *Medrobotics® Corporation Receives FDA Clearance for World's First and Only Flexible Transabdominal and Transthoracic Robotic Scope.* (2018).
25. Shademan A, Decker RS, Opfermann JD, Leonard S, Krieger A, Kim PC. Supervised autonomous robotic soft tissue surgery. *Sci Transl Med.* (2016) 8:337ra64. doi: 10.1126/scitranslmed.aad9398

2

Pharyngomalacia in Neonates: The Missed Issue

Mohammad Ashkan Moslehi*

Pediatric Interventional Pulmonology Division, Department of Pediatrics, School of Medicine, Shiraz University of Medical Sciences, Shiraz, Iran

Correspondence:
Mohammad Ashkan Moslehi
ashkanmoslehi@gmail.com

Background: Airway malacia (AM) is a weakness of the airway's frameworks making them collapsible during the respiratory phases. Although the larynx, trachea, and bronchus are the usual sites for malacia to occur, there is another important type of malacia that involves the pharynx. Pharyngomalacia (PM) or concentric pharyngeal wall inspiratory collapse (PWIC) is mostly missed during bronchoscopic evaluations in the neonates with noisy breathing because people are not aware of this condition.

Methods: This study aimed to evaluate the nasopharyngeal investigation among neonates suffering from noisy breathing. The retrospective study was undertaken to assess the frequency of PM and to propose indications for intervention in 100 neonates with noisy breathing. A thin fiberoptic bronchoscope was used to evaluate the upper airways under conscious status without any sedation in the neonates.

Results: A total of 100 neonates with noisy breathing from September 2015 to October 2018 were retrospectively analyzed. The most common presenting symptom was inspiratory stridor which was observed in 35 (92.1%) of cases. PM was diagnosed in 38 neonates (38%) including 27 (71%) males and 13 (29%) females. Seventeen (44.7%) cases had mild, 11 (28.9%) cases had moderate, and 10 (26.4%) cases had a severe type of PM. PM was more prominent at the velopharynx level in 15 (39.4%) cases, and it was accompanied by up to six synchronous airway abnormalities. The most frequent synchronous airway abnormality was laryngomalacia in 13 (34.3%).

Conclusion: PM is one of the causes of noisy breathing in infants. Since PM can be accompanied by the presence of other types of airway malacia, the issue becomes more complicated. On the other hand, lack of experience and facilities are two main causes for the accurate diagnosis and effective management among neonates. This study indicates that the investigation of pharynx is a missed part of the many workups that are used to diagnose the site of involvement in neonates with noisy breathing.

Keywords: neonates, stridor, pharyngomalacia, airway malacia, noisy breathing

INTRODUCTION

The upper airway is defined anatomically as the airway segment between the nostrils and trachea at the level of the thoracic inlet, including five compartments: the nasopharynx (functional during nasopharyngeal breathing), oropharynx cavity (functional during oropharyngeal breathing), the hypopharynx, the larynx, and upper third part of the trachea within the level of the thoracic inlet. Due to the parallel anatomic arrangement between the oral and nasal cavities, they are rarely the site of upper airway obstruction, except in cases of congenital malformation, massive head, and neck trauma and injuries from burns. Considering the pathophysiology of upper airway Obstruction (UAO), it is divided into dynamic (variable) and anatomical (fixed) obstruction. The major symptoms of UAO in neonates include noisy breathing and dyspnea. The severity of the symptoms directly depends on the severity of the obstruction. Noisy breathing in neonates is defined as unusual respiratory sounds during respiratory phases. The most important unusual sounds in neonates are stridor, wheezing, and snoring. Inspiratory stridor is the main symptom resulting from extra-thoracic airway partial obstruction. Differential diagnosis of stridor can be divided based on anatomical levels including supralaryngeal, laryngeal, and tracheal categories. Supralaryngeal causes of stridor consist of supralaryngeal causes which include vallecular cysts, thyroglossal cysts, and tongue dermoid or teratoma (1). Isolated pharyngomalacia is considered one of the causes in selected neonates with severe stridor (2). When the obstruction is acute and complete, such as bilateral choanal atresia, sudden dyspnea, or even suffocation may result at birth. But in chronic onset and uncompleted UAO, the neonate develops noisy breathing and dyspnea over time, especially during increased respiratory works such as feeding, crying, or sleeping in a prone position. The symptoms of dyspnea and noisy breathing are identical to those experienced with other types of airway malacia, such as tracheomalacia, bronchomalacia, or both. These similarities can lead to diagnostic confusion. Moreover, not all bronchoscopies looked at the pharynx for more investigation, and this makes pharyngomalacia a rarely diagnosed condition. This study was performed since the impact of PM as the major type of the UAO and its collaboration with other airway obstructions has not been well-understood yet.

MATERIALS AND METHODS

This retrospective study was done to investigate the role and the frequency of PM as a cause of noisy breathing in 100 neonates for 3 years. All records of neonates referred to our center with noisy breathing from September 2015 to October 2018 were included for reviewing. Bronchoscopy investigation is a routine investigation technique in neonates with noisy breathing that includes the following criteria: age <28 days, noisy breathing, dyspnea, cyanotic cough spells, aspiration and cyanotic spells during feeding, and recurrent apnea episodes. Aspiration is clinically defined as presenting choking, cyanosis, and apnea during feeding and is confirmed through fiberoptic endoscopic evaluation of swallowing (FEES) and barium swallow study (BSS). Exclusion criteria are as follows: age more than 1 month, parental disagreements, and no nasopharyngeal endoscopy examination.

The study was approved by the hospital ethical committee, and the parents or caregiver gave their informed consent to be enrolled in the study. Moreover, written informed consent was obtained from all the parents for both the publication and any accompanying images.

The assessment of upper airway dynamics was emphasized by using a thin (2.8 mm) flexible bronchoscope (Olympus Company, Japan) when the patients were on their spontaneous breathing with a nasal approach. Since different levels of sedation led to different dynamic and functional results and there was the possibility of interference of the results in the bronchoscopy evaluations, neither generalized anesthesia nor sedation was administered. For minimizing the possibility of airway irritation and spasm, lidocaine gel (2%) was applied all over the exterior surface of the FFB flexible bronchoscope. Based on the established protocol at the authors' department, a nasal cannula was inserted through one of the nostrils down to the nasopharynx to maintain oxygenation. No PEEP or positive ventilation was used at the time of endoscopy evaluations as it could interfere with the flaccidity of airway walls and the final reports. According to the bronchoscopy investigation, PM was defined in multiple sites as follows: from the level of the hard palate to the tip of the uvula (velopharynx), from the end of the uvula to the tip of the epiglottis (oropharynx), and finally from the tip of the epiglottis to the vocal cords (hypopharynx). As to the best of the author's knowledge, there were not any grading scales regarding the severity of obstruction in PM. Thus, the author used a new modified grading scale based on the one that has been used for adenoid hyperplasia and tracheomalacia depending on the present airway obstruction and severity of the symptoms. So, it has been graded as mild, moderate, and severe when an obstruction was <50%, between 50 and 75%, and more than 75% of the airway diameter, respectively.

To prove the exact role of PM in induced symptoms, positive pressure ventilation of 5 cm water was applied by closing the anesthesia bag valve and bypassing the obstruction level through using the nasopharyngeal tube. These maneuvers aborted the pharyngeal wall collapse and the symptoms. Patients affected by mild to severe PM benefited from supportive medical management while airway structural stability was expected with increasing age. The supportive care used included nasal washing with normal saline, nasopharyngeal mucosal gentle suctioning, antireflux positions, and therapy with oral proton-pump inhibitors (PPIs) like omeprazole, nasopharyngeal catheters, continuous positive airway pressure (CPAP), or bilevel positive airway pressure (BiPAP).

All patients underwent a follow-up program adjusted to individual patients' conditions and needs in terms of the different types of PM every 2–3 months for up to 3 years.

RESULTS

In a retrospective review of consecutive endoscopic evaluations and clinical data of 100 (48 female and 52 male) neonates with UAO, PM was diagnosed in 38 neonates (38%) including 25(65.8%) males and 13 (34.2%) females. The age of neonates at the time of endoscopy diagnosis was from 7 to 28 days after birth. With regard to the extent of PM, the number (present) of children with mild, moderate (**Figure 1**), and severe (**Figure 2**) were 17 (44.7%), 11 (28.9%), and 10 (26.4%), respectively. Based on the results of the bronchoscopy investigations, PM was most

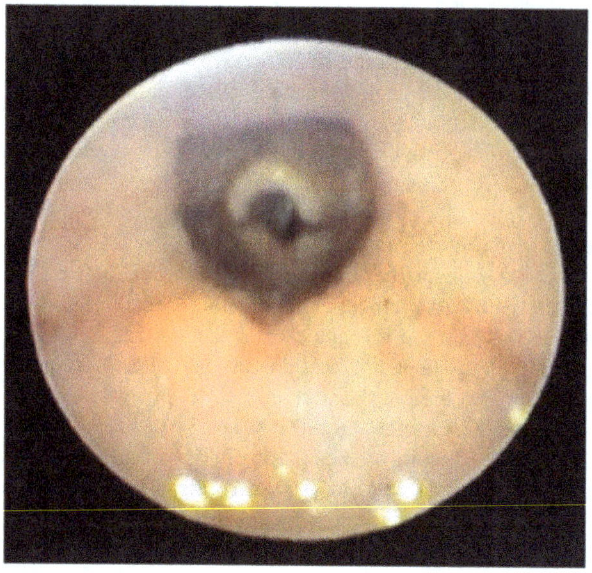

FIGURE 1 | Moderate PM.

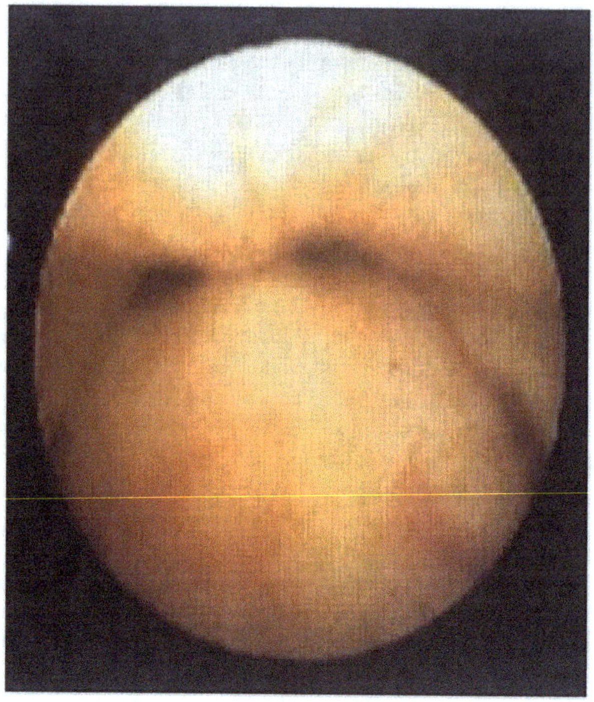

FIGURE 2 | Severe PM.

prominent at the velopharynx level 15 (39.4%) followed by hypopharynx 13 (34.2%), the whole length of pharynx 7 (18.4%), and oropharynx 3 (8%). The most common presenting symptoms were inspiratory stridor 35 (92.1%), cyanotic cough spell 27 (71%), aspiration and cyanotic spells during feeding 21 (55.2%), and recurrent apnea 18 (47.3%).

This study also showed that PM was accompanied by up to six synchronous airway abnormalities; the most frequent ones were laryngomalacia 13 (34.3%), tracheomalacia 12 (31.5%), bronchomalacia 6 (15.8%), larygotracheobronchomalacia 3 (8%), tracheoesophageal fistula (TEF) 2 (5.2%), and posterior laryngeal cleft 2 (5.2%). The results are presented in **Table 1**. Generalized hypotonia was the most common associated systemic finding 4 (12%). There were two neonates with Down syndrome and one with VACTER syndrome suffering from severe PM at the level of velopharynx.

Non-invasive positive ventilation devices including CPAP and BiPAP were used in 21 (55.3%) neonates with moderate to severe PM. The duration of use of these devices varied depending on the age and severity of the PM (mean, 7 ± 3.5 months). Four (10.5%) cases including one patient with VACTER, one with Down syndrome, one with posterior laryngeal cleft, and one with TEF underwent tracheostomy.

In the follow-up, 35 (92%) of the cases became asymptomatic from 10 to 24 months (mean, 18 ± 5 months) by using supportive care.

DISCUSSION

Noisy breathing is one of the most common indications for doing bronchoscopic investigations in neonates. UAO and LAO are the main causes of these abnormal breathing sounds. UAO is a potentially severe and life-threatening complication among neonates. Tracheomalacia is the most common congenital UAO among this age group (1). Its incidence seems to be underestimated but reported as about 1 in every 2,100 children (3). Most children are either asymptomatic or minimally symptomatic, and most cases involve posterior malacia of the trachea, with associated broad tracheal rings. On the other hand, PM is a dynamic obstruction of the air column proximal to the glottis during inspiration. The author's objective was to assess PM's incidence and its contribution to the symptoms of UAO and to propose indications for intervention.

As 38% of neonates had various types of pharyngomalacia, this study showed that there are some important misdiagnoses in previous studies regarding the causes of noisy breathing in neonates. A wide variety of PM exists that is often missed first, as the oral approach is the often-used routine bronchoscopy route for any investigations done by a pulmonologist. Secondly, most pediatric bronchoscopists may not be familiar with the anatomical and physiological aspects of the upper airways especially in the neonates and young infants. Thirdly, it is difficult to do the bronchoscopy setup in small neonates especially in the unstable ones, and lastly, neonatal bronchoscopy facilities are unavailable in many centers. Based on this study, male neonates were more prone to have PM than females. There is a scant research regarding the related issue in the literature. However, based on bronchoscopic investigations, this may be because male neonates have longer velopharynx compared with female neonates (4). Previously, laryngomalacia (87.2%), pharyngomalacia (33.3%), and tracheomalacia (10.3%) were

TABLE 1 | Detailed data.

Demographics	n = 38
Sex (male)	25 (65.8%)*
Sex (female)	13 (34.2%)*
Birth gestational age (weeks)	36 (25-41)+
Age at the time of bronchoscopy (days)	16 (7-28)+
Severity	
Mild	17 (44.7%)*
Moderate	11 (28.9%)*
Severe	10 (26.4%)*
Site of maximum involvement	
Velopharynx	15 (39.4%)*
Hypopharynx	13 (34.2%)*
Whole length of pharynx	7 (18.4%)*
Oropharynx	3 (8%)*
Symptoms	
Stridor	35 (92.1%)*
Cyanotic cough spell	27 (71%)*
Aspiration (cyanotic spells during feeding)	21 (55.2%)*
Recurrent apnea	18 (47.3%)*
Synchronous airway abnormalities	
Laryngomalacia	13 (34.3%)*
Tracheomalacia	12 (31.5%)*
Bronchomalacia	6 (15.8%)*
Larygotracheobronchomalacia	3 (8%)*
Tracheoesophageal fistula (TEF)	2 (5.2%)*
Posterior laryngeal cleft	2 (5.2%)*

**Frequency (percentage). +Median (min-max).*

reported as the three most prevalent findings on endoscopy of neonates with sleep apnea (5). PM was also reported as an under-recognized rare condition in patients with Down syndrome who had sleep apnea (6). Thus, PM may account for one of the major causes of obstructive sleep apnea. In the study by Shatz et al., the majority of children had obstruction related to pharyngeal hypotonia and collapse. They also mentioned that PM can lead to prolonged hospitalization and intensive care admission and may raise the difficulty in management issues (7). The severity of PM was measured through severe retractions and respiratory compromises like respiratory failure, apnea, cyanotic spells, the need for more respiratory supports depending on additional oxygen, extubation failure, choking spells while feeding, and poor weight gain. Moreover, as there were no standard severity grading scales especially in neonates, the author considers the percentage of stenosis as the described severity scales from mild to severe. According to this scaling, most of the cases had mild to moderate PM.

Similar to other types of airway malacia, PM seems to be a self-limiting condition and spontaneous recovery occurred within 36 months. Although mild PM is watched expectantly and anticipated to improve with time, there were more severe symptomatic PMs.When it occurs with other airway insults, it warrants interventions like non-invasive ventilatory supports (nasopharyngeal catheters, CPAP, bilevel instruments) and rarely may need surgery in some cases (8, 9).

In this study, most of the index cases (92%) became asymptomatic due to supportive care including antireflux position and therapy, the decrease of mucosal stickiness of the nasopharyngeal wall with nasal spray 10–15 min before feeding and 3–5 ml normal saline oral solution after feeding, gentle nasal suctioning, and small frequent feeding.

In neonates with compromised airway disorders where swallowing interrupts with normal smooth breathing, this causes sucking-swallowing discoordination (SSD) leading to aspiration although the exact incidence is not well-established (10, 11).

In this study, more than half of the patients had aspiration due to SSD clinically presented with cyanotic spells during feeding and was approved by FEES and BSS. Direct vision investigation with FEES study revealed that aspiration became effectively diminished by resolving the PM-induced partial obstruction using nasopharyngeal bypassing, gentle mucosal suctioning, and patient positioning with 30–45% of body (not neck flection) elevation.

Progressive and severe PM cases required a nasopharyngeal catheter for bypassing the stenotic level; CPAP or BiPAP form weeks to months. Four cases underwent tracheostomy procedures especially those with concomitant syndromes (VACTERL and Down syndromes). It seems the rest of the cases became asymptomatic as they were followed up until the time of publishing the data.

This study has some limitations including the nature of retrospective studies, lack of previous research studies on the topic, limited access to data, and a combination of abnormalities which on their own can cause noisy breathing.

The incidence of PM among neonates with UAO was beyond expectations in this study, and its role in UAO deserves greater recognition. This study also showed a combination of abnormalities, which on their own can cause noisy breathing. Its commonly associated abnormalities can include laryngeal clefts, TEF, and bronchomalacia. The current gold standard for the diagnosis of PM is a dynamic evaluation under direct vision through nasopharyngoscopy. A better diagnosis of PM will improve the treatment of UAO.

AUTHOR CONTRIBUTIONS

MM wrote the manuscript and approved it for publication.

REFERENCES

1. Kamran A, Jennings RW. Tracheomalacia and tracheobronchomalacia in pediatrics: an overview of evaluation, medical management, and surgical treatment. *Front Pediatr.* (2019) 7:512. doi: 10.3389/fped.2019.00512
2. Chan EY, Ng DK, Chow PY, Kwok KL. Pharyngomalacia as a cause of severe neonatal stridor. *Singapore Med J.* (2007) 48:e246–7.
3. Boogard R, Huijsmans SH, Pijnenburg, Tiddens HA, de Jongste JC, Merkus PJ. Tracheomalacia and bronchomalacia in children: incidence and patient characteristics. *Chest.* (2005) 128:3391–7. doi: 10.1378/chest.128.5.3391
4. Ronen O, Malhotra A, Pillar G. Influence of gender and age on upper-airway length during development. *Pediatrics.* (2007) 120:1028–34. doi: 10.1542/peds.2006-3433
5. Bandyopadhya A, Muston H, Slave JE, Jalou HE, Engle WA, DaftaryMS AS. Endoscopic airway findings in infants with obstructive sleep apnea. *J Pulm Respir Med.* (2018) 8:448 doi: 10.4172/2161-105X.100 0448
6. Shing YRL, Daniel KN, Pok YC, Ka LK. Obstructive sleep apnea syndrome secondary to pharyngolaryngomalacia in a neonate with down syndrome. *Int J Pediatr Otorhinolaryngol.* (2005) 69:919–21. doi: 10.1016/j.ijporl.2005.0 2.008
7. Shatz A, Goldberg S, Picard E, Kerem E. Pharyngeal wall collapse and multiple synchronous airway lesions. *Ann Otol Rhinol Laryngol.* (2004) 113:483–7. doi: 10.1177/000348940411300613
8. Froehlich P, Seid AB, Denoyelle F, Pransky SM, Kearns DB, Garabedian EN, et al. Discoordinate pharyngolaryngomalacia. *Int J Pediatr Otorhinolaryngol.* (1997) 14:9–18. doi: 10.1016/S0165-5876(96)01454-1
9. Schweiger C, Manica D, Becker CF, Abreu LSP, Manzini M, Sekine L, et al. Tracheostomy in children: a ten-year experience from a tertiary center in southern Brazil. *Braz J Otorhinolaryngol.* (2017) 83:627–32. doi: 10.1016/j.bjorl.2016.08.002
10. Thompson DM. Abnormal sensorimotor integrative function of the larynx in congenital laryngomalacia: a new theory of etiology. *Laryngoscope.* (2007) 117(Suppl. 114):1–33. doi: 10.1097/MLG.0b013e31804a5750
11. Simons JP, Greenberg LL, Mehta DK, Fabio A, Maguire RC, Mandell DL. Laryngomalacia and swallowing function in children. *Laryngoscope.* (2016) 126:478–84. doi: 10.1002/lary.25440

3

Primary Posterior Tracheopexy in Esophageal Atresia Decreases Respiratory Tract Infections

*E. Sofie van Tuyll van Serooskerken[1], Stefaan H. A. J. Tytgat[1,2], Johannes W. Verweij[1,2], Arnold J. N. Bittermann[2,3], Saskia Coenraad[2,3], Hubertus G. M. Arets[2,4], David C. van der Zee[1,2] and Maud Y. A. Lindeboom[1,2]**

[1] Department of Pediatric Surgery, Pediatric Wilhelmina Children's Hospital, University Medical Center Utrecht, Utrecht, Netherlands, [2] Congenital Esophageal and Airway Team Utrecht, Pediatric Wilhelmina Children's Hospital, University Medical Center Utrecht, Utrecht, Netherlands, [3] Department of Pediatric Otorhinolaryngology, Pediatric Wilhelmina Children's Hospital, University Medical Center Utrecht, Utrecht, Netherlands, [4] Department of Pediatric Pulmonology, Pediatric Wilhelmina Children's Hospital, University Medical Center Utrecht, Utrecht, Netherlands

***Correspondence:**
Maud Y. A. Lindeboom
m.y.a.lindeboom@umcutrecht.nl

Background: Esophageal atresia (EA) is often accompanied by tracheomalacia (TM). TM can lead to severe respiratory complaints requiring invasive treatment. This study aims to evaluate if thoracoscopic primary posterior tracheopexy (PPT) can prevent the potential sequelae of TM in patients with EA.

Methods: A cohort study including all consecutive EA patients treated between 2014 and July 2019 at the Wilhelmina Children's Hospital was conducted. Two groups were distinguished: (group 1) all EA patients born between January 2014 and December 2016 and (group 2) all EA patients born between January 2017 and July 2019, after introduction of PPT. In the latter group, PPT was performed in EA patients with moderate (33–66%) or severe (67–100%) tracheomalacia, seen during preoperative bronchoscopy. Group differences were assessed using the Fisher's exact test for bivariate variables and the Mann–Whitney *U*-test for continuous variables.

Results: A total of 64 patients were included in this study (28 patients in group 1; 36 patients in group 2). In group 2, PPT was performed in 14 patients. Respiratory tract infections (RTIs) requiring antibiotics within the first year of life occurred significantly less in group 2 (61 vs. 25%, $p = 0.004$). Brief resolved unexplained events (BRUEs) seemed to diminish in group 2 compared to group 1 (39 vs. 19%, $p = 0.09$).

Conclusion: Thoracoscopic primary posterior tracheopexy decreases the number of respiratory tract infections in EA patients. The clinical impact of reducing RTIs combined with the minimal additional operating time and safety of PPT outweighs the risk of overtreatment.

Keywords: esophageal atresia, tracheomalacia, bronchoscopy, thoracoscopy, posterior tracheopexy, brief resolved unexplained event, respiratory tract infection

INTRODUCTION

In up to 87% of patients, esophageal atresia (EA) can be associated with some form of tracheomalacia (TM) (1). TM can be caused by flaccidity of the cartilaginous anterior rings, a floppy posterior membrane, or both and may lead to a dynamic collapse of the tracheal lumen (2, 3). This collapse of the trachea can result in a wide spectrum of symptoms and sequelae ranging from mild complaints, such as stridor or wheezing, to brief resolved unexplained events (BRUEs) (3). Furthermore, collapse of the trachea may lead to an ineffective cough and impaired clearance of secretions, increasing the risk of respiratory tract infections (4, 5). In severe TM, invasive treatment might be warranted (6, 7). Surgical treatment of preference depends on the type of TM and includes aortopexy to lift the aortic compression on the anterior flaccid cartilaginous rings (3, 8), or posterior tracheopexy of the floppy membrane to prevent posterior tracheal intrusion (9). In a previous study, we have introduced a new approach in which a posterior tracheopexy is performed during the thoracoscopic correction of EA. Results showed this approach to be feasible (10).

The aim of this study is to evaluate if thoracoscopic primary posterior tracheopexy (PPT) can prevent the potential respiratory sequelae of tracheomalacia in patients with EA and concurrent TM.

METHODS

Study Design and Participants

A cohort study including all consecutive EA patients between January 2014 and July 2019 was conducted at the University Medical Center Utrecht, Wilhelmina Children's Hospital. The variables of interest were collected prospectively at standardized time points for all children according to standard clinical practice. The comparative design was applied after data collection. Patients were excluded for follow-up if they had died before the age of 1 year. In January 2017 thoracoscopic PPT for moderate or severe TM was introduced in our hospital. Two patient subgroups were distinguished: (group 1) all EA patients born between January 2014 and December 2016 and (group 2) all EA patients born between January 2017 and July 2019, after the introduction of PPT. Data of patients that underwent thoracoscopic PPT were prospectively collected.

Surgical Procedure

Since 2014 almost all infants with EA underwent a rigid bronchoscopy prior to surgery to evaluate the presence of TM and to exclude a proximal fistula. Since 2017, a standardized scoring system for TM has been introduced (11). Patients with moderate to severe tracheomalacia were eligible for PPT. Tracheal obstruction, evaluated by bronchoscopy, was defined as collapse of the tracheal wall at three different levels, the upper third, middle third, and lower third of the trachea (11). TM was considered moderate when the tracheal lumen collapsed 33–66% and severe when 67–100%. The surgical procedure of thoracoscopic PPT during esophageal repair has been described previously (10). In short, during the procedure for thoracoscopic esophageal repair, the posterior tracheal membrane is fixed to the anterior spinal ligament with one to three non-absorbable sutures (**Figure 1**), prior to the anastomosis of the esophageal ends (**Figure 2**).

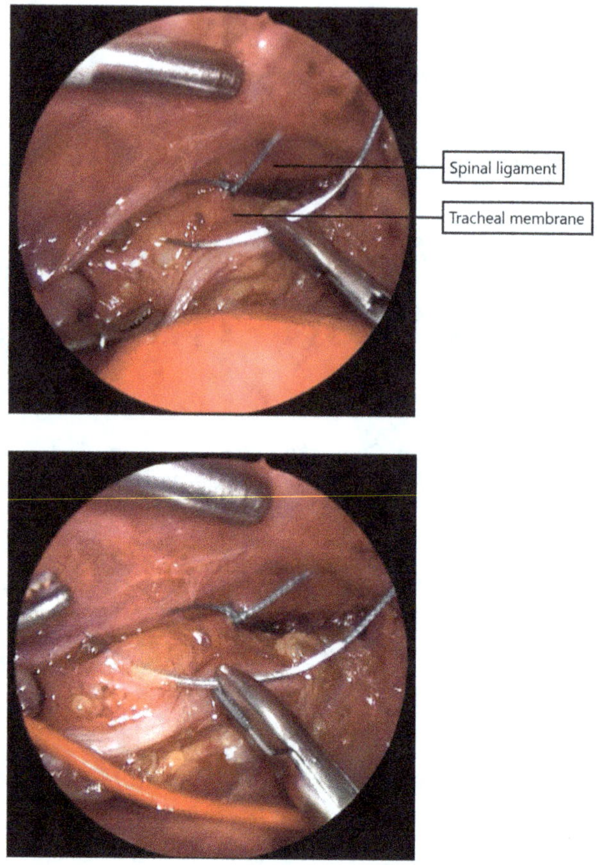

FIGURE 1 | The posterior tracheal membrane is fixed to the the anterior spinal ligament with one to three non-absorbable sutures.

Clinical Assessment

All baseline characteristics, including gender, type of EA and associated anomalies, and all surgical data including age at time of surgery, postoperative complications and length of hospital and NICU stay, were collected. Prospective data of patients that underwent PPT was obtained during standard EA follow-up in outpatient care at 4 weeks and 3, 6, 12 months of age.

Respiratory Outcome

Patients underwent standardized clinical assessment regarding respiratory symptoms. The primary outcome measures were respiratory symptoms, including respiratory tract infections (RTIs) requiring antibiotics within the first year of life and occurrence of BRUEs. Diagnosis of the RTIs was made by the pediatric pulmonologist. The pediatric pulmonologists based

---

Abbreviations: EA, esophageal atresia; TM, tracheomalacia; PPT, primary posterior tracheopexy; BRUE, brief resolved unexplained event; RTI, respiratory tract infection.

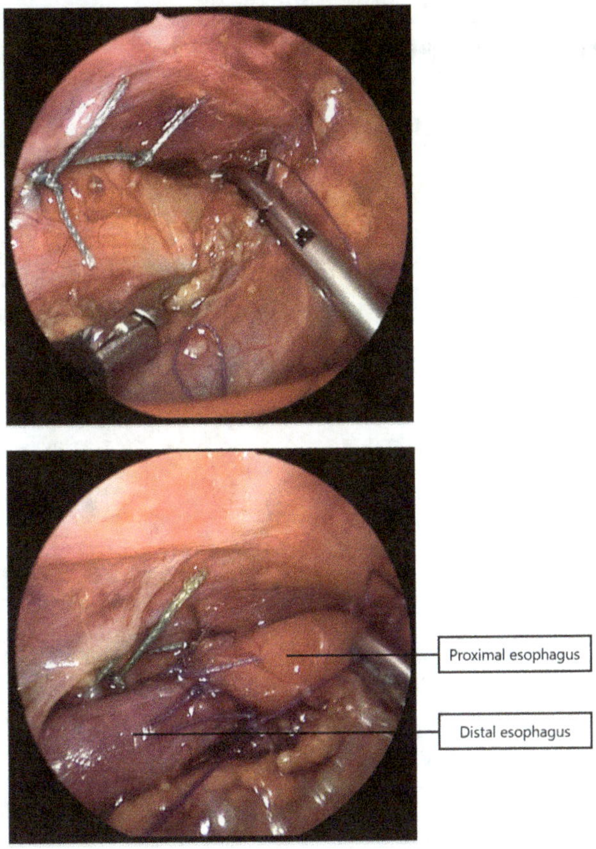

FIGURE 2 | After performing the tracheopexy, the proximal and distal esophagus are anastomosed.

TABLE 1 | Patient characteristics of group 1 and group 2.

Variable	Group 1 (2014–2016) $n = 28$	Group 2 (2017–2019) $n = 36$	*p*-value
Male	16 (57%)	24 (67%)	0.45
Gestational age (weeks)	39.2 (31.6–41.6)	37.3 (28.3–42.3)	0.08
Premature	7 (25%)	16 (44%)	0.12
Twin	3 (11%)	2 (6%)	0.65
Birthweight (g)	2,755 (1,585–4,170)	2,692 (1,050–3,950)	0.37
Apgar score			
1 min	8 (2–9)	9 (3–10)	0.17
5 min	9 (3–10)	9 (5–10)	0.48
Type EA			
A	3 (11%)	1 (3%)	0.38
B	1 (3.6%)	0	
C	23 (82%)	32 (89%)	
D	0	2 (5.6%)	
E	1 (3.6%)	1 (2.8%)	
Associated anomalies#			
Trisomy 21	2 (7%)	1 (3%)	0.57
VACTERL	6 (21%)	8 (22%)	1.0
Musculoskeletal	10 (36%)	15 (42%)	0.80
Urogenital	8 (29%)	5 (14%)	0.33
Cardiovascular	12 (43%)	15 (42%)	1.0
Gastrointestinal	4 (14%)	2 (6%)	0.40

EA, esophageal atresia.
All data are presented as median (range) or n (%).
#Some patients had multiple anomalies.

their decision on symptpoms and/or chest X-rays. Antibiotic treatment was prescribed by the pediatric pulmonologist. BRUE is defined as an event in which an infant younger than 1 year old presents with cyanosis, pallor, altered breathing, hypotonia or hypertonia and/or altered responsiveness (12).

Statistical Analysis

Continuous variables were presented as median and range and categorical data were presented as frequencies and percentage. To assess group differences for bivariate variables the Fisher's exact test was used. Group differences for continuous variables were assessed using the Mann-Whitney *U*-test. A $p < 0.05$ was considered significant. The analyses were performed with SPSS for Windows, version 25.0 (IBM Corp., Armonk, NY).

Ethical Approval

This cohort study was submitted to the UMCU Ethics Committee. No ethical approval was required according to the Medical Research Involving Human Subject Act. The study was carried out in accordance with the Declaration of Helsinki.

RESULTS

In total, 67 consecutive EA patients were admitted at the Wilhelmina Children's Hospital between January 2014 and July 2019. Three patients that died within the first weeks after birth were excluded from further analysis. One patient died before esophageal repair due to severe prematurity with pulmonary bleeding. Two patients died after esophageal repair due to causes unrelated to surgery (cardiac anomalies and cerebral abscesses). The 64 remaining patients were all evaluated in our outpatient clinic at 4 weeks and 3, 6, 12 months. The patients were divided into two groups: the first group, before the introduction of PPT, consisted of 28 consecutive patients admitted between 2014 and 2016 (group 1). The second group, after the introduction of PPT, consisted of 36 patients admitted between 2017 and 2019 (group 2). Patient characteristics were comparable between the two groups, as shown in **Table 1**.

In group 2, a PPT was performed in 14 patients (39%). Of these 14 patients, 12 patients (86%) had EA Gross type C, and 2 patients (14%) type D. Patient characteristics are presented in **Table 2**. There were no relevant significant differences between the no-PPT patients and the PPT patients within group 2.

TABLE 2 | Patient characteristics of group 2 (2017–2019).

Variable	No-PPT, $n = 22$	PPT, $n = 14$	*p*-value
Male	14 (64%)	10 (71%)	0.73
Gestational age (weeks)	36.7 (29.1–42.3)	38.4 (28.3–41.4)	0.35
Premature	12 (55%)	4 (29%)	0.18
Twin	2 (9%)	0 (0%)	0.51
Birthweight (g)	2,249 (1,220–3,950)	3,008 (1,050–3,550)	0.22
Apgar score			
1 min	9 (4–10)	8.5 (3–9)	0.84
5 min	9 (7–10)	9 (5–10)	0.74
Type EA			
A	1 (4.5%)	0	0.20
C	20 (91%)	12 (86%)	
D	0	2 (14%)	
E	1 (4.5%)	0	
Associated anomalies[#]			
Trisomy 21	1 (4.5%)	0	1.0
VACTERL	3 (14%)	5 (36%)	0.22
Musculoskeletal	10 (45.5%)	5 (36%)	0.73
Urogenital	0	5 (36%)	0.005*
Cardiovascular	9 (41%)	6 (43%)	1.0
Gastrointestinal	1 (4.5%)	1 (7%)	1.0

PPT, primary posterior tracheopexy; EA, esophageal atresia.
All data are presented as median (range) or n (%).
[#]Some patients had multiple anomalies.
**Indicating statistical significance.*

TABLE 3A | Surgical data of group 1 and group 2.

Variable (median, range)	Group 1 (2014–2016) $n = 28$	Group 2 (2017–2019) $n = 36$	*p*-value
Age at EA surgery (d)	3 (0–58)	3.5 (1–54)	0.17
NICU time (d)	9 (3–126)	8 (3–81)	0.91
LOS (d)	20 (10–159)	25.5 (10–178)	0.14
Leakage	3 (11%)	6 (17%)	0.72

EA, esophageal atresia; LOS, length of hospital stay.

Surgical Outcome

Overall analyses of group 1 and group 2 showed no significant differences in age at EA surgery, postoperative NICU time, length of hospital stay or anastomotic leakage between the two groups (**Table 3A**). In group 2, moderate to severe tracheal collapse was diagnosed in 13 patients (**Table 4**). In two patients with mild TM (20% tracheal collapse) on bronchoscopy, increased flaccidity of the posterior tracheal membrane was seen during thoracoscopy after ligation and transection of the distal tracheoesophageal fistula. Therefore, a PPT was also performed in these two patients. The middle and distal third of the trachea were most often affected with a median tracheal collapse of 50% (range 20–90%). Thoracoscopic PPT was uncomplicated and successful in all patients with a median of 2 sutures (range 1–3). Median time per suture was 6 min (range 4–12 min). Anastomotic leakage occurred in 21% and could be treated conservatively in all patients. There were no significant differences in surgical outcome between patients with or without PPT in group 2 (**Table 3B**).

Patients that underwent PPT were operated at a median age of 3.5 days (range 1–35 days). Surgery was postponed due to respiratory instability in one patient of group 2, a premature neonate of 1,050 g (28.7 weeks). One patient of group 2 was operated in an emergency setting because of a gastric perforation and pneumothorax that occurred during CPR shortly after birth.

TABLE 3B | Surgical data of group 2 (2017–2019).

Variable (median, range)	No-PPT, $n = 22$	PPT, $n = 14$	*p*-value
Age at EA surgery (d)	3.5 (1–54)	3.5 (1–35)	0.28
NICU time (d)	8 (3–81)	11 (3–59)	0.83
LOS (d)	24 (13–178)	28 (12–93)	0.81
Leakage	3 (14%)	3 (21%)	0.66

PPT, primary posterior tracheopexy; EA, esophageal atresia; LOS, length of hospital stay.

TABLE 4 | Tracheomalacia evaluated during bronchoscopy before EA repair in group 2.

Variable	Group 2 (2017–2019) $n = 36$
No TM	5 (14%)
TM mild	15 (42%)
TM moderate/severe	13 (36%)
No TM evaluation possible	3 (8%)

EA, esophageal atresia; TM, tracheomalacia.

TABLE 5 | Respiratory outcome in group 1 and group 2.

Variable	Group 1 (2014–2016) $n = 28$	Group 2 (2017–2019) $n = 36$	*p*-value
BRUE	11 (39%)	7 (19%)	0.09
RTI <1 year	17 (61%)	9 (25%)	0.004*

BRUE, brief resolved unexplained event; RTI, respiratory tract infection requiring antibiotics.
**Indicating statistical significance.*

Overall Respiratory Outcome

In group 1, 11 patients (39%) experienced at least one BRUE, compared to seven patients (19%) in group 2 ($p = 0.09$). RTIs requiring antibiotics within the first year of life occurred

TABLE 6 | Respiratory outcome in group 2 (2017–2019).

Variable	No-PPT, $n = 22$	PPT, $n = 14$	p-value
BRUE	6 (27%)	1 (7%)	0.21
RTI <1 year	6 (27%)	3 (21%)	1.0

PPT, primary posterior tracheopexy; BRUE, brief resolved unexplained event; RTI, respiratory tract infection requiring antibiotics.

significantly less often after introduction of PPT (group 1 vs. group 2; 61 vs. 25%, $p = 0.004$; **Table 5**).

In group 1, three patients underwent an aortopexy at the median age of 12 days (range 12–29). In two of these three patients, severe TM was evaluated preoperatively with bronchoscopy. In one patient after aortopexy, TM persisted and consequently a posterior tracheopexy was performed.

In group 2, redo tracheopexy was not warranted in any of the PPT-patients. Bronchoscopy was incomplete in three patients of group 2 and TM could not be evaluated, because spontaneous breathing during bronchoscopy was impaired due to ventilation problems. Of these three patients, one had to undergo a secondary posterior tracheopexy and another patient was treated by aortopexy.

Four patients, two in each group, all with multiple comorbidities, needed a tracheostomy. One patient with a tracheostomy and Down's syndrome in group 1, died during follow-up due to accidental decannulation.

Respiratory Outcome After PPT Introduction

Subgroup analysis of group 2 showed occurrence of BRUEs in one patient (7%) in the PPT-patients group vs. 6 patients (27%) in the no-PPT patients group (**Table 6**). This difference, however, was non-significant. The one patient with BRUEs after PPT had two tracheoesophageal fistulas (the distal fistula was located in the carina, and the proximal fistula in the middle part of the trachea) and a severe TM in the middle part of the trachea on preoperative bronchoscopy. Therefore, this patient underwent selective PPT only at the level of this middle part of the trachea. Postoperative bronchoscopy in this patient with multiple comorbidities, including a subglottic stenosis and retrognathia, revealed a severe TM in the distal part of the trachea.

RTIs requiring antibiotics within the first year were seen in 21% in the PPT-patients vs. 27% in the no-PPT patients group. One patient in the PPT-patient group experienced postoperative respiratory distress caused by a suture granuloma. After removal of the granuloma by bronchoscopy, no further respiratory problems occurred.

DISCUSSION

This is the first prospective study to evaluate respiratory outcome after thoracoscopic primary posterior tracheopexy in EA patients with tracheomalacia.

This novel PPT technique decreases the number of respiratory tract infections (RTIs) in EA patients with moderate or severe TM. The number of BRUEs also seemed to decrease after introduction of PPT, although this was not statistically significant. Furthermore, the PPT-procedure takes only short additional operative time and there were no differences in hospital length of stay, NICU stay and postoperative leakage between the PPT-group and the no-PPT group.

Respiratory morbidity in EA is very common during early childhood (13). EA patients often suffer from RTIs during the first year of life (14–17). This is in line with our findings, showing 61% of patients with RTIs within the first year of life before introduction of PPT. After the introduction of PPT, RTIs requiring antibiotics were significantly decreased in both EA patients that underwent a PPT, as well as the entire EA cohort (EA patients with and without PPT between 2017 and 2019). Therefore, selecting EA patients with moderate to severe TM for PPT improves the respiratory outcome of EA patients as a whole. In a previous study on PPT (18), a decrease in RTIs was not seen. However, results are difficult to compare, since this study compared preoperative data to postoperative data within a group of 18 patients and follow-up duration was shorter (5 months).

Another possibly life-threatening aspect of respiratory morbidity is posed by BRUEs. Although the decrease in number of BRUEs after the introduction of PPT from 39 to 19% seemed evident, it was not statistically significant. However, this may be explained by the small number of patients. In the study by Shieh et al. (18), a decrease in BRUEs was shown ($p = 0.049$). However, in this study, almost 30% of patients were re-operated for persistent collapse of the trachea.

In a previous study (10), we showed thoracoscopic PPT to be feasible and safe, with favorable short-term outcome. During the longer follow-up in this study, one patient experienced respiratory problems, caused by a suture granuloma. After bronchoscopic removal of the granuloma, no more respiratory problems had occurred. Flexible bronchoscopic visualization during posterior tracheopexy may prevent this type of complication from occurring. Therefore, this has now been implemented as routine procedure during PPT in our center. Moreover, this may also optimize positioning of the sutures in the tracheal wall.

In three patients, TM could not be evaluated due to ventilation difficulties during bronchoscopy. In these patients, PPT was not performed since the extent of TM was unknown. In this study, in two out of three patients, a secondary surgical intervention for severe TM was warranted. In these patients posterior tracheopexy was challenging because of multiple adhesions and risk of damaging the esophageal anastomosis. Therefore, median duration of secondary tracheopexy takes significantly longer than PPT (hours vs. minutes) and can be associated with complications (3, 10).

Attention for respiratory morbidity in EA patients, and especially for TM, has raised over the past few years (1, 19, 20). Therefore, routine preoperative rigid bronchoscopy is performed in all EA patients in the University Medical Center Utrecht, Wilhelmina Children's Hospital since 2015. The introduction of a standardized scoring system for TM in 2017 (11) by the dedicated congenital esophageal and airway team has led to increased awareness and improved recordings at our center.

A limitation of this study was that the rigid bronchoscopy was not repeated after PPT. In order to evaluate the effect of PPT, collapse of the trachea should be compared by rigid bronchoscopy before and after PPT. This would, however, require a second anesthesia for rigid bronchoscopy since spontaneous breathing is not possible directly after thoracoscopic EA repair and PPT. Therefore, our congenital esophageal and airway team has chosen not to evaluate the trachea by means of a second invasive procedure.

Although the data of the no-PPT patients was assessed retrospectively, the variables of interest were collected prospectively at standardized moments for all patients. Standardized questionnaires were not used, however, structured interviews regarding gastrointestinal and respiratory symptoms were conducted in every patient at our Congenital Esophageal and Airway outpatient clinic.

Another limitation is that no standardized scoring system was used during preoperative bronchoscopy in group 1. However, the baseline characteristics were similar within the two groups and therefore we expect that there are no significant differences on severity of tracheomalacia between the two groups.

Preferably, a prospective trial in EA patients with moderate or severe TM randomizing for PPT or no-PPT is needed to provide the best level of evidence. This comparative study shows the potential benefits of primary posterior tracheopexy in EA patients with concurrent moderate to severe tracheomalacia with a low complication rate.

CONCLUSIONS

In conclusion, this study shows that thoracoscopic primary posterior tracheopexy during esophageal atresia repair can significantly decrease respiratory tract infections that require antibiotics during the first year of life. The clinical impact of reducing respiratory tract infections combined with the relatively minimal additional operating time and safety of PPT may outweigh the risk of overtreatment. This, however, should be evaluated in an international, multicenter randomized controlled trial comparing PPT to no-PPT in neonates with EA.

Naturally, this advanced technique should only be performed in centers with a team of experienced pediatric upper GI- and airway surgeons, otolaryngologists, pulmonologists and anesthesiologists.

AUTHOR CONTRIBUTIONS

ESTS conceptualized and designed the study, collected the data, carried out the initial analysis, drafted the initial manuscript, and reviewed and revised the manuscript. ML conceptualized and designed the study, contributed to the writing, supervised the data collection and the progress, and reviewed and revised the manuscript. ST and DZ provided input to the study, supervised the data collection and the progress, and reviewed and revised the manuscript. JV, AB, SC, and HA reviewed the study design, contributed to the interpretation of data, and reviewed and revised the manuscript. All authors approved the final manuscript as submitted and agree to be accountable for all aspects of the work in ensuring that questions related to the accuracy or integrity of any part of the work are appropriately investigated and resolved.

REFERENCES

1. Cartabuke RH, Lopez R, Thota PN. Long-term esophageal and respiratory outcomes in children with esophageal atresia and tracheoesophageal fistula. *Gastroenterol Rep.* (2016) 4:310–4. doi: 10.1093/GASTRO/GOV055
2. Hysinger EB. Laryngomalacia, tracheomalacia and bronchomalacia. *Curr Probl Pediatr Adolesc Health Care.* (2018) 48:113–8. doi: 10.1016/J.CPPEDS.2018.03.002
3. Torre M, Carlucci M, Speggiorin S, Elliott MJ. Aortopexy for the treatment of tracheomalacia in children: review of the literature. *Ital J Pediatr.* (2012) 38:62. doi: 10.1186/1824-7288-38-62
4. Kamran A, Jennings RW. Tracheomalacia and tracheobronchomalacia in pediatrics: an overview of evaluation, medical management, and surgical treatment. *Front Pediatr.* (2019) 7:512. doi: 10.3389/fped.2019.00512
5. Sadreameli SC, Mcgrath-Morrow SA. Respiratory care of infants and children with congenital tracheo-oesophageal fistula and oesophageal atresia. *Paediatr Respir Rev.* (2016) 17:16–23. doi: 10.1016/j.prrv.2015.02.005
6. Hysinger EB, Panitch HB. Paediatric tracheomalacia. *Paediatr Respir Rev.* (2016) 17:9–15. doi: 10.1016/j.prrv.2015.03.002
7. Fraga JC, Jennings RW, Kim PCW. Pediatric tracheomalacia. *Semin Pediatr Surg.* (2016) 25:156–64. doi: 10.1053/j.sempedsurg.2016.02.008
8. Jennings RW, Hamilton TE, Smithers CJ, Ngerncham M, Feins N, Foker JE. Surgical approaches to aortopexy for severe tracheomalacia. *J Pediatr Surg.* (2014) 49:66–71. doi: 10.1016/j.jpedsurg.2013.09.036
9. Shieh HF, Smithers CJ, Hamilton TE, Zurakowski D, Rhein LM, Manfredi MA, et al. Posterior tracheopexy for severe tracheomalacia. *J Pediatr Surg.* (2017) 52:951–5. doi: 10.1016/j.jpedsurg.2017.03.018
10. Tytgat SHAJ, van Herwaarden-Lindeboom MYA, van Tuyll van Serooskerken ES, van der Zee DC. Thoracoscopic posterior tracheopexy during primary esophageal atresia repair: a new approach to prevent tracheomalacia complications. *J Pediatr Surg.* (2018) 53:1420–3. doi: 10.1016/j.jpedsurg.2018.04.024
11. Bairdain S, Smithers CJ, Hamilton TE, Zurakowski D, Rhein L, Foker JE, et al. Direct tracheobronchopexy to correct airway collapse due to severe tracheobronchomalacia: short-term outcomes in a series of 20 patients. *J Pediatr Surg.* (2015) 50:972–7. doi: 10.1016/j.jpedsurg.2015.03.016
12. Krishnan U, Mousa H, Dall'Oglio L, Homaira N, Rosen R, Faure C, et al. ESPGHAN-NASPGHAN guidelines for the evaluation and treatment of gastrointestinal and nutritional complications in children with esophageal atresia-tracheoesophageal fistula. *J Pediatr Gastroenterol Nutr.* (2016) 63:550–70. doi: 10.1097/MPG.0000000000001401
13. Beardsmore CS, MacFadyen UM, Johnstone MS, Williams A, Simpson H. Clinical findings and respiratory function in infants following repair of oesophageal atresia and tracheo-oesophageal fistula. *Eur Respir J.* (1994) 7:1039–47.
14. Leibovitch L, Zohar I, Maayan-Mazger A, Mazkereth R, Strauss T, Bilik R. Infants born with esophageal atresia with or without tracheo-esophageal fistula: short-and long-term outcomes. *Isr Med Assoc J.* (2018) 20:161–6.

15. Spoel M, Meeussen CJHM, Gischler SJ, Hop WCJ, Bax NMA, Wijnen RMH, et al. Respiratory morbidity and growth after open thoracotomy or thoracoscopic repair of esophageal atresia. *J Pediatr Surg.* (2012) 47:1975–83. doi: 10.1016/J.JPEDSURG.2012.07.044
16. Lacher M, Froehlich S, von Schweinitz D, Dietz HG. Early and long term outcome in children with esophageal atresia treated over the last 22 years. *Klin Pädiatr.* (2010) 222:296–301. doi: 10.1055/s-0030-1249610
17. Chetcuti P, Phelan PD. Gastrointestinal morbidity and growth after repair of oesophageal atresia and tracheo-oesophageal fistula. *Arch Dis Child.* (1993) 68:163–6. doi: 10.1136/adc.68.2.163
18. Shieh HF, Smithers CJ, Hamilton TE, Zurakowski D, Visner GA, Manfredi MA, et al. Posterior tracheopexy for severe tracheomalacia associated with esophageal atresia (EA): primary treatment at the time of initial EA repair versus secondary treatment. *Front Surg.* (2017) 4:80. doi: 10.3389/fsurg.2017.00080
19. Deboer EM, Prager JD, Ruiz AG, Jensen EL, Deterding RR, Friedlander JA, et al. Multidisciplinary care of children with repaired esophageal atresia and tracheoesophageal fistula; Multidisciplinary care of children with repaired esophageal atresia and tracheoesophageal fistula. *Pediatr Pulmonol.* (2016) 51:576–81. doi: 10.1002/ppul.23330
20. Conforti A, Valfrè L, Scuglia M, Trozzi M, Meucci D, Sgrò S, et al. Laryngotracheal abnormalities in esophageal atresia patients: a hidden entity. *Front Pediatr.* (2018) 6:401. doi: 10.3389/fped.2018.00401

4

Robot-Assisted Laparoscopic and Thoracoscopic Surgery: Prospective Series of 186 Pediatric Surgeries

Mario Navarrete Arellano [1] and Francisco Garibay González [2]*

[1] Hospital Central Militar, SEDENA, Mexico City, Mexico, [2] Department of Pediatrics, Hospital Militar de Especialidades de la Mujer y Neonatología, SEDENA, Mexico City, Mexico

Correspondence:
Mario Navarrete Arellano
drcirugiaroboticamx@gmail.com

Objective: We present the applications and experiences of robot-assisted laparoscopic and thoracoscopic surgery (RALTS) in pediatric surgery.

Materials and Methods: A prospective, observational, and longitudinal study was conducted from March 2015 to March 2018 that involved a non-random sample of a pediatric population that was treated with RALTS. The parameters examined were: gender, age, weight, height, diagnoses, surgical technique, elapsed time of console surgery, estimated bleeding, need for hemotransfusion, complications, surgical conversions, postoperative hospital stay, and follow-up. The Clavien-Dindo classification of complications was used. The surgical system used was the da Vinci model, Si version (Intuitive Surgical, Inc., Sunnyvale, CA. U.S.A), with measures of central tendency.

Results: In a 36-months period, 186 RALTS cases were performed, in 147 pediatric patients and an adult; 53.23% were male, and the remaining were female. The average age was 83 months, ranging from 3.5 to 204 months, plus one adult patient of 63 years. The stature was an average of 116.6 cm, with a range of 55–185 cm; the average weight was 26.9 kg, with a range of 5–102 kg; the smallest patient at 3.5 months was 55 cm in stature and weighed 5.5 kg. We performed 41 different surgical techniques, grouped in 4 areas: urological 91, gastrointestinal and hepatobiliary (GI-HB) 84, thoracic 6, and oncological 5. The console surgery time was 137.2 min on average, ranging from 10 to 780 min. Surgeon 1 performed 154 operations (82.8%), and the remainder were performed by Surgeon 2, with a conversion rate of 3.76%. The most commonly performed surgeries were: pyeloplasty, fundoplication, diaphragmatic plication, and removal of benign tumors, by area. Hemotransfusion was performed for 4.83%, and complications occurred in 2.68%. The average postoperative stay was 2.58 days, and the average follow-up was 23.5 months. The results of the 4 areas were analyzed in detail.

Conclusion: RALTS is safe and effective in children. An enormous variety of surgeries can be safely performed, including complex hepatobiliary, and thoracic surgery in small children. There are few published prospective series describing RALTS in the pediatric population, and most only describe urological surgery. It is important to offer children the advantages and safety of minimal invasion with robotic assistance; however, this procedure has only been slowly accepted and utilized for children. It is possible to implement a robust program of pediatric robotic surgery where multiple procedures are performed.

Keywords: robotic surgery, pediatric surgery, robotic urological surgery, robotic gastrointestinal surgery, robotic thoracic surgery, robotic oncological surgery, minimally invasive surgery, children

INTRODUCTION

Robotic surgery is one technology that has gained an enormous surge in use on adults. The general surgical applications have been quite varied in adults, but the technique has been particularly useful in urology for prostate surgery (1–4). There have been few reports that have been published for robotic general pediatric surgery (5–14). Thus, far, the largest number of procedures and publications have been produced for robotic urological pediatric surgery (15–34).

Trends in the literature indicate that pediatric robot-assisted minimally invasive surgery is continuing to be globally utilized (15–23, 31–34). Numerous case reports, case series, and comparative studies have unequivocally demonstrated that robotic surgery in children is safe (35). Robotic enhancements offer improvements to conventional minimal access surgery, permitting technical capabilities beyond existing threshold limits of human performance for surgery within the spatially constrained operative workspaces in children (15).

The first robotic procedure in children was fundoplication, were carried out by Meininger et al. in July 2000 and reported in April 2001 (36, 37).

If traditional laparoscopy is used, the reconstructive procedures are very challenging, and long periods of time are necessary to acquire the appropriate skills and confidence, vs. with RALS (robot-assisted laparoscopic surgery), the learning curve is shorter (31, 38–40).

In systematic investigations of databases of pediatric robot-assisted surgery, the global surgical conversion rate was 4.7% (7), other a net overall reported surgical conversion rate of 2.5% (15). Najmaldin and Antao (41) reported their initial 16-months experience with 50 abdominal procedures involving the gastrointestinal and hepatobiliary (GI-HB) and urological areas. Twelve different robotic surgical techniques were used, and the most frequent surgeries were fundoplication and pyeloplasty, with 6% conversions (41).

In published studies of pediatric robotic surgery, transoperative complications are infrequent, and in the postoperative period, the frequency varies from 0 to 15% (7, 41–43).

Minimally invasive surgery is commonly used for many applications in adult surgical oncology, including biopsy and resection of malignant disease in the chest and abdomen, and management of therapeutic complications. Because there has been an increasing availability of smaller instruments and equipment more suitable to the pediatric patient, for conventional laparo-thoracoscopy, there has been an increase in the use of these techniques with children. With robotic assistance there are also risks, among others, are port-site metastases and peritoneal spread, after resection due to minimal invasion of neoplasms (44, 45). The current status of robotic surgery for tumors in children is low volume usage, and globally a relatively static adoption (46–48).

There is a scarcity of publications from Latin American countries to date describing pediatric patients that have undergone robotic surgery. Secin et al. (49) conducted a survey among the main urologists working in public hospitals in Latin America, in 10 robotic programs based in 4 countries: 4 in Brazil, 3 in Mexico, 2 in Argentina, and 1 in Venezuela. In Venezuela, at the University Hospital of Caracas, 4 robotic surgeries had been performed in pediatric patients, with 2 pyeloplasties, one megacolon surgery, and one resection of an ovarian tumor that had been treated in the period from 2010 to 2012 (unpublished data). For adult patients, there are publications for various specialties (50–54).

The objective of this publication is to present the applications and our experience of RALTS in pediatric surgery.

MATERIALS AND METHODS

This prospective, observational and longitudinal study of the robotic surgeries performed on a pediatric population was conducted from March 2015 to March 2018. Our hospital is a public tertiary care facility, and the robotic surgery program includes several surgical specialties in adult and pediatric surgery. The diagnoses of the pathologies were made with laboratory, radiological, cabinet, and special studies according to the case.

Non-random samples were all treated with RALTS. The parameters recorded were gender, age, weight, height, diagnoses, surgical technique, elapsed time of console surgery, estimated bleeding, hemotransfusion, complications, conversions, postoperative hospital stay, and follow-up. Both authors (surgeons) initially performed some simple surgical techniques, and then advanced to more complex surgeries, with subsequent advancement to different points of the learning curve for robotic surgery.

The Clavien-Dindo classification of surgical complications was used (55, 56). The surgical system used was the da Vinci model, Si version (Intuitive Surgical, Inc., Sunnyvale, CA. U.S.A). We used 8-mm robotic instruments consisting of 2 or 3 robotic trocars according to the surgical technique, 8.5-mm or 12-mm robotic 30° lens for a three-dimensional camera, and a 5-mm trocar laparoscopic for one assistant.

In the following procedures, we used 3 robotic work arms: for urological surgery, in the Mitrofanoff procedure with or without augmentation cystoplasty; for GI-HB surgery, in fundoplications and in the biliodigestives; and in thoracic surgery, in lobectomies, and in oncological surgery, in 4 of the 5 procedures, the exception was the resection of the mediastinal teratoma. In the first 10 fundoplications, we used a 1-0 silk suture to elevate the liver, but after lesion of the left hepatic duct occurred, and we subsequently opted to use the third robotic instrument for that purpose. The docking charts for robotic surgery that are suggested for surgical techniques in adults were not applicable for children. Thus, at times, 3 cm of separation was required between each trocar when performing surgery on infants, due to the limited space in such a small patient.

The postoperative follow-up was at 8, 30, and 90 to 120 days, and then every 6 months. Between 90 and 120 days, radiographic and cabinet studies were carried out according to the treated pathology to evaluate the results. We used measures of central tendency. The analysis of the results was made based on the number of procedures. The data was entered into a spreadsheet in Microsoft Office Excel 2013 version.

In relation to ethical considerations of the study, being of an observational nature, it was not necessary to consent to enter the study to the patients. The Research Ethics Committee of the Hospital evaluated and approved the study. In Mexico, robot-assisted surgery complies with the records and regulations of the Mexican health authorities. In our institution, robotic surgery is routinely authorized for execution. In order to perform the medical-surgical procedures, we obtained the informed consent in writing from the parents or guardians and the adult patient.

TABLE 1 | Prospective series of 186 pediatric surgeries using RALTS.

Area	Procedures	*n* (%)
UROLOGICAL		
	Pyeloplasty	19
	Nephrectomy	18
	Ureteral reimplantation	17
	Mitrofanoff	6
	Nephroureterectomy	6
	Varicocelectomy	5
	Release of extrinsic obstruction	
	UP union	3
	Inguinal hernia repair	3
	Desderivation of ureterostomy and ureteral reimplantation	2
	Cystolithotomy	2
	Various*	10
	Subtotal	**91 (48.92)**
GI-HB		
	Primary fundoplication	38
	Redo fundoplication	13
	Cholecystectomy	11
	Gastrostomy	9
	Biliodigestive**	6
	Operation of malone	2
	Various***	5
	Subtotal	**84 (45.16)**
THORACIC		
	Diaphragmatic plication	3
	Lobectomy	2
	Bronchogenic cyst excision	1
	Subtotal	**6 (3.23)**
Oncological		
	Mediastinal teratoma	1
	Resection of carcinoid in stomach	1 (adult)
	Left radical nephrectomy	1
	Retroperitoneal lipoma	1
	Left adrenalectomy (pheochromocytoma)	1
	Subtotal	**5 (2.69)**

Ureteroureterostomy, augmentation cystoplasty, bladder neck closure, heminephrectomy with ureterectomy, perirenal abscess drainage, colostomy closure, enterovesical fistula closure, review of Mitrofanoff, ureterostomy, and ureteropyelography.

*** Roux-en-Y hepaticojejuno (5) or portojejuno (1) anastomosis reconstruction.*

**** Duodenoplasty with adherensiolysis, extraction of gastric trichobezoar, drainage, and debridement of recurrent retrohepatic abscess post-appendectomy, gastrojejunoanastomosis with Roux-en-Y and splenectomy.*

RESULTS

In a 36-months period, we performed 186 RALTS in 147 pediatric patients and one adult patient. Of the procedures, 53.23% (99) were in male, and the rest were female; the average age was 83 months, ranging from 3.5 to 204 months, plus one patient of 63 years. The average height was 116.6 cm, and ranged from 55 to 185 cm, with an average weight of 26.9 kg, ranging from 5 to 102 kg; the smallest patient was 3.5 months old with a height of 55 cm and weight 5.5 kg (**Supplementary Table 1**).

We performed 41 different surgical techniques, grouped in 4 areas: urological 91 (48.92%), GI-HB 84 (45.16%), thoracic 6 (3.23%), and oncological 5 (2.69%), as shown in **Table 1**. Our 3 most frequent urological procedures were pyeloplasty, nephrectomy, and ureteral reimplantation, totaling 54 and representing 59.34% of this area. GI-HB, primary fundoplication, redo-fundoplication, and cholecystectomy totaled 62 and represented 73.8% in this area. Diaphragmatic plication and lobectomy were the most frequent for thoracic surgery, and there were only isolated cases of oncological surgery.

Of the total procedures, the elapsed console surgery time was an average of 137.2 min, ranging from 10 to 780 min. Surgeon 1 performed 154 procedures (82.8%), and Surgeon 2 performed 32 procedures (17.2%). Global hemotransfusion occurred in 4.83%, and complications occurred in 2.68%, with a surgical conversion rate of 3.76%. The average postoperative stay was 2.58 days, and the average follow-up was 23.5 months.

There was a predominance of patients males in urological (62.6%), and oncological (80%), and a predominance of patients females in thoracic (66.6%) and GI-HB (53.5%). In relation to age, weight, and height, the smallest group of patients underwent thoracic procedures (14.5 months, 9.1 kg, 78.8 cm, average values), and the largest underwent GI-HB surgery (97.7 months, 29.7 kg, 125 cm, average values), intermediate average values those subjected to urological surgery (72.9 months, 20.3 kg, 110 cm), and oncological patients (57.3 months, 18 kg, 113 cm, average values). Patients of 10 kg or less were 12 of urological, 10 of GI-HB, 4 of thoracic and 1 of oncological procedures, totaling 27 cases, representing 14.5% of our casuistry.

The evolution of the console surgery times is exemplified by the most frequently performed procedures, which were urological, pyeloplasty, and GI-HB, primary fundoplication. Surgeon 1 consistently reduced the time required for surgery as the procedures continued to evolve and advance, of 227 min in the first pyeloplasty at 115 min in the procedure 19, and for primary fundoplication, it was reduced of 115 min in the first fundoplication at 56 min in the procedure 26 (**Supplementary Figures 1, 2**).

Of the three most frequently performed procedures by area, the following results were obtained. For urological procedures, 19 pyeloplasty surgeries were performed, with console surgery time of 183 min on average, 0% conversions, 5.2% complications (1 case), stay PO of 3.4 days, with a success rate of 100%. There were 18 nephrectomy surgeries, with console surgery time of 102 min on average, 0% conversions, 5.2% complications (1 case), and stay PO of 1.9 days. There were 17 units of ureteral reimplantation, with console surgery time of 139 min on average, 0% conversions, 0% complications, stay PO of 2.1 days, with 88.24% resolution of reflux; one patient with recurrent bilateral reflux was reoperated and reflux was resolved, with 100% secondary success.

Appendicovesicostomy or Mitrofanoff operation, we performed 6 of these procedures, without predominance of gender, with average age of 9.25 years, weight of 30.7 kg, height of 1.24 m, console surgery time of 262 min, estimated bleeding of 26 ml, with one conversion, and stay PO of 4.34 days. For one patient at 30 days PO, it was improperly manipulated and the Mitrofanoff was dismantled. This complication was not related to surgery, and thus, we can consider a success of 83.34%; open surgery was used for the reoperation, and at the follow-up, all the ducts were continent.

For GI-HB surgery, there were 38 primary fundoplication procedures, plus gastrostomy for feeding in 9 cases, with a console surgery time of 159 min on average, 5.26% conversions (2 cases), 5.26% complications (2 cases), stay PO of 2.4 days; at follow-up PO, there were 2 cases of partial dismantling of fundoplication and hiatal hernia (5.26%), at 11 and 24 months, with a follow-up PO of 17.7 months on average. There were 13 procedures of redo fundoplication (the two robotic cases with recurrence are included), with a console surgery time of 188 min on average, 7.7% conversions (1 case), 0% complications, and stay PO of 2.3 days, with a follow-up PO of 19.5 months on average. There were 11 cholecystectomy procedures, with a console surgery time of 53 min on average, 0% conversions, and 0% complications, with a stay PO of 1.5 days.

The results of 4 patients treated with choledochal cyst, 3 females and 1 male, with average age of 36 months, average weight of 15 kg, and average height of 94.2 cm. There were three cases of cyst type 1-A and one type 1-C; the size of the cyst was 8–12.5 cm, with an average of 9.6 cm. Minimally invasive surgery was performed, with the extracorporeal Roux-en-Y procedure assisted by laparoscopy, and resection of the cyst, cholecystectomy, and the hepaticojejunal anastomosis to Roux-en-Y was performed with robotic assistance. The average surgical times were 130 min with assistance by laparoscopy and 230 min for console surgery time, with an average of 32.5 ml of bleeding. There were no conversions or complications. The average PO stay was 4.7 days, with a 15-months follow-up, and the patients evolved asymptomatically.

For thoracic procedures, there were 3 procedures with diaphragmatic plication, with a console surgery time of 161.6 min on average, 0% conversions, 33.3% complications (1 case), and stay PO of 5.6 days. There were 2 lobectomy procedures, with a console surgery time of 314 min, 50% conversions (1 case), 0% complications, and stay PO of 3 days. There was 1 procedure of resection of a bronchogenic cyst, with console surgery time of 269 min, with no conversion, no complications, and stay PO of 3 days.

There were 5 isolated cases of oncological procedures (**Table 1**).

The estimated average bleeding in each area of procedures performed, in relation to the average weight of the patients, was as follows: blood loss was 6.1 ml/kg for oncological procedures, 2 ml/kg for thoracic, 1.3 ml/kg for urological, and 1.1 ml/kg for GI-HB. However, the highest number of hemotransfusions occurred during the GI-HB procedures, with 5 cases, against 4 cases of the remaining 3 areas of procedures.

There were 2 complications that occurred intraoperatively (IO) a lesion of the left hepatic duct when applying a suture point for traction and elevating the liver during a fundoplication, and rupture of a renal vein when trying to apply a staple during a nephrectomy. These complications were classified as IIIB and II, respectively, according to the Clavien-Dindo classification. The treatment of these complications was Roux-en-Y hepatico-yeyunostomy, and bleeding control and hemotransfusion, respectively.

There were 3 PO complications: (i) a urinoma in a patient with pyeloplasty, with readmission at 9 PO days, (ii) an enterovesical fistula in 2a., 1 week PO, in a patient with augmentation cystoplasty and colostomy closure, and (iii) prolonged drainage of pleural fluid (11 days) in a patient with diaphragmatic plication. According to the Clavien-Dindo classification, the first two corresponded to IIIb, and the third corresponded to I. The treatment of these complications consisted of percutaneous application of a multiproposite catheter for the first patient, a second surgery was performed for the second patient, and the last patient was hospitalized for 12 days to drain fluids.

The robotic procedures that required conversion, was to an open surgery. In the urological procedure, the conversion was required due to the technical difficulty in the appendicovesicostomy anastomosis. In the GI-HB procedures, the reasons for the 4 conversions were multiple intestinal adhesions, technical difficulty in 2 primary fundoplications with gastrostomy, and in a redo of a fundoplication. The reason for the conversion into a lobectomy was technical difficulty, and in the radical nephrectomy, it was difficult to identify the anatomy when dividing the horseshoe kidney.

The longest average PO stay of 4.33 days occurred in patients that underwent a thoracic procedure. In the other 3 areas, the PO stays were 2.48 days in GI-HB, 2.58 days in urological and 2.6 days in oncological. The average PO follow-up among the patients in the 4 areas of surgical procedures was very similar, between 24.5 and 31.4 months, with a range between 7 and 43 months overall (**Supplementary Table 2**).

DISCUSSION

The robotic surgery program began in our hospital in November 2014, and pediatric surgery was incorporated in March 2015. The first procedures with robotic assistance were performed on the pediatric population on March 23, 2015, after Surgeon 1 received training and certification as a console surgeon of the da Vinci surgical system, with previous experience in open surgery and conventional laparo-thoracoscopy. Recommendations were followed to perform some less complex cases and progress toward highly complex procedures, with subsequent integration into the Hospital Committee of Robotic Surgery.

In our experience, the order of frequency of the procedures, from highest to lowest by area, was urological, GI-HB, and thoracic (**Table 1**), which coincides with what has previously been reported (15). There are numerous reports that the most frequent urological procedure performed is pyeloplasty, and the most frequent GI-HB surgery performed is fundoplication, which varies between lobectomy, ligation of the ductus arteriosus, and mediastinal masses in the reports of thoracic procedures, which are aspects that also coincide with our treated pediatric population (5–7, 15).

During the 18 years that have elapsed since the first 2 fundoplications were carried out (36, 37), more than 70 different surgical techniques have been published. Cundy et al. performed a 2013 systematic literature search for all reported cases of robotic surgery in children during an 11-year period. During this time, 137 articles reported 2,393 procedures in 1,840 patients, and the most prevalent gastrointestinal, genitourinary, and thoracic procedures were fundoplication, pyeloplasty, and lobectomy, respectively (15). These 3 previous robotic surgical techniques represented 46.55% and genitourinary procedures 59.92% of the total surgeries, confirming that the greatest amount of these types of published studies are in the field of urology (16–34).

In 11-years period (April 2001 to March 2012), the published literature reporting robotic surgery in children, categorized by study design, comprises 34% case reports, 52% case series, and 14% non-randomized comparative studies (n = 220 publications), and the study design was prospective in only 6% of non-randomized comparative studies. As well, 79% of these 220 publications originated from the United States, and the remainder were from 17 other countries, with 14% from Europe, 4% from the Middle East, and 3% from Asia (15).

Qualitatively, we find that with complex and laborious procedures, the time of console surgery is longer as compared to standard open surgery, but we agree that robotic surgery enables more refined hand-eye coordination, superior suturing skills, better dexterity, and precise dissection. It is achieved by the characteristics of robotic surgical platforms that include motion scaling, greater optical magnification, 3D and stereoscopic vision, increased articulated instrument tip dexterity, tremor filtration, operator-controlled camera movement, and elimination of the fulcrum effect (15), and all of this translates into greater safety for patients and advantages for the surgeon.

Considering the examples of 19 procedures of pyeloplasty (with an average of 183 min) and 38 procedures of primary fundoplication plus gastrostomy for feeding in 9 cases (an average of 159 min) as the most frequently performed procedures, our console surgery times are very satisfactory when comparing them with what was reported by other authors as 221 and 170 min, respectively, without including added procedures (7). In a meta-analysis of fundoplication, 6 series of patients were included for a total of 135 patients that underwent robotic fundoplication surgery (with some cases of gastrostomy), and the average console surgery time was 168.3 min, with 3% conversions, 8.9% complications, and 5.31 days PO stay (57).

Robotic ureteral reimplantation for the treatment of pediatric vesicoureteral reflux should be reclassified as a complex reconstructive procedure in pediatric urology. Over the past decade, higher than expected complication rates and suboptimal reflux resolution rates at some centers have been reported. The robotic ureteral reimplantation results have widely varied, with reflux resolution from 77 to 100% and complications from 0 to 12.5% (58). Using a standard technique to improve reimplantation results that was modified according to Gundeti et al. (59), we obtained results with 0% complications, primary success of 88.24%, and secondary success of 100%.

Although it is recommended that a surgeon perform a minimum of one robotic operation per week, it is important to emphasize that 15 to 30 robotic procedures should be performed to achieve optimal console surgery times, according to the type of procedure. Then, the use of this technology can become profitable. The period during which a surgeon finds that the procedures are more difficult, take longer, and there is potentially a higher rate of complications and less effectiveness due to inexperience, which is called the learning curve (60). The use of robot assistance dramatically decreases the learning curve, because overcome the limitations of conventional laparoscopy (31, 38–40). Our console surgery times have evolved in 19 pyeloplasties and in 26 fundoplications, with a decrease of 50% and of almost 52%, respectively.

Robotic assistance has special applications in complex and reconstructive surgery. By areas, urological: pyeloplasty, ureteral reimplantation, augmentation cystoplasty, and Mitrofanoff procedure; GI-HB: revision fundoplication and hiatal hernia and biliary-digestive correction; thoracic tumors: tumor excision and thymectomy; and oncological: resection of tumors of selected cases. For all these procedures, from the open technique, we jump to robotic surgery.

Because of the limitations, conventional laparoscopic surgery in pediatric surgery has been primarily limited to simple or extirpative surgery, more complex or reconstructive surgery by laparoscopy, can only be performed by a limited number of highly qualified surgeons (61).

Since the publication of the initial experience of robotic-assisted laparoscopic ileocistoplasty and the appendicovesicostomy of Mitrofanoff by Gundeti et al (62), it was shown that is a safe, feasible and effective procedure (62). Of the urological surgery, is one of the most complex procedures, in a publication of the retrospective cohort consisted of 18 patients, with mean age of 11 years, console surgery time of 494 min, stay PO of 5.2 days, continence in 94.4%, Clavien-Dindo grade 1 complications in 5 patients and grade IIIb in 2 patients (63).

The patients with neural tube defects may also require redo surgery at the bladder neck for persistent incontinence or any of these procedures with creation of a Malone antegrade continence enema (64, 65).

In a series of cases, retrospectively evaluated for open appendicovesicostomy and robotic, the comparison did not reveal significant differences in the number of acute complications or reoperations between the groups (66).

Our results are satisfactory with the Mitrofanoff, of 6 procedures, one conversion, and all the ducts were continent to follow up.

A multi-center analysis was performed in the United States regarding the complications and conversions in a large cohort of pediatric patients (880 procedures) that underwent robotic urological surgery to 90-day PO. There were with 41 (4.8%) Grade IIIa and Grade IIIb complications, and one patient (0.1%) had a grade IVa complication. Intraoperative visceral injuries secondary to robotic instrument exchange and traction injury were seen in four patients (0.5%), with subsequent conversion to an open procedure. Grade I and II complications were seen in 59 (6.9%) and 70 (8.2%) patients, respectively. The overall 90-day complication rate was similar to those appearing in reports of laparoscopic and open surgical procedures. A total of 14 (1.6%) surgeries were converted to an open or pure laparoscopic procedure (67).

Complications of robotic surgery in urology in a single institution, with 10 different types of procedures performed in included 136 patients, 11 total complications (8.1%): 2 grade I (1.5%), 7 grade II (5.1%), and 2 grade IIIb (1.5%). Complications included ileus in 2 patients, port site infection in 2, urinary leak in 2, urinary retention in 2, urinary tract infection in 2, and stent migration in 1 (43).

There are few reports of minimally assisted surgery by robot for the treatment of choledochal cyst (68–72). Currently, the standard treatment is open surgery. The first cases of resection of choledochal cyst with robotic assistance were reported by Lee et al. (70) and Woo et al. (71).This treatment method is safe and effective, it is associated with earlier postoperative feeding and discharge from the hospital, technically robotic-assistance facilitates performing the biliodigestive anastomosis and for pediatric choledochal cyst showed results comparable to those for open surgery, and thus, is considered to be a valid and alternative surgery for this pathology (71, 72).

A recent systematic review that included a total of 86 patients, 7 patients experienced conversion to open surgery, and the surgery success rate was 91.9%. The hospitalization time was 8.8 days. Eight patients had biliary fistula, one patient had anastomotic stenosis, and one patient had wound dehiscence (73).

The results in the 4 cases that we treat of choledochal cyst confirm the safety and efficacy of this surgical alternative, with 0% complications and conversions.

There are benefits and limitations of using robotic surgery for children with cancer (74), it is feasible for the surgical treatment of tumors in pediatric patients and only isolated adverse events have been reported for malignant tumors, such as tumor spillage and residual disease (45). The current status of robotic surgery for tumors in children is low volume usage, in a relatively static global state of adoption and when applied the oncological surgical principles must be respected (46, 47).

In pediatrics, urologic oncology cases are often managed with open surgery, but is feasibility of using the robotic approach in carefully selected cases, and safely and effectively adapted adult robotic techniques for genitourinary oncology cases in children and young adults (48).

Our experience with robotic-assisted surgery for oncological procedures is limited, with only isolated cases to date. However, the results have been satisfactory, with only one conversion and 0% complications in 5 cases. It is only a matter of time before appropriate cases arise, and we will be going forward in this area with robotic surgery.

Hemotransfusion occurred in 4.83% of the procedures we performed. The average calculation per/kg of weight of estimated bleeding was minimal, and the highest number of hemotransfusions was in the GI-HB procedures, with 5 cases consisting of 4 fundoplications and the case of duodenoplasty with adherensiolysis that merited conversion to open. Complications occurred in 2.68% (5 cases), two IO and three PO. In published reports, rates are very variable, with complications occurring in 8 cases (3%) of 274 robotic procedures during the first 6 years of experience in a London hospital (42). Other reported with 50 abdominal procedures involving the gastrointestinal and hepatobiliary (GI-HB) and urological areas, twelve different robotic surgical techniques were used, there was 6% conversions (41).

In systematic investigations of databases containing information on robot-assisted surgery in children, the global complications ranged from 0 to 15% (7).

Our global conversion rate of 3.76% did not significantly differ from that reported by Cundy et al. (15), with 2.5% overall; by area of procedures, the conversion rates of gastrointestinal, genitourinary, and thoracic procedures were 3.9, 1.3, and 10%, respectively (15). Our conversion rates of the same areas were 4.76, 1.09, and 16.6%, respectively. In their first 100 robotic surgeries, Meehan and Sandler (5) reported conversions of 13.48% in non-urological abdominal procedures and 18.18% in thoracic surgeries. For 96 robotic procedures, De Lambert (2013) reported a conversion rate of 3.1%, which corresponds to patients in the groups of general surgery, urologic surgery, and thoracic surgery (6). A systematic database search was performed that included data from all published reports until October 2007 (31 studies and 513 patients), and the conversion rate for all pediatric robotic procedures was 4.7% (7).

We have not been presented with malfunctions of the robot during the procedures.

There are very few publications of pancreatic pathology in children, treated with a robotic approach, we find only case reports (75–77).

There are approximately 60 da Vinci systems in hospitals in Latin America to date, and there are few that are used to perform surgery on children. The costs of technology, consumables, and maintenance are the main obstacles in Latin American countries that prevent robotic surgery from being practiced more widely. The situation is more adverse in private hospital institutions, because insurance companies only approve a few cases of robotic surgery for adult patients, and children are regularly not approved.

We consider viable, if there is enough experience in Pediatric Surgeons, to implement a robust program of robotic surgery where multiple procedures are performed and after overcoming the learning curve, with efficiency, effectiveness and safety to be used in the complex cases of the different areas of Pediatric surgery is a way to maintain the volume of cases and reduce costs by using robotic assistance routinely in conjunction with other surgical specialties.

The biggest obstacles preventing the use of robotic surgery on a pediatric population are the learning curve, technical limitations, the size of the robotic instruments, and the inconvenience, the costs (78, 79). The manufacturer of the da Vinci surgical robot recommends an 8-cm distance between each port. This is impossible to achieve in neonatal cases (79). This technical limitation, we overcome it have used a 3-cm separation between each trocar, and we have performed various procedures in younger infants with no problems.

There are very few studies that evaluate its cost (30) in an integral way and consider a multitude of factors in addition to the surgical event. The most important factor in Latin American countries is cost, which limits the adoption of robotic surgery.

The outcomes of RALTS are comparable to open surgery and conventional laparoscopic surgery and demonstrate continued improvement with experience. Outcomes can become more cost-efficient if shorter operative times are achieved, and with marketing competition, by providing less expensive robotic systems and instruments. Robotic surgery is suitable in the pediatric practice, which necessitates fine dissections and sutures in narrow anatomical spaces. The results of robotic surgery in the field of pediatrics are encouraging (80).

Our data and other series demonstrate that the short- and long-term morbidity associated with robotic surgery is low in a pediatric population, even during the learning period (44). This information allows affirmation that robot-assisted laparoscopic surgery is safe and efficient in the pediatric population. Although open surgery is still the gold standard for many pediatric diseases, there is a chance to change this view due to the inherent advantages in reconstructive surgery that can be attained with robot-assisted laparoscopy (81). We fully share this vision and consider that children, like adults, should have the opportunity and receive the benefits of RALTS.

CONCLUSION

RALTS is safe and effective in children. An enormous variety of surgeries can be safely performed including complex surgical cases, even in small children. There are few published prospective series describing pediatric RALTS, since most are only urological.

This technology has only been slowly adopted for use in children. Pediatric Surgeons must advocate for the benefit of our patients and overcome the obstacles to increase the adoption and more widely disseminate its use.

The present prospective series reporting pediatric robotic surgery is the first in Latin America, and its results are very satisfactory, which allows us to affirm that we have accumulated favorable experiences and that we can offer our pediatric patients the benefits and advantages of robotic surgery.

It is possible to implement a robust program of pediatric robotic surgery where multiple procedures are performed.

AUTHOR CONTRIBUTIONS

MNA contributed to the prospective registration of all the information, designed the data spreadsheet for Microsoft Office Excel 2013 version, performed 154 procedures, performed patient follow-up, analyzed the published information (references), analyzed the experimental results, and compared them with the published data, and wrote the manuscript. FGG contributed information to the prospective registry pertaining to the 32 procedures that he performed, and also obtained follow-up information from the patients.

REFERENCES

1. Atug F, Castle EP, Woods M, Srivastav SK, Thomas R, Davis R. Transperitoneal versus extraperitoneal robotic-assisted radical prostatectomy: is one better than the other? *Urology.* (2006) 68:1077–81. doi: 10.1016/j.urology.2006.07.008
2. Mikhail AA, Orvieto MA, Billatos ES, Zorn KC, Gong EM, Brendler CB, et al. Robotic-assisted laparoscopic prostatectomy: first 100 patients with one year of follow-up. *Urology.* (2006) 68:1275–9. doi: 10.1016/j.urology.2006.08.1060
3. Khaira HS, Bruyere F, Malley PJ, Peters JS, Costello AJ. Does obesity influence the operative course or complications of robot-assisted laparoscopic prostatectomy. *Brit J Urol Int.* (2006) 98:1275–8. doi: 10.1111/j.1464-410X.2006.06488.x
4. Tseng TY, Kuebler HR, Cancel QV, Sun L, Springhart WP, Murphy BC, at al. Prospective health-related quality-of-life assessment in an initial cohort of patients undergoing robotic radical prostatectomy. *Urology.* (2006) 68:1061–6. doi: 10.1016/j.urology.2006.06.017
5. Meehan JJ, Sandler A. Robotic surgery: a single- institutional review of the first 100 consecutive cases. *Surg Endosc.* (2008) 22:177–82. doi: 10.1007/s00464-007-9418-2

6. de Lamberg G, Fourcade L, Centi J, Fredon F, Braik K, Szwarc C, et al. How to successfully implement a robotic pediatric surgery program: lessons learned after 96 procedures. *Surg Endosc.* (2013) 27:2137–44. doi: 10.1007/s00464-012-2729-y
7. Sinha SK, Haddad M. Robot-assisted surgery in children: current status. *J Robotic Surg.* (2008) 1:243–6. doi: 10.1007/s11701-007-0054-6
8. Alqahtani A, Albassam A, Zamakhshary M, Shoukri M, Altokhais T, Aljazairi A, et al. Robot-assisted pediatric surgery: how far can we go? *World J Surg.* (2010) 34:975–8. doi: 10.1007/s00268-010-0431-6
9. Al-Bassam A. Robotic-assisted surgery in children: advantages and limitations. *J Robot Surg.* (2010) 4:19–22. doi: 10.1007/s11701-010-0181-3
10. Camps JI. The use of robotics in pediatric surgery: my initial experience. *Pediatr Surg Int.* (2011) 27:991–6. doi: 10.1007/s00383-011-2901-9
11. Marhuenda C, Giné C, Asensio M, Guillén G, Martínez Ibáñez V. Robotic surgery: first pediatric series in Spain. *Cir Pediatr.* (2011) 24:90–2.
12. Ballouhey Q, Villemagne T, Cros J, Szwarc C, Braik K, Longis B, et al. A comparison of robotic surgery in children weighing above and below 15.0 kg: size does not affect surgery success. *Surg Endosc.* (2015) 29:2643–50. doi: 10.1007/s00464-014-3982-z
13. Bütter A, Merritt N, Dave S. Establishing a pediatric robotic surgery program in Canada. *J Robot Surg.* (2017) 11:207–10. doi: 10.1007/s11701-016-0646-0
14. Mattioli G, Pini Prato A, Razore B, Leonelli L, Pio L, Avanzini S, et al. Da Vinci robotic surgery in a pediatric hospital. *J Laparoendosc Adv Surg Tech A.* (2017) 27:539–45. doi: 10.1089/lap.2016.0390
15. Cundy TP, Shetty K, Clark J, Chang TP, Sriskandarajah K, Gattas NE, et al. The first decade of robotic surgery in children. *J Pediatr Surg.* (2013) 48:858–86. doi: 10.1016/j.jpedsurg.2013.01.031
16. Lee RS, Retik AB, Borer JG, Peters CA. Pediatric robot assisted laparoscopic dismembered pyeloplasty: comparison with a cohort of open surgery. *J Urol.* (2006) 175:683–67. doi: 10.1016/S0022-5347(05)00183-7
17. Passerotti CC, Nguyen HT, Eisner BH, Lee RS, Peters CA. Laparoscopic reoperative pediatric pyeloplasty with robotic assistance. *J Endourol.* (2007) 21:1137–40. doi: 10.1089/end.2007.9929
18. Volfson IA, Munver R, Esposito M, Dakwar G, Hanna M, Stock JA. Robot-assisted urologic surgery: safety and feasibility in the pediatric population. *J Endourol.* (2007) 21:1315–8. doi: 10.1089/end.2007.9982
19. Peters CA. Robotically assisted surgery in pediatric urology. *Urol Clin North Am.* (2004) 31:743–52. doi: 10.1016/j.ucl.2004.06.007
20. Lee RS, Passerotti CC, Cendron M, Estrada CR, Borer JG, Peters CA. Early results of robot assisted laparoscopic lithotomy in adolescents. *J Urol.* (2007) 177:2306–10. doi: 10.1016/j.juro.2007.01.178
21. Franco I, Dyer LL, Zelkovic P. Laparoscopic pyeloplasty in the pediatric patient: hand sewn anastomosis versus robotic assisted anastomosis: is there a difference? *J Urol.* (2007) 178:1483–6. doi: 10.1016/j.juro.2007.06.012
22. Yee DS, Shanberg AM, Duel BP, Rodriguez E, Eichel L, Rajpoot D. Initial comparison of robotic-assisted laparoscopic versus open pyeloplasty in children. *Urology.* (2006) 67:599–602. doi: 10.1016/j.urology.2005.09.021
23. Casale P. Robotic pediatric urology. *Curr Urol Rep.* (2009) 10:115–8. doi: 10.1007/s11934-009-0021-z
24. Christman MS, Casale P. Robot-assisted bladder diverticulectomy in the pediatric population. *J Endourol.* (2012) 26:1296–300. doi: 10.1089/end.2012.0051
25. Bansal D, Cost NG, Bean CM, Riachy E, Defoor WR Jr, Reddy PP, et al. Comparison of pediatric robotic-assisted laparoscopic nephroureterectomy and laparoendoscopic single-site nephroureterectomy. *Urology.* (2014) 83:438–42. doi: 10.1016/j.urology.2013.08.066
26. Mason MD, Anthony Herndon CD, Smith-Harrison LI, Peters CA, Corbett ST. Robotic-assisted partial nephrectomy in duplicated collecting systems in the pediatric population: techniques and outcomes. *J Pediatr Urol.* (2014) 10:374–9. doi: 10.1016/j.jpurol.2013.10.014
27. Liu DB, Ellimoottil C, Flum AS, Casey JT, Gong EM. Contemporary national comparison of open, laparoscopic, and robotic-assisted laparoscopic pediatric pyeloplasty. *J Pediatr Urol.* (2014) 10:610–5. doi: 10.1016/j.jpurol.2014.06.010
28. Esposito C, Masieri L, Steyaert H, Escolino M, Cerchione R, La Manna A, et al. Robot-assisted extravesical ureteral reimplantation (revur) for unilateral vesico-ureteral reflux in children: results of a multicentric international survey. *World J Urol.* (2018) 36:481–8. doi: 10.1007/s00345-017-2155-9
29. Kawal T, Srinivasan AK, Chang J, Long C, Chu D, Shukla AR. Robotic-assisted laparoscopic ureteral re-implant (RALUR): can post-operative urinary retention be predicted? *J Pediatr Urol.* (2018) 14:323.e1–5. doi: 10.1016/j.jpurol.2018.05.010
30. Varda BK, Wang Y, Chung BI, Lee RS, Kurtz MP, Nelson CP. Has the robot caught up? National trends in utilization, perioperative outcomes, and cost for open, laparoscopic, and robotic pediatric pyeloplasty in the United States from 2003 to 2015. *J Pediatr Urol.* (2018) 14:336.e1–8. doi: 10.1016/j.jpurol.2017.12.010
31. Garcia I, Salas de Armas IA, Pimpalwar A. Current trends in pediatric robotic surgery. *Bangladesh J Endosurg.* (2014) 2:15–28. doi: 10.3329/bje.v2i1.19589
32. Monn MF, Bahler CD, Schneider EB, Whittam BM, Misseri R, Rink RC, et al. Trends in robot-assisted laparoscopic pyeloplasty in pediatric patients. *Urology.* (2013) 81:1336–41. doi: 10.1016/j.urology.2013.01.025
33. Sukumar S, Roghmann F, Sood A, Abdo A, Menon M, Sammon JD, et al. Correction of ureteropelvic junction obstruction in children: national trends and comparative effectiveness in operative outcomes. *J Endourol.* (2014) 28:592–8. doi: 10.1089/end.2013.0618
34. Varda BK, Johnson EK, Clark C, Chung BI, Nelson CP, Chang SL. National trends of perioperative outcomes and costs for open, laparoscopic and robotic pediatric pyeloplasty. *J Urol.* (2014) 191:1090–5. doi: 10.1016/j.juro.2013.10.077
35. Cundy TP. *Clinical Application and Evaluation of Robot-Assisted Surgery in Children* (Thesis 2014). Avaliable online at: https://spiral.imperial.ac.uk/bitstream/10044/1/.../1/Cundy-TP-2015-PhD-Thesis.pdf
36. Meininger D, Byhahn C, Markus BH, Heller K, Westphal K. Total endoscopic Nissen fundoplication with the robotic device "da Vinci" in children. Hemodynamics, gas exchange, and anesthetic management. *Anaesthesist.* (2001) 50:271–5. doi: 10.1007/s001010051001
37. Meininger DD, Byhahn C, Heller K, Gutt CN, Westphal K. Totally endoscopic Nissen fundoplication with a robotic system in a child. *Surg Endosc.* (2001) 15:1360. doi: 10.1007/s00464-001-4200-3
38. Westebring-van der Putten EP, Goossens RHM, Jakimowicz JJ, Dankelman J. Haptics in minimally invasive surgery—a review. *Minimally Invas Ther.* (2008) 17:3–16. doi: 10.1080/13645700701820242
39. Braumann C, Jacobi CA, Menenakos C, Ismail M, Rueckert JC, Mueller JM. Robotic-assisted laparoscopic and thoracoscopic surgery with the da Vinci system: a 4-year experience in a single institution. *Surg Laparosc Endosc Percutan Tech.* (2008) 18:260–6. doi: 10.1097/SLE.0b013e31816f85e5
40. Vereczkel A, Bubb H, Feussner H. Laparoscopic surgery and ergonomics: it's time to think of ourselves as well. *Surg Endosc.* (2003) 17:1680–2. doi: 10.1007/s00464-003-9020-1
41. Najmaldin A, Antao B. Early experience of tele-robotic sugery in children. *Int J Med Robot Comp Assist Surg.* (2007) 3:199–202. doi: 10.1002/rcs.150
42. Gattas N, Smith C, Alizai NK, Wyk V, Sellors J, Whiteley S, et al. Short and long term complications of robotic abdominal surgery in children. In: *Presented at the 5th Hamlyn Symposium on Medical Robotics*, London, United Kingdom, July 1–2, (2012), 11. Avaliable online at: http://ubimon.doc.ic.ac.uk/Hamlyn2012/public/Hamlyn_2012_proceedings_2.pdf
43. Bansal D, Defoor WR Jr, Reddy PP, Minevich EA, Noh PH. Complications of robotic surgery in pediatric urology: a single institution experience. *Urology.* (2013) 82:917–20. doi: 10.1016/j.urology.2013.05.046
44. Cribbs RK, Wulkan ML, Heiss KF, Gow KW. Minimally invasive surgery and childhood cancer. *Surg Oncol.* (2007) 16:221–8. doi: 10.1016/j.suronc.2007.09.002
45. Cundy TP, Marcus HJ, Clark J, Hughes-Hallett A, Mayer EK, Najmaldin AS, et al. Robot-assisted minimally invasive surgery for pediatric solid tumors: a systematic review of feasibility and current status. *Eur J Pediatr Surg.* (2014) 24:127–35. doi: 10.1055/s-0033-1347297
46. Bentas W, Wolfram M, Bräutigam R, Binder J. Laparoscopic transperitoneal adrenalectomy using a remote-controlled robotic surgical system. *J Endourol.* (2002) 16:373–6. doi: 10.1089/089277902760261419
47. Meignan P, Ballouhey Q, Lejeune J, Braik K, Longis B, Cook AR, et al. Robotic-assisted laparoscopic surgery for pediatric tumors: a bicenter experience. *J Robot Surg.* (2018) 12:501–8. doi: 10.1007/s11701-017-0773-2

48. Varda BK, Cho P, Wagner AA, Lee RS. Collaborating with our adult colleagues: a case series of robotic surgery for suspicious and cancerous lesions in children and young adults performed in a free-standing children's hospital. *J Pediatr Urol.* (2018) 14:182.e1–8. doi: 10.1016/j.jpurol.2018.01.003
49. Secin FP, Coelhjo R, Gardiner JM, Salcedo JGC, Puente R, Martínez L, et al. Robotic surgery in public hospitals of Latin-America: a castle of sand? *World J Urol.* (2018) 36:595–601. doi: 10.1007/s00345-018-2227-5
50. Terra RM. Thymic minimally invasive surgery: state of the art across the world: Central-South America. *J Vis Surg.* (2017) 14:124. doi: 10.21037/jovs.2017.07.13
51. Mota Filho FHA, Sávio LF, Sakata RE, Ivanovic RF, Nunes da Silva NA, Soares MR, et al. Robot-assisted single port radical nephrectomy and cholecystectomy: description and technical aspects. *Int Braz J Urol.* (2018) 44:202–3. doi: 10.1590/s1677-5538.ibju.2016.0560
52. Poffo R, Toschi AP, Pope RB, Montanhesi PK, Santos RS, Teruya A, et al. Robotic cardiac surgery in Brazil. *Ann Cardiothorac Surg.* (2017) 6:17–26. doi: 10.21037/acs.2017.01.01
53. Machado MA, Makdissi FF, Surjan RC, Abdalla RZ. First robotic-assisted laparoscopic liver resection in Latin America. *Arq Gastroenterol.* (2009) 46:78–80. doi: 10.1590/S0004-28032009000100019
54. Machado MA, Makdissi FF, Surjan RC, Abdalla RZ. Robotic resection of intraductal neoplasm of the pancreas. *J Laparoendosc Adv Surg Tech A.* (2009) 19:771–5. doi: 10.1089/lap.2009.0164
55. Dindo D, Demartines N, Clavien PA. Classification of surgical complications: a new proposal with evaluation in a cohort of 6336 patients and results of a survey. *Ann Surg.* (2004) 240:205–13. doi: 10.1097/01.sla.0000133083.54934.ae
56. Clavien PA, Barkun J, de Oliveira ML, Vauthey JN, Dindo D, Schulick, et al. The Clavien-Dindo classification of surgical complications: five-year experience. *Ann Surg.* (2009) 250:187–96. doi: 10.1097/SLA.0b013e3181b13ca2
57. Cundy TP, Harling L, Marcus HJ, Athanasiou T, Darzi AW. Meta-analysis of robot-assisted versus conventional laparoscopic fundoplication in children. *J Ped Surg.* (2014) 49:646–52. doi: 10.1016/j.jpedsurg.2013.12.014
58. Baek M, Koh ChJ. Lessons learned over a decade of pediatric robotic ureteral reimplantation. *Investig Clin Urol.* (2017) 58:3–11. doi: 10.4111/icu.2017.58.1.3
59. Gundeti MS, Boysen WR, Shah A. Robot-assisted laparoscopic extravesical ureteral reimplantation: technique modifications contribute to optimized outcomes. *Eur Urol.* (2016) 70:818–23. doi: 10.1016/j.eururo.2016.02.065
60. Bach Ch, Miernik A, Schönthale M. Training in robotics: the learning curve and contemporary concepts in training. *Arab J Urol.* (2014) 12:58–61. doi: 10.1016/j.aju.2013.10.005
61. De Naeyer G, Schatteman P, Carpentier P, Mottrie A. Learning curve in robotic surgery: review of the literature (RALP, RAPN, and RARC). *World J Urol.* (2013) 31:455–61.
62. Gundeti MS, Acharya SS, Zagaja GP, Shalhav AL. Paediatric robotic-assisted laparoscopic augmentation ileocystoplasty and Mitrofanoff appendicovesicostomy (RALIMA): feasibility of and initial experience with the University of Chicago technique. *BJU Int.* (2011) 107:962–9. doi: 10.1111/j.1464-410X.2010.09706.x
63. Famakinwa OJ, Rosen AM, Gundeti MS. Robot-assisted laparoscopic mitrofanoff appendicovesicostomy technique and outcomes of extravesical and intravesical. *Eur Urol.* (2013) 64:831–6. doi: 10.1016/j.eururo.2013.05.007
64. Gargollo PC, Granberg C, Gong E, Tu D, Whittam B, Dajusta D. Complex robotic lower urinary tract surgery in patients with history of open surgery. *J Urol.* (2019) 201:162–8. doi: 10.1016/j.juro.2018.06.017
65. Murthy P, Cohn JA, Selig RB, Gundeti MS. Robot-assisted laparoscopic augmentation ileocystoplasty and mitrofanoff appendicovesicostomy in children: updated interim results. *Eur Urol.* (2015) 68:1069–75. doi: 10.1016/j.eururo.2015.05.047
66. Grimsby GM, Jacobs MA, Gargollo PC Comparison of complications of robot-assisted laparoscopic and open appendicovesicostomy in children. *J Urol.* (2015) 194:772–6. doi: 10.1016/j.juro.2015.02.2942
67. Dangle PP, Akhavan A, Odeleye M, Avery D, Lendvay T, Koh CJ, et al. Ninety-day perioperative complications of pediatric robotic urological surgery: a multi-institutional study. *J Pediatr Urol.* (2016) 12:102.e1–6. doi: 10.1016/j.jpurol.2015.08.015
68. Chang EY, Hong YJ, Chang Hk, Oh JT, Han SJ. Lessons and tips from the experience of pediatric robotic choledochal cyst resection. *J Laparoendosc Adv Surg Tech.* (2012) 22:609–14. doi: 10.1089/lap.2011.0503
69. Alizai NK, Dawrant MJ, Najmaldin AS. Robot-assisted resection of choledochal cysts and hepatojejunostomy in children. *Pediatr Surg Int.* (2014) 30:291–4. doi: 10.1007/s00383-013-3459-5
70. Lee H, Hirose S, Bratton B, Farmer D. Initial experience with complex laparoscopic biliary surgery in children: biliary atresia and choledochal cyst. *J Pediatr Surg.* (2004) 39:804–7. doi: 10.1016/j.jpedsurg.2004.02.018
71. Woo R, Le D, Albanese CT, Kim SS. Robot-assisted laparoscopic resection of a type I choledochal cyst in a child. *J Laparoendosc Adv Surg Tech.* (2006) 16:179–83. doi: 10.1089/lap.2006.16.179
72. Kim NY, Chang EY, Hong YJ, Park S, Kim HY, Bai SJ, et al. Retrospective assessment of the validity of robotic surgery in comparison to open surgery for pediatric choledochal cyst. *Yonsei Med J.* (2015) 56:737–43. doi: 10.3349/ymj.2015.56.3.737
73. Wang XQ, Xu SJ, Wang Z, Xiao YH, Xu J, Wang ZD, et al Robotic-assisted surgery for pediatric choledochal cyst: case report and literature review. *World J Clin Cases.* (2018) 6:143–9. doi: 10.12998/wjcc.v6.i7.143
74. Meehan JJ. Robotic surgery for pediatric tumors. *Cancer J.* (2013) 19:183–8. doi: 10.1097/PPO.0b013e318289486c
75. Hu MG, Xiao YH, Song DD, Zhao GD, Liu YZ, Wang Z, et al. First experience of robotic spleen-preserving distal pancreatectomy in a child with insulinoma. *World J Surg Oncol.* (2017) 15:199. doi: 10.1186/s12957-017-1265-6
76. Liang M, Jiang J, Dai H, Hong X, Han X, Cong L, et al. Robotic enucleation for pediatric insulinoma with MEN1 syndrome: a case report and literature review. *BMC Surg.* (2018) 18:44. doi: 10.1186/s12893-018-0376-5
77. Lalli R, Merritt N, Schlachta CM, Bütter A. Robotic-assisted, spleen-preserving distal pancreatectomy for a solid pseudopapillary tumour in a pediatric patient: a case report and review of the literature. *J Robot Surg.* (2019) 13:325–9. doi: 10.1007/s11701-018-0835-0
78. Herron DM, Marohn M. A *Consensus Document on Robotic Surgery.* SAGES, (2007). Avaliable online at: https://www.sages.org/publications/guidelines/consensus-document-robotic-surgery/
79. Bruns NE, Soldes OS, Ponsky TA. Robotic surgery may not "make the cut" in pediatrics. *Front Pediatr.* (2015) 3:1–3. doi: 10.3389/fped.2015.00010
80. Chaussy Y, Becmeur F, Lardy H, Aubert D. Robot-assisted surgery: current status evaluation in abdominal and urological pediatric surgery. *J Laparoendosc Adv Surg Tech.* (2013) 23:530–8. doi: 10.1089/lap.2012.0192
81. Kibar Y, Yalcin S, Kaya E, Kopru B, Ebiloglu T, Ergin G, et al. Our experiences with robot- assisted laparoscopic surgery in pediatric patients: the first case series from Turkey. *Turk J Urol.* (2017) 43:355–60. doi: 10.5152/tud.2017.88303

5

Tracheomalacia and Tracheobronchomalacia in Pediatrics: An Overview of Evaluation, Medical Management and Surgical Treatment

*Ali Kamran and Russell W. Jennings**

Department of General Surgery, Harvard Medical School, Boston Children's Hospital, Boston, MA, United States

Correspondence:
Russell W. Jennings
russell.jennings@childrens.harvard.edu

Tracheobronchomalacia (TBM) refers to airway collapse due to typically excessive posterior membrane intrusion and often associated with anterior cartilage compression. TBM occurs either in isolation or in association with other congenital or acquired conditions. Patients with TM typically present non-specific respiratory symptoms, ranging from noisy breathing with a typical barking cough to respiratory distress episodes to acute life-threatening events and recurrent and/or prolonged respiratory infections. There are no definitive standardized guidelines for the evaluation, diagnosis, and treatment of TBM; therefore, patients may be initially misdiagnosed and incorrectly treated. Although milder cases of TBM may become asymptomatic as the diameter of the airway enlarges with the child, in cases of severe TBM, more aggressive management is warranted. This article is an overview of the clinical presentation, evaluation, diagnosis, medical management, and surgical treatment options in pediatric tracheomalacia.

Keywords: tracheomalacia, tracheobronchomalacia, aortopexy, tracheopexy, tracheobronchopexy

INTRODUCTION

Tracheomalacia (TM) refers to an excessive increase in compliance of the trachea, such that the airway is more susceptible to dynamic and/or static collapse; this is distinguishable from intrinsic airway stenosis caused by mural problems such as complete tracheal rings. TM may be localized or generalized. The mainstem bronchi may also be affected, which is referred to as tracheobronchomalacia (TBM). Less commonly, the mainstem bronchi and/or their distal divisions at the lobar or segmental level are affected alone, which is known as bronchomalacia (BM) (1–5).

The causes of airway malacia can be broadly divided into those congenital conditions that are associated with an excessively compliant or collapsible airway and those where the airway cartilage is found to be normal but is malformed due to a secondary or acquired cause. Tracheomalacia is the most common congenital tracheal abnormality with a reported incidence of 1 in 2,100 children (6), which is likely an underestimation given a wide spectrum of non-specific symptoms that are initially misdiagnosed (7). Primary or congenital TM/TBM can be found alone or in conjunction with other genetic and congenital disorders (5, 8, 9). Given the common origin of the trachea and esophagus during embryologic development, TM/TBM is a common respiratory problem in children who have esophageal atresia with or without tracheal-esophageal fistula (EA/TEF) (10–14). TM/TBM may also be associated with other airway and lung pathologies, such as laryngomalacia, laryngeal

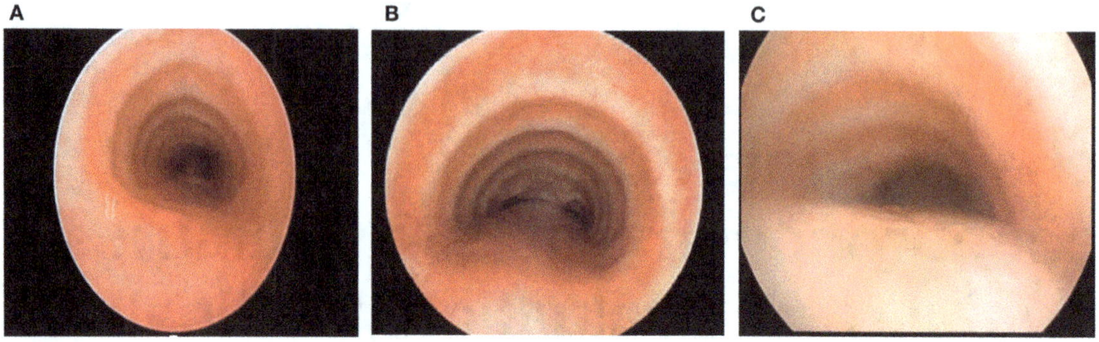

FIGURE 1 | (A) Tracheal structure with normal C-shape rings. **(B)** U-shaped rings with a wider posterior membrane, demonstrating posterior intrusion. **(C)** Bow-shaped rings with a broad posterior membrane and severe posterior intrusion.

clefts, bronchopulmonary dysplasia, or cystic fibrosis (7, 15, 16). The airway malacia can be acquired from cartilage malformation caused by external compression from vascular abnormalities, such as vascular ring, pulmonary sling, or aberrant subclavian artery, or other mediastinal masses (17–20). Prolonged intubation, chronic infections, or inflammatory conditions may also cause TM/TBM (21–23).

ANATOMY

The normal trachea and main bronchi are supported by relatively rigid C-shaped cartilages anteriorly and laterally, and a short pliable posterior membrane (5). Changes in pressure, in part, determine the airway diameter during the respiratory cycle. The pliable posterior membrane moves inward during expiration, narrowing the airway and accelerating the airflow and mucus clearance. In a healthy person, the decrease in airway diameter is negligible and typically not more than 10–20% even with coughing, although some adult studies have shown up to 50% posterior intrusion with coughing by airway imaging and CT scans (24, 25). In patients with TM/TBM, the physiological narrowing of the airway is accentuated during expiration, and in severe cases, a clinically obvious airway collapse occurs predominantly when the expiratory effort is increased, such as during coughing or crying. The airway collapse may be attributable to the dynamic posterior intrusion and/or combined with a region of fixed anterior collapse. If the entire cartilage ring configures in an upside-down U shape or even bow shape, the posterior membrane is broader and more dynamic and intrudes into the airway lumen during expiration and periods of increased intra-thoracic pressure (**Figure 1**) (14). Also, intrinsic weakness of cartilages can have a profound effect on airway compliance; in the worst cases resulting in severe airway collapse at rest or with minimal exhalation effort. Anterior compression is typically caused by blood vessels such as the aorta or innominate artery, which may alter the shape of the cartilages even if they have normal strength leading to fixed anterior airway collapse.

SYMPTOMS AND SIGNS

Clinical presentation of TM/TBM includes a range of non-specific respiratory symptoms, depending on the location, extent, and severity of the airway collapse. Many children with TM/TBM do not show symptoms until age 2–3 months (5, 26, 27). However, in cases with long-segment TM/TBM, symptoms may begin at birth (27). In some patients, TM/TBM becomes apparent soon after repair of EA/TEF when they cannot be extubated (27). A barking cough with expiratory rhonchi or inspiratory stridor may be present in most patients with TM/TBM. The extensive airway collapse can lead to ineffective cough and reduced clearance of secretions. As a result, patients with TM/TBM are at increased risk of frequent upper respiratory infections, prolonged recovery from an upper respiratory infection, and recurrent or persistent pneumonia (24, 28–31). Also, the airway obstruction often results in insufficient ventilation; therefore, patients may experience exercise intolerance, hypoxic episodes, or apneic events (5, 6, 27, 28). The symptoms can be worsened by any activities or conditions that increase the intrathoracic pressure and the patient's respiratory efforts, including activities such as coughing, crying, Valsalva maneuvers, feeding, forced expiration, or lying supine (5, 27).

DIAGNOSIS AND EVALUATION

There is no definitive standardized guideline for diagnosis and evaluation of TM/TBM. The diagnosis should be suspected by a clinical history of signs and symptoms that would be suggestive of TM/TBM, including barky cough, noisy breathing, recurrent pneumonia, prolonged pulmonary infection, feeding difficulties with dyspnea, cough, and aspiration, transient respiratory distress requiring positive pressure, oxygen dependence, ventilator dependence, blue spells, and apparent life-threatening events (ALTEs) (27, 28). Patients with apneic events require careful cardiac and neurologic evaluations to exclude these causes. Esophageal abnormalities, including strictures and tracheoesophageal fistulas, as well as gastroesophageal reflux, must be ruled out (27).

For the most accurate diagnosis of TM/TBM, direct visualization is achieved through flexible and rigid endoscopy, including laryngoscopy, tracheoscopy, and bronchoscopy (13, 24, 30, 31). Three-phase dynamic bronchoscopy is considered the gold standard for the diagnosis of TM/TBM. The first phase occurs while the patient is shallow breathing, which reveals the basic anatomy of the airway as well as compression, cartilage malformation, and secretion accumulation. It may also show vocal cord motion, depending on the depth of anesthesia. Vocal cord motion may be altered and even markedly depressed, sometimes differently on each vocal cord, with small amounts of anesthesia; this must be taken into consideration during the exam (13). The second phase is to induce coughing and Valsalva maneuvers while observing the entire airway, which reveals the maximum dynamic airway collapse as well as the secretion accumulation that gets displaced from the distal airways and comes into the larger airways. This phase is critical for identifying TM/TBM. The third phase is to distend the airways to 40–60 cm of water after aspirating all secretions out, which reveals the structures and lesions that may not normally be seen. This phase allows the identification of tracheoesophageal fistula (TEF), tracheal diverticulum, and aberrant bronchi (29) as well as regions of fixed compression. There are no standard criteria for establishing the diagnosis of TM/TBM endoscopically; however, most surgeons consider a more than 50% dynamic narrowing in the airway lumen with forced exhalation or coughing to diagnose TM/TBM (27). The majority of children with symptomatic TM/TBM have more than 75% airway collapse of one or more

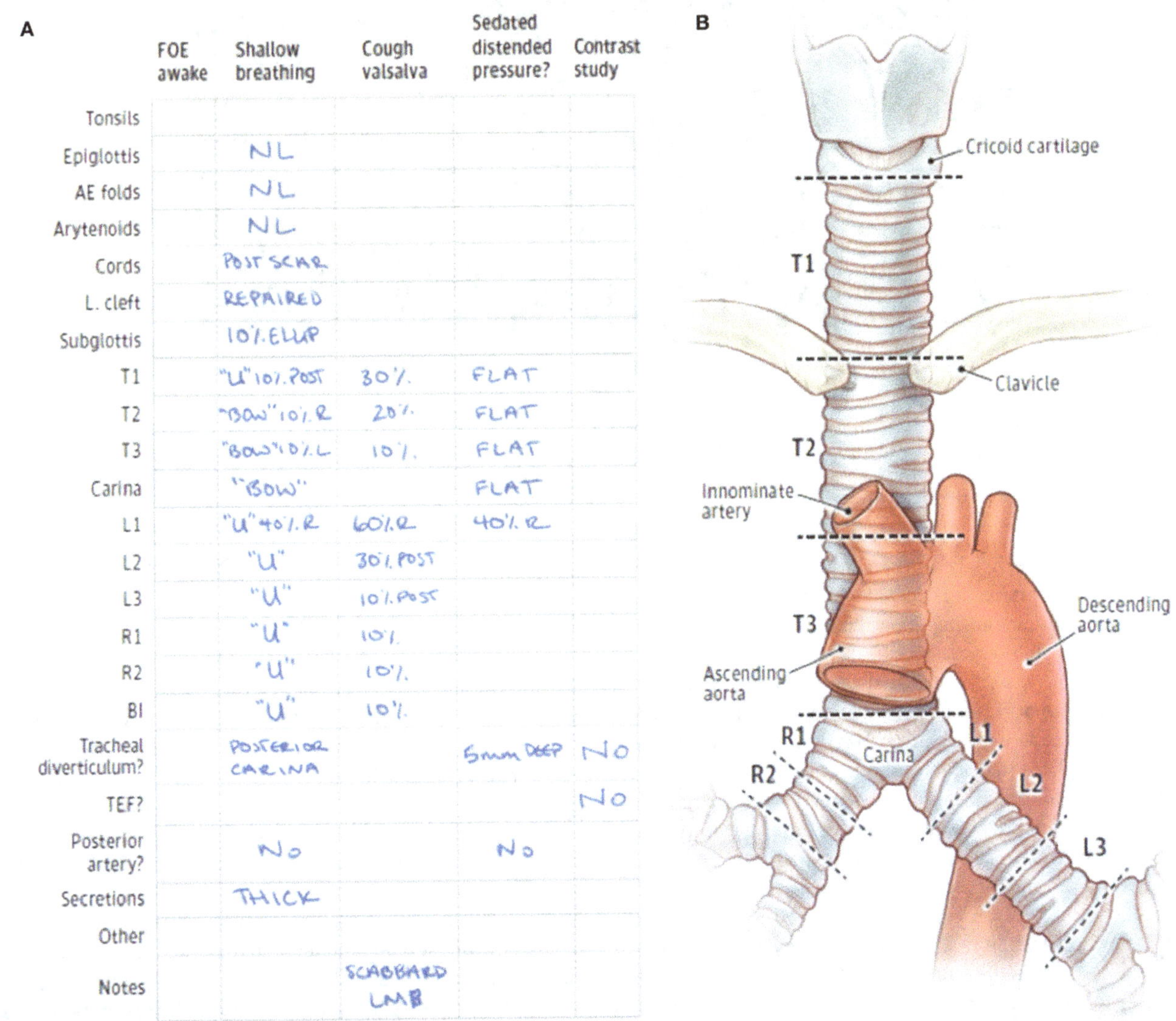

A

	FOE awake	Shallow breathing	Cough valsalva	Sedated distended pressure?	Contrast study
Tonsils					
Epiglottis		NL			
AE folds		NL			
Arytenoids		NL			
Cords		POST SCAR			
L. cleft		REPAIRED			
Subglottis		10% ELLIP			
T1		"U" 10% POST	30%	FLAT	
T2		"BOW" 10% R	20%	FLAT	
T3		"BOW" 10% L	10%	FLAT	
Carina		"BOW"		FLAT	
L1		"U" 40% R	60% R	40% R	
L2		"U"	30% POST		
L3		"U"	10% POST		
R1		"U"	10%		
R2		"U"	10%		
BI		"U"	10%		
Tracheal diverticulum?		POSTERIOR CARINA		5mm DEEP	NO
TEF?					NO
Posterior artery?		NO		NO	
Secretions		THICK			
Other					
Notes			SCABBARD LMB		

FIGURE 2 | (A) Standardized form for documentation of 3-phase bronchoscopic findings. **(B)** Anatomic divisions of the trachea and mainstem bronchi to facilitate classification and description of tracheobronchomalacia. FOE, fiberoptic examination; AE, aryepiglottic; L cleft, laryngeal cleft; T1, trachea level 1; T2, trachea level 2; T3, trachea level 3; L1, left mainstem bronchus level 1; L2, left mainstem bronchus level 2; L3, left mainstem bronchus level 3; R1, right mainstem bronchus level 1; R2, right mainstem bronchus level 2; BI, bronchus intermedius; TEF, tracheoesophageal fistula; R, right-sided; L, left-sided; LMB, left mainstem bronchus; NL, normal; ELLIP, elliptical cricoid; U, U-shaped rings; BOW, bow-shaped rings [Illustration was adapted from Choi et al. (14) Copyright 2019 by American Medical Association].

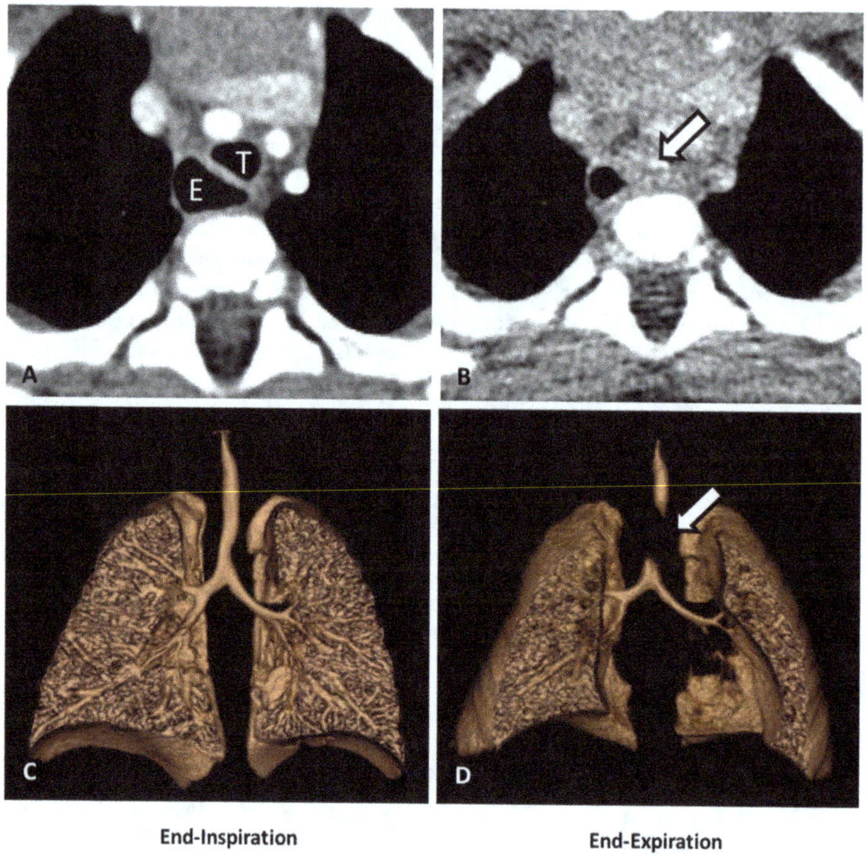

FIGURE 3 | Dynamic airway CT scan with 3-D reconstruction. **(A)** CT scan (cross-sectional view): partial collapse of the mid trachea (T) and dilated esophageal dilation (E) at end-inspiration. **(B)** CT (cross-sectional view): complete collapse of the mid trachea (arrow) at end-expiration. **(C)** 3-D reconstruction of the airways: partial collapse of the mid trachea at end-inspiration. **(D)** 3-D reconstruction of the airways: complete collapse of the mid trachea at end-expiration (arrow).

regions with forced exhalation or coughing, and those with recurrent pulmonary infections typically have complete collapse of one or more regions, causing impaired mucus clearance from the airway distal to that region.

Our team routinely uses a standardized reporting system for bronchoscopic evaluation based on anatomic regions and the severity of airway collapse. The airway has different surrounding structures throughout its course in the mediastinum. Taking these differences into account is important for a complete assessment of the airway as well as better communication with other providers. Anatomic regions are classified into the upper (T1), middle (T2), and lower (T3) trachea; and right and left mainstem bronchi. T1 is the upper third of the trachea, located above the clavicles and up to the cricoid cartilage (extrathoracic trachea). T2 is the middle third of the trachea, located below the clavicles to the takeoff of the innominate artery, which can usually be easily visualized during bronchoscopy. T3 is the lower third of the trachea, including the carina and the takeoff of the two mainstem bronchi. The right mainstem is divided into the proximal and distal right mainstem (R1, R2), and the left mainstem is divided into the proximal, middle, and distal left mainstem (L1, L2, L3). For each of these regions, we determine the percentage of airway narrowing and contribution of anterior collapse and/or posterior intrusion (13, 14) (**Figure 2**) as well as note any other airway distortion (such as lateral intrusion) or other airway lesions such as masses, cobblestoning, fistulas, etc.

In recent years, dynamic airway evaluation and angiography using a contrast-enhanced multidetector computed tomography (MDCT) with two-dimensional (2D) and three-dimensional (3D) reconstructions have become an important modality to aid in the evaluation of thoracic anomalies in pediatric patients (13, 14) (**Figure 3**). The dynamic airway evaluation can be performed in two phases of end-inhalation and end-exhalation (paired end-inspiratory and end-expiratory). Younger patients (usually under 6 years of age) may require sedation with laryngeal mask or intubation, but older patients can hold their breath (20, 32). Deep inhalation or breathe holding with 20 cm of water airway pressure is performed during the inspiration phase, and the exhalation phase is done with maximal exhalation or with zero airway pressure. The changes in the caliber of large airways are compared at both end-inspiration and end-expiration to identify the location of the TM/TBM caused by external compression (20, 33), but may not identify the severity of dynamic airway collapse due to the zero airway pressure used (as opposed to high end-expiratory pressures during coughing). Posterior membrane intrusion may create a "frown-sign" during forced exhalation (34). CT angiogram with 3-D reconstructions helps to evaluate vascular anomalies, if present, and the airway anatomic relationships to surrounding vasculatures. We also use a modified dynamic CT angiogram to identify the artery of Adamkiewicz to avoid injury to the spinal cord during surgery. MDCT study provides important information about the location and extent of TM/TBM, as well as the surrounding intra-thoracic structures and anomalies. This information helps surgeons to better understand the region of TM/TBM and the relevant surrounding structures, such as the location of the aorta and the innominate artery relative to the trachea, and the presence of any vascular anomaly that might alter the surgical plan. However, it is important to understand that a dynamic MDCT tends to markedly underestimate the degree of airway collapse (13, 27), and therefore, it cannot be used to "rule out" TM/TBM and needs to be employed in combination with diagnostic 3-phase bronchoscopy.

Other studies that are helpful in the preoperative assessment include an esophagram to assess swallowing, strictures, and aspiration, a ventilation-perfusion (V/Q) scan to assess lung performance, and an echocardiogram to confirm acceptable heart function prior to undergoing a large surgery (31). A newer study is the nuclear clearance study, which can assess the function of the esophagus, emptying of the stomach, aspiration, and tracheal clearance.

MEDICAL MANAGEMENT

Many physicians have the opinion that symptoms may improve within a few years without surgical intervention. All patients affected by mild to severe TM/TBM may benefit from medical management. The mainstay of medical management while awaiting airway structural stability is the optimization of the ciliary clearance of secretions since the cough clearance mechanism is thwarted by airway collapse (24, 28–31). In order to optimize airway clearance, ipratropium bromide (Atrovent) is administered to minimize the secretions without thickening the secretions as may occur with glycopyrronium bromide (Robinul). Normal saline or hypertonic saline is also nebulized to thin the secretions as much as possible. We have many patients with clinical signs of cough and recurrent respiratory infections who are effectively managed on a clearance regimen and can avoid surgery. Pulmonary hygiene (formerly referred to as pulmonary toilet) and chest physiotherapy to help with mucociliary clearance, as well as control of gastroesophageal reflux (GER) to minimize aspiration of inflammatory gastric contents, are also encouraged. In patients with a history of EA/TEF, the concern for esophageal dysmotility with stagnation and bacterial or fungal overgrowth and/or GER and the need for fundoplication must be seriously considered. Concerns for recurrent or congenital tracheoesophageal fistula leading to airway contamination should be investigated. In our opinion, routine and aggressive or continuous use of corticosteroids should be avoided due to the risks of cartilage degradation and progressive tracheomalacia. Continued exposure to steroids may cause tissue weakening and progressive small airway collapse. In addition, enthusiastic use of steroids can lead to Cushingoid appearance and adrenal suppression.

There is little evidence for the benefit of bronchodilators and muscarinic agents in patients with TM/TBM. While bronchodilators are widely used for wheezy patients with reactive airway disease, administrating a beta-agonist may worsen TM/TBM by reducing the tone of airway smooth muscle, resulting in a more pliable posterior membrane (35). On the contrary, muscarinic agonists such as bethanechol and methacholine can directly stimulate the airway smooth muscle and increase the posterior membranous tone (35). However, there is no evidence supporting the clinical efficacy of pharmacologic stimulation of airway muscle tone in patients with dynamic airway collapse caused by the posterior intrusion of the membranous component.

In the past, the initial approach in patients with severe TM/TBM was the placement of a tracheostomy and long-term mechanical ventilation. Tracheostomy is not a risk-free procedure, particularly in small infants, requiring changes in the size and length of the tracheostomy tube as the child grows. Even after successful tracheostomy placement, this approach may be associated with risk of tracheal injury, inflammation-causing granulation tissue, tracheo-arterial fistula formation, tracheal stenosis, tracheal pouch formation, tracheo-esophageal fistula formation, tracheal plugging, accidental decannulation, delayed vocalization, and difficulty with decannulation as the placement of the tracheal tube does not address the problem of the collapsible airway distal to the end of the tracheostomy tube. In addition, secondary TM and tracheal fibrosis from the presence of the tracheostomy may occur. In patients with TM/TBM that extends beyond the tip of the tracheostomy tube, the utility of the tracheostomy is to be questioned since the patient will still require positive airway pressures and may continue to have blue spells and recurrent infections that can cause progression of the TM/TBM.

SURGICAL TREATMENT

A common misconception is that children outgrow TM/TBM. The truth is that TM/TBM is typically a congenital malformation of the tracheal cartilages and can sometimes slowly get less clinically serious over time, but TBM does not resolve on its own and can even get worse with age. Surgical treatment is reserved for the most severe cases and must be specific to the type and location of the TM/TBM in each patient based on the detailed diagnostic assessment protocol. All the associated conditions, such as cartilage deformation, vascular anomalies, mediastinal masses, tracheoesophageal fistula, abnormal airway branching as well as chest wall and spine deformity, should also be taken into account. Each operation needs to be customized to the airway anatomy, including decisions about the desired anatomic relationships of the trachea to the esophagus and major vasculature. Surgical options for the treatment of TM/TBM include pexy procedures (anterior

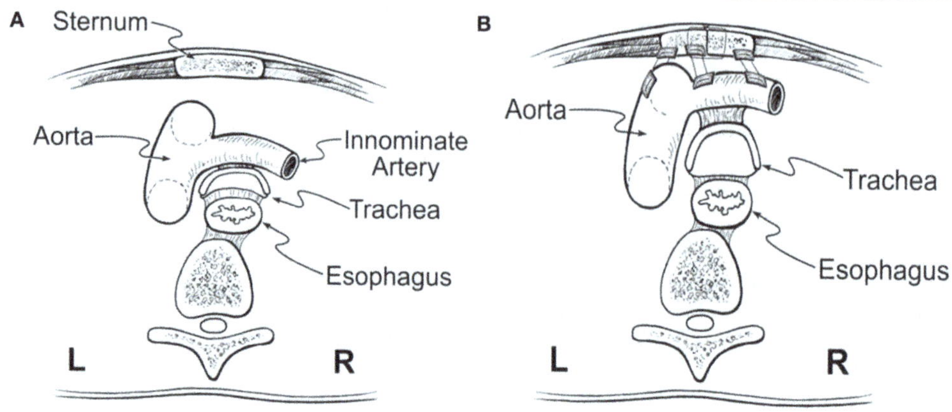

FIGURE 4 | Anterior aortopexy. **(A)** Anterior collapse of the trachea, caused by compression of the aorta. **(B)** Anterior aortopexy with suspension of both the ascending aorta and the innominate artery to the posterior surface of the sternum using pledgeted horizontal mattress sutures. This image was illustrated by Dr. John Foker and published with his permission.

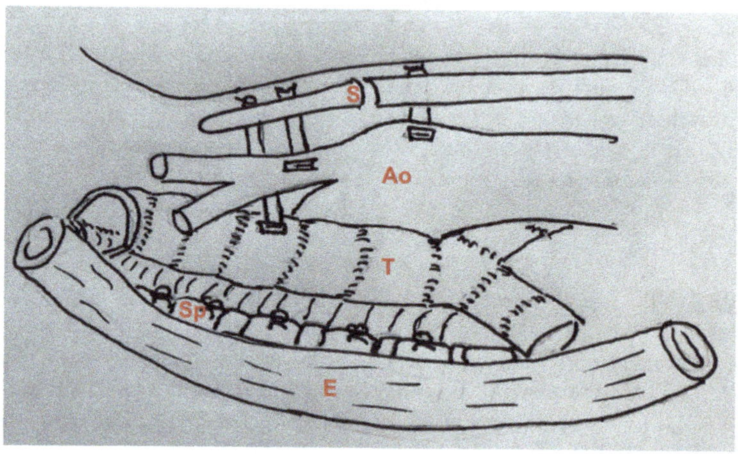

FIGURE 5 | Posterior and anterior tracheopexy combined with anterior aortopexy. S, sternum; Ao, aorta; T, trachea; Sp, spine; E, esophagus.

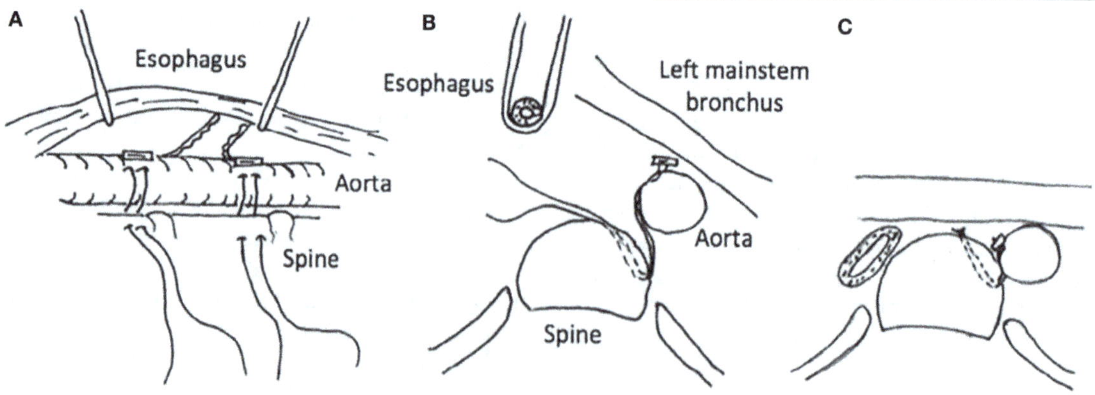

FIGURE 6 | Posterior descending aortopexy. **(A)** Anatomic relationships of the descending aorta to the esophagus and the spine. **(B)** Cross-sectional view: the esophagus is rotated to the right and the descending aorta is moved to the left and secured to the side of the spine as posteriorly as necessary to relieve posterior pressure off the left mainstem bronchus. **(C)** Descending aortopexy sutures are tied, relieving left mainstem posterior intrusion and compression between the descending aorta and the pulmonary artery.

aortopexy, anterior and/or posterior tracheopexy, anterior and/or posterior mainstem bronchopexy, posterior descending aortopexy), tracheal resection and end-to-end anastomosis or slide tracheoplasty, and placement of external splints and internal stents either absorbable or permanent (36).

Tracheomalacia has historically been addressed with anterior aortopexy. This technique was derived from the operation described by Gross in 1948 to treat the innominate artery compression syndrome and was popularized by Filler et al. (37). Through the anterior approach, after removing the thymus, the ascending aorta or aortic arch and innominate artery pulled anteriorly and then sutured to the posterior surface of the sternum (30, 38) (**Figure 4**). The airway is loosely attached anteriorly to the major vessels by areolar tissue. Aortopexy relieves the anterior compression and supports the anterior wall of the trachea through tension on the areolar tissue. This technique can also be used to suspend the pulmonary artery, innominate artery, or pericardium if the anterior airway collapse persists (31). However, aortopexy does not directly address the airway pathologies associated with TM/TBM. Anterior aortopexy may not be a sufficient strategy in the patients with dynamic airway collapse caused by the posterior intrusion of the membranous component, which is the major contributor to airway collapse in many pediatric cases. In a recent meta-analysis, aortopexy was effective in clinically improving more than 80% of children; however, 8% showed no improvement, 4% showed worsening of their symptoms, and 6% died (30).

To address this problem, our group developed anterior and posterior tracheobronchopexy to directly address anterior airway collapse and posterior membranous intrusion, respectively (28, 31, 39). Anterior tracheobronchopexy supports the anterior wall of the trachea and/or main bronchi to the sternum and anterior chest wall, whereas the posterior tracheobronchopexy fixes the posterior membrane to the anterior longitudinal spinal ligament (**Figure 5**). Tracheobronchopexy is done under direct bronchoscopic guidance to confirm the precision of suture placement by providing tracheal luminal visualization during suture placement and to avoid full-thickness sutures. To achieve optimal airway patency, patients may require airway procedures from both posterior and anterior approaches. The posterior work is preferred to be done first, allowing adequate scarring of the posterior tracheal membrane before pulling the anterior trachea in the opposite direction with anterior aortopexy and anterior tracheopexy. Our group has recently reviewed our first 98 patients who underwent posterior tracheobronchopexy through an open approach, proving bronchoscopic and clinical evidence of improvement in airway collapse (29). More recently, we have performed posterior tracheobronchopexy through thoracoscopic and robotic approaches for the treatment of TM/TBM in select individuals (40).

The effectiveness of posterior tracheobronchopexy can be limited if compression of the mainstem bronchus from the descending aorta is noted. The posterior descending aortopexy can be used to relieve left mainstem posterior intrusion and compression between the descending aorta and the pulmonary artery (41) (**Figure 6**). The posterior descending aortopexy can be performed from either the right or the left side. Most commonly, it is performed from the right side in patients with a left aortic arch as other airway work can be performed through the same incision. After mobilizing of the descending aorta, the posterior descending aortopexy is performed by passing autologous pericardial (or other tissue such as pleural or scar tissue) pledgeted polypropylene sutures to secure the aorta to the side of the spine, and as posteriorly as necessary to relieve posterior pressure off the left mainstem bronchus (41). This posterior movement of the aorta may necessitate dividing one or more intercostal arteries, and preoperative MDCT helps to avoid risking injury to the artery of Adamkiewicz.

The pediatric trachea tolerates less anastomotic tension but is more mobile than the adult trachea. Tracheal resection with either end-to-end anastomosis or as a slide tracheoplasty may be indicated in patients with some types of short-segment TBM, such as the congenital absence of cartilage or severe cartilage deformation. However, this approach is not widely used because TBM rarely affects a short segment of the trachea or bronchus.

Internal airway stents have been attempted to treat severe tracheobronchial stenosis or tracheobronchomalacia; however, the use of this technique in children has been limited due to serious complications including migration or fracture, erosion into nearby structures, formation of granulation tissue, difficult removal, and the need for additional dilations or stents, especially with patient growth (42–45). Therefore, this approach has fallen out of the favor but is still considered in highly selected patients with life-threatening airway obstruction who have failed other therapeutical strategies or in whom the risk-benefit analysis points to internal stent placement.

External splinting may offer airway support as an alternative to internal stenting in selected patients with life-threatening TM/TBM. External splints with autologous materials and prosthetic materials have been used to stabilize the malacic or deformed airway. Implantation of external prosthetic splint has raised concerns in terms of long-term effects and complications, including infection and erosion into nearby structures (46). An external splint made from the molded resorbable plate can be sutured around the airway, providing temporary airway support with full resorption predicted to occur within 1–3 years (47). This hopefully allows enough time for the cartilages to reform in a more favorable shape and allows for the growth of the airway in the pediatric patient. Interesting work in this field has been performed by Dr. Green's group in Michigan. They introduced both resorbable and permanent custom-printed external splints for the treatment of severe tracheobronchomalacia (47–50). Using a CT scan and custom software with 3-D reconstruction of the airways, a polycaprolactone or nylon splint is created and then secured around the trachea or bronchus to keep the airway open. A recent study published by this group reported the clinical efficacy of the 3D-printed bioresorbable airway splint device in a series of critically ill children with severe tracheobronchomalacia (50). The Esophageal and Airway Treatment (EAT) Center has been using the moldable bioresorbable plates (RapidSorb, Synthes CMF) to make intra-operative customized external splints in patients found to have airway compression or deformation not alleviated by anterior or posterior airway pexy placement. Many of these patients had complex airways which also required slide tracheoplasty or bronchoplasty, and/or anterior and posterior tracheobronchopexy.

CONCLUSIONS

Tracheobronchomalacia is a clinically challenging condition, frequently undiagnosed or misdiagnosed in pediatrics, and includes many airway pathologies that cause either fixed or dynamic airway narrowing. Patients are best assessed and managed by a multidisciplinary team in centers specializing in complex pediatric airway disorders. The treatment plan should be individualized with a thorough approach to the underlying pathology and clinical concerns. All patients warrant aggressive medical management. For those children considered candidates for surgical intervention, three-phase dynamic bronchoscopy, and dynamic airway CT showing the position of vessels and other important landmarks in the mediastinum are helpful in surgical planning.

AUTHOR CONTRIBUTIONS

AK and RJ: study conception and design and critical revision. AK: drafting of the manuscript.

REFERENCES

1. Baxter JD, Dunbar JS. Tracheomalacia. *Ann Otol Rhinol Laryngol.* (1963) 72:1013–23. doi: 10.1177/000348946307200415
2. Masters IB, Chang AB, Patterson L, Wainwright C, Buntain H, Dean BW, et al. Series of laryngomalacia, tracheomalacia, and bronchomalacia disorders and their associations with other conditions in children. *Pediatr Pulmonol.* (2002) 34:189–95. doi: 10.1002/ppul.10156
3. Masters IB, Zimmerman PV, Chang AB. Longitudinal quantification of growth and changes in primary tracheobronchomalacia sites in children. *Pediatr Pulmonol.* (2007) 42:906–13. doi: 10.1002/ppul.20681
4. Tan JZ, Ditchfield M, Freezer N. Tracheobronchomalacia in children: review of diagnosis and definition. *Pediatr Radiol.* (2012) 42:906–15. doi: 10.1007/s00247-012-2367-5
5. Carden KA, Boiselle PM, Waltz DA, Ernst A. Tracheomalacia and tracheobronchomalacia in children and adults: an in-depth review. *Chest.* (2005) 127:984–1005. doi: 10.1378/chest.127.3.984
6. Boogard R, Huijsmans SH, Pijnenburg, Tiddens HA, de Jongste JC, Merkus PJ. Tracheomalacia and bronchomalacia in children: incidence and patient characteristics. *Chest.* (2005) 128:3391–7. doi: 10.1378/chest.128.5.3391
7. Fischer AJ, Singh SB, Adam RJ, Stoltz DA, Baranano CF, Kao S, et al. Tracheomalacia is associated with lower FEV1 and *Pseudomonas* acquisition in children with CF. *Pediatr Pulmonol.* (2014) 49:960–70. doi: 10.1002/ppul.22922
8. Holinger PH, Johnston KC, Zimmermann AA. Congenital malformations of the trachea, bronchi, and lung. *Trans Ann Meet Am Bronchoesophageol Assoc.* (1952) 58:67–8.
9. Hysinger EB, Panitch HB. Paediatric tracheomalacia. *Paediatr Respir Rev.* (2016) 17:9–15. doi: 10.1016/j.prrv.2015.03.002
10. Wailoo MP, Emery JL. Normal growth and development of the trachea. *Thorax.* (1982) 37:584–7. doi: 10.1136/thx.37.8.584
11. Wailoo MP, Emery JL. The trachea in children with tracheoesophageal fistula. *Histopathology.* (1979) 3:329–38. doi: 10.1111/j.1365-2559.1979.tb03014.x
12. Emery JL, Haddadin AJ. Squamous epithelium in respiratory tract of children with trachea-esophageal fistula. *Arch Dis Child.* (1971) 46:236–42. doi: 10.1136/adc.46.247.236
13. Ngerncham M, Lee EY, Zurakowski D, Tracy DA, Jennings R. Tracheobronchomalacia in pediatric patients with esophageal atresia: comparison of diagnosis laryngoscope/bronchoscopy and dynamic airway multidetector computed tomography. *J Pediatr Surg.* (2015) 50:402–7. doi: 10.1016/j.jpedsurg.2014.08.021
14. Choi S, Lawlor C, Rahbar R, Jennings R. Diagnosis, classification, and management of pediatric tracheobronchomalacia: a review. *JAMA Otolaryngol Head Neck Surg.* (2019) 145:265–75. doi: 10.1001/jamaoto.2018.3276
15. Hysinger EB, Friedman NL, Padula MA, Shinohara RT, Zhang H, Panitch HB, et al. Tracheobronchomalacia is associated with increased morbidity in bronchopulmonary dysplasia. *Ann Am Thorac Soc.* (2017) 14:1428–35. doi: 10.1513/AnnalsATS.201702-178OC
16. Strychowsky JE, Rahbar R. Laryngotracheoesophageal clefts. *Semin Pediatr Surg.* (2016) 25:128–31. doi: 10.1053/j.sempedsurg.2016.02.005
17. Valletta EA, Pregarz M, Bergamo-Andreis IA, Boner AL. Tracheoesophageal compression due to congenital vascular anomalies. *Pediatr Pulmonol.* (1997) 24:93–1053.
18. Horvath P, Hucin B, Hruda J, Sulc J, Brezovský P, Tuma S, et al. Intermediate to late results of surgical relief of vascular tracheobronchial compression. *Eur J Cardiothorac Surg.* (1992) 6:366–71. doi: 10.1016/1010-7940(92)90174-V
19. Backer LC, Mavroudis C, Rigsby CK, Holinger LD. Trends in vascular ring surgery. *J Thorac Cardiovasc Surg.* (2005) 129:1339–47. doi: 10.1016/j.jtcvs.2004.10.044
20. Lee EY, Zurakowski D, Waltz DA, Mason KP, Riaz F, Ralph A, et al. MDCT evaluation of the prevalence of tracheomalacia in children with mediastinal aortic vascular anomalies. *J Thorac Imaging.* (2008) 23:258–65. doi: 10.1097/RTI.0b013e31817fbdf7
21. Shaha AR, Burnett C, DiMaio T, Jaffe BM. An experimental model for the surgical correction of tracheomalacia. *Am J Surg.* (1991) 162:417–20. doi: 10.1016/0002-9610(91)90162-7
22. Campbell AH, Young IF. Tracheobronchial collapse—a variant of obstructive respiratory disease. *Br J Dis Chest.* (1963) 57:174–81. doi: 10.1016/S0007-0971(63)80049-2
23. Benjamin B. Tracheomalacia in infants and children. *Ann Otol Rhinol Laryngol.* (1984) 93:438–42. doi: 10.1177/000348948409300503
24. Deacon JWF, Widger J, Soma MA. Paediatric tracheomalacia—a review of clinical features and comparison of diagnostic imaging techniques. *Int J Pediatr Otorhinolaryngol.* (2017) 98:75–81. doi: 10.1016/j.ijporl.2017.04.027
25. Boiselle PM, O'Donnell CR, Bankier AA, Ernst A, Millet ME, Potemkin A, et al. Tracheal collapsibility in healthy volunteers during forced expiration: assessment with multidetector CT. *Radiology.* (2009) 252:255–62. doi: 10.1148/radiol.2521081958
26. Maeda K. Pediatric airway surgery. *Pediatr Surg Int.* (2017) 33:435–43. doi: 10.1007/s00383-016-4050-7
27. Fraga JC, Jennings RW, Kim PC. Pediatric tracheomalacia. *Semin Pediatr Surg.* (2016) 25:156–64. doi: 10.1053/j.sempedsurg.2016.02.008
28. Bairdain S, Zurakowski D, Baird CW, Jennings RW. Surgical treatment of tracheobronchomalacia: a novel approach. *Paediatr Respir Rev.* (2016) 19:16–20. doi: 10.1016/j.prrv.2016.04.002
29. Shieh HF, Smithers CJ, Hamilton TE, Zurakowski D, Visner GA, Manfredi MA, et al. Posterior tracheopexy for severe tracheomalacia. *J Pediatr Surg.* (2017) 52:951–5. doi: 10.1016/j.jpedsurg.2017.03.018
30. Torre M. Aortopexy for the treatment of tracheomalacia in children: review of the literature. *Ital J Pediatr.* (2012) 38:1–9. doi: 10.1186/1824-7288-38-62
31. Jennings RW, Hamilton TE, Smithers CJ, Ngerncham M, Feins N, Foker JE. Surgical approaches to aortopexy for severe tracheomalacia. *J Pediatr Surg.* (2014) 49:66–71. doi: 10.1016/j.jpedsurg.2013.09.036
32. Lee EY, Boiselle PM. Tracheobronchomalacia in infants and children: multi- detector CT evaluation. *Radiology.* (2009) 252:7–22. doi: 10.1148/radiol.2513081280
33. Pan W, Peng D, Luo J, et al. Clinical features of airway malacia in children: a retrospective analysis of 459 patients. *Int J Clin Exp Med.* (2014) 7:3005–12.

34. Roy AK, Roy M, Kerolus G. Recurrent dyspnea and wheezing—pulmonary function test and dynamic computed tomography may unfold the diagnosis of tracheobronchomalacia. *J Community Hosp Intern Med Perspect.* (2017) 7:303–6. doi: 10.1080/20009666.2017.1383119
35. Panitch HB, Keklikian EN, Motley RA, Wolfson MR, Schidlow DV. Effect of altering smooth muscle tone on maximal expiratory flows in patients with tracheomalacia. *Pediatr Pulmonol.* (1990) 9:170–6. doi: 10.1002/ppul.1950090309
36. Svetanoff WJ, Jennings RW. Updates on surgical repair of tracheobronchomalacia. *J Lung Health Dis.* (2018) 2:17–23.
37. Filler RM, Rosselo P, Lebowitz R. Life-threating anoxic spells caused by tracheal compression after repair of esophageal atresia: correction by surgery. *J Pediatr Surg.* (1976) 41:739–48. doi: 10.1016/0022-3468(76)90098-1
38. Morabito A, MacKinnon E, Alizai N, Asero L, Bianchi A. The anterior mediastinal approach for management of tracheomalacia. *J Pediatr Surg.* (2000) 35:1456–8. doi: 10.1053/jpsu.2000.16413
39. Bairdain S, Smithers CJ, Hamilton TE, Zurakowski D, Rhein L, Foker JE, et al. Direct tracheobronchopexy to correct airway collapse due to severe tracheobronchomalacia: short-term outcomes in a series of 20 patients. *J Pediatr Surg.* (2015) 50:972–7. doi: 10.1016/j.jpedsurg.2015.03.016
40. Kamran A, Hamilton TE, Zendejas B, Nath B, Jennings RW, Smithers CJ, et al. Minimally invasive surgical approach for posterior tracheopexy to treat severe tracheomalacia: lessons learned from initial case series. *J Laparoendosc Adv Surg Tech A.* (2018) 28:1525–30. doi: 10.1089/lap.2018.0198
41. Shieh HF, Smithers CJ, Hamilton TE, Zurakowski D, Visner GA, Manfredi MA, et al. Descending aortopexy and posterior tracheopexy for severe tracheomalacia and left mainstem bronchomalacia. *Semin Thorac Cardiovasc Surg.* (2018) 31:479–85. doi: 10.1053/j.semtcvs.2018.02.031
42. Wallis C, McLaren CA. Tracheobronchial stenting for airway malacia. *Paediatr Respir Rev.* (2018) 27:48–59. doi: 10.1016/j.prrv.2017.09.002
43. Antón-Pacheco JL. Tracheobronchial stents in children. *Semin Pediatr Surg.* (2016) 25:179–85. doi: 10.1053/j.sempedsurg.2016.02.011
44. Nicoli T. Airway stents in children. *Pediatr Pulmonol.* (2008) 43:330–44. doi: 10.1002/ppul.20790
45. Valerie EP, Durrant AC, Forte V, Wales P, Chait P, Kim PC. A decade of using intraluminal tracheal/bronchial stents in the management of tracheomalacia and/or bronchomalacia: is it better than aortopexy? *J Pediatr Surg.* (2005) 40:904–7. doi: 10.1016/j.jpedsurg.2005.03.002
46. Shieh HF, Jennings RW. Three-dimensional printing of external airway splints for tracheomalacia. *J Thorac Dis.* (2017) 9:414–16. doi: 10.21037/jtd.2017.02.53
47. Morrison RJ, Sengupta S, Flanangan CL, Ohye RG, Hollister SJ, Green GE. Treatment of severe acquired tracheomalacia with a patient specific, 3D-printed, permanent tracheal splint. *JAMA Otolaryngol Head Neck Surg.* (2017) 143:523–5. doi: 10.1001/jamaoto.2016.3932
48. Zopf DA, Hollister SJ, Nelson ME, Ohye RG, Green GE. Bioresorbable airway splint created with a three-dimensional printer. *N Engl J Med.* (2013) 368:2043–5. doi: 10.1056/NEJMc1206319
49. Zopf DA, Flanagan CL, Wheeler M, Hollister SJ, Green GE. Treatment of severe porcine tracheomalacia with a 3-dimensionally printed, bioresorbable, external airway splint. *JAMA Otolaryngol Head Neck Surg.* (2014) 140:66–71. doi: 10.1001/jamaoto.2013.5644
50. Les AS, Ohye RG, Filbrun AG. 3D-printed, externally-implanted, bioresorbable airway splints for severe tracheobronchomalacia. *Laryngoscope.* (2019) 129:1763–71. doi: 10.1002/lary.27863

6

Hidden Infection in Asymptomatic Congenital Lung Malformations

*Chenyu Liu[1], Xuejiao Yu[2], Kaisheng Cheng[1], Dengke Luo[1], Miao Yuan[1], Taozhen He[1] and Chang Xu[1]**

[1] Department of Pediatric Surgery, West China Hospital of Sichuan University, Chengdu, China, [2] Department of Clinical Pathology, West China Hospital of Sichuan University, Chengdu, China

Correspondence:
Chang Xu
huaxixuchang@163.com

Background: Whether to operate on asymptomatic patients with congenital lung malformations (CLMs) remains controversial. Our study intended to find out the proportion of hidden infection in CLMs and its effect on surgery, to provide help for the management of asymptomatic CLMs patients.

Methods: A retrospective review of the medical records of patients with asymptomatic CLMs from January 2011 to December 2020 was performed in our center. Selected asymptomatic patients were divided into a non-hidden infection group (NHI) and a hidden infection group (HI).

Results: A total of 581 asymptomatic CLMs patients were included in this study. Thirty-two percent of asymptomatic CLMs patients had hidden infection in the lesion. Among various CLMs diseases, intralobular pulmonary sequestration had the highest percentage of hidden infection (48.8%). With age, the proportion of HI gradually increased. Patients in the HI and NHI groups were 223 and 121. The incidence of pleural adhesion and focal abscess in the HI group were 14.9 and 7.4%. Statistical significances were shown between the two groups in intraoperative blood loss ($p = 0.002$), operation time ($p = 0.045$), chest tube drainage time ($p < 0.001$), postoperative hospital stay ($p < 0.001$), and air leak ($p = 0.012$).

Conclusion: The proportion of HI detected by postoperative pathological results was high and they could increase the difficulty and risk of surgery. Therefore, early surgery may be a more appropriate choice for the management of asymptomatic CLMs patients.

Keywords: congenital lung malformations, hidden infection, congenital pulmonary airway malformation, bronchopulmonary sequestration, lobectomy, children

INTRODUCTION

With the development of ultrasound technology and the frequent use of prenatal screening, the incidence of congenital lung malformations (CLMs) has been increasing in recent years (1, 2). Therefore, pediatric surgeons will encounter more asymptomatic CLMs patients. Over the past few decades, the understanding of the disease has deepened, but controversy still exists (3). The greatest controversy was whether to perform surgical treatment on asymptomatic CLMs patients

(4). Surgeons who did not support surgery believed that the trauma caused by surgery was relatively large, the rate of malignant transformation was low, a long-term follow-up would be more beneficial, and surgical intervention should be performed until symptoms appeared (5–7). Doctors who supported surgery believed that early surgery not only had a lower risk of postoperative complications but also had good postoperative lung function compensation in children. Duaa et al. showed that the postoperative exercise capacity of the patients was close to the normal children (8). The researches result from multiple centers have proved that postoperative lung function can be compensated to the normal level (9–11). And most importantly, the surgery eliminates the risk of infection and malignant transformation (12, 13). Such a large controversy makes it difficult for pediatric surgeons to choose strategies for children with asymptomatic CLMs.

Different studies had controversies about the proportion of asymptomatic patients who eventually developed symptoms. Wong et al. showed that 86% of asymptomatic patients eventually developed symptoms, with a median age of two years old (14). However, Thompson et al. found that only 13% of patients eventually developed symptoms through long-term clinical observation (15), which was the core argument over the management of the disease. If the proportion of patients with symptoms is low, conservative management seems to be better; if the proportion of patients with symptoms is high, early surgery may be better, because if the surgery is performed when symptoms occur, the risk and difficulty of surgery, length of hospital stay, and postoperative complications would greatly increase (12, 16). Infection is the most common complication of CLMs, and it is also the focal point for managing asymptomatic CLMs. Past studies have usually focused on children with symptomatic infection but have ignored children with hidden infection. Therefore, the real proportion of infection may be greatly underestimated. For the first time, our study retrospectively analyzed medical records through a large sample size of asymptomatic CLMs patients to provide help for clinical decision making.

TABLE 1 | Characteristics of the study population.

Variables		AP	AH
Gender	Female	232	69 (29.7%)
	Male	349	117 (33.5%)
Basic illness	CPAM	367	103 (28.1%)
	ILS	121	59 (48.8%)
	ELS	67	16 (23.9%)
	BC	14	5 (35.7%)
	CLE	12	3 (25.0%)
Total		581	186 (32.0%)

AP, aymptomatic CLMs patients; AH, asymptomatic CLMs patients who had hidden infection; CPAM, congenial pulmonary airway malformation; ILS, intralobar pulmonary sequestration; BC, bronchial cyst; ELS, congenital lobar emphysema.

TABLE 2 | Characteristics of hidden infection in patients with CPAM or ILS.

Variables	CPAM		ILS	
	AP	AH	AP	AH
Lobe				
LUL	49	12 (24.5%)	2	2 (100%)
LLL	101	37 (36.6%)	71	42 (59.2%)
RUL	46	10 (21.7%)	3	1 (33.3%)
RML	14	4 (28.6%)	2	0
RLL	134	29 (21.6%)	33	13 (39.4%)
ML	23	11 (47.8%)	1	1 (100%)
Stocker type				
0	0	0		
1	130	46 (35.4%)		
2	186	47 (25.3%)		
3	39	6 (15.4%)		
4	12	4 (33.3%)		
Total	367	103 (28.1%)	121	59 (48.8%)

LUL, left upper lobe; LLL, left lower lobe; RUL, right upper lobe; RML, right middle lobe; RLL, right lower lobe; ML, multiple lobes.

MATERIALS AND METHODS

This retrospective study was approved by the Ethics Committee of West China Hospital of Sichuan University (file no. 2021-1306). We reviewed the cases of CLMs in our center from January 2011 to December 2020. Patient information and surgery-related information were retrieved from the electronic medical record system. Pathological pictures were obtained from slide scanner systems or reacquired original pathology slides from the pathology slide library. All specimens were routinely stained with hematoxylin and eosin. If the existence of inflammatory cell infiltration was uncertain, immunohistochemistry would be added (LCA, CD3, CD4, CD8, CD15, CD16, or CXCR were used for staining). The pathology pictures were reviewed by two senior pathologists, a third expert was invited when the opinions were inconsistent. The inclusion criteria for hidden infection were patients who had no symptoms related to CLMs since birth but had a pathologically significant number of inflammatory cell infiltration (neutrophils, macrophages, or lymphocytes) under the microscope. Exclusion criteria were CLMs patients who developed symptoms, age >14 years old or missing clinical data. Pathologists and surgeons worked independently, they did not know each other's results until all the work was done.

Since 2011, multiple surgical methods have been performed in our center, to ensure the consistency of the baseline, asymptomatic patients with CPAM or IPS who underwent thoracoscopic lobectomy were selected to evaluate the impact of hidden infection on surgery. Selected asymptomatic patients were divided into a non-hidden infection group (NHI) and a hidden infection group (HI). Appearances of lesion abscesses and pleural adhesions in the HI group were then recorded through surgical records.

Differences were compared using Pearson's chi-square test for non-continuous data, Wilcoxon test for continuous non-parametric data, and Student's t-test or Fisher's exact test for continuous parametric data. $p < 0.05$ was considered

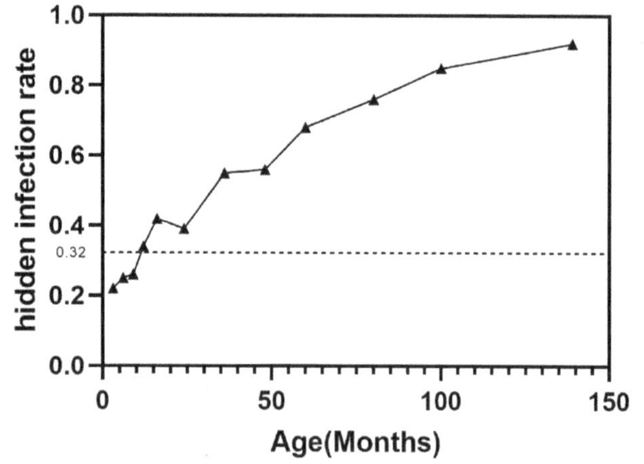

FIGURE 1 | The proportion of hidden infections gradually increased with age.

statistically significant. SPSS 26.0 statistical software was used for statistical analyses.

RESULTS

A total of 581 asymptomatic CLMs patients met the criteria. The characteristics of the study population were shown in **Table 1**. A total of 186/581 (32%) asymptomatic CLMs patients had hidden infection in the lesion. Hidden infections that can be detected only by H&E staining accounted for 169/186 (90.9%) cases, different immunohistochemical methods were used in 17/186 cases (9.1%). The rate of hidden infection in males was higher than that in females (33.5% vs 29.7%), but the difference was not statistically significant (p = 0.338). The characteristics of CPAM and ILS in different lung lobes and stocker classification (17) were shown in **Table 2**. CLMs lesions located in the left lower lobe or multiple lung lobes had a relatively high proportion of hidden infection. Among CPAM classified by Stocker, the proportion of type 1 CPAM has the highest rate of hidden infection (35.4%). The rates of hidden infection in asymptomatic CLMs patients of different ages were plotted as a line graph (**Figure 1**). With age, the proportion of hidden infections in the lesions of asymptomatic patients increased.

Patients in the HI and NHI groups were 223 and 121. Through retrospective analysis of surgical records, intraoperative and postoperative comparisons of the two groups were shown in **Table 3**. The proportions of pleural adhesions and lesion abscesses in the HI group were 14.9% (18/121) and 7.4% (9/121). The differences in basic illness (p = 0.084) and sex (p = 0.319) were not statistically significant between the NHI group and the HI group. Five patients were converted to open in the HI group, while none were in the NHI group. There were statistical differences in operation time (p = 0.045), blood loss (p = 0.002), chest tube duration ($p < 0.001$), and postoperative hospital stay ($p < 0.001$) between the two groups. According to the Clavien–Dindo postoperative complications classification (18), no statistical difference was shown in patients with no

TABLE 3 | Characteristics of asymptomatic patients with CPAM or ILS who underwent thoracoscopic lobectomy.

Variables		NHI (n = 223)	HI (n = 121)	p
Basic illness	CPAM	167	80	0.084
	ILS	56	41	
Age (month)		8 (6–72)	10 (6–76)	0.048
Sex	Male	141	83	0.319
	Female	82	38	
Conversion to open		0	5	
Operation time (min)		57 (52–76)	61 (55–85)	0.045
Blood loss (ml)		5 (5–15)	10 (5–15)	0.002
Major bleeding		0	0	
Blood transfusions		13	9	0.560
Chest tube duration (day)		2.1 ± 1.2	2.7 ± 1.0	<0.001
Postoperative hospital stay (day)		3 (3–5)	4 (4–5)	<0.001
Air leak		11	15	0.012
Clavien–Dindo classification	None	71 (31.8%)	32 (26.4%)	0.179
	I	117 (52.5%)	43 (35.5%)	0.002
	II	35 (15.7%)	41 (33.9%)	<0.001
	IIIa/b	0	5 (4.1%)	
	IV/V	0	0	

complications (p = 0.179) between the two groups but were in grade I (p = 0.002) and II ($p < 0.001$) complications.

DISCUSSION

In our study, patients with hidden infection accounted for 32% of all asymptomatic CLMs patients, and the real proportion of infection in CLMs may be greatly underestimated. Compared with previous studies, our study systematically described the proportion of hidden infection on CLMs through a large series and evaluated the impact of HI on surgery. HI would increase the difficulty and risk of surgery and cause more surgical complications, so early surgery may be a better choice for asymptomatic CLMs patients.

Computed tomography (CT) is currently the most commonly used method for diagnosing CLMs disease after birth, and it has unique advantages compared to ultrasound or MRI (19, 20). In some asymptomatic patients, infection in the lesion could be found through preoperative CT, manifesting as fluid retention in the lesion, which appeared to be lung abscess (**Figure 2**). However, imaging tests cannot always detect this phenomenon, the pathogens in the lesions were not yet powerful to cause symptoms and imaging changes but could manifest in pathology (**Figure 3**). Neutrophil infiltration often represents acute infection, and macrophage or lymphocyte infiltration always represents chronic infection. Long-term chronic infection was more common in the HI group. Pelizzo et al. found that 50% (3/6) of asymptomatic CPAM patients had chronic inflammation through histopathologic examination (21). Durelle et al. found that eighteen asymptomatic CLMs patients (26%) had the microscopic disease (22). Microbial evidence has been suggested in asymptomatic CPAM infants for bacteria and fungi (*Pneumocystis jirovecii*, which is often found in

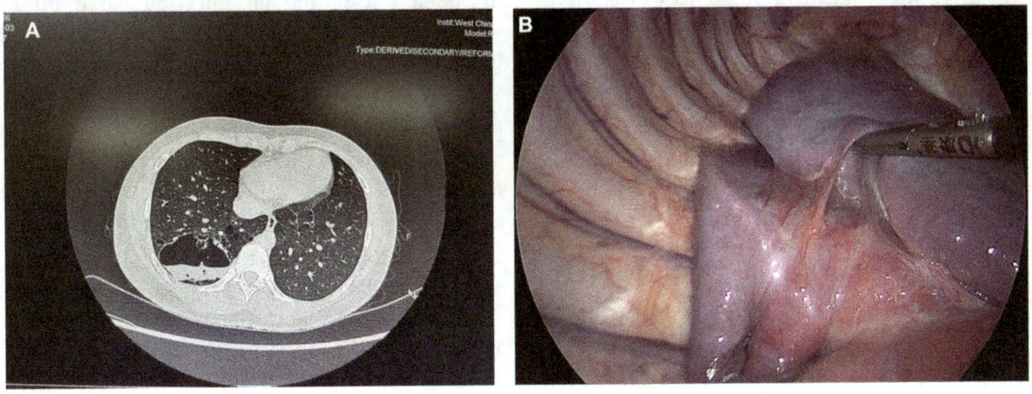

FIGURE 2 | (A) A typical CPAM patient with an abscess in the lesion. **(B)** Pleural adhesion in a 7-year-old asymptomatic CPAM patient. These two pictures showed the special situations in asymptomatic CLMs patients.

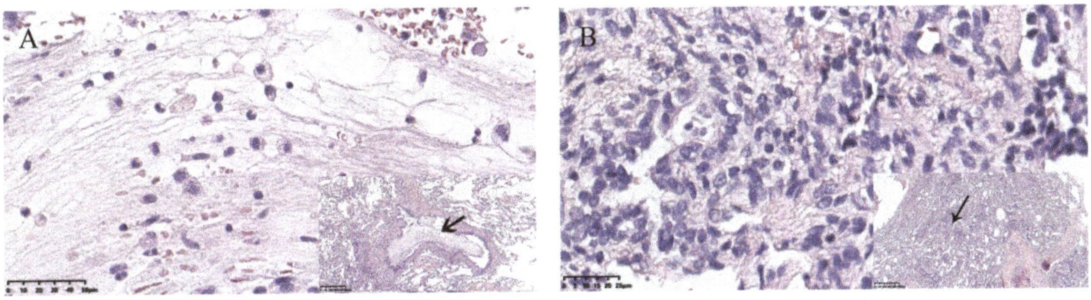

FIGURE 3 | (A) Neutrophil infiltration, which always indicates acute inflammation. Viscous exudate in the bronchioles was also found. **(B)** Lymphocyte infiltration, representing chronic infection, and thickening of blood vessel walls could also be seen.

immunodeficient patients) (23). Mycobacteria in CLMs lesions have also been reported by several studies (24–26). These opportunistic infections were unlikely to occur in the normal lung, it indicated that there could be immunodeficiency limited in the CLMs lesions, which made the CLMs lesions prone to infection, but the patients did not develop any symptoms. This may be the reason for the high rate of hidden infections in our study, it could also explain the reason of the increasing chance of developing an apparent infection with age.

Different types of CLMs diseases showed different proportions of hidden infections. ILS often appears as lung infection or other CLMs-related symptoms. Zhang et al. showed that up to 71% of ILS patients developed an infection (27). Our study also found that ILS had the highest proportion of hidden infection among various CLMs diseases, while ELS was lower. This was probably because ILs is always connected to normal lung tissue and communicate with the vitro environment, and easier to be invaded by microorganisms. Our study showed that the proportions of asymptomatic infections involving the left lower lobe or multiple lung lobes were higher in children with CPAM. Therefore, when the routine postnatal CT examinations of asymptomatic CPAM patients find that the lesions are located in the above positions, pediatric surgeons should be particularly vigilant. There was an obstruction hypothesis about the etiology of CPAM, which was believed to be the obstruction of the trachea and bronchus in different regions caused the occurrence of CPAM (28). Stocker type 1 CPAM manifests as a cyst diameter greater than 5 mm, so it is also called macrocystic type CPAM (29). Macrocystic CPAM tends to accumulate gas or liquid due to poor drainage and large cavities, which may be the reason why type 1 CPAM is susceptible to hidden infection. A study from Japan showed that the proportion of patients with CLMs-related symptoms gradually increased with age, similar to their research results. Our study found that the proportion of hidden infections also gradually increased with age (30). Older patients were often admitted to the hospital because of symptoms, and the remaining asymptomatic patients had a higher proportion of hidden infections, which indicated that CLMs may have the characteristics of asymptomatic stage and symptomatic stage, patients with hidden infections would gradually develop symptoms as they age.

In our study, patients with hidden infections sometimes presented with pleural adhesions or empyema. Mineo et al. showed that the existence of these two situations may enhance the difficulty and risk of surgery (31). In our study, patients in the HI group had a higher operative time, intraoperative blood loss, and postoperative drainage time and a higher risk of postoperative complications than those in the NHI group. Although no patients had Clavien–Dindo grade IV/V complications, such as organ failure and death, there were statistical differences in grade I–III complications between the two groups, suggesting that more serious complications occurred in the HI group. The hidden infection could lead to larger surgical injury and more exudates, causing longer drainage time and hospital stay, meanwhile, enhancing the risk of air leakage.

Postoperative air leak is the most common complication of thoracic surgery. In our center, the criteria for removing the chest tube are no obvious bubble exudates in the water-sealed bottle when the baby cries, and postoperative CT (X-rays for ELS and BC which the surgery does not involve lung parenchyma) shows good lung recruitment without obvious pneumothorax or pleural effusion. In patients with hidden infections, the surgery was more likely to cause more exudates and leakage in tiny airways or alveoli, resulting in prolonged postoperative drainage time and increasing suffering for the young patients. It is believed that thoracotomy could lead to musculoskeletal deformities (32) and cause acute or chronic pain. Five patients in the HI group experienced conversion to open, while the NHI group did not. Tong et al. found that the most common reason for conversions was vascular injury (33). Pleural adhesion or abscess shielded the pulmonary arteries or veins, increasing the risk of vascular damage during thoracoscopic lobectomy and finally leading to conversions. Therefore, early surgery has a lower risk of hidden infection, reducing the difficulty and risk of surgery, more importantly, eliminating the risk of overt infection and malignant transformation.

With the increasing understanding of CLMs and the maturity of pediatric thoracic surgery, the number of centers supporting surgery on asymptomatic patients has gradually increased in recent years (28, 34). Based on the above reasons, in our center, we also recommend that children with asymptomatic CLMs prenatally diagnosed should undergo thoracoscopic surgery between 6 months and 1 year of age. At this age, children can tolerate the surgery and anesthesia well (35), and the lung can continue to develop to get better compensation (36). Future research should focus on the analysis of the microbial population in the lesion of hidden infection based on next-generation sequencing and immunological research to clarify the mechanism of hidden infection in CLMs patients. Our research was only a single-center retrospective study and lacked monitoring of postoperative lung function. It was unknown whether there was a difference in the long-term prognosis of patients between the NHI and HI groups, but for the first time, our study aimed at the hidden infection of CLMs through a large sample size and analyzed the influence of hidden infection on the operation, which may help pediatric surgeons make clinical decisions about whether to perform an early surgical intervention on asymptomatic CLMs patients.

CONCLUSION

We performed a retrospective study on hidden infections of CLMs. The proportion of hidden infections detected by pathology was high, they increased the difficulty and risk of surgery. Therefore, early surgery may be a more appropriate choice for the management of asymptomatic CLMs patients.

AUTHOR CONTRIBUTIONS

CL participated in the whole research process. XY provided pathological support. KC, DL, MY, and TH participated in data collection and graph production. CX provided guidance and supervised the conduct of research. All authors read and approved the final manuscript.

ACKNOWLEDGMENTS

Thank all the members of the team from West China Hospital of Sichuan University who made efforts to this study.

REFERENCES

1. Stocker LJ, Wellesley DG, Stanton MP, Parasuraman R, Howe DT. The increasing incidence of foetal echogenic congenital lung malformations: an observational study. *Prenat Diagn.* (2015) 35:148–53. doi: 10.1002/pd.4507
2. Zobel M, Gologorsky R, Lee H, Vu L. Congenital lung lesions. *Semin Pediatr Surg.* (2019) 28:150821. doi: 10.1053/j.sempedsurg.2019.07.004
3. Wong KKY, Flake AW, Tibboel D, Rottier RJ, Tam PKH. Congenital pulmonary airway malformation: advances and controversies. *Lancet Child Adolesc Health.* (2018) 2:290–7. doi: 10.1016/S2352-4642(18)30035-X
4. Annunziata F, Bush A, Borgia F, Raimondi F, Montella S, Poeta M, et al. Congenital lung malformations: unresolved issues and unanswered questions. *Front Pediatr.* (2019) 7:239. doi: 10.3389/fped.2019.00239
5. Criss CN, Musili N, Matusko N, Baker S, Geiger JD, Kunisaki SM. Asymptomatic congenital lung malformations: is nonoperative management a viable alternative?. *J Pediatr Surg.* (2018) 53:1092–7. doi: 10.1016/j.jpedsurg.2018.02.065
6. Hsieh CC, Chao AS, Chang YL, Kuo DM, Hsieh TT, Hung HT. Outcome of congenital cystic adenomatoid malformation of the lung after antenatal diagnosis. *Int J Gynaecol Obstet.* (2005) 89:99–102. doi: 10.1016/j.ijgo.2004.11.031
7. Ng C, Stanwell J, Burge DM, Stanton MP. Conservative management of antenatally diagnosed cystic lung malformations. *Arch Dis Child.* (2014) 99:432–7. doi: 10.1136/archdischild-2013-304048
8. Dunn A, Pearce K, Callister R, Collison A, Morten M, Mandaliya P, et al. Exercise capacity is not decreased in children who have undergone lung resection early in life for congenital thoracic malformations compared to healthy age-matched children. *Pediatr Pulmonol.* (2017) 52:1340–8. doi: 10.1002/ppul.23772
9. Dincel A, Yilmaz Yegit C, Ergenekon AP, Erdem Eralp E, Gokdemir Y, Kiyan G, et al. Long-term respiratory outcomes of post-op congenital lung malformations. *Pediatr Int.* (2021) 63:704–9. doi: 10.1111/ped.14488
10. Naito Y, Beres A, Lapidus-Krol E, Ratjen F, Langer JC. Does earlier lobectomy result in better long-term pulmonary function in children with congenital lung anomalies? A prospective study. *J Pediatr Surg.* (2012) 47:852–6. doi: 10.1016/j.jpedsurg.2012.01.037
11. Tocchioni F, Lombardi E, Ghionzoli M, Ciardini E, Noccioli B, Messineo A. Long-term lung function in children following lobectomy for congenital lung

malformation. *J Pediatr Surg.* (2017) 52:1891–7. doi: 10.1016/j.jpedsurg.2017.08.059

12. Kapralik J, Wayne C, Chan E, Nasr A. Surgical versus conservative management of congenital pulmonary airway malformation in children: a systematic review and meta-analysis. *J Pediatr Surg.* (2016) 51:508–12. doi: 10.1016/j.jpedsurg.2015.11.022
13. Style CC, Cass DL, Verla MA, Cruz SM, Lau PE, Lee TC, et al. Early vs late resection of asymptomatic congenital lung malformations. *J Pediatr Surg.* (2019) 54:70–4. doi: 10.1016/j.jpedsurg.2018.10.035
14. Wong A, Vieten D, Singh S, Harvey JG, Holland AJA. Long-term outcome of asymptomatic patients with congenital cystic adenomatoid malformation. *Pediatr Surg Int.* (2009) 25:479–85. doi: 10.1007/s00383-009-2371-5
15. Thompson AJ, Sidebotham EL, Chetcuti PAJ, Crabbe DCG. Prenatally diagnosed congenital lung malformations-A long-term outcome study. *Pediatr Pulmonol.* (2018) 53:1442–6. doi: 10.1002/ppul.24119
16. Elhattab A, Elsaied A, Wafa T, Jugie M, Delacourt C, Sarnacki S, et al. Thoracoscopic surgery for congenital lung malformations: does previous infection really matter?. *J Pediatr Surg.* (2021) 56:1982–7. doi: 10.1016/j.jpedsurg.2021.01.036
17. Stocker JTJH. Congenital pulmonary airway malformation: a new name for and an expanded classification of congenital cystic adenomatoid malformation of the lung. *Histopathology.* (2002) 41:424–30.
18. Dindo D, Demartines N, Clavien P-A. Classification of surgical complications: a new proposal with evaluation in a cohort of 6336 patients and results of a survey. *Ann Surg.* (2004) 240:205–13. doi: 10.1097/01.sla.0000133083.54934.ae
19. Mon RA, Johnson KN, Ladino-Torres M, Heider A, Mychaliska GB, Treadwell MC, et al. Diagnostic accuracy of imaging studies in congenital lung malformations. *Arch Dis Child Fetal Neonatal Ed.* (2019) 104:F372–7. doi: 10.1136/archdischild-2018-314979
20. Zirpoli S, Munari AM, Primolevo A, Scarabello M, Costanzo S, Farolfi A, et al. Agreement between magnetic resonance imaging and computed tomography in the postnatal evaluation of congenital lung malformations: a pilot study. *Eur Radiol.* (2019) 29:4544–54. doi: 10.1007/s00330-019-06042-w
21. Pelizzo G, Barbi E, Codrich D, Lembo MA, Zennaro F, Bussani R, et al. Chronic inflammation in congenital cystic adenomatoid malformations. An underestimated risk factor?. *J Pediatr Surg.* (2009) 44:616–9. doi: 10.1016/j.jpedsurg.2008.10.064
22. Durell J, Thakkar H, Gould S, Fowler D, Lakhoo K. Pathology of asymptomatic, prenatally diagnosed cystic lung malformations. *J Pediatr Surg.* (2016) 51:231–5. doi: 10.1016/j.jpedsurg.2015.10.061
23. Till H, Kashofer K, Laje P, ElHaddad A, Warncke G, Gorkiewicz G, et al. Microbial evidence in congenital pulmonary airway malformations of young asymptomatic infants. *J Laparoendosc Adv Surg Tech A.* (2019) 29:685–7. doi: 10.1089/lap.2017.0456
24. Ikegame S, Nagamatsu Y, Nagata N, Kazumi Y, Mitarai S, Iwasaki Y, et al. Congenital cystic adenomatoid malformation in adulthood complicated by Mycobacterium celatum infection. *Intern Med.* (2012) 51:2203–7. doi: 10.2169/internalmedicine.51.7848
25. Kim YJ, Kim DY, Seo JW, Lee SA, Hwang JJ, Kim HJ, et al. A case of congenital cystic adenomatoid malformation infected with mycobacterium avium-intracellulare complex. *Tuberc Respir Dis.* (2013) 74:28–31. doi: 10.4046/trd.2013.74.1.28
26. Yatera K, Izumi M, Imai M, Ikegami T, Miyazaki N, Kido M. Intralobar sequestration with tuberculous infection confined to the sequestrated lung. *Respirology.* (2005) 10:685–8. doi: 10.1111/j.1440-1843.2005.00770.x
27. Zhang N, Zeng Q, Chen C, Yu J, Zhang X. Distribution, diagnosis, and treatment of pulmonary sequestration: report of 208 cases. *J Pediatr Surg.* (2019) 54:1286–92. doi: 10.1016/j.jpedsurg.2018.08.054
28. Leblanc C, Baron M, Desselas E, Phan MH, Rybak A, Thouvenin G, et al. Congenital pulmonary airway malformations: state-of-the-art review for pediatrician's use. *Eur J Pediatr.* (2017) 176:1559–71. doi: 10.1007/s00431-017-3032-7
29. Adzick NS, Harrison MR, Glick PL, Golbus MS, Anderson RL, Mahony BS, et al. Fetal cystic adenomatoid malformation: prenatal diagnosis and natural history. *J Pediatr Surg.* (1985) 20:483–8. doi: 10.1016/s0022-3468(85)80470-x
30. Kuroda T, Nishijima E, Maeda K, Fuchimoto Y, Hirobe S, Tazuke Y, et al. Clinical features of congenital cystic lung diseases: a report on a nationwide multicenter study in Japan. *Eur J Pediatr Surg.* (2016) 26:91–5. doi: 10.1055/s-0035-1566095
31. Mineo TC, Pompeo E, Rogliani P, Villaschi S, Pistolese C, Simonetti G. Thoracoscopic reduction pneumoplasty for severe emphysema: do pleural adhesions affect outcome?. *Thorac Cardiovasc Surg.* (1999) 47:288–92. doi: 10.1055/s-2007-1013160
32. Lam FKF, Lau C-T, Yu MO, Wong KKY. Comparison of thoracoscopy vs. thoracotomy on musculoskeletal outcomes of children with congenital pulmonary airway malformation (CPAM). *J Pediatr Surg.* (2021) 56:1732–6. doi: 10.1016/j.jpedsurg.2021.01.028
33. Tong C, Li T, Huang C, Ji C, Liu Y, Wu J, et al. Risk factors and impact of conversion to thoracotomy from 20,565 cases of thoracoscopic lung surgery. *Ann Thorac Surg.* (2020) 109:1522–9. doi: 10.1016/j.athoracsur.2019.12.009
34. Esposito C, Bonnard A, Till H, Leva E, Khen-Dunlop N, Zanini A, et al. Thoracoscopic management of pediatric patients with congenital lung malformations: results of a European multicenter survey. *J Laparoendosc Adv Surg Tech A.* (2021) 31:355–62. doi: 10.1089/lap.2020.0596
35. Eber E. Antenatal diagnosis of congenital thoracic malformations: early surgery, late surgery, or no surgery?. *Semin Respir Crit Care Med.* (2007) 28:355–66. doi: 10.1055/s-2007-981656
36. Mullassery D, Smith NP. Lung development. *Semin Pediatr Surg.* (2015) 24:152–5. doi: 10.1053/j.sempedsurg.2015.01.011

7

Current Concepts in Pediatric Robotic Assisted Pyeloplasty

Ramphis A. Morales-López [1,2], *Marcos Pérez-Marchán* [1,2] *and Marcos Pérez Brayfield* [1,2*]

[1] *Division of Urology, Department of Surgery, University of Puerto Rico School of Medicine, San Juan, PR, United States,*
[2] *HIMA-San Pablo Group, Caguas, PR, United States*

***Correspondence:**
Marcos Pérez Brayfield
mperezb1@yahoo.com

Robotic surgery in pediatric urology has been gaining popularity since its introduction almost two decades ago. Robotic assisted pyeloplasty is the most common robotic procedure performed in pediatric urology. Advances in robotic technology, instrumentation, patient care and surgical expertise have allowed the correction of ureteropelvic junction (UPJ) obstruction in most patients using this minimally invasive technique. The excellent experience with robotic assisted pyeloplasty has challenged other approaches as a new standard for the treatment of UPJ obstruction. In this review, we will describe the technique as it relates to the different robotic platforms, review the surgical experience and compare its results to other surgical approaches. Also, we will discuss patient and parent satisfaction, cost and financial considerations, along with evaluating the future of robotic surgery in the treatment of UPJ obstruction.

Keywords: pediatric urology, robotics, pyeloplasty, UPJ obstruction, children

INTRODUCTION

Despite its recent beginnings, robotic assisted surgery has been progressing in the treatment of many conditions in pediatric urology. Since the introduction of laparoscopic pyeloplasty in 1993 in adults and 2 years later in the pediatric population, minimally invasive laparoscopic approach for the treatment of ureteropelvic junction obstruction (UPJO) became an evident viable option. In 1994, the first robotic system used in the urological practice known as AESOP was introduced. Later, the evolution of these devices would bring the Zeus system and finally the Da Vinci system while continuously increasing their precision and effectivity (1). This new surgical approach was embraced by doctors throughout the US and promoted a statistical increase in use throughout the country (2).

When compared to classical laparoscopic surgery, robotic assistance offers several benefits. Tremor cancellation, three-dimensional vision and 7° of freedom allow the surgeon to optimally perform in confined working spaces such as those found during pediatric surgery while executing precise and delicate movements with ease (3). In 2002, the first pediatric robotic procedure performed was the robotic laparoscopic pyeloplasty (4). The high incidence of UPJO combined with the surgeons' previous experience with the laparoscopic approach naturally made it a pioneer procedure for robotics in pediatric urology.

Until now, the gold standard method for treating UPJO is open dismembered pyeloplasty with a success rate between 90 and 100%. Laparoscopic pyeloplasty had gain popularity but it struggled to be adopted by many pediatric urologists because of its technical difficulty and tedious learning curve. However, robotic assisted laparoscopic pyeloplasty (RALP) had all the advantages of the laparoscopic approach with an ease of use and a much shorter learning curve. This allows some surgeons to transition from open pyeloplasty to a minimally invasive robotic approach without any previous laparoscopic experience. RALP has been the most commonly reported robotic procedure in children to date (5). In this review, we will describe the technique as it relates to the different robotic platforms, review the surgical experience over the last 5 years and compare its results to other surgical approaches. Also, we will discuss patient and parent satisfaction, cost and financial considerations, along with evaluating the future of robotic surgery in the treatment of UPJ obstruction.

BACKGROUND

UPJO is a common cause of pediatric hydronephrosis occurring in 1 per 1,000–2,000 newborns (6). Widespread use of antenatal ultrasonography (US) and the increase availability of postnatal imaging have resulted in earlier and more frequent diagnosis of hydronephrosis. UPJO is found more commonly in boys than in girls with up to 67% of cases involving the left kidney, and up to 10% seen bilaterally (7). Renal dysplasia, multicystic dysplastic kidney, duplicated renal collecting system where the lower pole UPJ is usually the obstructed segment; horseshoe kidney; and ectopic kidney have been found in association with UPJO. The etiology can be described as lesions that involve the UPJ intrinsically, lesions that are extrinsic or a combination of both.

The initial postnatal evaluation is performed with a renal/bladder US in order to determine the presence of pelvocalyceal dilation with or without renal cortical thinning. The most widely used grading systems of the severity of hydronephrosis on US are the Society of Fetal Urology (SFU) system and the Anterior/Posterior (AP) diameter of the renal pelvis. In 2014, a multidisciplinary consensus group developed the urinary tract dilation (UTD) classification system pertinent to antenatal and postnatal evaluation. The new classification incorporated the following six US parameters: AP renal pelvis diameter (APD), calyceal dilation, renal parenchymal thickness, renal parenchymal appearance, bladder abnormalities, and ureteral abnormalities (8).

Diuretic renography is the most widely used non-invasive technique to determine the severity and functional significance of UPJ obstruction (9). Technetium-99 m mercaptoacetyltriglycerine (^{99m}Tc-MAG3) is the ideal tracer for the pediatric population. One of the most useful measurements in diuretic renography is the estimate of differential renal function. This is considered significant when it is <40%. This percentage usually is well-correlated with the half-life (T1/2) washout curve.

Other than US and MAG3 renal scan there are other imaging and diagnostic tests also less commonly utilized for diagnosis of UPJO. Magnetic resonance imaging has been used by some center as their study of choice to evaluate UPJO (10). Developments in magnetic resonance imaging (MRI) technology have made it possible to image kidneys while assessing anatomy, renal transit times as well as intracellular metabolic parameters independent of blood flow and tubular function.

Indications for surgical interventions are ipsilateral UPJO with <40% of differential renal function (DRF) on diuretic renography, bilateral severe UPJO with renal parenchymal atrophy, obstructive pattern on diuretic renography with abdominal mass, urosepsis, or cyclic flank pain with or without vomiting and recurrent UTI under antibiotic prophylaxis.

Robotic Assisted Laparoscopic Pyeloplasty (RALP)

RALP is now a well-established method of correcting UPJO (5). It has the advantage of being able to help overcome the difficulties encountered with laparoscopic dissecting and suturing. The basic principle is similar to that of laparoscopic pyeloplasty but facilitated by 3-D imaging and the help of an articulated instrument. The operative technique has evolved to the point where RALP can be successfully performed in most pediatric patients. Some limitations could be encountered in infants <5 mo. or patients with a small abdominal cavity due to the limited available working space.

Positioning

The procedure starts with a crucial element for success: proper positioning of the patient. The patient is positioned at the edge of the table with the arms resting on a folded arm board. This will allow the robot arms to use their full range without table interference. Our preferred patient position is the 45° or modified flank position. This position with the use of the table rotation allow access and trocar placement in a near supine position avoiding potential complications. Also, this position allows for the intraabdominal contents to move away from the surgical site. We use two large jelly rolls to support the patient's back with the upper arm placed across the body in a praying position. The lower leg is bended at a 90° angle and the upper leg is straight. It is of outmost importance that the patient is well-padded specially between the legs, arms, and face. The patient is secured to the table with wide tape across the arms and shoulders, chest, hip, knee, and ankles. Care is taken not to place tape directly on patient's skin. With the help of the anesthesiologist, proper positioning, and adequate access to the patient's airway and IV lines are confirmed before the start of the procedure.

Initial Access, Insufflation, and Trocar Placement

With the table tilted away from the surgeon' side, the access is performed on a nearly flat patient. Our preferred approach is percutaneous using the Veress needle. Others have preferred the open Hassan technique for smaller children (11). After CO_2 insufflation to 8–10 mmHg, a 5 mm optical trocar is placed under direct vision in the infraumbilical position allowing easy and safe access. The port position for robotic assisted laparoscopic pyeloplasty will be in straight line for most patients using the DaVinci Xi system (**Figure 1**). The 8 mm robotic trocars are placed under direct vision with the last trocar replacing the infraumbilical trocar. With the DaVinci Xi, the trocar should have at least 3 cm of separation in order to avoid robotic arms collision. Other have described the best trocar position for the Si system which needs to be modified depending on the patient's size. Several options include straight line, triangulation, and HIDES (12). The HIDES trocar positioning allows for better cosmetic results with an infraumbilical port and 2 additional

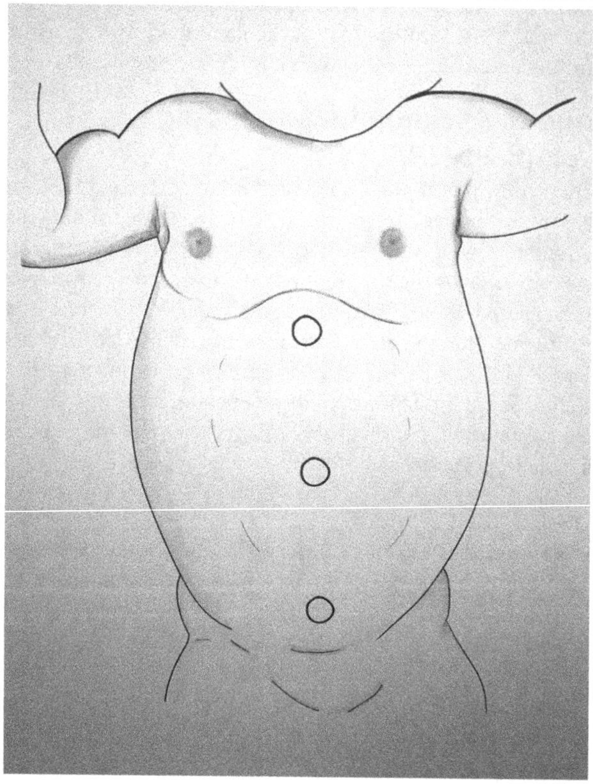

FIGURE 1 | DaVinci Xi port placement for RALP (Drawing by Carla Fernandez).

lower abdominal ports. "Burping" of all ports will give additional intraabdominal space needed in order to successfully perform the procedure on smaller children.

Docking With Si and Xi Systems

RALP requires the Xi robotic system to be docked at a 90° angle to the patient at the level of the infraumbilical port (camera site). We preferred to keep the robot at an established position and rotate the arms of the robot to adjust to the surgical site without moving the operating table. This allows the head of the patient to remain in the standard position and close to the anesthesiologists. Alternatively, the table could be rotated 180° to allow docking without rotation of the robotic arms. With the Si robotic system, the robot will need to be repositioned to come in a straight line with the camera site, trocar and the surgical site. As an example, the HIDES port placement the robot will dock from the inferolateral position (13).

Surgical Technique and Stent

Cystoscopy with a retrograde pyelogram can be performed selectively at the start of the procedure. Indication for cystoscopy with retrograde pyelogram included complex anatomy (ectopic/horseshoe kidney) and need to clarify preoperative testing. Our preferred surgical technique for the corrections of UPJO is the dismembered pyeloplasty. The procedure follows the same surgical principles described in the laparoscopic pyeloplasty (14). Instruments used during the procedure include: 2 dissecting forceps, scissors, 2 needle drivers, and a suction device. The approach to the UPJ area can be transmesenteric for left sided UPJO or with medial mobilization of the colon for Right sided UPJO and with selected complicated left sided UPJO. Caution is needed during the initial dissection of the UPJ area to avoid injury to a lower pole crossing vessels. Tethered stitches using 3-0 prolene on a CT needle can be placed to the renal pelvis and proximal ureter to help with exposure and ease of the operation. We preferred to place a stent in all patients undergoing robotic assisted pyeloplasty. The stent can be placed in an antegrade or retrograde fashion depending on the surgeon's preference.

Postop Care and Follow up

Indwelling urethral catheter is removed on POD # 1. Most patients are discharged within 24 h if they are able to void, tolerate diet and have adequate pain control. The ureteral stent is removed 6 weeks after the operation. Renal and bladder ultrasound is performed at 2 weeks., 3 mo., and 6 mo. post operatively. MAG-3 renal scan is reserved for symptomatic patients or significant residual hydronephrosis after 3 mo. follow up. Asymptomatic patients with residual hydronephrosis and good renal interval growth are followed with a renal and bladder ultrasound until resolution.

EXPERIENCE AND RESULTS

We retrospectively reviewed our experience with RALP using the DaVinci Xi robotic platform. We identified 41 patients with a mean age of 10.9 years (7 mo.−17 years). Ten patients were <1 year of age. Left RALP was performed in 27 patients and a right pyeloplasty in 14 patients. All procedures were performed using a transperitoneal approach. Our mean operative time was 135 min with a mean hospital stay of 1.5 days. The overall success rate for our series was 95%. Two patients had persistent SFU IV hydronephrosis requiring redo laparoscopic pyeloplasty and balloon dilatation, respectively. Four patients had post-operative complications including stent pain in 2 and non-obstructive small renal stone in 2. None of the patients less than a year of age had any complications. Residual hydronephrosis was identified in 29% of the patients.

Multiple authors have reported strong series with RALP (**Table 1**). A series of studies performed over the last decade show that when compared to open and laparoscopic pyeloplasty, the robotic assisted procedure has performed well in the treatment of UPJO (**Table 2**). These studies have shown comparable success rates with no statistically significance between the modalities.

In comparison to open or laparoscopic pyeloplasty, robotic pyeloplasty typically exhibit shorter hospital stay and less use of medication for pain management following the procedure (4). The only consistent negative variable has been the longer operative times exhibited by the robotic approach as compared to other modalities. Operative times seems to improve in center with high volume and surgeon's experience.

TABLE 1 | Series of reported robotic-assisted laparoscopic pyeloplasty cases.

Author	Procedure	# of pts	Mean age (yrs)	Laterality UPJ	Approach	Mean op time (min)	Hospital stay (days)	Complications	Success rate (%)
Kutikov et al. (15)	RALP	9	0.47	n/a	Transperitoneal	122.8	1.4	n/a	78
Avery et al. (16)	RALP	60	0.61	Bilateral (2)	Transperitoneal	232	1	7	91
Asensio et al. (17)	RALP	5	10.59	n/a	Transperitoneal	144	2.6	n/a	100
Olsen et al. (18)	RALP	65	7.9	n/a	Retroperitoneal	146	2	11	100
Minnillo et al. (19)	RALP	155	10.5	n/a	n/a	198.5	1.9	17	96
Singh et al. (20)	RALP	34	12	n/a	n/a	105	n/a	2	97
Atug et al. (21)	RALP	7	13	n/a	Transperitoneal	184	1.2	1	100
Franco et al. (22)	RALP	15	11.9	n/a	Transperitoneal	223	n/a	4	n/a
Perez-Brayfield	RALP	41	10.2	Right (14), Left (27)	Trans	135	1.5	5	95%

TABLE 2 | Series of reported cases comparing open pyeloplasty, laparoscopic pyeloplasty, and robotic-assisted laparoscopic pyeloplasty.

Author	Procedure (OP, LAP, RALP)	# of patients	Mean age (yrs)	Laterality UPJ	Approach	Mean operative time (min)	Hospital stay (days)	Complications	Success rate (%)
Barbosa et al. (23)	RALP	58	7.2	Bilateral (10)	Transperitoneal	n/a	n/a	1	76.9
	OP	154	1.2	n/a	n/a	n/a	n/a	7	67.9
Yee et al. (24)	RALP	8	11.5	n/a	n/a	363	2.4	1	100
	OP	8	9.8	n/a	n/a	248	3.3	0	87.5
Subotic et al. (25)	OP	8	9.8	n/a	n/a	248	3.3	0	87.5
Lee et al. (26)	RALP	33	7.9	n/a	n/a	219	2.3	1	94
	OP	33	7.6	n/a	n/a	181	3.5	0	100
Song et al. (27)	OP	30	8.5	Right (8), Left (22)	Transperitoneal	192.5	6.6	4	96.7
	LP	30	10.5	Right (6), Left (24)	Transperitoneal	197.4	5.8	4	89.7
	RALP	10	11	Right (3), Left (7)	Transperitoneal	254.1	3.2	1	100
Cundy et al. (28)	OP vs. RALP	157,166	7, 8.1	n/a	n/a	RALP (Longer OT)	RALP (shorter HS)	5, 9	88.5, 87.3
	LP vs. RALP	97, 151	6.5, 10	n/a	n/a	no significant diff.	RALP (shorter HS)	10, 10	96.9, 99.3
Salö et al. (29)	OP	92	6.2	Right (38), Left (54)	n/a	167	4.4	25	92
	RALP	31	8.3	Right (10), Left (21)	Retro (15), Trans (16)	249	3.4	9	94

COSTS AND CONSIDERATIONS

Several studies have delved into the evaluation of costs of the treatment options for UPJO. Some studies have even suggested a 2.7 time increase in cost in RALP as compared to other modalities of UPJO (30). In 2017 Jacobs et al. (31) published a cost analysis study in adult patients showing fairly similar costs for open pyeloplasty ($22,421) as compared to minimally invasive pyeloplasty ($22,843). Varda and colleagues evaluated the national trends of UPJO treatment modalities in children including analysis of the available data on cost (32). They reported evidence of an increasing trend toward utilization of minimally invasive pyeloplasty over open pyeloplasty. In the study, minimally invasive modalities had an increased cost with a significant increase in price related to RALP. Operating room costs were by far the greatest contributor to costs, with robotic supplies being the largest contributor to the rising cost. For example, when comparing laparoscopic vs. robotic approaches there was an average increase in costs of over $3,000.

In another study, Varda et al. again demonstrated an increased utilization of the RALP in children (33). They showed that within a 12-year period there was a persistent higher cost when RALP was compared with open pyeloplasty. The increased cost in RALP over open pyeloplasty persisted as the cost of operating room equipment for robotic cases remained high even when considering the cost associated with longer hospital stays related to open surgery. High volumes of RALP may be required for institutions to profit from the procedures as total investment cost is divided between an increased number of procedures performed. An estimated three to five robotic cases per week are necessary to profit from robotic surgery, which is a clear limitation for pediatric centers no matter their size (34). Reaching the required number of cases needed will be a challenge to children's hospitals with low to mid volume RALP programs.

Based on our analysis and personal experience there appears to be clear evidence that there is in fact a higher cost to RALP as compared to open and laparoscopic approaches. Published data seems to suggest than even with shorter length of stay attributed to RALP as compared to other treatment modalities, the high cost of training, maintenance and materials point to a greater cost as compared to other modalities. In the near future innovation in technology, robotic market competition and market tendencies may see a further normalization of RALP costs that could be comparable to other treatment options.

Parental Capital Gains

Other than the inherent cost analysis necessary for the evaluation and comparison of the treatment modalities of UPJO, there is also a further economic impact related to UPJO treatment as it pertains to parental gains/losses in the pediatric population. A 2011 study by Behan and colleagues evaluated the human capital gains associated to RALP in children (35). An evaluation of 44 patients most of which underwent RALP as compared to open approach was done retrospectively, in which indirect expenses to each procedure was estimated using already published financial models. Although parental work loss is sometimes used as the greatest variable to capital gains/loss other data was analyzed to evaluate the procedures. The results showed that the overall cost savings that are a result of decrease hospital length of stay for RALP may help compensate for the added operative costs previously alluded to. This study suggested that RP is associated with decreased lost parental wages and savings attributed to shorter length of stay, but the results are extremely dependent on the overall costs and amortization related to the robot. Prospective large center studies would be of great value to truly assess the impact of this variable in the treatment modalities of UPJO.

Satisfaction

In the pediatric population satisfaction is not merely based on patient satisfaction and outcomes, but also related to parental satisfactions. Freilich et al. evaluated parental satisfaction based on a modified Glasgow Children's Benefit Inventory (36). Groups of open and RALP were compared based in most part to the responses of the questionnaire. Overall the results of the study showed that even when objective success of surgery were similar between groups (i.e., decreased hydronephrosis on imaging, improved renal scan measures), RALP was favored overall by parents. In regard to specific variables such as postoperative pain, speed to normal activity, speed of return to normal sports, surgery incision scar, impact of surgery on parental life, burden of postop visits/studies, and overall satisfaction, parents seemed to find a greater difference between actual results and expected results within the robotic wing. Based on this study there is increased satisfaction when RALP is undertaken especially in regards to cosmesis and recovery, but expectations as compared to actual results are almost always improved notwithstanding the type of treatment modality employed.

The effect of cosmesis takes greater impact when novel treatment techniques are utilized within the endoscopic treatment realm. For example, hidden incision endoscopic surgery (port sites at level of a Pfannenstiel incision) did show greater satisfaction from patients and parents in regard to cosmetic results in a series of 12 patients published by Gargollo in 2011 (37). In our experience endoscopic approaches are preferred by parents based on the reported considerations as well.

Benefits vs. Risks

Apart from patient benefits like reduced pain, improved cosmetic results, shorter hospitalization, and rapid convalescence there are also added technical benefits to robotic surgery. Extensive published data exists on the benefits of magnified three-dimensional vision, the advantage of having an increased number of working arms, reduced tremors, and overall improved ergonomics. These qualities are an upside on robotic surgery when compared to both open and conventional laparoscopic approaches.

In a review of 5,400 laparoscopic cases performed Peters reported an overall complication rate of 5.4% (38). The greatest predictor of complication rate was surgeon experience.

Braga et al. published a systematic review and metanalysis of RALP vs. conventional laparoscopic approaches (39). RALP showed improved operative time reduction, and a significantly shorter stay at the hospital, but no statistical significance was found with regards to the rates of complications between the treatment modalities. The effects of reduced morbidity in robotic surgery, especially within the pediatric population, is also apparent due to a trend to its utilization in redo cases (40). Up to this point when compared to conventional laparoscopy there is no clear or definitive decrease in morbidity in RALP, especially in experienced hands.

Future of Robotic Pyeloplasty

The future of RP seems to lie both on achieving greater utilization of the currently described technique as well as in the development of new techniques and technology. Single ports, smaller surgical sites, telesurgery, and hidden surgical incisions all seem to be in development and may show promise as they become more available.

Further miniaturization of robotic arms, especially in the form of table mounted systems, will allow for increased dexterity (4). Baek et al. published data regarding the use of 5 mm instruments for RALP in children of different ages (infants and non-infants). Utilization of smaller port sites allowed for safe intervention of RALP in infant children with similar results when compared to older children (41). Improvement in the 5 mm instrument and miniaturization of the robotic arms will facilitate RALP in the smaller infant patients (4).

Another area of particular interest is further development of force-feedback mechanisms to the surgeon that can compensate for the lack of tactile feedback in robotic cases. This in conjunction with newer technologies like virtual reality and augmented reality may not only change robotic surgery as a whole but may also improve education in robotic surgery including RALP.

CONCLUSION

RALP is safe, effective, and well-accepted by surgeons, patients and their parents. There are real concerns regarding the longer operative times and cost associated with this procedure. As surgeons become better trained and have more experience with this technology operative time and associated cost should reduce significantly. Also, as more companies develop additional robotic technology, competition should produce more affordable robotic systems and instrumentations directly reducing the overall cost to the health systems. In the near future, RALP could become our new gold standard in the treatment of UPJO or at least be an equal to the open approach pyeloplasty.

AUTHOR CONTRIBUTIONS

RM-L, MP-M and MPB contributed in all aspects of the manuscript including research, writing, and editing of manuscript.

REFERENCES

1. Passerotti C, Peters CA. Pediatric robotic-assisted laparoscopy: a description of the principle procedures. *Sci World J.* (2006) 6:2581–8. doi: 10.1100/tsw.2006.399
2. Ekin RG, Celik O, Ilbey YO. An up-to-date overview of minimally invasive treatment methods in ureteropelvic junction obstruction. *Cent Eur J Urol.* (2015) 68:245–51. doi: 10.5173/ceju.2015.543
3. Orvieto MA, Large M, Gundeti MS. Robotic paediatric urology. *BJUJ Int.* (2012) 110:2–13. doi: 10.1111/j.1464-410X.2011.10877.x
4. Kearns JT, Gundeti MS. Pediatric robotic urology surgery—2014. *J Indian assoc Pediatr Surg.* (2014) 19:123–8. doi: 10.4103/0971-9261.136456
5. Howe A, Kozel Z, Palmer L. Robotic surgery in pediatric urology. *Asian J Urol.* (2017) 4:55–67. doi: 10.1016/j.ajur.2016.06.002
6. Vemulakonda V, Wilcox D, Crombleholme T, Bronsert M, Kempe A. Factors associated with age at pyeloplasty in children with ureteropelvic junction obstruction. *Pediatr Surg Int.* (2015) 31:871–7. doi: 10.1007/s00383-015-3748-2
7. Park JM, Bloom DA. The pathophysiology of UPJ obstruction. *Curr Consept Urol Clin North Am.* (1998) 25:161–9. doi: 10.1016/S0094-0143(05)70004-5
8. Nguyen HT, Benson CB, Bromley B, Campbell JB, Chow J, Coleman B, et al. Multidisciplinary consensus on the classification of prenatal and postnatal urinary tract dilation (UTD classification system). *J Pediatr Urol.* (2014) 10:982–98. doi: 10.1016/j.jpurol.2014.10.002
9. Faure A, London K, Smith GHH. Early mercaptoacetyltriglycine(MAG-3) diuretic renography results after pyeloplasty. *BJU Int.* (2016) 118:790–6. doi: 10.1111/bju.13512
10. Parikh K, Hammer M, Kraft K, Ivančić V, Smith EA, Dillman JR. Pediatric ureteropelvic junction obstruction: can magnetic resonance urography identify crossing vessels? *Pediatr Radiol.* (2015) 45:1788–95. doi: 10.1007/s00247-015-3412-y
11. Jiang X, Anderson C, Schnatz PF. The safety of direct trocar versus veress needle for laparoscopic entry: a meta-analysis of randomized clinical trials. *J Laparoendos Adv Surg Tech.* (2012) 22:362–70. doi: 10.1089/lap.2011.0432
12. Hong YH, DeFoor WR, Reddy PP, Schulte M, Minevich EA, VanderBrink BA, et al. Hidden incision endoscopic surgery (HIdES) trocar placement for pediatric robotic pyeloplasty: comparison to traditional port placement. *J Robot Surg.* (2018) 12:43–7. doi: 10.1007/s11701-017-0684-2
13. Iranmanesh P, Morel P, Buchs NC, Pugin F, Volonte F, Kreaden US, et al. Docking of the da vinci si surgical system® with single-site technology. *Int J Med Robot Comput Assist Surg MRCAS* (2013) 9:12–6. doi: 10.1002/rcs.1481
14. Cao H, Zhou H, Liu K, Ma L, Liu D, Tao T, et al. A modified technique of paraumbilical three-port laparoscopic dismembered pyeloplasty for infants and children. *Pediatr Surg Int.* (2016) 32:1037–45. doi: 10.1007/s00383-016-3958-2
15. Kutikov A, Resnick M, Casale P. Laparoscopic pyeloplasty in the infant younger than 6 months - Is it technically possible? *J Urol.* (2006) 175:1477–79. doi: 10.1016/S0022-5347(05)00673-7
16. Avery DI, Herbst KW, Lendvay TS, Noh PH, Dangle P, Gundeti MS, et al. Robot-assisted laparoscopic pyeloplasty: multi-institutional experience in infants. *J Pediatr Urol.* (2015) 11:139.e1-5. doi: 10.1016/j.jpurol.2014.11.025
17. Asensio M, Gander R, Royo GF, Lloret J. Failed pyeloplasty in children: Is robot-assisted laparoscopic reoperative repair feasible? *J Pediatr Urol.* (2015) 11:69.e1–6. doi: 10.1016/j.jpurol.2014.10.009
18. Olsen LH, Rawashdeh YF, Jorgensen TM. Pediatric robot assisted retroperitoneoscopic pyeloplasty: a 5-year experience. *J Urol.* (2007) 178:2137–41. doi: 10.1016/j.juro.2007.07.057
19. Minnillo BJ, Cruz JAS, Sayao RH, Passerotti CC, Houck CS, Meier PM, et al. Long-term experience and outcomes of robotic assisted laparoscopic pyeloplasty in children and young adults. *J Urol.* (2011) 185:1455–60. doi: 10.1016/j.juro.2010.11.056
20. Singh O, Gupta SS, Hastir A, Arvind NK. Laparoscopic dismembered pyeloplasty for ureteropelvic junction obstruction: experience with 142 cases in a highvolume center. *J Endourol.* (2010) 24:1431–34. doi: 10.1089/end.2010.0002
21. Atug F, Woods M, Burgess SV, Castle EP, Thomas R. Robotic assisted laparoscopic pyeloplasty in children. *J Urol.* (2005) 174(4 Pt 1):1440–42. doi: 10.1097/01.ju.0000173131.64558.c9
22. Franco I, Dyer LL, Zelkovic P. Laparoscopic pyeloplasty in the pediatric patient: hand sewn anastomosis versus robotic assisted anastomosis–is there a difference? *J Urol.* (2007) 178:1483–6. doi: 10.1016/j.juro.2007.06.012
23. Barbosa JA, Kowal A, Onal B, Gouveia E, Walters M, Newcomer J, et al. Comparative evaluation of the resolution of hydronephrosis in children who underwent open and robotic-assisted laparoscopic pyeloplasty. *J Pediatr Urol.* (2013) 9:199–205. doi: 10.1016/j.jpurol.2012.02.002
24. Yee DS, Shanberg AM, Duel BP, Rodriguez E, Eichel L, Rajpoot D. Initial comparison of robotic-assisted laparoscopic versus open pyeloplasty in children. *Urology* (2006) 67:599–602. doi: 10.1016/j.urology.2005.09.021
25. Subotic U, Rohard I, Weber DM, Gobet R, Moehrlen U, Gonzalez R. A minimal invasive surgical approach for children of all ages with ureteropelvic junction obstruction. *J Pediatr Urol.* (2012) 8:354–8. doi: 10.1016/j.jpurol.2011.07.004
26. Lee RS, Retik AB, Borer JG, Peters CA. Pediatric robot assisted laparoscopic dismembered pyeloplasty: comparison with a cohort of open surgery. *J Urol.* (2006) 175:683–7. doi: 10.1016/S0022-5347(05)00183-7
27. Song SH, Lee C, Jung J, Kim SJ, Park S, Park H, et al. A comparative study of pediatric open pyeloplasty, laparoscopy-assisted extracorporeal pyeloplasty, and robot-assisted laparoscopic pyeloplasty. *PLoS ONE* (2017) 12:e0175026. doi: 10.1371/journal.pone.0175026
28. Cundy T, Harling L, Hughes-Hallett A, Mayer EK, Najmaldin AS, Athanasiou T, et al. Meta-analysis of robot-assisted vs conventional laparoscopic and open pyeloplasty in children. *BJU Int.* (2014) 114:582–94. doi: 10.1111/bju.12683
29. Salö M, Sjöberg Altemani T, Anderberg M, Salö M, Sjöberg Altemani T. Pyeloplasty in children: perioperative results and long-term outcomes of robotic-assisted laparoscopic surgery compared to open surgery. *Pediatr Surg Int* (2016). 32:599–607. doi: 10.1007/s00383-016-3869-2
30. Link RE, Bhayani SB, Kavoussi LR. A prospective comparison of robotic andlaparoscopic pyeloplasty. *Ann Surg.* (2006) 243:486–91. doi: 10.1097/01.sla.0000205626.71982.32
31. Jacobs BL, Seelam R, Lai JC, Hanley JM, Wolf JS, Hollenbeck BK, et al. Cost analysis of treatments for ureteropelvic junction obstruction. *J Endourol.* (2017) 31:204–9. doi: 10.1089/end.2016.0722

32. Varda BK, Johnson EK, Clark C, Chung BI, Nelson CP, Chang SL. National trends of perioperative outcomes and costs for open, laparoscopic and robotic pediatric pyeloplasty. *J Urol.* (2014) 191:1090–5. doi: 10.1016/j.juro.2013.10.077
33. Varda BK, Wang Y, Chung BI, Lee RS, Kurtz MP, Nelson CP, et al. Has the robot caught up? National trends in utilization, perioperative outcomes, and cost for open, laparoscopic, and robotic pediatric pyeloplasty in the United State from 2003 to 2015. *J Pediatric Urol.* (2018) 14:336.e1–336.e8. doi: 10.1016/j.jpurol.2017.12.010
34. Palmer KJ, Lowe GJ, Coughlin GD, Patil N, Patel VR. Launching a successful robotic surgery program. *J Endourol.* (2008) 22:819–24. doi: 10.1089/end.2007.9824
35. Behan JW, Kim SS, Dorey F, De Filippo RE, Chang AY, Hardy BE, et al. Human capital gains associated with robotic assisted laparoscopic pyeloplasty in children compared to open pyeloplasty. *J Urol.* (2011) 186:1663–7. doi: 10.1016/j.juro.2011.04.019
36. Freilich DA, Penna FJ, Nelson CP, Retik AB, Nguyen HT. Parental satisfaction after open versus robot assisted laparoscopic pyeloplasty: results from modified glasgow children's benefit inventory survey. *J Urol.* (2010) 183:704–8. doi: 10.1016/j.juro.2009.10.040
37. Gargollo PC. Hidden incision endoscopic surgery: description of technique, parental satisfaction and applications. *J Urol.* (2011) 185:1425–32. doi: 10.1016/j.juro.2010.11.054
38. Peters CA. Complications in pediatric urological laparoscopy: results of a survey. *J Urol.* (1996) 155:1070–3. doi: 10.1016/S0022-5347(01)66394-8
39. Braga LH, Pace K, DeMaria J, Lorenzo AJ. Systematic review and meta-analysis of robotic-assisted versus conventional laparoscopic pyeloplasty for patients with ureteropelvic junction obstruction: effect on operative time, length of hospital stay, postoperative complications, and success rate. *Eur Urol.* (2009) 56:848–57. doi: 10.1016/j.eururo.2009.03.063
40. Reddy MN, Nerli RB. The laparoscopic pyeloplasty: is there a role in the age of robotics? *Urol Clin North Am.* (2015) 42:43–52. doi: 10.1016/j.ucl.2014.09.004
41. Baek M, Silay M, Au Jk, Huang GO, Elizondo RA, Puttmann KT, et al. Does the use of 5 mm instruments affect the outcomes of robot-assisted laparoscopic pyeloplasty in smaller working spaces? A comparative analysis of infants and older children. *J Pediatr Urol.* (2018) 14:537.e1–537.e6. doi: 10.1016/j.jpurol.2018.06.010

8

The Important Role of Endoscopy in Management of Pediatric Pseudomembranous Necrotizing Tracheitis

*Xiling Wu, Lei Wu and Zhimin Chen**

Department of Pulmonology, The Children's Hospital, Zhejiang University School of Medicine, National Clinical Research Center for Child Health, Hangzhou, China

Correspondence:
Zhimin Chen
zmchen@zju.edu.cn

Pseudomembranous necrotizing tracheitis is a rare, but life-threatening cause of central airway obstruction. Here, we reported three cases of pediatric pseudomembranous necrotizing tracheitis. The infectious etiologies were *Staphylococcus aureus* secondary to influenza A virus *and Aspergillus fumigatus*. Endoscopy was used in diagnosis and management of all patients and two patients survived. The improvement in mortality rate of these diseases need early recognition and prompt treatment with mechanical debridement by endoscope and early initiation of broad spectrum antibiotics. Endoscopy is a promising tool to diagnose and remove the pseudomembrane, therefore relieving central airway obstruction.

Keywords: necrotizing tracheitis, endoscopy, airway obstruction, mechanical debridement, pediatric

INTRODUCTION

Pseudomembranous necrotizing tracheitis is a rare, but life-threatening cause of central airway obstruction. Common infectious etiologies included bacterial, fungal, and/or viral infection(s) (1). The risk fact was bacterial infection secondary to influenza virus and long-term use of hormones or antibiotics. Patients usually have hoarseness, cough, dyspnea, wheezing and inspiratory stridor. Diagnosis requires a comprehensive endoscopic examination and biopsy (2). Endoscopy (flexible or rigid) has a very important role in both diagnosis and management of pseudomembranous necrotizing tracheitis. Once patients exhibit signs and symptoms of airway obstruction, mechanical debridement by endoscopy is necessary (2). A delay in treatment can significantly worsen the patient's prognosis. Here, we report three cases of pediatric pseudomembranous necrotizing tracheitis. Endoscopy was used to remove the pseudomembrane in all patients and two patients survived.

CASE PRESENTATION

Case 1

A 20-month-old girl presented at our hospital with a history of cough and fever for 2 days, and shortness of breath for 1 day. She also had hoarseness. On admission she was short of breath and exhibited laryngeal stridor. Physical examination revealed that there was no wheezing in both lungs. Computed tomography (CT) demonstrated inflammation in the left lower lobe. Her initial laboratory tests results were as follow: hemoglobin 11.6 g/dL, WBC14.11 $\times$ 10^9 /L, platelet count of 272 $\times$ 10^9 /L, and C-reactive protein (CRP) of 63 mg/L. On the first night of admission, laryngoscope was performed and revealed mucous edema of the larynx. Her situation deteriorated quickly, subsequently requiring intubation. However, her oxygen saturation was still unstable and the airway pressure was high during mechanical ventilation. She received tracheal tube replacement, during which brown solid matter measuring ~1 cm was drawn from her trachea (**Figures 1A,B**). After tube replacement, her airway pressure decreased and her situation improved after 2 days of meropenem and methylprednisolone treatment Mechanical ventilation was changed to a face mask. Both WBC count and CRP level subsequently decreased to within normal ranges. Sputum bacterial cultures showed a small amount of methicillin-sensitive *Staphylococcus aureus* (MSSA) grow. Sputum antigen testing of influenza (A and B), parainfluenza (I, II, and III), respiratory syncytial virus, adenovirus was negative, and the tuberculin skin test was non-reactive. On day 4, fiberoptic bronchoscopdy showed substantial white matter attached to the anterior commissure of the larynx and trachea (**Figures 2A1,A2**). Biopsy was performed for pathologic evaluation. Histologic evaluation of biopsy samples revealed flaky necrotic tissue and massive neutrophil infiltration (**Figure 3A**). On day 5, CT showed a slight high-density cord-like image ~2 cm below the vocal cord and pneumonia in the left lower lobe (**Figure 4A**). Pathogen detection including fungi, viruses, and bacteria was negative.

The patient had cyanosis and shortness of breath after a gust of coughing on the evening of day 6 after admission. Oxygen saturation decreased to 69%. She had convuls after 2 min and her heart rate decreased with oxygen saturation of 60–70%. We performed tracheal intubation and cardiopulmonary resuscitation. X-ray showed pneumothorax in bilateral lungs and the patient died within 3 h.

To further clarify the causative pathogen, DNA from necrotic tissue was extracted using the DNA Extraction Kit (Omega Bio-Tech Co., Ltd) and determined to be positive for *S. aureus* by the *Staphylococcus aureus* Real Time PCR Kit (Shanghai ZJ Bio-Tech Co., Ltd.).

Case 2

A 28-month-old girl was admitted with a history of fever and cough for 4 days and progressive shortness of breath for 3 days. Her sputum was brown. Upon admission, she was short of breath and irritable with positive tri-retraction sign. Bilateral respiratory sounds were decreased with rhonchus. Routine blood routine examination revealed WBC of 11.71 × 10^9/L and CRP of 93 mg/L. X-ray showed inflammation in bilateral lungs (**Figure 4B**). The patient was hoarseness, shortness of breath, restlessness and the blood gas indicated the decrease of oxygen saturation. She was diagnosed with acute laryngitis with three degrees of laryngeal obstruction, type I respiratory failure, and pneumonia. On the first day of admission, laryngoscopy was performed, which revealed substantial yellowish-white pus in the trachea. Respiratory failure rapidly progressed, subsequently requiring intubation. Bronchoscopy was performed and revealed substantial yellowish-white pus attached to the trachea and right main bronchus (**Figures 2B1,B2**). Biopsy was then performed (**Figure 1C**). Alveolar lavage fluid tests indicated the following: lymphocytes 8%, neutrophils 30%, macrophages 63%, and eosinophils <1%. Histologic evaluation revealed fibrin necrotic exudates (**Figure 3B**). Sputum analysis for viral antigens revealed influenza A positivity. Lavage fluid culture was positive for *S. aureus*. Pathogen detection for fungus or other bacteria was negative. The patient was treated with meropenem, vancomycin, and methylprednisolone. Oseltamivir was also given. Bronchoscopy was performed four times to remove the pseudomembrane and her condition improved. However, on day 8 of admission, her oxygen saturation decreased and she was suspected of having mucous membrane exfoliation. A white sputum bolt sample measuring 2.5 cm was removed by rigid microscopy and the patient's oxygen saturation increased to within normal ranges.

On day 10, the patient's tracheal tube was removed and bronchoscopy was performed seven consecutive times. The tenth bronchoscopic examination showed clear reduction in endotracheal secretion and the mucous membrane was a normal color. On day 32, she was discharged from our hospital.

Case 3

A 19-month-old girl presented at our hospital with a history of recurrent fever and cough for 2 weeks. She was diagnosed

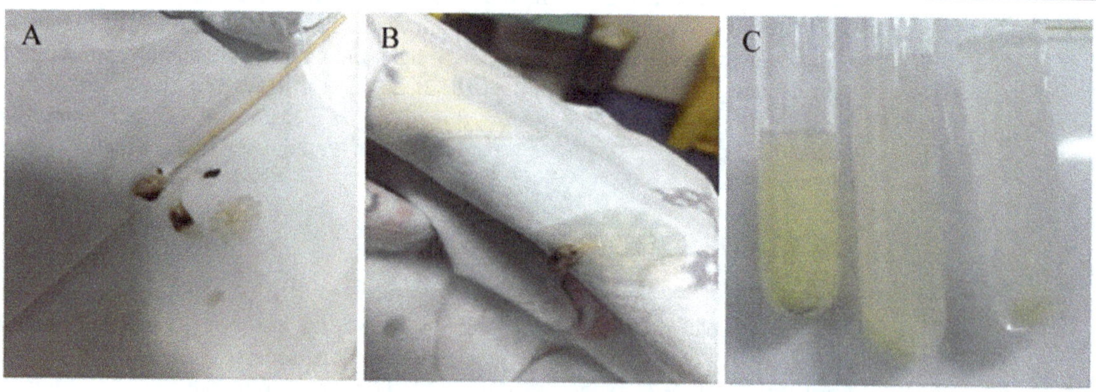

FIGURE 1 | Images of airway secretions or mucous exudates for cases 1 and 2. **(A,B)** Case 1, **(C)** Case 2.

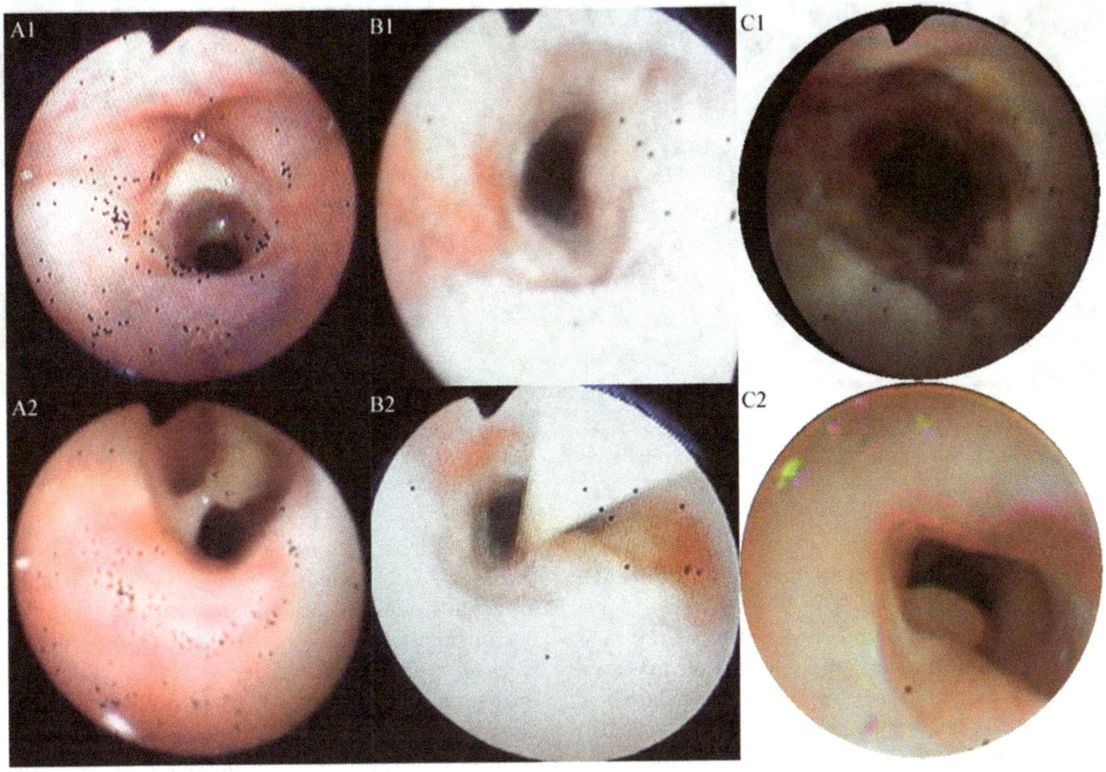

FIGURE 2 | Trancheal bronchoscopy images for the three cases. **(A,B)** Cases 1 **(A1,A2)** and 2 **(B1,B2)** showed substantial purulent secretion and necrotic mucosa. **(C)** Case 3 showed necrotic mucosa during acute phase **(C1)** and irregularly shaped trachea and granulation during the recovery phase **(C2)**.

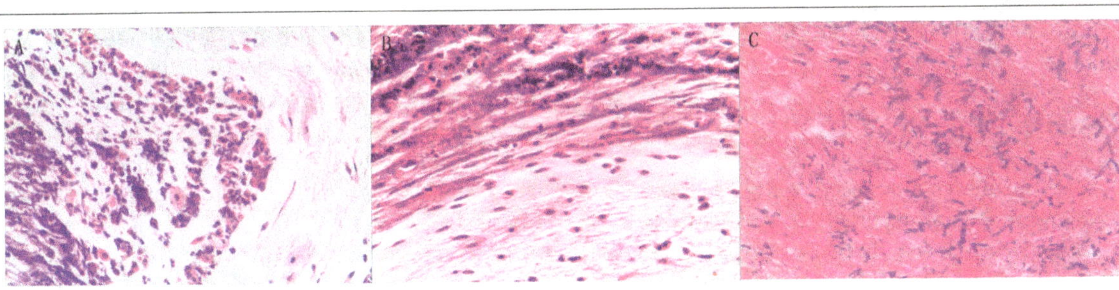

FIGURE 3 | Pathologic results of tracheal biopsy for the three cases. **(A)** Case 1 exhibited neutrophil infiltration and fibrinoid necrosis. **(B)** Case 2, it showed fibrinoid necrosis and purulent cells. **(C)** Case 3 demonstrated fibrinoid exudation and substantial *Aspergillus* load. (Hematoxylin and eosin staining, 200 × magnification).

with pneumia by a local hospital and had received azithromycin, ceftriaxone, and methylprednisolone treatment. However, her fever and cough persisted. Upon admission at our hospital, her respiratory rate was 70 breaths/min and body temperature was 39.7°C. Her eyelids were swollen and she had a needle-like rash over her entire body. Chest examination revealed crackles in two lung fields. Laboratory examinations revealed WBC count of 2.5×10^9/L, normocytic anemia (hemoglobin of 10.1 g/dL), thrombocytosis (platelet count of 75×10^9/L), and elevated CRP of 28 mg/L. CT demonstrated inflammation in the lungs and pleural effusion. We suspected infection by a drug-resistant microorganism and administered imipenem and methylprednisolone therapy. On day 9, her condition deteriorated and her respiratory rate increased with frequent cyanosis. The patient subsequently received tracheal intubation and mechanical ventilation. Because we could not exclude the possibility of methicillin-resistant *S. aureus* (MRSA) infection, vancomycin was administered. However, her oxygen saturation was only about 80%. X-ray showed interstitial emphysema, mediastinal emphysema, and subcutaneous emphysema in the lungs. She then received extracorporeal membrane oxygenation for 5 days. On day 22, bronchoscopy was performed, which revealed substantial purulent secretion and necrotic areas throughout the tracheal mucosa (**Figure 2C1**). Her condition improved and her tracheal tube was removed. Histologic evaluation showed inflammatory necrotic tissue

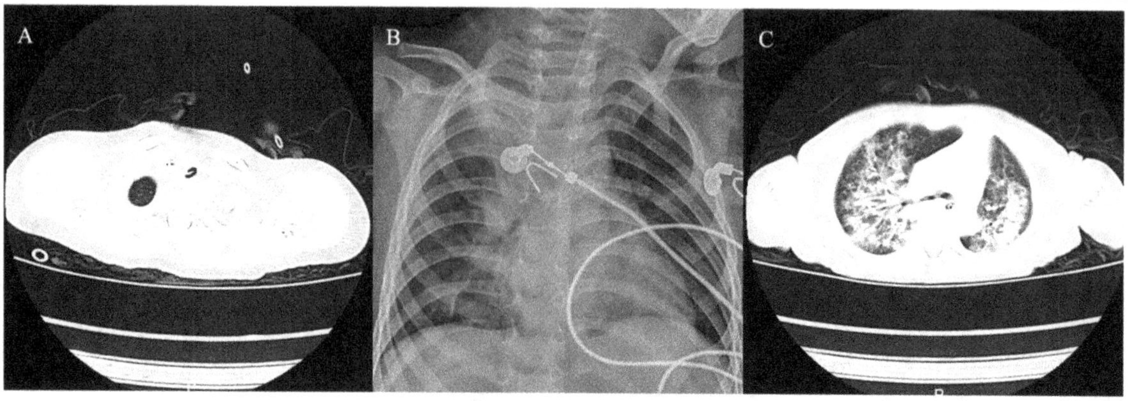

FIGURE 4 | Imaging findings of the three cases. **(A)** Case 1 showed membranous material that was strongly adherent to the tracheal wall. **(B)** Case 2 showed inflammation in bilateral lungs. **(C)** Case 3 had local stenosis of right main bronchus.

and *Aspergillus fumigatus* infection (**Figure 3C**). Repeat CT showed local stenosis of right main bronchus (**Figure 4C**) and a cavity formed near the pleura in the right lower lung. She subsequently received voriconazole, caspofungin, and amphotericin B treatment. Bronchoscopy was performed seven times to remove the pseudomembrane. The last bronchoscopic examination during hospitalization showed tracheal stenosis and granulation (**Figure 2C2**). On day 44, she was discharged from our hospital and received oral voriconazole for 6 months. The last bronchoscopic examination showed persistence of some mucosal irregularities. CT taken 1 year after discharge showed almost complete absence of lung inflammation.

All patients were previously healthy and had no significant family history.

DISCUSSION

Pediatric pseudomembranous necrotizing tracheitis is rare. The disease was first reported as a complication of prolonged assisted ventilation in newborns in 1983 (3). Despite mucosal trauma from mechanical ventilation, mucosal damage from an antecedent viral infection may contribute to the pathogenesis of this disease (4, 5). The most common infectious etiologies reported were *Corynebacterium diphtheria, Corynebacterium pseudodiphtheriticum, S. aureus, Bacillus cereus, Pseudomonas aeruginosa, Aspergillus species, and Haemophilus influenza* (2, 5, 6). Opportunistic infection occurs in immunosuppressed patients such as those with hematologic malignancies, organ transplantation, or neutropenia (7). Pseudomembranous necrotizing tracheitis can also be a rare extra-intestinal manifestation of ulcerative colitis in children (8). This disease should be differentiated from acute laryngitis, epiglottitis, foreign body inhalation, and obstructive fibrinous tracheal pseudomembrane (9).

Bacterial bronchitis primarily affects preschool and early school-aged children, however, cases of children with necrotizing tracheitis are rarely reported (10). We searched the PubMed and Embase databases for articles published until December 30, 2019, using the following search terms: (necrotic OR necrotizing OR pseudomembranous OR aspergillus) AND (tracheitis OR tracheobronchitis). Neonatal necrotizing tracheitis was excluded. We only found seven cases of pediatric necrotizing tracheitis (**Table 1**). The exact incidence is unknown. All cases presented with high fever, cough, inspiratory stridor, hoarseness, and tachypnea. All patients had acute deterioration characterized by severe upper airway obstruction.

In the present report, all patients were girls aged 1–3 years old. The first two patients got ill in the spring, while the third fell ill in the summer. The infectious etiologies of the three cases were MSSA secondary to influenza A virus, and *Aspergillus* sp. However, the mechanism by which these infections progressed to necrotizing tracheitis was not entirely clear. Although community-acquired *S. aureus* strains isolated from the first two patients were sensitive to methicillin, the strains likely had stronger virulence than the typical MSSA strains. Case 2 had coinfection of influenza A virus and *S. aureus*. These organisms are known to have destructive synergism. For instance, *S. aureus* strain was shown to secret proteases capable of enhancing influenza infectivity and pathogenicity in the respiratory tract5. In case 3, Aspergillus infection may have resulted from the patinet's long-term use of antibiotics and hormones, and neutropenia. The course of disease for *Aspergillus* infection is longer and the prognosis is relatively poorer than other etiologies.

Imaging features of pseudomembranous necrotizing tracheitis include circumferential thickening of the trachea, tracheal stenosis, and diffuse haziness and irregularity of the tracheal wall (13). The CT scan of case 1 showed membranous material compatible with endoluminal densities that was strongly adherent to the tracheal wall below the vocal cord. All cases had radiological findings suggestive of pneumonia.

Microscope images can aid in the correct diagnosis of patients with complex respiratory conditions of similar presentation (1, 14). Bronchoscopic findings consisted of membranous plaques, thick respiratory secretions, ulceration, or denudation

TABLE 1 | Cases of children with necrotizing tracheitis.

Number	Age	Sex	Etiology	Basic disease	Imaging	Endoscopic findings	Prognosis	Country	Reference
1	3m	F	Unknown	Tetralogy of Fallot and absent pulmonary valve, a radical cure	Strong stenosis was supposed at the truncus intermedius	The mucosa was red with some scabs and the lumen was narrow with a lot of secretions	Died	Japan	(11)
2	8m	M	Unknown	No	Left lung was hyperinflation with mediastinal shifting	There were swelling, bleeding, necrosis, and scab in tracheal and bronchial mucosa	Well	Portugal	(12)
3	9y	F	Influenza A and methicillin-resistant *staphylococcus aureus*	No	Chest X-ray revealed there was bilateral patchy infiltration	Copious dark and cloudy secretions, ragged, and severely edematous with adherent fibrinous debris and patchy plaques	Died	USA	(13)
4	5y	F	Aspergillosis	Fanconi anemia	CT of the thorax revealed bibasilar pulmonary opacities	A white exophytic lesion was in the tracheal	Died	Colombia	(14)
5	9y	F	Aspergillosis	Chronic myelogenous leukemia,hematopoietic cell transplantation	Chest X-ray was normal. Lateral neck films showed subglottic airway narrowing with soft tissue fullness of the glottis and subglottic areas	There were an erythematous and edematous supraglottis and extensive pseudomembranous and obstructive tracheitis, an estimated 50–60% of the entire tracheal lumen was filled	Died	USA	(15)
6	16y	F	Unknown	Ulcerative colitis	Not mentioned	There were mucous ulceration and white plaques along tracheal	Well	Portugal	(8)
7	7y	F	Influenza A-H1N1 combined with *staphylococcus aureus*	No	Chest X-ray showed there was inflammation in the right lung	There were black and yellow necrotic substances in the main airway, accompanied by hemorrhage and a large amount of yellow purulent substances	Died	China	(16)

of airway mucosa (15). Endoscopy (flexible or rigid) also has an important role in both tracheal and bronchial tissue sampling for microscopic analysis and culture, and helps to avert the need for intubation (17). Treatment in the acute phase of the illness frequently requires insertion of an endotracheal tube into the inflamed airway, which may lead to the subsequent development of mucosal shedding and subglottic stenosis. Once a patient exhibited signs and symptoms of central airway obstruction, he or she often needs immediate bronchoscopic intervention to restore airway patency (2). Rigid bronchoscopy is the safest treatment modality, both for confirming and relieving airway obstruction in patients with acute respiratory failure (18, 19). It can maintain airway open, diagnose quickly and relieve airway obstruction in time. When the patient deteriorated or his vital signs were unstable, rigid bronchoscopy will be the first choice.

Given the concern about early scar formation and recurrent airway obstruction, it has been suggested that early flexible bronchoscopy should be performed in patients with evidence of severe tracheitis (2). In this report, repeated resection of pseudomembranous was often carried out under flexible bronchoscopy.

Case 1 was our first experience of necrotizing tracheitis. The patient only received endoscopic examination twice. When her situation worsened, her parents refused intervention by rigid endoscopy. She subsequently died of profound mucosal sloughing, which almost completely obstructed the main airway. The other two cases received endoscopic examination and mechanical debridement several times and showed a significantly improved prognosis. Therefore, awareness and early recognition and therapeutic intervention are essential to improved prognosis and prevent progression to respiratory failure in pediatric pseudomembrance necrotizing tracheitis.

Broad-spectrum intravenous antibiotic therapy should be initiated as soon as the clinical diagnosis is made. A third-generation cephalosporin agent combined with a beta-lactamase resistant penicillin is appropriate for first-line therapy (20). If MRSA is suspected, then vancomycin or linezolid should be chosen. Antibiotic coverage should also be modified according to culture. Voriconazole is currently the first choice for the treatment of invasive aspergillosis (7). Corticosteroids treatment remains controversial. However, based on the rationale that they reduce airway inflammation and oedema, it was used in most of patients (21).

CONCLUSION

Pseudomembrance necrotizing tracheitis should be considered in children who present with an acute, life-threatening upper airway obstruction. Improvement in the mortality rate of this disease requires early recognition and prompt treatment with mechanical debridement by endoscopy and early initiation of broad-spectrum antibiotic therapy.

AUTHOR CONTRIBUTIONS

ZC supervised research work. XW and LW participated in collecting information of three cases and searched for literatures. They contributed equally to this work. All authors participated in the interpretation of the data. All authors read and approved the final manuscript.

ACKNOWLEDGMENTS

We thank Weizhong Gu and Wei Li for their assistance.

REFERENCES

1. Gabrilovich MI, Huff MD, McMillen SM, Quinter C. Severe necrotizing tracheobronchitis from panton-valentine leukocidin-positive MRSA Pneumonia Complicating Influenza A-H1N1-09. *J Bronchology Interv Pulmonol.* (2017) 24:63–6. doi: 10.1097/LBR.0000000000000314
2. Guerrero J, Mallur P, Folch E, Keyes C, Stillman IE, Gangadharan SP, et al. Necrotizing tracheitis secondary to corynebacterium species presenting with central airway obstruction. *Respir Care.* (2014) 59:e5–8. doi: 10.4187/respcare.02150
3. Metlay LA, Macpherson TA, Doshi N, Milley JR. A new iatrogenous lesion in newborns requiring assisted ventilation. *N Eng J Med.* (1983) 309:111–2. doi: 10.1056/NEJM198307143090214
4. Colt HG, Morris JF, Marston BJ, Sewell DL. Necrotizing tracheitis caused by corynebacterium pseudodiphtheriticum: unique case and review. *Rev Infect Dis.* (1991) 13:73–6. doi: 10.1093/clinids/13.1.73
5. Yamazaki Y, Hirai K, Honda T. Pseudomembranous Tracheobronchitis caused by methicillin-resistant *Staphylococcus aureus. Scand J Infect Dis.* (2002) 34:211–3. doi: 10.1080/00365540110077083
6. Khan MS, Przebinda AS, Claros-Sorto J, Porter A. Pseudomembranous tracheobronchitis: a rare presentation of pseudomonas aeruginosa infection. *J Bronchology Interv Pulmonol.* (2016) 23:319–22. doi: 10.1097/LBR.0000000000000300
7. Fernándezruiz M, Silva JT, Sanjuan R, De DB, Garcíaluján R, Lópezmedrano F, et al. Aspergillus tracheobronchitis: report of 8 cases and review of the literature. *Medicine.* (2012) 91:261–73. doi: 10.1097/MD.0b013e31826c2ccf
8. Nunes IS, Abreu M, Corujeira S, Oliveira J, Tavares M, Rocha C, et al. Tracheitis - A rare extra-intestinal manifestation of ulcerative colitis in children. *GE Port J Gastroenterol.* (2016) 23:259–63. doi: 10.1016/j.jpge.2016.03.002
9. Yildirim BB, Karalezli A, Hasanoglu HC, Kandemir O. Obstructive fibrinous tracheal pseudomembrane. *J Bronchology Interv Pulmonol.* (2012) 19:129–31. doi: 10.1097/LBR.0b013e31824f525f
10. Almutairi B, Kirk V. Bacterial tracheitis in children: approach to diagnosis and treatment. *Paed Child Health.* (2004) 9:25–30. doi: 10.1093/pch/9.1.25
11. Kawata H, Shimazaki Y, Kadoba K, Nakano S, Matsuda H. Necrotizing tracheobronchitis following radical repair in tetralogy of Fallot with absent pulmonary valve–a case report. *Nihon Kyobu Geka Gakkai Zasshi.* (1994) 42:924–30.
12. Sztajnbok J, Waetge AP, Escobar AM, Grisi SJ. Necrotizing tracheobronchitis in an infant. *J Pediatr.* (1997) 73:349. doi: 10.2223/JPED.552
13. Sharp JK, Hereth J, Fasanello J. Bronchoscopic findings in a child with pandemic novel H1N1 influenza A and methicillin-resistant *Staphylococcus aureus. Pediatr Pulmonol.* (2011) 46:92–5. doi: 10.1002/ppul.21306
14. Restrepo-Gualteros SM, Jaramillo-Barberi LE, Rodríguez-Martínez CE, Camacho-Moreno G, Nino G. Invasive pulmonary aspergillosis: a case report. *Biomedica.* (2016) 35:171–6. doi: 10.7705/biomedica.v35i2.2357
15. Gauguet S, Madden K, Wu J, Duncan C, Lee GS, Miller T. Case report of a child after hematopoietic cell transplantation with acute aspergillus tracheobronchitis as a cause for respiratory failure. *Case Rep Pediatr.* (2016) 2016:9676234. doi: 10.1155/2016/9676234
16. Fang X, Cao L. [A case of necrotic tracheobronchitis caused by severe H1N1 combined with *Staphylococcus aureus* infection]. *Zhonghua Er Ke Za Zhi.* (2019) 57:229–31. doi: 10.3760/cma.j.issn.0578-1310.2019.03.016
17. Le X, Jain P, O'Brien S. Aspergillus pseudomembranous necrotizing tracheitis. *Am J Hematol.* (2013) 88:242. doi: 10.1002/ajh.23332
18. Sehgal IS, Dhooria S, Bal A, Aggarwal AN, Behera D, Agarwal R. Obstructive fibrinous tracheal pseudomembrane after endotracheal intubation. *Resp Care.* (2016) 2011:69–71. doi: 10.4187/respcare.04662
19. Bua J, Trappan A, Demarini S, Grasso D, Schleef J, Zennaro F. Neonatal necrotizing tracheobronchitis. *J Pediatr.* (2011) 159:699–699.e1. doi: 10.1016/j.jpeds.2011.04.043
20. Mandal A, Kabra SK, Lodha R. Upper airway obstruction in children. *Indian J Pediatr.* (2015) 82:737–44. doi: 10.1007/s12098-015-1811-6
21. Tebruegge M, Pantazidou A, Thorburn K, Riordan A, Round J, De Munter C, et al. Bacterial tracheitis: a multi-centre perspective. *Scand J of Infect Dis.* (2009) 41:548–57. doi: 10.1080/00365540902913478

9

Interdisciplinary Radical "En-Bloc" Resection of Ewing Sarcoma of the Chest Wall and Simultaneous Chest Wall Repair Achieves Excellent Long-Term Survival in Children and Adolescents

Alireza Basharkhah[1], Herwig Lackner[2], Anna Karastaneva[2], Marko Bergovec[3], Stephan Spendel[4], Christoph Castellani[1], Erich Sorantin[5], Martin Benesch[2], Bernadette Liegl-Atzwanger[6], Freyja-Maria Smolle-Jüttner[7], Christian Urban[2], Michael Höllwarth[1], Georg Singer[1] and Holger Till[1]*

[1] Department of Pediatric and Adolescent Surgery, Medical University of Graz, Graz, Austria, [2] Division of Pediatric Hematology-Oncology, Department of Pediatrics and Adolescent Medicine, Medical University of Graz, Graz, Austria, [3] Department of Orthopedics and Trauma, Medical University of Graz, Graz, Austria, [4] Division of Plastic, Aesthetic and Reconstructive Surgery, Department of Surgery, Medical University of Graz, Graz, Austria, [5] Division of Pediatric Radiology, Department of Radiology, Medical University of Graz, Graz, Austria, [6] Diagnostic and Research Center of Pathology, Medical University of Graz, Graz, Austria, [7] Division of Thoracic and Hyperbaric Surgery, Department of Surgery, Medical University of Graz, Graz, Austria

***Correspondence:**
Georg Singer
georg.singer@medunigraz.at

Introduction: Ewing sarcomas of the chest wall, historically known as "Askin tumors" represent highly aggressive pediatric malignancies with a reported 5-year survival ranging only between 40 and 60% in most studies. Multimodal oncological treatment according to specific Ewing sarcoma protocols and radical "en-bloc" resection with simultaneous chest wall repair are key factors for long-term survival. However, the surgical complexity depends on tumor location and volume and potential infiltrations into lung, pericardium, diaphragm, esophagus, spine and major vessels. Thus, the question arises, which surgical specialties should join their comprehensive skills when approaching a child with Ewing sarcoma of the chest wall.

Patients and Methods: All pediatric patients with Ewing sarcomas of the chest wall treated between 1990 and 2020 were analyzed focusing on complete resection, chest wall reconstruction, surgical complications according to Clavien-Dindo (CD) and survival. Patients received neo-adjuvant chemotherapy according to the respective Ewing sarcoma protocols. Depending on tumor location and organ infiltration, a multi-disciplinary surgical team was orchestrated to perform radical en-bloc resection and simultaneous chest wall repair.

Results: Thirteen consecutive patients (seven boys and six girls) were included. Median age at presentation was 10.9 years (range 2.2–21 years). Neo-adjuvant chemotherapy (n = 13) and irradiation (n = 3) achieved significant reduction of the median tumor volume (305.6 vs. 44 ml, $p < 0.05$). En-bloc resection and simultaneous chest wall reconstruction was achieved without major complications despite multi-organ involvement. Postoperatively, one patient with infiltration of the costovertebral joint and laminectomy required surgical re-intervention (CD IIIb). 11/13 patients were treated with clear resections margins (R1 resection in one patient with infiltration of the costovertebral joint and marginal resection < 1 mm in one child with multiple pulmonary metastases). All patients underwent postoperative chemotherapy; irradiation was performed in four children. Two deaths occurred 18 months and 7.5 years after diagnosis, respectively. Median follow-up for the remaining patients was 8.8 years (range: 0.9–30.7 years). The 5-year survival rate was 89% and the overall survival 85%.

Conclusion: EWING specific oncological treatment and multi-disciplinary surgery performing radical en-bloc resections and simultaneous chest wall repair contribute to an improved survival of children with Ewing sarcoma of the chest wall.

Keywords: Askin tumor, Ewing sarcoma, chest wall reconstruction, tumor resection, multimodal therapy, chemotherapy

INTRODUCTION

Ewing sarcomas arising in the chest wall (historically known as Askin tumors) are small round cell sarcomas, molecularly defined by gene fusions involving one member of the FET family of genes and a member of the ETS family of transcription factors (1). They mainly arise from ribs, but paravertebral, sternal and scapular localizations have also been reported (2). In 1979, Askin et al. were the first ones to describe them in children, adolescents and young adults with a female preponderance (3, 4). Over the years, it became obvious that Askin tumor does not represent an separate tumor entity. In contrast, molecular studies showed identical molecular findings as seen in Ewing Sarcoma. Therefore, the terminology Askin tumor/primitive neuroectodermal tumor is not recommended by the resent WHO classification of bone and soft tissue tumors (1).

Clinically, children usually present late with a chest wall mass, chest pain or respiratory distress due to an intrathoracic mass (5). Unspecific symptoms such as fever, enlarged superficial lymph nodes, decreased general condition and nocturnal sweat may occur (6). Rarely, patients initially present with pathological fracture or metastasis related symptoms (7). Diagnostics reveal location and volume of the primary tumor as well as infiltrations e.g., into vertebral column, lung, pericardium, diaphragm or esophagus. Differential diagnoses include the group of undifferentiated small round cell sarcomas of bone and soft tissue, neuroblastoma, lymphoma, small-cell carcinoma, rhabdomyosarcoma, monophasic synovial sarcoma, and desmoplastic small round cell tumor.

Interdisciplinary and multimodal treatment of Ewing sarcoma is guided by the appropriate EWING protocols (8, 9). Aggressive treatment regimen have been shown to lead to longer relapse-free survival (6). Radical "en-bloc" resection remains crucial facing multiple challenges such as infiltrations e.g., into lung, spine, pericardium or diaphragm. Simultaneous chest wall reconstruction remains similarly challenging when covering large defects with prosthetic materials and viable tissue to prevent instability, flailing and infections. Thus, the question arises, which surgical specialties should build one team and join their comprehensive skills when approaching a child with Ewing Sarcoma of the chest wall. The present study elucidates the surgical and oncological outcome of children with Ewing Sarcoma of the chest wall treated by a multidisciplinary team of surgical specialists orchestrated according to the individual anatomical complexity.

PATIENTS AND METHODS

Following approval of the local ethics committee (EK 33-191 ex 20/21), we performed a retrospective analysis of all patients with Ewing Sarcoma of the chest wall treated at the Departments of Pediatric and Adolescent Surgery and Pediatrics and Adolescent Medicine between January 1990 and December 2020.

Patients received pediatric oncological management according to the currently valid protocol. Depending on the surgical complexity, a multidisciplinary surgical team was orchestrated to achieve radical "en-bloc" resections and simultaneous chest wall reconstructions. Pediatric surgeons or thoracic surgeons mainly performed en-bloc resections including resections of pulmonary, diaphragmatic, pericardial and esophageal infiltrations (**Figure 1**). They also inserted the prosthetic patches into the defect. Orthopedic surgeons took the lead for partial resection of a vertebral body and hemilaminectomy in one case with infiltration of the transverse process. Finally, plastic surgeons were responsible for covering the prosthetic patch with a muscle flap.

The diagnosis of Ewing Sarcoma of the chest wall was confirmed based on histological, immunohistochemical and molecular findings. Patient data were analyzed for presentation, tumor characteristics, oncological treatment, surgical outcome, surgical complications according to Clavien-Dindo (10), long-term follow-up and overall, progression free and relapse free survival.

RESULTS

From 1990 to 2020, 13 patients (n = 7 male, n = 6 female) underwent interdisciplinary multimodal therapy for Ewing

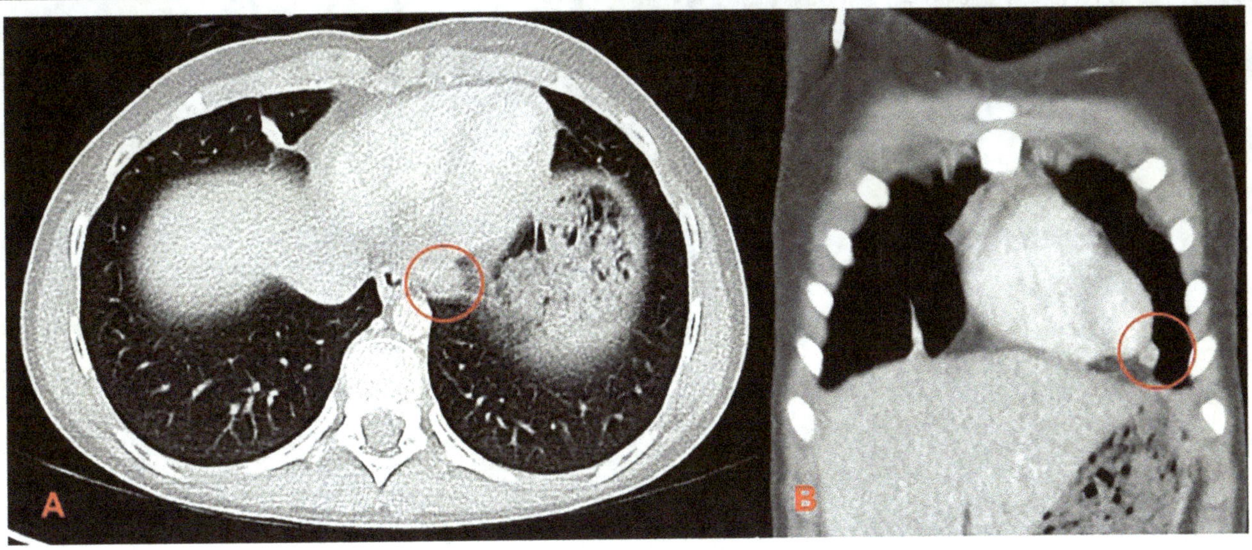

FIGURE 1 | Preoperative CT revealing multiple metastases: **(A)** shows a paraesophageal metastasis (red circle) and **(B)** demonstrates a pericardial metastasis (red circle). Both were removed surgically during initial resection (Patient #13).

Sarcoma of the chest wall. The median age of the patients at the time of presentation was 10.9 years ranging from 2.2 to 21 years.

Clinically, eight patients reported increasing thoracic pain. Three children had been treated for pneumonia. In two patients, the parents accidentally detected a thoracic swelling. One boy suffered from pneumothorax after a bout of laughter. Other unspecific symptoms included nocturnal sweating, fever, reduced general condition and collapse.

All patients underwent chest radiographs, bone scan, CT and MRI examinations revealing thoracic masses and the typical lytic bone destructions or cortical affection. Malignant pleural effusion was detected in four children, pleural seeding in three. At the time of presentation, two patients had pulmonary metastases. Detailed clinical data are presented in **Table 1**.

Neoadjuvant Treatment

All patients underwent diagnostic biopsies. On H&E morphology the tumors were composed of uniform small round tumor cells with fine chromatin, inconspicuous nuclei and scant clear or eosinophilic cytoplasm. The individual tumor cells were evenly spaced. Immunohistochemical examination revealed a strong membranous CD99 staining in all tumors. Tumors in the differential diagnosis were excluded using a broad immunohistochemical panel of antibodies. Molecular analyses were performed in 11/13 cases. Depending on the year of diagnosis FISH, RT-PCR and Archer fusion plex sarcoma panel were performed to confirm the diagnosis of Ewing Sarcoma. One boy had an additional tri-/tetrasomy of chromosome 8.

Chemotherapy was administered in all patients, i.e., two patients in the early nineties were treated according to the CESS 86 (11) and EICESS 92 (12), four and six according to the Euro-E.W.I.N.G. 99 (8) and EWING 2008 (9) protocols, respectively. In one patient (date of diagnosis 2009) initially diagnosed as desmoplastic round cell tumor, the diagnosis was revised after the patient developed a pulmonary metastasis. She was initially treated according to CWS 2002 (13) and postoperatively according to EURO-EWINGS 99. Three patients underwent irradiation additionally to their neoadjuvant chemotherapy due to malignant pleural effusion and pleural carcinosis.

Neo-adjuvant chemotherapy and irradiation led to a statistically significant reduction of the tumor volume from a median of 305.6 ml (ranging from 32 to 814 ml) to 44 ml (ranging from 2 to 215 ml) ($p < 0.001$, Wilcoxon Test) (**Table 2**).

Perioperative Course

En-bloc resection and simultaneous chest wall reconstruction was achieved in all cases without major complications despite multi-organ involvement. The affected rib and at least two adjacent ribs was removed in continuity with all infiltrations. Additional distant lesions were excised as well. In one case, orthopedic surgeons successfully performed partial vertebral body resection and hemilaminectomy for infiltrations into the transverse process (**Figure 2**). Pediatric and plastic surgeons could cover all chest wall defects with a prosthetic patch and muscle flaps. Postoperatively, the patient with infiltration of the costovertebral joint and hemi-resection of one vertebral body developed a liquor fistula requiring surgical intervention (placement of a lumbar drainage; CDC IIIb).

Table 2 summarizes detailed information concerning procedure, specialists of the team, chest wall reconstruction and short-term complications (30 days) according to CDC.

Histologically, complete resection was achieved in 11/13. R1 resection was found in one patient with infiltration of the costovertebral joint. Marginal resection of <1 mm was found in one child with multiple pulmonary metastases (**Table 3**).

Histologic evaluation of the tumor resection specimen after multimodal treatment revealed no viable appearing tumor cells in 9 cases therefore classifying them as Salzer-Kuntschik I grade

TABLE 1 | Clinical data of 13 patients treated with Askin tumors between 1990 and 2020.

ID	Year of diagnosis	Age	Sex	Primary tumor	Side	Complexity of disease
1	1990	7	M	6th–7th	Right	Adherent to lung
2	1994	21	M	8th	Right	Pleura, adherent to diaphragm
3	2001	16.5	M	6th	Right	Malignant pleural effusion
4	2001	2.5	F	11th	Right	Adherent to diaphragm
5	2001	10.5	M	4th	Right	Adherent to lung
6	2001	18	F	9th	Left	adherent to diaphragm
7	2009	12	F	4th–6th	Right	Left lower lobe, malignant pleural effusion
8	2012	16.5	M	7th	Left	Malignant pleural effusion, tumor embolism, adherent to diaphragm and the lung lower lobe
9	2014	11	M	4th	Left	Malignant pleural effusion, adherent to the lung lower and upper lobe
10	2017	3	F	7th	Left	Adherent to vertebral body and transverse process
11	2018	8	M	3th	Right	Adherent to lung
12	2019	9	F	6th	Right	Pleura
13	2020	11.5	F	3th	Left	Pleura, left lower lobe, diaphragmatic, paraesophageal, pericardial

of regression. In one case the regression grade was III (<10% vital tumor cells) and in the three remaining patients there were more than 50% vital tumor cell (regression grade V) (14).

All patients underwent adjuvant chemotherapy. Additional postoperative irradiation was administered in four cases, due to the above-mentioned marginal resection ($n = 2$), malignant pleural effusion ($n = 1$) and pulmonary metastases ($n = 1$). One patient with a histological confirmed invasion of tumor into a small pulmonary artery and malignant pleural effusion (patient #8) refused the advised radiotherapy.

Long-Term Outcome and Sequelae

Overall survival rate with multimodal therapy is 85% at a median follow-up of 8.8 years (ranging from 0.9 to 30.7 years). The 5-year survival rate is 89%. The median progression free survival was 7 years (range: 0.4–30.7 years). While one patient is still under the primary therapy and one patient passed away during primary therapy, the median relapse free survival in the remaining 11 patients was 8 years (0.4–30 years).

Eight out of the 13 patients had an uneventful oncological follow-up without signs of relapse or sequelae (**Table 3**). Patient #10, who required partial vertebral body resection developed postoperative scoliosis. A local relapse 2 years later necessitated radiotherapy. Three years after the primary diagnosis, a metastasis was found in the cervical vertebral column (C2) and she is currently under chemotherapy and radiotherapy. Two further patients had postoperative complications: Patient #1 developed postoperative scoliosis and pulmonary restriction with a tumor free interval of 30 years and patient #9 suffers from pulmonary restriction at a tumor free interval of 6.5 years.

Two patients died. In Patient #2 pulmonary metastasis occurred 5 years after the initial diagnosis. The metastasis was resected and chemotherapy including high-dose chemotherapy with autologous stem cell support was administered. However, two further relapses occurred, and he passed away 7.5 years after the initial diagnosis.

Patient #7 who initially presented with pleural effusion and pulmonary metastasis in the contralateral lower lobe developed six bilateral lung metastases later. Despite resection via sternotomy, chemotherapy and radiation the girl suffered from multiple recurrent metastases in both lungs and died 18 months after the first diagnosis.

DISCUSSION

With an aggressive multimodal interdisciplinary team approach with "targeted" surgical specialists we achieved an 85% overall survival rate at a median follow-up of 8.8 years and a 5-year survival rate of 89%. Two of the 13 patients treated during the last 30 years died 18 months and 7.5 years after diagnosis, respectively. Two patients are still under therapy.

Ewing sarcoma of the chest wall usually have a poor prognosis. Triarico et al. have reported a series of 9 patients with "Askin tumors," and their 5-year survival was 60% at a median follow-up of 53.1 months (15). Five-year survival of patients with localized extra-skeletal Ewing sarcomas has been described with 69.7% (16). Additionally, the overall survival rate after a median follow-up of 28 months was 45% in a study by Laskar (17).

Poor prognosis has been associated with tumor diameters > 5 cm, LDH levels > 240 U/l and late stage diagnosis (4). In another study, patients with poor histological response to chemotherapy and positive surgical margins had significantly worse event-free survival (18). Laskar et al. have shown that age at diagnosis higher than 18 years, poor response to induction chemotherapy, and presence of pleural effusion are indicators of inferior survival (17).

Cornerstones of current treatment protocols include neo-adjuvant chemotherapy, radical "en-bloc" resection

TABLE 2 | Treatment of 13 patients with Askin tumors.

ID	Preoperative therapy	Initial tumor volume (ml)	Tumor volume after CTX (ml)	Procedure performed	Surgical team	Material used for reconstruction	Complications CDC in 30 days
1	CESS 86/irradiation	32	4	Resection of the dorsal part of the 6th, the entire 7th rib, the transverse process and partial resection of the lung lower lobe	PS		
2	EICESS 92/irradiation	810	215	Partial resection of the 7th–9th ribs with adherent diaphragm	TS	Corium flap plastic and m. latissimus dorsi flap at a later time point autologous transplantation of the contralateral 7th rib and m. rectus abdominis flap at a later time point	
3	EURO EWING 99	148	2	Partial resection of the 5th–7th ribs	PS, OT	Vicryl® mesh and m. latissimus dorsi flap	
4	EURO EWING 99	246.5	16	Partial resection of the 10th–12th ribs with adherent diaphragm	PS, PL	Vicryl® mesh and m. latissimus dorsi flap	
5	EURO EWING 99	813.7	15.2	Partial resection of the 3rd–5th ribs with adherent lung	PS	Goretex® patch, Vicryl® mesh	
6	EURO EWING 99	199	5.2	Partial resection of the 8th–10th ribs with adherent diaphragm	PS	Goretex® patch, Vicryl® mesh	
7	CWS 2002 pilot	216	88.6	Partial resection of the 4th–7th ribs	PS	Tutomesh® plastic and m. latissimus dorsi flap	
8	EWING 2008	175	8.8	Partial resection of the 5th–9th ribs with adherent diaphragm and the lung lower lobe	OT, TS	Gore® Dualmesh®, Prolene® Mesh m. latissimus dorsi flap	
9	EWING 2008	310	37	Partial resection of the 3rd–7th ribs and the adherent lung lower and upper lobe	PS, TS, PL	Prolene® Mesh m. latissimus dorsi flap	
10	EWING 2008	72	15	Partial resection of 6th–8th with partial vertebral body resection/hemilaminectomy, resection of the transverse process and dorsal root ganglia	PS, OT, PL	Prolene® Mesh m. latissimus dorsi flap and m. trapezius	Liquor fistula lumbar drainage
11	EWING 2008	83	5.4	Partial resection of 2nd–4th ribs and adherent lung	PS, OT, PL	Prolene® Mesh m. pectoralis flap	
12	EWING 2008/ irradiation	53.1	2	Partial resection of the 4th–6th and pleural metastases	PS, OT, PL	Prolene® Mesh m. latissimus dorsi flap	
13	EWING 2008	814	158	Partial resection of the 1st–5th ribs with metastases to pericardium, lung, diaphragm	PS, OT, PL	Prolene® Mesh m. latissimus dorsi flap	

CTX, chemotherapy; PS, Pediatric Surgery; OT, Orthopedic Surgery; PL, Plastic Surgery; TS, Thoracic Surgery; CDC, Clavien-Dindo Classification.

and chest wall reconstruction as well as adjuvant chemotherapy/radiotherapy (19, 20).

Neo-adjuvant chemotherapy has been shown to prolong survival rates (21, 22). This may be attributed to the formation of a pseudo-capsule, which reduces the risk of intraoperative tumor rupture and tumor cell dissemination (21, 23, 24). By shrinking tumor volume it decreases vascularity and vulnerability and improves feasibility of complete removal with negative microscopic margins (4, 25–27). In our study, we confirmed the efficacy of neo-adjuvant chemotherapy with a significantly reduced tumor volume following preoperative chemotherapy (**Table 2**). Moreover, Demir et al. reported that neo-adjuvant chemotherapy significantly increased the complete resection rate with 5-year survival rates with or without neo-adjuvant therapy of 77 and 37%, respectively (28).

Following neo-adjuvant chemotherapy, complete "en-bloc" resection of the primary lesion and simultaneous reconstruction of the defect is mandatory. Radical surgical resection is associated with better survival; patients with complete resection have a higher 5-year survival rate compared to patients who had an incomplete resection (28). The surgical complexity primarily depends not only on tumor location and volume, but also on the extent of infiltrations into lung, pericardium, diaphragm, esophagus or spine. Thus, the question arises, which surgical

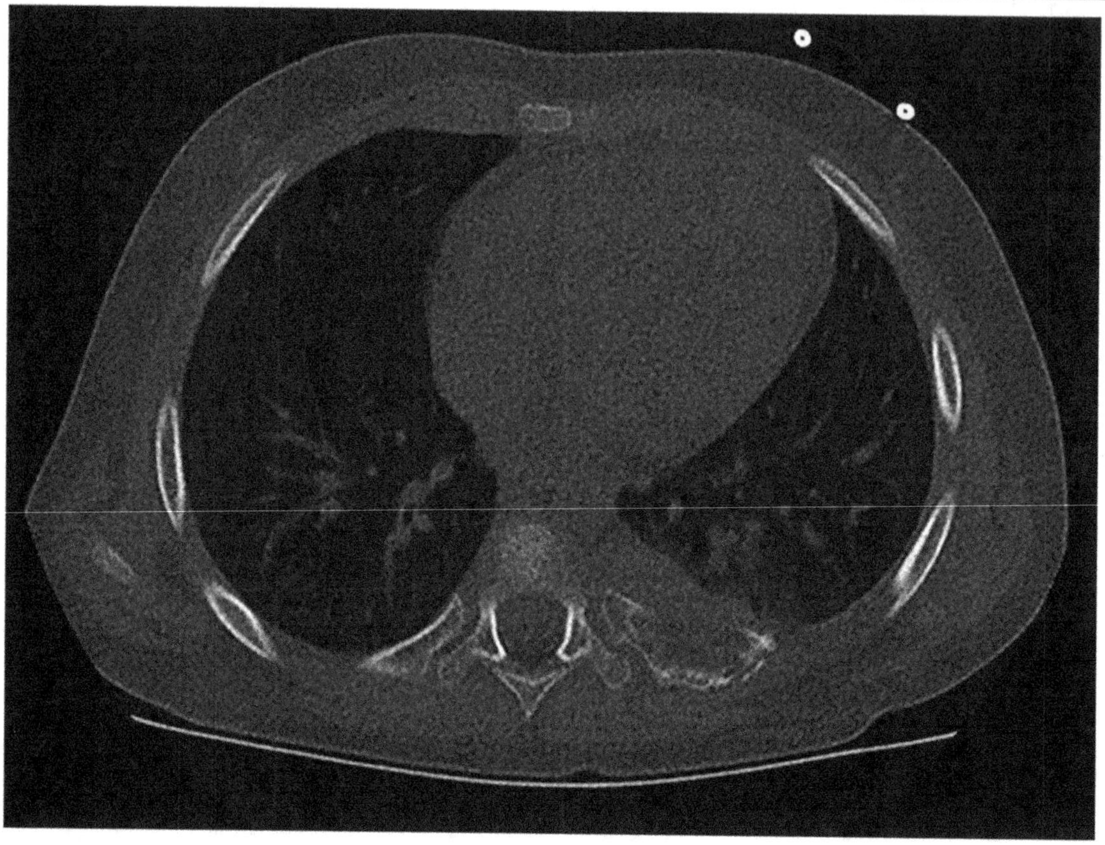

FIGURE 2 | Tumor arising from the paravertebral dorsal portion of the left 7th rib with infiltration of the transverse process and vertebral body. This extent required en bloc resection of the ribs 6–8 and additional removal of the costovertebral joint and hemilaminectomy (patient #10).

TABLE 3 | Outcome and complications of 13 patients treated with Askin tumors.

ID	Local resection status	Grade of regression	Postoperative therapy (CTX/irradiation)	Auto-PSCTx	Relapses	Outcome years	Sequelae
1	R0	1	+/–		–	30.7	Scoliosis, pulmonary restriction
2	R0	1	+/–	+	Lung/local	†7.5	
3	R0	1	+/+	–	–	20	
4	R0	1	+/–	–	–	19.9	
5	R0	3	+/–	–	–	19.5	
6	R0	1	+/–	–	–	19.4	
7	R0	5	+/+	+	Lung bilateral	†1.5	
8	R0	1	+/refused	+	–	8.8	
9	R0	1	+/–	+	–	7	Pulmonary restriction
10	R1	5	+/+	–	Local/cervical	3.4	Scoliosis
11	R0	1	+/–	–	–	2.9	
12	R0	1	+/–	+	–	1.2	
13	Marginal	5	+/+	+	–	0.9	

CTX, chemotherapy; PSCTx, peripheral stem cell transplantation. † deceased.

specialists should build one team and join their comprehensive skills when approaching a child with Ewing sarcoma of the chest wall. In the literature, there are some reports about the team approach (6, 15, 29), but the studies report lower survival rates than those achieved in ours. We orchestrated the team according to the surgical complexity and organ involvement, targeting "en-bloc" resection with a preferably macroscopic safety margin of 1 cm. This strategy is technically more demanding when the first and second rib have to be removed. Care should be taken to avoid injury of subclavian vessels and brachial plexus.

Simultaneously, all distant metastases within the ipsilateral thoracic cavity must be managed requiring pulmonary, cardiac, esophageal and diaphragmatic expertise. In our setting pediatric surgeons or thoracic surgeons faced these challenges successfully with minor complications. Finally, simultaneous repair of the chest wall defect requires distinct surgical finesse. A variety of materials is available to cover the defect. This includes synthetic meshes, bioprosthetic materials, stainless-steel bars, osseo-integrated titanium systems, autografts, homografts or porcine or bovine xenografts. In 2020, Smelt et al. described the successful application of personalized three-dimensional (3D)-printed chest wall prostheses made of methylmetacrylate covered by expanded polytetrafluoroethylene for patients undergoing chest wall resection and reconstruction (30). However, due to residual growth and development, the choice of the optimal material is a major consideration in the pediatric and adolescent population. The material should be malleable enough to conform to the shape of the chest wall, rigid enough to prevent paradoxical motion and protective for the intrathoracal organs. Additionally, it should be durable, non-allergenic, non-toxic, biologically inert and radiolucent (31, 32). One advantage of synthetic meshes used in our patients is their permeability, which minimizes the amount of postoperative pleural effusion. The mesh is sutured tautly to the surrounding tissue allowing ingrowth of connective tissue and incorporation of the mesh into the body (33). Most centers also insert a prosthetic patch into the skeletal defect and cover it with viable tissue like a muscular flap. This dual layer technique offers the advantage that well-vascularized tissue facilitates integration of the underlying material into the surrounding tissue thereby minimizing the risk of infections (34). In our series no infection of the patches or flaps occurred.

Nevertheless, long-term sequelae such as scoliosis cannot always be prevented. In our series, two of the 13 patients developed scoliosis. In a recently published report, Marqués et al. describe the successful operative correction of four pediatric patients with scoliosis secondary to extensive chest resections due to Askin tumors (35). Moreover, female patients should be also observed regarding mammary sequelae. However, due to the rarity of the disease there is no real recommendation for mammary reconstruction in affected female patients.

Local relapse represents a major negative factor for mortality (36). Christiansen et al. described a series of 8 patients, in which 4 out of 5 patients with relapse died (6). In our series, we found similar mortality rates as two out of three patients with relapses died and the third one is still under treatment. In 2013, we have already published our experience with seven patients with Ewing sarcoma of the chest wall. We were able to achieve a 5-year survival rate of 86% and an overall survival of 71% (22). By adding another 6 patients in the current report, we support this relatively high survival rate.

Postoperative irradiation was applied in four of the patients. In two of them due to viable tumor cells with Salzer-Kuntschik grade V regression and marginal resection, in one boy with a malignant pleural effusion and in one girl with multiple pulmonary metastases. Patient #8 refused the recommended postoperative radiotherapy. Radiotherapy should only be reserved for individual patients with unfavorable non metastatic tumors or for patients with a high risk of recurrence, such as in an incomplete resection or viable tumor (26, 37), due to the late effects related to radiotherapy such as chest wall deformities, pulmonary fibrosis and risk of secondary malignancies (19).

Limitations of the present study include the relatively low number of patients and the short observation period of four patients (patients 10–13). However, due to the rarity of Ewing sarcomas in general and the location chest wall in particular large series in children and adolescents concentrating on the surgical approach are scarce in the literature.

In conclusion, Ewing sarcoma specific oncological (neo)adjuvant treatment and multi-disciplinary surgery performing radical en-bloc resections and simultaneous chest wall repair contribute to an improved long-time survival of children and adolescents with Ewing sarcoma of the chest wall.

AUTHOR CONTRIBUTIONS

AB, CC, GS, and HT analyzed the data, wrote the manuscript and performed the statistics. AB, HL, AK, MBer, SS, CC, ES, MBen, BL-A, F-MS-J, CU, MH, and HT operated, treated and examined the patients and critically reviewed the manuscript. All authors contributed to the article and approved the submitted version.

REFERENCES

1. Flechter C. *WHO Classification of Soft Tissue and Bone Tumours.* (2020). Lyon: International Agency for Research on Cancer.
2. Jürgens H, Bier V, Harms D, Beck J, Brandeis W, Etspuler G, et al. Malignant peripheral neuroectodermal tumors. A retrospective analysis of 42 patients. *Cancer.* (1988) 61:349–57. doi: 10.1002/1097-0142(19880115)61:2<349::AID-CNCR2820610226>3.0.CO;2-0
3. Askin FB, Rosai J, Sibley RK, Dehner LP, Mcalister WH. Malignant small cell tumor of the thoracopulmonary region in childhood: a distinctive clinicopathologic entity of uncertain histogenesis. *Cancer.* (1979) 43:2438–51. doi: 10.1002/1097-0142(197906)43:6<2438::AID-CNCR2820430640>3.0.CO;2-9
4. Zhang KE, Lu R, Zhang P, Shen S, Li X. Askin's tumor: 11 cases and a review of the literature. *Oncol Lett.* (2016) 11:253–6. doi: 10.3892/ol.2015.3902
5. Devi LP, Kumar R, Kalita JP, Khonglah Y, Handique A. Locally advanced Askin's tumour in a child-a rare case report and review of the literature. *Indian J Surg Oncol.* (2015) 6:288–91. doi: 10.1007/s13193-015-0422-z
6. Christiansen S, Semik M, Dockhorn-Dworniczak B, Rotker J, Thomas M, Schmidt C, et al. Diagnosis, treatment and outcome of patients with Askin-tumors. *Thorac Cardiovasc Surg.* (2000) 48:311–5. doi: 10.1055/s-2000-7874
7. Laine M, Ghorfi IA, Lambatten D, Kettani F, Abid A. Rapidly fatal Askin's tumor: a case report and literature review. *Pan Afr Med J.* (2014) 18:104. doi: 10.11604/pamj.2014.18.104.4549
8. Juergens C, Weston C, Lewis I, Whelan J, Paulussen M, Oberlin O, et al. Safety assessment of intensive induction with vincristine, ifosfamide,

doxorubicin, and etoposide (VIDE) in the treatment of Ewing tumors in the EURO-E.W.I.N.G. 99 clinical trial. *Pediatr Blood Cancer.* (2006) 47:22–9. doi: 10.1002/pbc.20820

9. Dirksen U, Brennan B, Le Deley MC, Cozic N, Van Den Berg H, Bhadri V, et al. High-dose chemotherapy compared with standard chemotherapy and lung radiation in Ewing sarcoma with pulmonary metastases: results of the European Ewing Tumour Working Initiative of National Groups, 99 Trial and EWING 2008. *J Clin Oncol.* (2019) 37:3192–202. doi: 10.1200/JCO.19.00915
10. Dindo D, Demartines N, Clavien PA. Classification of surgical complications: a new proposal with evaluation in a cohort of 6336 patients and results of a survey. *Ann Surg.* (2004) 240:205–13. doi: 10.1097/01.sla.0000133083.54934.ae
11. Jurgens H, Bier V, Dunst J, Harms D, Jobke A, Kotz R, et al. The German Society of Pediatric Oncology Cooperative Ewing Sarcoma Studies CESS 81/86: report after 6 1/2 years. *Klin Padiatr.* (1988) 200:243–52. doi: 10.1055/s-2008-1033716
12. Paulussen M, Ahrens S, Braun-Munzinger G, Craft AW, Dockhorn-Dworniczak B, Dorffel W, et al. EICESS 92 (European Intergroup Cooperative Ewing's Sarcoma Study) - preliminary results. *Klin Padiatr.* (1999) 211:276–83. doi: 10.1055/s-2008-1043800
13. Seitz G, Urla C, Sparber-Sauer M, Schuck A, Vokuhl C, Blank B, et al. Treatment and outcome of patients with thoracic tumors of the Ewing sarcoma family: a report from the Cooperative Weichteilsarkom Studiengruppe CWS-81, −86, −91, −96, and −2002P trials. *Pediatr Blood Cancer.* (2019) 66 (Suppl. 3):e27884. doi: 10.1002/pbc.27884
14. Salzer-Kuntschik, M, Delling, G, Beron, G, and Sigmund, R. (1983). Morphological grades of regression in osteosarcoma after polychemotherapy - study COSS 80. *J Cancer Res Clin Oncol.* 106:21–4. doi: 10.1007/BF00625047
15. Triarico S, Attina G, Maurizi P, Mastrangelo S, Nanni L, Briganti V, et al. Multimodal treatment of pediatric patients with Askin's tumors: our experience. *World J Surg Oncol.* (2018) 16:140. doi: 10.1186/s12957-018-1464-9
16. Applebaum MA, Worch J, Matthay KK, Goldsby R, Neuhaus J, West DC, et al. Clinical features and outcomes in patients with extraskeletal Ewing sarcoma. *Cancer.* (2011) 117:3027–32. doi: 10.1002/cncr.25840
17. Laskar S, Nair C, Mallik S, Bahl G, Pai S, Shet T, et al. Prognostic factors and outcome in Askin-Rosai tumor: a review of 104 patients. *Int J Radiat Oncol Biol Phys.* (2011) 79:202–7. doi: 10.1016/j.ijrobp.2009.10.039
18. Tural D, Molinas Mandel N, Dervisoglu S, Oner Dincbas F, Koca S, Colpan Oksuz D, et al. Extraskeletal Ewing's sarcoma family of tumors in adults: prognostic factors and clinical outcome. *Jpn J Clin Oncol.* (2012) 42:420–6. doi: 10.1093/jjco/hys027
19. Shamberger RC, Laquaglia MP, Krailo MD, Miser JS, Pritchard DJ, Gebhardt MC, et al. Ewing sarcoma of the rib: results of an intergroup study with analysis of outcome by timing of resection. *J Thorac Cardiovasc Surg.* (2000) 119:1154–61. doi: 10.1067/mtc.2000.106330
20. Van Den Berg H, Van Rijn RR, Merks JH. Management of tumors of the chest wall in childhood: a review. *J Pediatr Hematol Oncol.* (2008) 30:214–21. doi: 10.1097/MPH.0b013e318162bd54
21. Sawin RS, Conrad EU 3rd, Park JR, Waldhausen JH. Preresection chemotherapy improves survival for children with Askin tumors. *Arch Surg.* (1996) 131:877–80. doi: 10.1001/archsurg.1996.01430200087015
22. Basharkhah A, Pansy J, Urban C, Hollwarth ME. Outcomes after interdisciplinary management of 7 patients with Askin tumor. *Pediatr Surg Int.* (2013) 29:431–6. doi: 10.1007/s00383-013-3272-1
23. Dunst J. The role of radiotherapy in the local treatment of Ewing's sarcoma. *Praxis.* (1995) 84:1148–51.
24. Zimmermann T, Blutters-Sawatzki R, Berghauser KH, Christiansen H, Padberg W. Primitive neuroectodermal tumor. *Chirurg.* (1997) 68:732–7. doi: 10.1007/s001040050262
25. Picci P, Rougraff BT, Bacci G, Neff JR, Sangiorgi L, Cazzola A, et al. Prognostic significance of histopathologic response to chemotherapy in nonmetastatic Ewing's sarcoma of the extremities. *J Clin Oncol.* (1993) 11:1763–9. doi: 10.1200/JCO.1993.11.9.1763
26. Saenz NC, Hass DJ, Meyers P, Wollner N, Gollamudi S, Bains M, et al. Pediatric chest wall Ewing's sarcoma. *J Pediatr Surg.* (2000) 35:550–5. doi: 10.1053/jpsu.2000.0350550
27. Veronesi G, Spaggiari L, De Pas T, Solli PG, De Braud F, Catalano GP, et al. Preoperative chemotherapy is essential for conservative surgery of Askin tumors. *J Thorac Cardiovasc Surg.* (2003) 125:428–9. doi: 10.1067/mtc.2003.198
28. Demir A, Gunluoglu MZ, Dagoglu N, Turna A, Dizdar Y, Kaynak K, et al. Surgical treatment and prognosis of primitive neuroectodermal tumors of the thorax. *J Thorac Oncol.* (2009) 4:185–92. doi: 10.1097/JTO.0b013e318194fafe
29. Parikh M, Samujh R, Kanojia RP, Mishra AK, Sodhi KS, Bal A. Peripheral primitive neuroectodermal tumor of the chest wall in childhood: clinico-pathological significance, management and literature review. *Chang Gung Med J.* (2011) 34:213–7.
30. Smelt J, Pontiki A, Jahangiri M, Rhode K, Nair A, Bille A. Three-dimensional printing for chest wall reconstruction in thoracic surgery: building on experience. *Thorac Cardiovasc Surg.* (2020) 68:352–6. doi: 10.1055/s-0039-1678611
31. Mahabir RC, Butler CE. Stabilization of the chest wall: autologous and alloplastic reconstructions. *Semin Plast Surg.* (2011) 25:34–42. doi: 10.1055/s-0031-1275169
32. Seder CW, Rocco G. Chest wall reconstruction after extended resection. *J Thorac Dis.* (2016) 8:S863–S871. doi: 10.21037/jtd.2016.11.07
33. Sanna S, Brandolini J, Pardolesi A, Argnani D, Mengozzi M, Dell'amore A, et al. Materials and techniques in chest wall reconstruction: a review. *J Vis Surg.* (2017) 3:95. doi: 10.21037/jovs.2017.06.10
34. Gapany C, Raffoul W, Zambelli PY, Joseph JM. Latissimus dorsi muscle-flap over Gore-Tex patch for coverage of large thoracic defects in paediatric Ewing sarcoma. *Pediatr Blood Cancer.* (2009) 52:679–81. doi: 10.1002/pbc.21848
35. Marques C, Pizones J, Sanchez-Marquez JM, Martin-Baldan M, Fernandez-Baillo N, Sanchez Perez-Grueso FJ. Surgical treatment of scoliosis developed after extended chest wall resection due to Askin tumor during childhood. *Spine Deform.* (2019) 7:180–5. doi: 10.1016/j.jspd.2018.06.016
36. Takanami I, Imamura T, Naruke M, Kodaira S. Long-term survival after repeated resections of Askin tumor recurrences. *Eur J Cardiothorac Surg.* (1998) 13:313–5. doi: 10.1016/S1010-7940(98)00005-0
37. Dou X, Yan H, Wang R. Treatment of an Askin tumor: a case report and review of the literature. *Oncol Lett.* (2013) 6:985–9. doi: 10.3892/ol.2013.1488

10

Robotic Approach to Creation of Continent Catheterisable Channels—Technical Steps, Current Status and Review of Outcomes

Ramnath Subramaniam [1,2,3*]

[1] *Consultant Paediatric Urologist, Leeds Teaching Hospitals NHS Trust, Leeds, United Kingdom,* [2] *Department of Paediatric Urology, University of Leeds, Leeds, United Kingdom,* [3] *Department of Paediatric Urology, University of Ghent, Ghent, Belgium*

***Correspondence:**
Ramnath Subramaniam
R.Subramaniam@leeds.ac.uk

Purpose: To report the current status of Robotic approach to creation of Catheterisable channel (CC) with the author's personal experience compared to published literature on technical steps, follow up, and outcomes.

Methods: CC data was extracted from the prospective database set up for all Robotic pediatric urology procedures performed by the author at his institution. A literature search was then performed to look at the evidence base.

Results: Eighteen consecutive cases (8M:7F) of Robotic approach to creation of CC was identified and included. All attempted cases were successfully completed without any conversion to open approach. Median age at surgery was 10.75 years (IQR 6.9–16.5); Median OT 197 min (IQR 131–295) with concomitant procedures in 4 cases. Appendix was used in 14 cases as CC conduit and distal ureter in 4 cases. Median Length of stay (LOS) was 2.75 days (IQR 2–6) and Median FU 27.3 m. Whilst FU duration is comparable to published series, average OT and LOS was much lower in this series. The LOS in this robotic series is much lower than the author's experience with open approach (2.75 vs. 5.8 days). No major complications postoperatively except for one exit site wound infection managed conservatively. None of the CC have been revised in this series and all channels are patent with 12 F or 14 F admissible catheter size. There were no cases of incontinence related to technique of creation of CC and no incidence of exit site stomal stenosis with use of ACE stopper until channel matures and Clean intermittent catheterisation (CIC) is established.

Conclusion: Robotic approach to CC is feasible, safe with excellent outcomes and minimum morbidity. Robotic complex bladder reconstructive surgery offers some advantages to children compared to open approach but is only currently performed in few tertiary centers with expertise.

Keywords: catheterisable channel, robotic approach, pediatric urology, outcomes - health care, current status

INTRODUCTION

Congenital and acquired affections to the bladder can lead to poor bladder emptying with attendant consequences of recurrent urinary tract infections, damage to renal upper tracts, and incontinence. Two vital landmark developments in the management of bladder emptying include Clean intermittent catheterization (CIC) per urethra introduced by Lapides in 1970s (1) and subsequent extension of this concept by Mitrofanoff to create catheterisable channel (CC) using appendix to facilitate bladder drainage when CIC per urethra is not feasible (2). Up until recently, open surgical approach was favored by most pediatric urologists with few reports of laparoscopic assisted attempt to create the channel. Robotics has recently provided an alternative with enhanced minimally invasive option in creating such channels with its attendant benefits (3, 4), not least to the surgeon due to ergonomics (5). This article looks at the author's personal experience with the Robotic approach, description of technical steps, and a review of published literature as regards potential benefits, current status and outcomes.

METHODS

The methodology in this paper is set in two parts. The first is the patient series from the author's personal experience and the second is the review of literature to ascertain outcomes when possible and define the current status of Robotic approach to CC comparing different studies along with the author's experience.

Patient Database

A prospective database collating all information with regards to author's personal experience with Robotic approach to all procedures in pediatric urology was set up since 2013. Informed and written consent was obtained from the patients or their legal guardian in this study. Information related to creation of CC within this database was extracted and analyzed. A comparison to Length of stay (LOS) with similar group of cases with an open approach was made to calculate cost analysis together with patient level cost (PLICS) data from the author's institution. Formal ethical committee is not required for this type of audit.

Literature Search

A search was done from Institutional library resources using terms "Robotic," "Mitrofanoff" and "Catheterisable channel" and restricted to pediatric age group.

TECHNICAL STEPS IN THE CREATION OF THE CC

The technical steps described below are the author's preferred approach recognizing there might be variations amongst other surgeons to the approach. At the outset, it is important to note that the author's preferred exit site for CC is right iliac fossa; some other surgeons might prefer the umbilicus. The robotic platform mentioned in this series is the Si Da Vinci system.

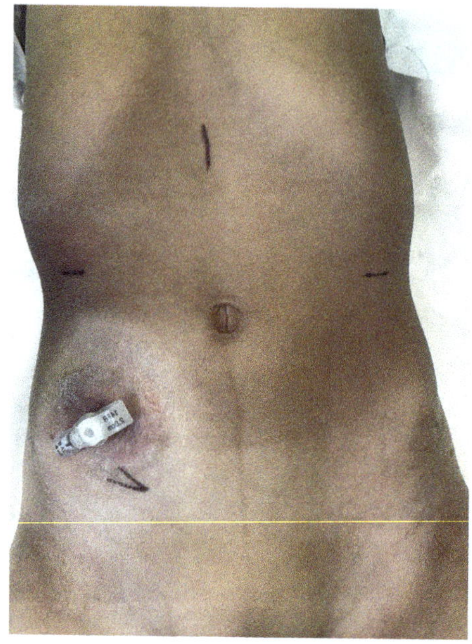

FIGURE 1 | Preoperative picture of a patient with caecostomy button *in situ* for bowel washouts. Port sites are marked- 12 Camera port in epigastrium; two 8 mm working ports on the respective hypochondrium; Exit site at right iliac fossa.

Patient and Robot Positioning

Patient is placed supine on the operating table with extreme side docking of the robot from the left side. The right side therefore is available for exit site incision and placement of large step port to facilitate retrieval of the channel into the exit site. This assumes appendix or the right ureter as the chosen conduit for the CC. Side docking, often to the extreme is a useful maneuver in pediatric patients and has the advantages of leaving the patient supine on the table and the robot can be docked from either side (6). This is particularly important in small theaters where space can be a constraint given that existing theaters do not cater for the footprint of Robotic surgical equipment.

Port Sites

The 12 mm camera port is placed in the midline of epigastric region to stay as far away as possible from target organs, namely the appendix and bladder. Two 8 mm working ports are placed in the right and left hypochondrium. The exit site is marked up with a "V"; this will eventually be used for the VQ plasty to facilitate skin lined stoma at exit site (**Figure 1**). During the procedure, a large (10–12 mm) step port is placed through the base of the exit site incision. This facilitates retrieval of the CC onto the exit site. Given the complex needs for these group of patients, particularly with bowel affection for e.g., Spina bifida cases, often they have a caecostomy in place for bowel management. In the author's institution, the caecostomy is fashioned with a button for washouts (if not effective per rectum). In the **Figure 1**, the child has a caecostomy button placed previously.

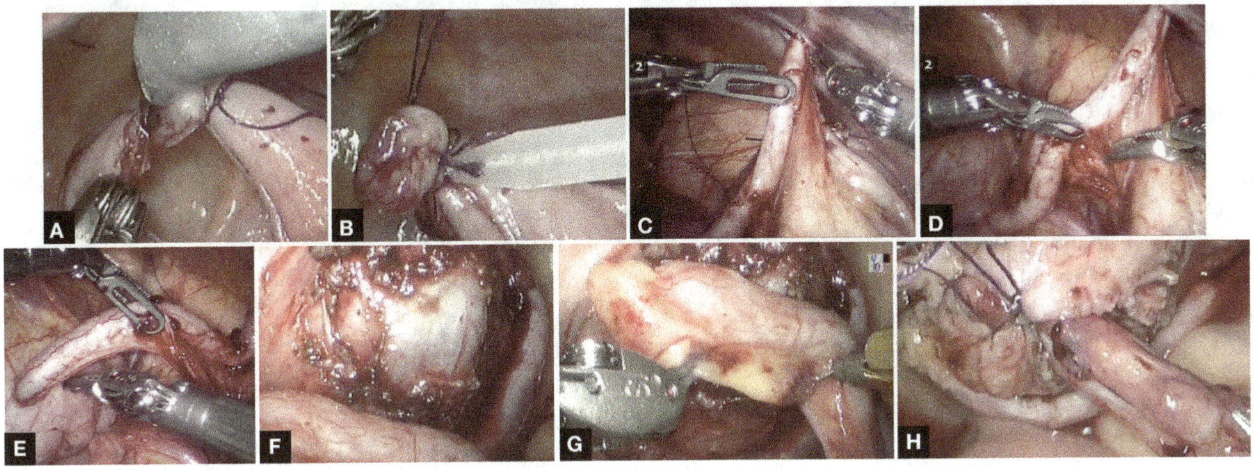

FIGURE 2 | The technical steps in the creation of CC is shown in this series of pictures. Note not all pics are from the same case study but does represent the relevant individual steps in the procedure. **(A)** Appendix divided from caecum with ligature at caecal base. **(B)** Endoloop to secure the caecal stump further. **(C)** Appendix routed into exit site. **(D)** Ensuring vascular pedicle on its mesentery is not under tension and adequately mobilized. **(E)** Appropriately sized Foley catheter inserted into appendix. **(F)** Adequately sized detrusorotomy performed. **(G)** Typically, a 4:1 ratio of detrusorotomy to length of appendix ensures continence to channel. **(H)** Extravesical implantation of the appendix completed.

Conduits for the Channel

It is generally agreed that appendix raised on its vascular pedicle is the best available conduit. The author has used the ureter in selected cases when a dilated tortuous ureter is available and there is no associated vesicoureteric reflux; when a nephroureterectomy has been performed for appropriate clinical indication or appendix is not available. The other option is to create a conduit with small bowel (Monti procedure); the author has no personal experience with this option by the Robotic approach. The outcomes from author's experience with appendix and ureter are detailed in the Results section.

Procedure

Once the ports are placed, the steps in creation of CC are illustrated in **Figure 2**. The appendix is mobilized on its vascular pedicle and divided from the caecum with a ligature and endoloop to secure the caecal stump. This is done through the step port placed by the assistant at the exit site. The appendix is then retrieved through the step port and an appropriately sized foley's catheter is placed into the lumen of the appendix. Typically, a 12 F catheter is placed, although in some cases, it might have to be a 10 F catheter, whilst some can accommodate 14 F catheter. However, this can later be sized up (if required) via fluoroscopy when CC is mature and established. Peritoneum over the bladder is opened and bladder mobilized and anchored with stay sure to the abdominal wall. A detrusorotomy is then performed to create a detrusor defect in the posterior wall of the bladder and facilitate extravesical implantation of the appendix. An incision at the proximal end of the detrusorotomy is made and the tip of the appendix is opened to allow the Foley catheter to be inserted into the bladder lumen and the balloon is inflated. The length of detrusor defect should be a minimum of 4:1 ratio in comparison to the width of the appendix. The appendix is anastomosed to bladder mucosa with 50 PDS sutures followed by the detrusor wrap using interrupted 40 PDS sutures, making sure that some stitches do incorporate the appendix to maintain the tunnel length within the detrusor. The peritoneum is then reposited making sure the CC is extraperitoneal. VQ-plasty is performed to fashion a skin lined exit site for the CC. The CC is accessible for CIC typically after 6 weeks once it is mature.

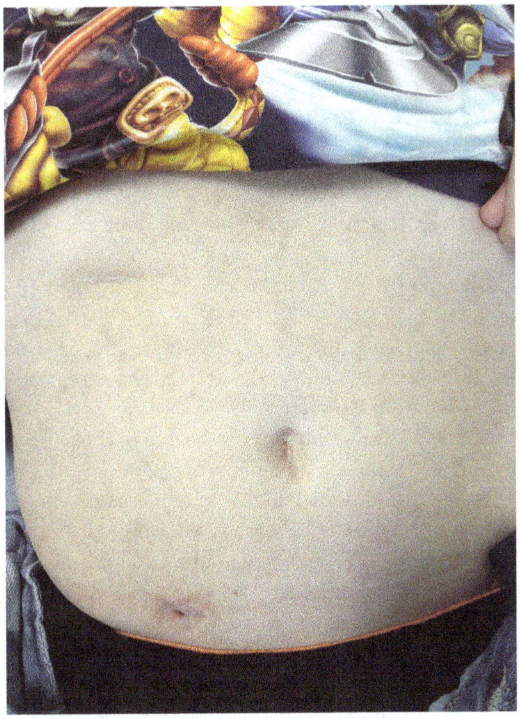

FIGURE 3 | Postoperative appearance of a child 6 months after creation of CC.

Post-operative Phase

All port sites are infiltrated with local anesthetic and none of the patients in this series have had epidural catheter for pain relief. The patients are allowed liquids the same afternoon with full feeds established shortly thereafter. The patients are discharged home with Foley catheter *in situ* via the CC. The Clinical nurse specialist supervises home care and starts CIC in ~6 weeks postop. A typical postoperative appearance of the CC approximately 6 months after the procedure is shown in **Figure 3**.

RESULTS

In this series, 18 children underwent procedure "Robotic approach to creation of CC." The demographic details for each of these patients are as shown in **Table 1**. All procedures attempted by Robotic approach were successfully completed and there were no open conversions. Literature search produced 6 relevant and comparable published reports summarized in **Table 2**, all retrospective studies from a total of 6 centers across USA. There is one multicenter series reporting an experience of 88 cases involving 5 tertiary children's hospital (12). Three papers highlighted in gray within **Table 2** are progressive reports over time from the same center in Chicago (led by Gundeti) (8–10). There is only one comparable series of CC procedure alone (7); all others have a mix of concomitant enterocystoplasty (EC). This makes the comparison challenging; nevertheless, the author has made an attempt to draw relevant conclusions from all the possible literature search yields.

Salient features from the author's series are the following:

a. Prospectively collected and analyzed data from a single surgeon series.
b. Exclusive report of Robotic approach to creation of CC without EC.
c. Median Operating time (OT) 197 min, much lower than 323 min from comparable series (Others have reported mean OT as 347 min for CC alone).
d. All patients in the author's series have had their CC exit site stoma sited at the iliac fossa.
e. No conversion to open and no immediate postoperative complications from the CC except one wound infection.
f. Median LOS is 2.75 days; lower than reported multicenter series at 5.2 days. Comparatively, average LOS for open cases in the authors institution was 5.8 days. As per PLICS data, average bed occupancy in the children's ward is ~£300/day. Therefore, with an average saving of £1,000 per patient episode from this series, that makes a saving of ~£15–18 K for the hospital by using the Robotic approach in this series alone.
g. Median FU is 27.3 months with the longest FU at 60 months and the average for the first 13 cases is 36.6 months i.e., over 3 years. All channels are patent currently with no incidence of exit site stomal stenosis. All patients use ACE stopper, the use of which has eliminated stomal stenosis as reported by the author in a previous publication many years ago (13).
h. Experience with using ureter in selected cases for CC conduit; out of 4 children with ureteric mitrofanoff (all boys), 2 of them (50%) complain of transient pain when catheter enters the bladder.
i. Three children have had some difficulty in accessing the CC at the very end toward its entry into the bladder at variable periods during FU. They underwent endoscopy to evaluate the channel ensuring patency and admitting 12 F catheter easily. One child who had 10 F catheter intraoperatively had interventional radiology support to upscale the catheter to 12 F, 4 months after the procedure.

DISCUSSION

This is a report of 18 consecutive cases with Robotic approach to creation of CC and is the first such report from a center outside the USA. Much of the published experience with the use of robot in pediatric urology is with pyeloplasty and upper tract procedures such as nephrectomy or heminephrectomy (3, 4, 14–17). Increasingly, the indications are expanding with reports on the use of robot for ureteric reimplantation (18–20).

The first description of the use of robot for creation of CC is a case report in 2004 (21). It then took a further 5 years before the publication of a series from a single center (7) and literature search for similar experience with the Robotic approach yields only a handful of published material, testifying that the experience with the use of robot for bladder reconstructive surgery is limited to few centers at this point in time. Moreover, the published material from some of the centers have a combination of EC together with CC, making the process of drawing definite conclusions at best challenging. Nevertheless, there are important points to highlight from the collective experience with common themes, variations in technique, and reported outcomes.

There is not a lot to dwell on indications for the procedure, fairly well-recognized and similar with the author's experience and published literature; and the age range at which surgery is performed is well-matched.

Technical Aspects of the Creation of CC

In children, port placements are key to successful completion of the procedure by the robotic approach, because the recommended 8–10 cm distance between ports in adults is not realistically achievable. The author routinely places three ports, one for the camera, and two working ports corresponding to three arms of the robot as is the preference for other surgeons in published literature except for Grimsby et al. (11) where they prefer a 4th arm is deployed for assistance. In a pediatric program, the 4th arm is pretty much redundant for majority of the procedures. Some suggest use of a 5 mm laparoscopic port to exchange sutures (7), but the author relies on the assistants to exchange sutures via the working port, which of course needs excellent team effort. The author cannot emphasize enough the role of a well-trained first assistant as regards efficiency and minimizing the need for additional port in an already cramped set up. The benefits of side docking in pediatric robotic program and alluded to in the technical aspects earlier in the report has been published elsewhere (6).

TABLE 1 | Summary of the author's experience with Robotic approach to creation of CC.

		Comments
No of cases (Gender)	18 (8M:7F)	Consecutive cases with Robotic approach
Median age at op (IQR)	10.75 (6.9–16.5)	Clinical indication–neurogenic (10) valve bladder (3) and others (5)
No of ports	3	Additional Step port at exit site to retrieve channel
Median OT (IQR)	197 min (131–295)	4 concomitant procedures–1 nephroureterctomy; 1 caecostomy button for bowel management; 1 proximal ureter reimplant with distal ureter as CC; 1 detrusorotomy (autoaugmentation)
Exit site VQ plasty	18	4 had caecostomy button *in situ* pre-op and 1 had concomitant caecostomy button inserted during this episode.
Channel size (Foley catheter)	10 F–1	10 F channel was later upscaled to 12 F by interventional radiology team after 4 months.
	12 F–13	
	14 F–4	
Channel conduit	14 appendix and 4 distal ureter	(When Ureters used for CC- 1 had nephroureterectomy and 3 others had proximal ureteric reimplant)
Conversion to open	0	
Median LOS (IQR)	2.75 (2–6)	Comparative open cases LOS 5.8 days
Complications post op	1	1 Wound infection at exit site; managed conservatively with antibiotics; No revision of CC in this series.
Median FU	27.3 m	Longest FU is 60 m; in total first 13 patients have a median FU of 36.6 months. Last 5 patients have relatively short FU of <12 m.
Stomal stenosis	0	All patients use ACE stopper post op until channel matures in few months and CIC pattern established
Channel patency	18	3 patients had difficulty in accessing channel at entry into bladder; endoscopy confirmed no issues and 12 F Foley inserted easily. No sub-fascial channel issues.

CC, Catheterisable channel; FU, Follow up; OT, Operating time; LOS, Length of stay in hospital post-op.

One important difference in this series is where the ports are placed. The author places the camera 12 mm port at the midline in the epigastric region and two ports on the hypochondrium to stay further away from the target organs, bladder, and appendix. In comparison, all the other surgeons (in published literature) place the ports much closer to the target organs with the camera port at the umbilicus. It is also worth noting that the ureter has been used as a conduit in selected cases in this series, the use of which has raised some observations and is further explained in the outcomes section Follow up and Outcomes.

It appears in those published series in **Table 2**; the exit site is preferentially the umbilicus whilst the author routinely sites the exit stoma in the iliac fossa. The use of step port to retrieve the conduit onto the exit site is another variation in the author's practice. It is difficult to know for sure, but it appears that the author's technique described earlier has contributed to a much lower median OT at <200 min compared to >300 min in other reported series (7, 22).

Incidence of concomitant EC is high in the reports especially from Chicago group (9, 10, 22) and the multicenter report (12) where there is a 15% incidence of EC and 39% incidence of bladder neck procedures (BNP). Therefore, this series is matched and comparable only to the report from Boston group Nguyen et al. (7) with regards to creation of CC without concomitant EC. It is interesting to note when comparing open and Robotic approach to CC, Grimsby et al. in their series report an incidence of concomitant EC is 54% in the open group vs. 3% in the Robotic group (11). This could be explained by the complexity of adding EC to the procedure at the same setting, given that the Chicago group led by Gundeti report mean OT at 623 min with EC compared to 347 with CC alone (8–10). To put into perspective, that is over 10 h of operating with EC, one of the main reasons for the limited experience with such complex reconstructive procedures.

In this series, the site of implantation of the CC in to the bladder is in the posterior wall with the bladder hitched up ensuring straight run off to the exit site. Interestingly, Famakinwa et al. from the Chicago group (9) mention the difference in implantation site if the CC is performed concomitantly with EC; the anterior wall is preferred if CC is done alone and the posterior wall if combined with EC.

Postoperative Phase and Complications

Murthy et al. have highlighted the advantages of using the robot in this procedure with reduced hospital stay and eliminating the need for epidural (10), which the author is in complete agreement.

The average LOS is much lower in the author's series at 2.75 days compared to 5.2 days in the multicenter series (12). In the healthcare setting within the UK, LOS is crucial to costs and by reducing the LOS with robotic approach compared to open (2.7 vs. 5.8 days as explained in the results section), significant savings have been made

TABLE 2 | Summary of published articles on robotic approach to CC.

References	CC	EC	No of CC cases (MedianAge at surgery)	Summary of findings (All retrospective reviews from USA and vast majority of cases in these series had umbilical exit site stoma)
Nguyen et al. (7)	Yes	No	10 (11.9 y)	Mean OT 323 min; one conversion to open; Median Hosp stay 5 days; Median FU 14.2 m; one open revision due to urine leakage post op; minor channel incontinence 2 cases. Comparison with open cases-no difference
Wille et al. (8)	Yes	Yes (5)	11 (10.4 y)	Reports from same center over time; mean OT 494 min; 639 with EC and 347 min without EC; Median FU 24.2 m; Robot advantages: reduced hospital stay and eliminates epidural. Minimum recommended detrusor wrap length 4 cm. Appendix on anterior wall if without EC; otherwise posterior wall.
Famakinwa et al. (9)	Yes	Yes (10)	18 (11.7 y)	
Murthy et al. (10)	Yes	Yes (15)	11 (11 y)	
Grimsby et al. (11)	Yes	Yes	39 (9.1 y)	Comparison of complications between open (28) cases; 54% EC in open cases and 3% in Robotic; Median FU 2.7 y; no significant difference in complication rates between open and robotic; 3 Clavien III complications in Robotic series.
Gundeti et al. (12)	Yes	Yes (15%)	88 (10.4 y)	Multi center series; Mean FU 29.5 m; LOS 5.2 days; 29.5% complication rate; 6 Clavien III; 12% CC revision rate; Mean detrusor length 3.9 cm ± 1.0.

CC, Catheterisable channel; EC, Enterocystoplasty; FU, Follow up; OT, Operating time; LOS, Length of stay in hospital post-op. Gray shaded rows indicate progressive over time reports from same institution.

in the author's series. This is important when it comes to working collaboratively with the management to realize the feasibility of a robotic program as also observed by others (23). Differences in healthcare worldwide could explain the paucity of reports linked to affordability from centers outside USA.

In this series, there has been no conversion to open and no major immediate postoperative complications except for an exit site wound infection in one case unlike a reported 29.5% complication rate with 6 Clavien III episodes from the multicenter series (12). It must be noted that they had concomitant 17% EC and 39% BNP. However, Grimsby et al. also reported 3 Clavien III complications in the Robotic group of their series (11). Nguyen et al. report one conversion to open in their series with 10 cases with one post-op urinary leak (7).

Follow Up and Outcomes

The mean FU is 27.3 m in this series and is comparable to the FU in the multicenter study of 29.5 m (12). The longest FU in this series is 60 months and the first 13 cases have over 3 years FU. This should be sufficient time to look at outcomes given that majority of the revisions occur in the first 24 months (24, 25). Although this point is highlighted by Nguyen et al. in their report, their FU of just 14.2 m is relatively short (7). There have been no revisions of the CC or the exit site in this series. This is significant compared to 12% CC revision rate in the multicenter study (12). Grimsby et al. report ~30% reoperation rates in both open and Robotic groups, although the reasons behind them is varied (11). They also have had 10% incontinence rates in the robotic group. It is difficult to know from the available reports whether the CC incontinence was technique related or due to other factors such as bladder dynamics.

There was no incidence of incontinence attributable to the technical aspects of CC in this series and it is worth mentioning the emphasis by the author on a minimum ratio of 4:1 when constructing then channel. The length of detrusor wrap is recognized as an important factor by others with a recommended length of 4 cm to ensure continence (8, 12). The author prefers to relate it to the width of the appendix akin to the principle with a ureteric reimplantation procedure.

It is important to mention that 4 boys in this series have had distal ureter as a CC conduit and 2 of them (50%) have reported considerable transient pain at point of entry into the bladder and 2 other boys (50%) in this series use the ureteric CC with no discomfort. This is also the author's experience with open cases and therefore now re-evaluating the use of ureter.

The author has published previously his experience with ACE stopper in the postoperative period (13) and this practice has continued over the years with stomal stenosis virtually eliminated and as is the case in this series. Wille et al. have reported 3 exit site revisions in their series of 11 cases (27%) (8). There is no incidence of CC access issues at sub-fascial plane in this series or other series with Robotic approach compared to reports by Indiana group who have the largest experience with CC using the open approach (26). Plausible explanation could be the direct alignment of the channel from within the abdomen with the robotic approach.

Summary

This is the first report of Robotic approach to CC from outside of USA with comparable outcomes and together with the collective experience from published literature albeit from few centers establishes the role of Robotics in creation of CC. There are common themes with some variation in technical aspects but the main advantages being reduced hospital stay and avoiding the need for invasive pain relief such as epidural compared to open approach. The series in this report has the lowest mean OT and LOS, both contributing to cost savings from a healthcare economic model point of view. The experience with robotic approach is limited to tertiary centers currently but there is sufficient expertise to allow other aspiring centers to take advantage of and avail the proctorship to facilitate safe introduction of complex reconstructive surgery into their individual Robotic program (27). This can only enhance the quality of care provided over time within pediatric urology.

AUTHOR CONTRIBUTIONS

The author confirms being the sole contributor of this work and has approved it for publication.

REFERENCES

1. Lapides J, Diokono AC, Lowe BS, Kalish MD. Follow up on unsterile, intermittent self-catheterization. *J Urol.* (1974) 111:184. doi: 10.1016/S0022-5347(17)59922-X
2. Mitrofanoff P. Trans-appendicular continent cystostomy in the management of the neurogenic bladder. *Chir Pédiatrique* (1980) 21:297–305.
3. Orvieto MA, Large M, Gundeti MS. Robotic paediatric urology. *BJU Int.* (2012) 110:2–13. doi: 10.1111/j.1464-410X.2011.10877.x
4. Howe A, Kozel Z, Palmer L. Robotic surgery in pediatric urology. *Asian J Urol.* (2017) 4:55–67. doi: 10.1016/j.ajur.2016.06.002
5. Esposito C, Ghoneimi AE, Yamataka A, Rothenberg S, Bailez M, Ferro M, et al. Work-related upper limb musculoskeletal disorders in paediatric laparoscopic surgery. A multicenter survey. *J Pediatr Surg.* (2013) 48:1750–6. doi: 10.1016/j.jpedsurg.2013.01.054
6. Subramaniam R. Current use of and indications for robot-assisted surgery in paediatric urology. *Eur Urol Focus* (2018) 4:662–4. doi: 10.1016/j.euf.2018.08.020
7. Nguyen HT, Passerotti CC, Penna FJ, Retik AB, Peters CA. Robotic assisted laparoscopic mitrofanoff appendicovesicostomy: preliminary experience in a pediatric population. *J Urol.* (2009) 182:1528–34. doi: 10.1016/j.juro.2009.06.055
8. Wille MA, Zagaja GP, Shalhav AL, Gundeti MS. Continence outcomes in patients undergoing robotic assisted laparoscopic mitrofanoff appendicovesicostomy. *J Urol.* (2011) 185:1438–43. doi: 10.1016/j.juro.2010.11.050
9. Famakinwa OJ, Rosen AM, Gundeti MS. Robot-assisted laparoscopic mitrofanoff appendicovesicostomy technique and outcomes of extravesical and intravesical approaches. *Eur Urol.* (2013) 64:831–6. doi: 10.1016/j.eururo.2013.05.007
10. Murthy P, Cohn JA, Selig RB, Gundeti MS. Robot-assisted laparoscopic augmentation ileocystoplasty and mitrofanoff appendicovesicostomy in children: updated interim results. *Eur Urol.* (2015) 68:1069–75. doi: 10.1016/j.eururo.2015.05.047
11. Grimsby GM, Jacobs MA, Gargollo PC. Comparison of complications of robot-assisted laparoscopic and open appendicovesicostomy in children. *J Urol.* (2015) 194:772–6. doi: 10.1016/j.juro.2015.02.2942
12. Gundeti MS, Petravick ME, Pariser JJ, Pearce SM, Anderson BB, Grimsby GM, et al. A multi-institutional study of perioperative and functional outcomes for pediatric robotic-assisted laparoscopic Mitrofanoff appendicovesicostomy. *J Pediatr Urol.* (2016) 12:386.e1–e5. doi: 10.1016/j.jpurol.2016.05.031
13. Subramaniam R, Taylor C. The use of an antegrade continence enema stopper in catheterizable channels virtually eliminates the incidence of stomal stenosis: preliminary experience. *J Urol.* (2009) 181:299–301. doi: 10.1016/j.juro.2008.09.038
14. Cundy TP, Harling L, Hughes-Hallett A, Mayer EK, Najmaldin AS, Athanasiou T, et al. Meta-analysis of robot-assisted vs conventional laparoscopic and open pyeloplasty in children. *BJU Int.* (2014) 114:582–94. doi: 10.1111/bju.12683
15. Spinoit A-F, Radford A, Ashraf J, Gopal M, Subramaniam R. Modified tubularized incised plate urethroplasty in distal hypospadias repair: stepwise technique with validated functional and cosmetic outcome. *J Pediatr Urol.* (2017) 13:86–7. doi: 10.1016/j.jpurol.2016.09.014
16. Silay MS, Spinoit AF, Undre S, Fiala V, Tandogdu Z, Garmanova T, et al. Global minimally invasive pyeloplasty study in children: results from the pediatric urology expert group of the european association of urology young academic urologists working party. *J Pediatr Urol.* (2016) 12:229. e1–7. doi: 10.1016/j.jpurol.2016.04.007
17. Monn MF, Bahler CD, Schneider EB, Whittam BM, Misseri R, Rink RC, et al. Trends in robot-assisted laparoscopic pyeloplasty in pediatric patients. *Urology* (2013) 81:1336–1341. doi: 10.1016/j.urology.2013.01.025
18. Esposito C, Masieri L, Steyaert H, Escolino M, Cerchione R, La Manna A, et al. Robot-assisted extravesical ureteral reimplantation (revur) for unilateral vesico-ureteral reflux in children: results of a multicentric international survey. *World J Urol.* (2018) 36:481–8. doi: 10.1007/s00345-017-2155-9
19. Boysen WR, Akhavan A, Ko J, Ellison JS, Lendvay TS, Huang J, et al. Prospective multicenter study on robot-assisted laparoscopic extravesical ureteral reimplantation (RALUR-EV): outcomes and complications. *J Pediatr Urol.* (2018) 14:262.e1–6. doi: 10.1016/j.jpurol.2018.01.020
20. Marchini GS, Hong YK, Minnillo BJ, Diamond DA, Houck CS, Meier PM, et al. Robotic assisted laparoscopic ureteral reimplantation in children: case matched comparative study with open surgical approach. *J Urol.* (2011) 185:1870–5. doi: 10.1016/j.juro.2010.12.069
21. Pedraza R, Weiser A, Franco I. Laparoscopic appendicovesicostomy (Mitrofanoff procedure) in a child using the da Vinci robotic system. *J Urol.* (2004) 171:1652–3. doi: 10.1097/01.ju.0000116066.72132.9a
22. Wille MA, Jayram G, Gundeti MS. Feasibility and early outcomes of robotic-assisted laparoscopic Mitrofanoff appendicovesicostomy in patients with prune belly syndrome. *BJU Int.* (2012) 109:125–9. doi: 10.1111/j.1464-410X.2011.10317.x
23. Murthy PB, Schadler ED, Orvieto M, Zagaja G, Shalhav AL, Gundeti MS. Setting up a pediatric robotic urology program: a USA institution experience. *Int J Urol.* (2018) 25:86–93. doi: 10.1111/iju.13415
24. Welk BK, Afshar K, Rapoport D, MacNeily AE. Complications of the catheterizable channel following continent urinary diversion: their nature and timing. *J Urol.* (2008) 180(Suppl. 4):1856–60. doi: 10.1016/j.juro.2008.03.093
25. Jacobson DL, Thomas JC, Pope J, Tanaka ST, Clayton DB, Brock JW, et al. Update on continent catheterizable channels and the timing of their complications. *J Urol.* (2017) 197:871–6. doi: 10.1016/j.juro.2016.08.119
26. Szymanski KM, Lopez PJ, Corbetta JP, Reed F, Ruiz J, Pullin Y, et al. Do anterior catheterizable urinary channels have fewer complications than posterior channels? An international cohort study. *J Pediatr Urol.* (2018) 14:48.e1–7. doi: 10.1016/j.jpurol.2017.06.020
27. Bowen DK, Lindgren BW, Cheng EY, Gong EM. Can proctoring affect the learning curve of robotic-assisted laparoscopic pyeloplasty? Experience at a high-volume pediatric robotic surgery center. *J Robot Surg.* (2017) 11:63–7. doi: 10.1007/s11701-016-0613-9

11

Surgical Management of Anterior Glottic Webs

I-Chun Kuo [1,2] *and Michael Rutter* [1*]

[1] *Division of Pediatric Otolaryngology, Aerodigestive and Esophageal Center, Cincinnati Children's Hospital Medical Center, Cincinnati, OH, United States,* [2] *Department of Otolaryngology-Head and Neck Surgery, Chang Gung Memorial Hospital, Taoyuan, Taiwan*

Correspondence:
Michael Rutter
mike.rutter@cchmc.org

Congenital webs are rare and represent <5% of all congenital laryngeal anomalies. They are usually a partial laryngeal atresia rather than a true web, and present as a thick and fibrotic web with subglottic extension and associated subglottic stenosis. All patients with a congenital anterior glottic web should be evaluated for chromosome 22q11.2 deletion syndrome. Management strategies are mainly based on the severity of airway obstruction and the anatomical extension of the webs. Simple division of the web endoscopically may be adequate for rare thin webs, however, an open approach is usually warranted for thick glottic webs regardless of Cohen grades. Open repair can be either with keel placement or reconstruction of the anterior commissure.

Keywords: congenital glottic web, congenital subglottic stenosis, laryngeal keel, laryngeal atresia, anterior commissure

Laryngeal webs are either acquired or congenital. Congenital webs are uncommon and represent fewer than 5% of congenital laryngeal anomalies. Congenital webs result from a disruption of autolysis of the laryngotracheal groove during 10th week of embryogenesis. Congenital webs vary in size and thickness based on the interruption of the embryologic recanalization process. Therefore, most congenital webs are a form of laryngeal atresia rather than a true web, and present as a thick and fibrotic web with subglottic extension resulting a subglottic stenosis with a small cricoid. In lateral xenography of the airway, the appearance is termed a "subglottic sail" (**Figure 1**). Anterior glottic webs are the most common type and comprise more than 95% of cases (1).

While there is no single defined gene that results in congenital glottic webbing, there is a significant association between anterior glottic webs and chromosome 22q11.2 deletion syndrome (velocardiofacial syndrome and DiGeorge syndrome). Approximately 65% of patients presenting with an anterior glottic web will have chromosome 22q11.2 deletion syndrome (2–5), and as the web may be the only early manifestation, it is recommended to refer all patients with congenital anterior glottic webs for genetic assessment.

Children born with congenital webs always have an abnormal or even absent cry at birth, and may present with airway obstruction, according to the thickness and location of webs. In an infant presenting with significant airway compromise in the first few days of life, the web is likely severe, and will require emergent airway intervention. Infants are remarkably tolerant of congenital airway compromise, and even patients with severe glottic webbing may initially show only mild airway symptoms, which then exacerbate over the first few months of life. Airway symptoms of severe webbing including biphasic stridor and retractions, which exacerbate when upset or feeding. In more severe cases, failure to thrive, apnea, and cyanosis are characteristic.

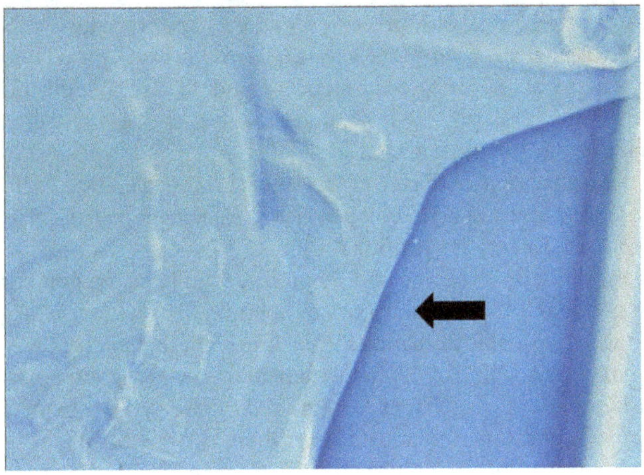

FIGURE 1 | "Subglottic sail" appearance in xenograph.

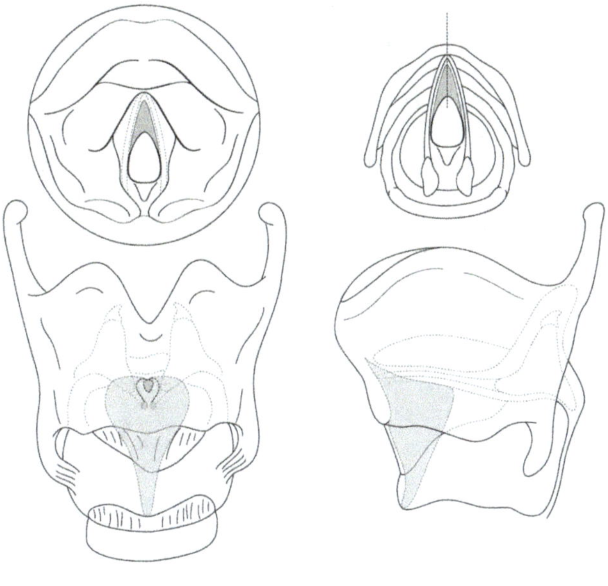

FIGURE 2 | The laryngeal web with subglottic extension appears as a "subglottic sail".

Initial evaluation should include awake flexible laryngoscopy to excludeother pathologies, such as laryngomalacia or vocal cord palsy. For definitive evaluation rigid bronchoscopy is recommended, with both the severity of the web and its subglottic extension being assessed. Flexible bronchoscopy offers an excellent view of the anterior commissure, and is therefore complimentary; whereas rigid bronchoscopy better evaluates the degree of subglottic stenosis, and angled (70°) telescopes may provide superior images of the web. In children with a severe web, bronchoscopy should be performed with care, to avoid further compromising an already compromised airway, and spontaneous ventilation with the infant maintaining his or her own airway is preferable to intubation or emergent tracheotomy (6).

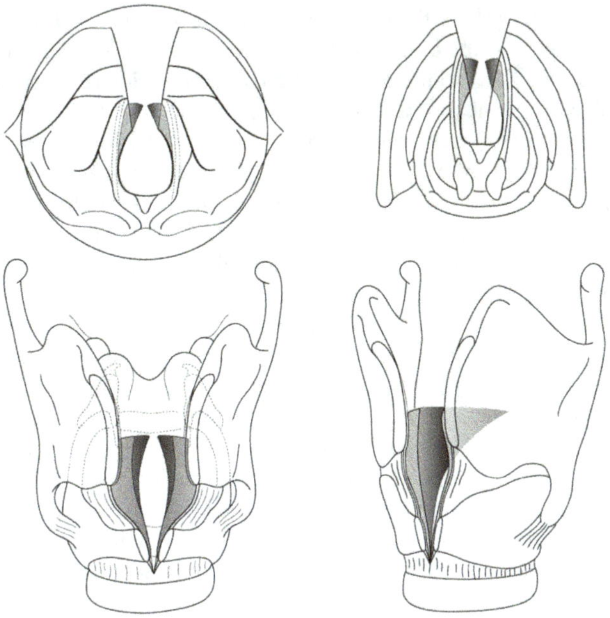

FIGURE 3 | The laryngofissure is down and through the cricoid cartilage.

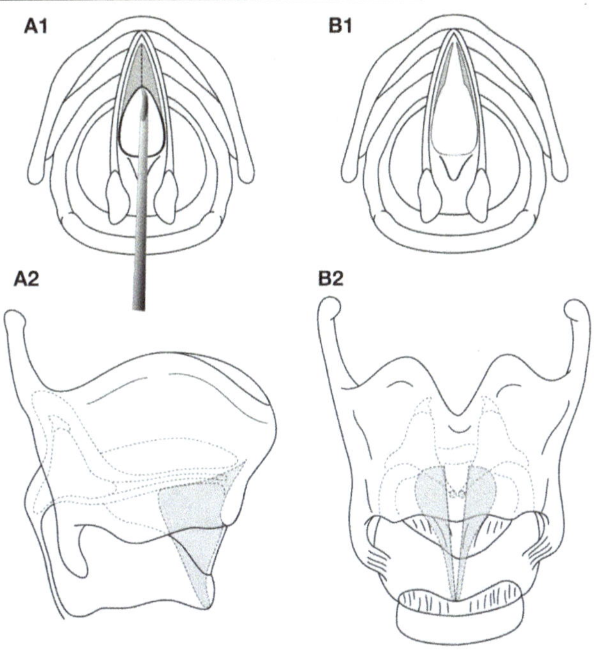

FIGURE 4 | (A1,A2,B1,B2) Endoscopic division of an anterior glottic web.

Management strategies are mainly based on the severity of airway obstruction and the anatomical extension of the webs (7). The anterior glottic webs are classified by the percentage of vocal cord involvement and the presence of subglottic extension which postulated by Cohen (8) in 1985.

According to the Cohen classification, a type 1 glottic web is a thin web with <35% of glottic involvement. Type 2 involves 35~50% of glottis. A type 3 web, has a 50~75% glottic involvement with anterior cricoid cartilage extension resulting in subglottic stenosis (SGS) formation. And a type 4 web involves 75~90% of the glottis with cricoid extension and associated SGS.

Infants with a type 1 web may present no respiratory symptoms but hoarseness whereas type 2 web causes mild airway symptoms and a weak cry. For a rare true gossamer-thin anterior glottic web, it may never be formally diagnosed, as intubation for airway stabilization may lyse the web and completely resolve the problem. In the rare thin type 1 and 2 anterior webs, simple division of the web endoscopically with a cold instrument (ex. sickle knife) is simple and effective, usually with the baby suspended on a small Lindholm laryngoscope. Excision can also be done with CO2 or KTP laser. Topical application of mitomycin-C is aimed to reduce scar formation, but evidence suggests that mitomycin-C may delay instead of preventing restenosis (9). Whereas, for thick glottic webs regardless of Cohen grades, open approach is usually warranted instead of endoscopic methods (10) as these webs have a strong tendency to recur after endoscopic division.

The timing for repair is mainly based on the severity of airway symptoms. For a severely compromised airway, intervention may either be early repair or tracheotomy placement with late repair. For mild or moderate webs without clinical airway compromise, late repair is preferable. A larger larynx makes surgery technically much easier. Late repair is typically performed by age 4 years, to improve voice quality before school age. Repair may be performed as a single- or double-staged procedure, depending on the experience of intensive care facilities and whether a tracheostomy is already present. A double-stage procedure with a suprastomal stent left in for a longer period is usually warranted for more severe subglottic stenosis, and in 22q11.2 deletion syndrome, especially the DiGeorge variant, post-operative edema may be a feature for months.

External approaches can be either reconstruction of the anterior commissure or open keel placement open. Open keel placement is reasonable for a severely scarred web (congenital or acquired) and requires a complete laryngofissure to adequately expose the larynx by splitting the thyroid cartilage under endoscopic guidance for ensuring midline approach. To facilitate meticulous midline placement of the laryngofissure, we recommend partially incising (grooving) the thyroid cartilage between the superior and inferior thyroid notches. When the web involves the subglottis as a "sail" (**Figure 2**) extending to the lower border of the cricoid cartilage, the laryngofissure is carried through the cricoid cartilage (**Figure 3**). To evaluate whether an anterior cartilage graft is required, a segment of age-appropriate endotracheal tube is placed through the split cricoid. If the subglottis cannot close comfortably over the endotracheal tube, a graft is used to repair the associated subglottic stenosis. The graft is inserted at cricoid level with its superior aspect being the upper border of the cricoid cartilage, and an appropriate size laryngeal keel is trimmed and inserted between the upper border of the anterior cricoid graft (if such a graft is present) to the superior thyroid notch. For preventing epiglottic petiole prolapse, the keel should be placed below the petiole insertion.

The infraglottic part of the keel should extend far enough to cover the raw split edges of the web, but should not about the

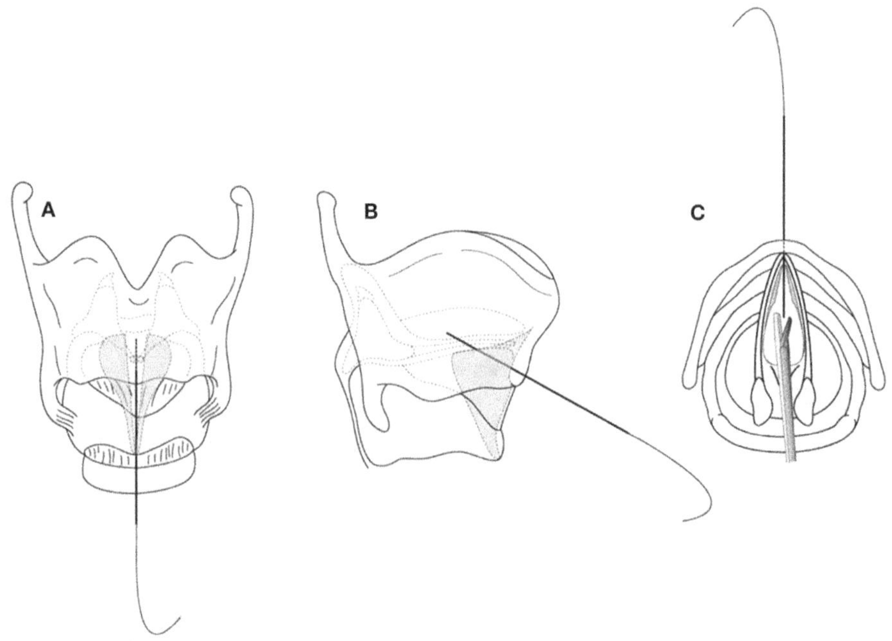

FIGURE 5 | (A–C) The suture to secure the web is passed into the larynx from externally.

mucosa of the posterior glottis. The keel is sutured into place with a complex suture technique. The airway is then closed with either single- or double-stage procedure. The keel is usually removed within 2 weeks, with longer stenting periods used for more severe webs. Another open procedure with laryngofissure is required for stent removal. Laryngofissure closure requires laterally placed mattress sutures.

There is an endoscopic alternative for laryngeal keel placement which is technically more challenging. It is ideal for minor webs whether congenital or acquired. Tracheotomy or intubation may not be necessarily required. This technique involves initially suspending the larynx with a laryngoscope, and endoscopically dividing the web with a sickle knife (**Figure 4**). With the patient still suspended, the neck is then prepped, and a small horizontal incision is made over the thyroid cartilage. A 4.0 Prolene suture on a small straight (Keith) needle is then passed through the midline of the lower thyroid cartilage, below the web, and visualized in the airway. The assistant then grasps the needle with a laparoscopic needle holder, and withdraws the needle from the mouth (**Figure 5**). The surgeon then places a hollow large bore needle through the midline of the upper thyroid cartilage, above the web until it is visualized in the airway. Next, an appropriate laryngeal keel (typically a thin piece of silastic sheet) is used to cover the raw surfaces of the web and passes the straight needle though the inferior and superior borders of the keel in the midline. The small needle is then placed into the lumen of the large bore hollow needle and withdrawn back into the neck incision (**Figure 6**). The suture is secured over a segment of an intravenous cannula, with multiple suture. The keel is removed 7 to 14 days later, with the neck incision being partially reopened to remove the suture securing the keel (6).

An alternative approach is open reconstruction of the anterior commissure, without a keel. Once the laryngofissure is done, if the mucosa at the cut edge overlying the vocal cord is suitably mobile, pexing sutures are used to attach it to the cut edge of the thyroid cartilage, recreating an anterior commissure. 6.0 PDS suture is recommended, on double armed BV-1 needles, with these being placed through the mucosal edge, and then through the thyroid cartilage near the edge of the laryngofissure

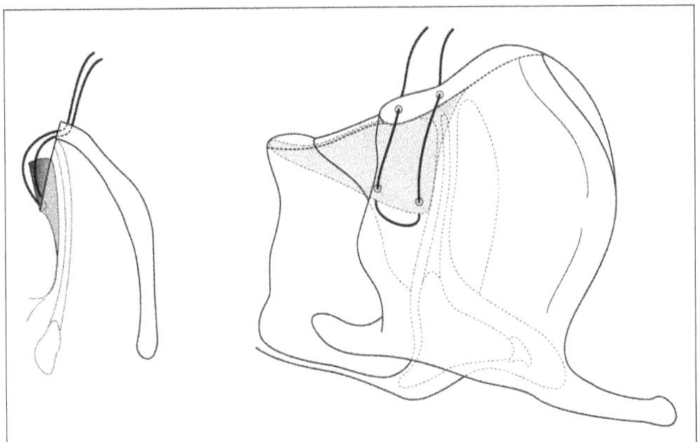

FIGURE 7 | The suture is placed as a mattress fashion.

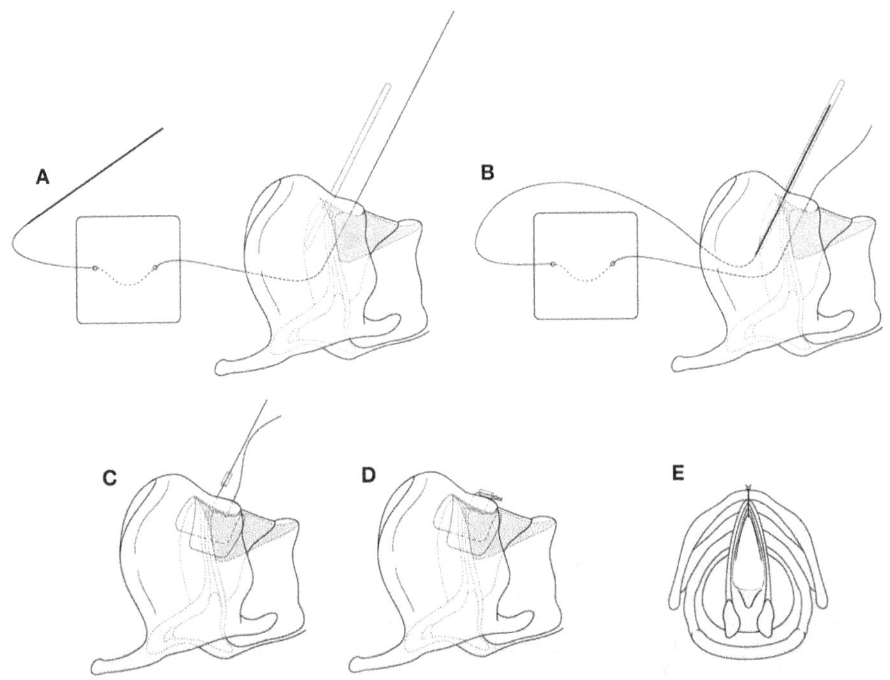

FIGURE 6 | (A–E) The silastic keel is inserted on the securing suture, and the suture is passed through a hollow angiocath to exit the larynx, and tied to secure the keel.

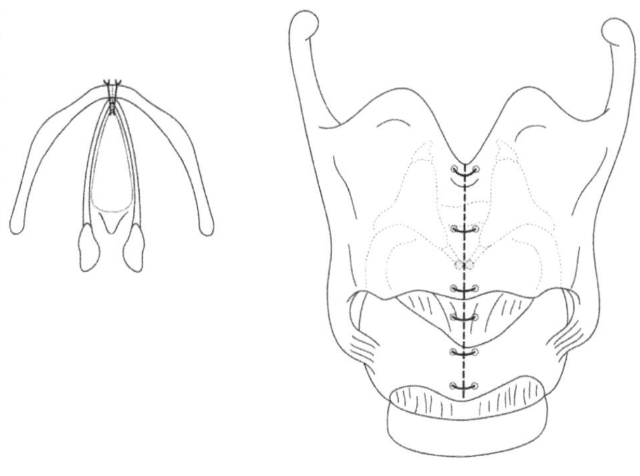

FIGURE 8 | After the pexing sutures are done separately each side, close the larygofissure.

at the level of the vocal ligament (**Figure 7**). This ligament lies at the junction of the lower third and upper two thirds of the laryngofissure in an infant. The suture is secured as a mattress fashion. A second pexing suture is placed below the initial suture to further mucosalize the raw incised edge of the web (**Figure 8**). The same procedure is then performed on the opposite vocal ligament. A segment of age-appropriate endotracheal tube is then placed into airway to determine whether an anterior cartilage graft will be needed for the subglottis. The airway is then closed, with intubation for 2 to 5 days (if this is a single stage procedure). This technique requires mobile vocal mucosa to achieve the mobility to "pex" the vocal cord mucosa back up to the thyroid cartilage, hence it is not suitable as a salvage procedure for a previously injured or operated web with scar formation. The mobile mucosa may provide a better long-term vocal outcome for its potential mucosal wave for vibration.

Options for cartilage grafts include thyroid alar and costal cartilage. Thyroid alar is useful for infants, and may be obtained from a superior lateral thyroid alar margin. Costal cartilage is an alternative choice and usually preferable for severe cases.

Total laryngeal atresia generally results in congenital high airway obstructive syndrome (CHAOS) unless there is a concomitant tracheoesophageal fistula. CHAOS is usually a pre-natal diagnosis on ultrasound and magnetic resonance imaging (11) with fetus presenting hydrops, everted diaphragms, mega-trachea, or prune belly syndrome. If recognized prenatally, ex-utero intrapartum treatment (EXIT) procedure to tracheostomy should be planned. As laryngeal atresia patients do not like to have a laryngeal lumen, and as the cricoid tends to be very small, repair is difficult. Repair is recommended after 4 years of age by cricotracheal resection with a complete laryngofissure. A prolonged postoperative stenting for at least more than 6 months is recommended. More than one procedure is typically necessary to achieve decannulation.

The selection of surgical management is usually surgeon dependent. Etiology of laryngeal web doesn't have impact on the choice of surgical procedure and the treatment outcome, whether it is congenital or iatrogenic (12). Surgeons make their decision based on their experience, and the judgement of the severity and complexity for the webs that they are facing. Some surgeons tend to start with endoscopic approach, and preserve open management as salvage procedures for failure cases. Advocators address the issue as open airway reconstruction is usually invasive and may have surgical and/or donor site morbidity. However, Alkan et al. reported higher re-adhesion/recurrence rate is correlated to higher Cohen Classification (12), for type 3/4 laryngeal webs lacking soft tissue for repair, direct open procedures may offer better surgical outcomes. Also, previous laser procedures tend to result in a complicated airway and have negative influence on following open surgical outcomes and more revisions (13).

For the past decades, both endoscopic and open procedures fail to provide promising results. The latest published case series, reported as high as 76 and 89% of recurrence rate for endoscopic and open approach, respectively (14). It once again emphasized the clinical and surgical challenging of laryngeal webs.

In summary, most congenital laryngeal webs are thick, thus open repair is warranted for an optimal outcome. It is recommended that all patients with congenital webs to be tested for 22q11.2 deletion syndrome. Scarred webs, whether congenital or acquired, are better managed with a keel placement, either open or endoscopic. Recreation of an anterior commissure with mobile mucosa of laryngeal webs by open reconstruction may provide a better voice quality even for severe congenital webs.

AUTHOR CONTRIBUTIONS

All authors listed have made a substantial, direct and intellectual contribution to the work, and approved it for publication.

REFERENCES

1. Izadi F, Delarestaghi MM, Memari F, Mohseni R, Pousti B, Mir P. The butterfly procedure: a new technique and review of the literature for treating anterior laryngeal webs. *J Voice.* (2010) 24:742–9. doi: 10.1016/j.jvoice.2009.03.005
2. Fokstuen S, Bottani A, Medeiros PF, Antonarakis SE, Stoll C, Schinzel A. Laryngeal atresia type III (glottic web) with 22q11.2 microdeletion: report of three patients. *Am J Med Genet.* (1997) 70:130–3. doi: 10.1002/(SICI)1096-8628(19970516)70:2<130::AID-AJMG5>3.0.CO;2-1
3. McElhinney DB, Jacobs I, McDonald-McGinn DM, Zackai EH, Goldmuntz E. Chromosomal and cardiovascular anomalies associated with congenital laryngeal web. *Int J Pediatr Otorhinolaryngol.* (2002) 66:23–7. doi: 10.1016/S0165-5876(02)00184-2
4. Miyamoto RC, Cotton RT, Rope AF, Hopkin RJ, Cohen AP, Shott SR, et al. Association of anterior glottic webs with velocardiofacial syndrome (chromosome 22q11.2 deletion). *Otolaryngol Head Neck Surg.* (2004) 130:415–7. doi: 10.1016/j.otohns.2003.12.014

5. Sacca R, Zur KB, Crowley TB, Zackai EH, Valverde KD, McDonald-McGinn DM. Association of airway abnormalities with 22q11.2 deletion syndrome. *Int J Pediatr Otorhinolaryngol.* (2017) 96:11–4. doi: 10.1016/j.ijporl.2017.02.012
6. Scadding G, Bull P, Graham J. *Laryngeal Webs Subglottic Hemangiomas.* Pediatric ENT. Berlin, Heidelberg: Springer (2007).
7. Goudy S, Bauman N, Manaligod J, Smith RJ. Congenital laryngeal webs: surgical course and outcomes. *Ann Otol Rhinol Laryngol.* (2010) 119:704–6. doi: 10.1177/000348941011901010
8. Cohen SR. Congenital glottic webs in children. A retrospective review of 51 patients. *Ann Otol Rhinol Laryngol Suppl.* (1985) 121:2–16. doi: 10.1177/00034894850940S601
9. Smith ME, Elstad M. Mitomycin C and the endoscopic treatment of laryngotracheal stenosis: are two applications better than one?. *Laryngoscope.* (2009) 119:272–83. doi: 10.1002/lary.20056
10. Chen J, Shi F, Chen M, Yang Y, Cheng L, Wu H. Web thickness determines the therapeutic effect of endoscopic keel placement on anterior glottic web. *Eur Arch Otorhinolaryngol.* (2017) 274:3697–702. doi: 10.1007/s00405-017-4689-2
11. Ryan G, Somme S, Crombleholme TM. Airway compromise in the fetus and neonate: prenatal assessment and perinatal management. *Semin Fetal Neonatal Med.* (2016) 21:230–9. doi: 10.1016/j.siny.2016.03.002
12. Alkan U, Nachalon Y, Vaisbuch Y, Katz O, Hamzany Y, Stern Y. Treating paediatric anterior glottic web: single-centre experience of 20 patients with comparison among techniques. *Clin Otolaryngol.* (2017) 42:893–7. doi: 10.1111/coa.12749
13. de Trey LA, Lambercy K, Monnier P, Sandu K. Management of severe congenital laryngeal webs - a 12 year review. *Int J Pediatr Otorhinolaryngol.* (2016) 86:82–6. doi: 10.1016/j.ijporl.2016.04.006
14. Lawlor CM, Dombrowski ND, Nuss RC, Rahbar R, Choi SS. Laryngeal Web in the Pediatric Population: Evaluation and Management. *Otolaryngol Head Neck Surg.* (2020) 162:234–40. doi: 10.1177/0194599819893985

12

The Role of Video-Assisted Thoracoscopic Surgery in Pediatric Oncology

Giovanna Riccipetitoni, Mirko Bertozzi, Marta Gazzaneo, Alessandro Raffaele and Fabrizio Vatta*

Department of Pediatric Surgery, Fondazione Istituti di Ricovero e Cura a Carattere Scientifico (IRCCS) Policlinico San Matteo, University of Pavia, Pavia, Italy

***Correspondence:**
Giovanna Riccipetitoni
g.riccipetitoni@gmail.com;
giovanna.riccipetitoni@unipv.it

Aim: Video-assisted thoracoscopic surgery (VATS) has been widely used in the last decades. Nevertheless, the pros and cons of thoracoscopy vs. open surgery in pediatric oncology are still under debate. In literature, VATS has been applied for both diagnostic and ablative surgery to treat neurogenic tumors, thymic neoplasms, lung tumors and metastases, germ cell tumors, lymphoproliferative diseases, and other rare tumors. Recent reviews described excellent outcomes in pediatric oncology as well as in the treatment of adult lung cancer, with a significantly higher rate of mortality and complication in thoracotomy compared to VATS. We reviewed our experience on thoracoscopy in pediatric malignancy and compared it to the literature.

Materials and Methods: This was a retrospective cohort-study of pediatric oncological patients who underwent VATS at our institution from 2007 to 2020, and a review of the recent literature on the topic.

Results: A total of 43 procedures were performed on 38 oncological patients (18 males, 20 females). Median age was years 7.72 (0.35–18.6). Diagnosis: 10 neurogenic tumors, nine hematological diseases, five metastases, four lypoblastomas, three thymic pathologies, three germ cell tumors, two pleuropneumoblastomas, two myofibroblastic tumors, one myoepithelial carcinoma, one liposarcoma, and three suspected oncological mass. In three cases, a 3D model was elaborated to better plan the surgical approach. Diagnostic biopsies were 22 (51.1%), and ablative surgeries, 21 (48.9%). One neurogenic tumor was resected with the Da Vinci Robot. Median operative time was 120 min (30–420). A drain was left in place in 20 (46.5%) for a median of 4 days. Median length of hospitalization was 5 days (1–18). One case (2.3%) was converted (intraoperative bleeding). There were three post-operative complications (7.0%): one pneumonia, one pleural effusion, and one diaphragmatic paralysis (need for plication). Results were compared to recent literature, and morbidity and conversion rate were comparable to reviewed publications.

Conclusion: VATS represents a valuable tool for diagnostic and therapeutic procedures in pediatric oncology. Nonetheless, it is a challenging technique that should be performed by expert surgeons on oncological and mini-invasive surgery. Three-dimensional reconstruction can optimize the pre-operative planning and guarantee a safer and more targeted treatment. Finally, the advent of robotics-assisted surgery represents a new challenge that may further implement the advantages of VATS.

Keywords: thoracoscopy, pediatrics, oncology, mini-invasive surgery, robotic-assisted thoracoscopic surgery

INTRODUCTION

Minimally invasive surgery (MIS), including thoracoscopy, has been widely applied in the last few decades and has now become the gold standard approach for a variety of procedures for both adults and children (1–3).

The advantages of MIS compared to the open approach are well-known, as it reduces tissue trauma, decreases post-operative pain, shortens hospital stay, and guarantees better cosmetic and long-term functional results (4, 5). Moreover, among of the most important benefits of thoracoscopy are the virtually non-existing musculoskeletal complications such as chest wall deformities, rib fusion, shoulder girdle weakness, and scoliosis, which can occur in up of 30% of pediatric patients undergoing thoracotomy (6, 7).

Nevertheless, video-assisted thoracoscopic surgery (VATS) still represents a challenge due to the limitation of working space, the smaller body size of children, reduced tactile feedback, and the lack of three-dimensional vision.

As far as it concerns pediatric oncology, in the last decades, many reports and experiences have been published on the use of thoracoscopy to diagnose and resect intrathoracic neoplasms. Nonetheless, the role of VATS is still considered a developing field and no consensus exists regarding the details of its application. Specific limitations are an even lower exposure in pediatric oncological cases compared to general thoracoscopic pathologies and the inability to perform digital palpation.

In the last years, robotics has been applied to perform a wide variety of procedures, including thoracic surgery (8). Nonetheless, very few reports describe the use of robotics in pediatric oncological thoracic surgery and its use is not yet validated.

The aim of this study is to review our experience in VATS and robotics-assisted thoracoscopy in pediatric malignancy and to compare it to the most recent literature.

MATERIALS AND METHODS

We performed a retrospective review of all pediatric oncological patients who underwent video-assisted thoracoscopic surgery (VATS) and robotics-assisted thoracoscopic surgery (RATS) at our Institution from 2007 to 2020.

Patients over 20 years old and/or with thoracic pathologies treated with thoracotomy or endoscopic procedures were excluded.

We analyzed demographic data, including age at surgery, sex, pathology, and possible comorbidities; operation time (OT); length of hospital stays (LHS); perioperative complications; and post-operative outcomes. All complications were classified according to the Clavien–Dindo classification and graded from I to V. If present, length of chest drain aspiration was evaluated.

A specific search was performed in scientific database (PUBMED, MEDLINE, and EMBASE) to compare our experience with the most recent literature on the field. We selected articles reporting thoracoscopy in oncological pediatric patients between 2014 and March 2021 using the following key-words: (pediatric) or (children) and (thoracoscopy) or (VATS) and (oncology) or (tumor).

Inclusion criteria were:

- Articles published between January 2014 and March 2021
- Articles written in English
- Articles focusing on VATS in pediatric oncology
- Median/mean age <18 years old
- Case series with more than 10 patients
- Articles where data concerning demographics, surgical indications, complication rate, and conversion rate were clearly deductible

All data were elaborated using the statistical software "R", version 3.4.1.

Descriptive statistics was used to present findings, and quantitative variables were expressed as median (range) to express our data. Data elaborated from the literature review were expressed as median (range) or mean ± standard deviations depending on the reference found in the original articles.

Surgical Methods

Under general anesthesia, lung collapse has been achieved by single-lung ventilation. We routinely used a double lumen endotracheal tube in adolescent patients, mainly for ablative procedures. In small children (more than 6 months of age), we adopted a standard endotracheal intubation associated to the use of an endobronchial blocker. Low-pressure CO_2 insufflation (4–5 mmHg; flow 0.5 L/min) was employed in infants <6 months or when a quick biopsy of anterior mediastinal tumors was required. NIRS and BIS brain-monitoring were applied according to the age of the patients.

Patients were placed in lateral decubitus, with an angle ranging from 60 and 90° to 120°, depending on the mass localization.

A 10-mm one-trocar operative optic was employed for biopsy in three cases (one germ cell tumor, one pleuropneumoblastoma, and one myofibroblastic inflammatory tumor).

A three-trocar technique was adopted in most of the remaining cases, positioned according to the characteristics of the lesion. The optic (5 or 10 mm) was placed in the typical mid-axillary position under the shoulder angle, whereas the operative trocars were placed in a triangulation fashion anteriorly or posteriorly depending on the site of the mass.

In small children, a 3-mm operative trocar technique with 5-mm optic was carried out to perform biopsies, whereas in ablative surgery, one 5-mm operative trocar was reserved for Ligasure® or other vessel sealers. In recent cases, a 3-mm vessel sealer has been used, allowing a 3-mm operative VATS also for ablative procedures.

Pulmonary resection was safely performed with staplers (5 or 12 mm), which required an additional trocar. Specimens were retrieved using a 5 mm Endobag.

Regarding the use of chest drain, we tried to avoid drainage placement in diagnostic biopsies, except in case of complications such as intraoperative bleeding. A drain was normally applied at the end of any ablative surgery.

When possible, an early extubation of the patients was made a few hours after the VATS procedure.

About RATS, we performed one procedure using the Da-Vinci SI® Robot for a mass located on the supero-posterior mediastinum. Optic trocar was positioned in the sixth intercostal space on the midaxillary line. Operative trocars were positioned 8 cm away from the optic, in the fifth intercostal space on the anterior axillary line, and in the seventh intercostal space on the paravertebral line, respectively. Finally, a 5-mm auxiliary trocar was placed in the fourth intercostal space on the anterior axillary line.

RESULTS

A total of 43 procedures were performed on 38 oncological patients (18 males, 20 females). Median age was 7.72 (0.35–18.6). Patients were grouped according to diagnosis, and we observed high prevalence of neurogenic tumors and hematologic diseases, as shown in **Table 1**.

We performed diagnostic biopsies in 22 cases (51.1%), compared to 21 cases of ablative surgeries (48.9%); 42 out of 43 procedures were completed by VATS technique (97.7%); only one patient required an open conversion (2.3%).

The procedures were carried out by single-lung ventilation using a double-lumen endotracheal tube in 14 adolescent patients, and standard endotracheal intubation associated to the use of an endobronchial blocker was adopted in 16 cases. In the remaining 13 cases, lung collapse was obtained with low-pressure CO_2 insufflation.

One patient with growing ganglioneuroblastoma intermixed of the supero-posterior mediastinum in a 7-years-old girl with Horner's syndrome and positive image-defined risk factor (IDRF) (symptomatic encased subclavian vessels) was operated with the Da-Vinci SI® Robot-assisted thoracoscopic surgery. The robotic approach was chosen to achieve a safer and more precise dissection.

In the whole series, median OT was 120 min (30–420): 90 for diagnostic biopsies, 190 for ablative surgery.

Overall, a thoracic drain was left in place in 20 cases, for a median length of 4 days.

Only three diagnostic procedures required chest drainage due to intraoperative bleeding (one germ cell tumor), pneumothorax (one pleuropneumoblastoma), and pleural effusion (one myofibroblastic inflammatory tumor). As for ablative surgeries, a chest tube was positioned in 17 out of 21 procedures.

Median LHS was 5 days (1–18).

In two cases, we observed intraoperative bleeding (4.7%): one biopsy of a germ cell tumor managed thoracoscopically and one lung resection for nephroblastoma metastasis which required conversion to open surgery. The conversion rate to open surgery was 2.3% in the whole series.

In our series, we observed three post-operative complications (7.0%): one pneumonia (Clavien Dindo: grade II) 2 weeks after biopsy for a germ cell tumor; one pleural effusion a week after resection of a posterior mediastinal ganglioneuroma, which required a re-insertion of a thoracic drain for a further 7 days (IIIb); and one persistent right diaphragmatic paralysis after the excision of a giant cystic lymphangioma, treated with a laparoscopic diaphragmatic plication (IVa) 1 year later, which required intensive care assistance.

No tumor upstaging or trocar site recurrences occurred.

An advanced 3D virtual reconstruction and printing technology was recently applied in three complex cases (multiple immature teratoma metastases, multiple cystic lesions after pleuro-pneumoblastoma excision, vessel encasement in IDRF-positive ganglioneuroblastoma intermixed).

A review of the most recent literature on the topic was performed. From a total of 229 articles, seven were included in the review according to the inclusion criteria (**Table 2**) (9–15).

All papers were retrospective reviews and analyzed VATS to perform either tumor biopsy, ablative surgery, or both. A total of 423 children were included in the review, with a median age of 8.8 years. Among pulmonary lesions, metastases resulted as the most common indication for surgery. On the other hand, in case of a mediastinal lesion, neurogenic tumor was the most represented group. Conversion rate ranged from 0 to 15.1%, most commonly due to intraoperative bleeding or difficult dissection of the mass due to strong adhesions. Complications occurred in 2.1–20% of cases, pneumothorax being the most common post-operative one. No articles reported port-site recurrences, intraoperative tumor rupture, or tumor upstaging. Average LHS ranged from 2 to 10 days.

DISCUSSION

VATS in pediatric oncological surgery represents a great surgical achievement but still faces many challenges. Alongside the limitations of the technique, there are no guidelines on the details of the use of VATS or its contraindications. However, its application is expanding, and the experience reported in literature is growing.

Our study presents a large cohort of oncological patients undergoing VATS and proves the feasibility and effectiveness of the use of MIS in pediatric oncology; 97.7% of cases in our series were successfully treated by thoracoscopy.

As far as it concerns the use of VATS for diagnostic procedures, MIS has been effectively used to perform mediastinal mass biopsies as well as pulmonary masses (10, 13, 16–18). Reported advantages of thoracoscopy are the possibility

TABLE 1 | Summarized data of all oncological patients undergoing VATS (in chronological order).

ID*	Sex	Year	Age (y)	Pre-op Imaging	Diagnosis	Localization	Side	Intervention	Operative Time (min)	Peri-op compli-cations	Conversion	Drain (days)	LHS (days)	Post-op complications	Type of complication (Clavien Dindo Classification)
JM	M	2007	14.00	TC	Germ cell tumor	Complete invasion of all hemithorax	R	Biopsy (1 trocar)	30	No	No	No	2	No	
VG	M	2007	14.00	TC	T-cell lymphoma	Anterior mediastinum	L	Biopsy	60	No	No	No	3	No	
BL	F	2008	3.00	TC	Germ cell tumor	Complete invasion of all hemithorax	L	Biopsy	90	Yes (bleeding)	No	Yes (4)	7	No	
GD	M	2009	1.00	TC	Pleuropulmonary blastoma	Superior and medium lobe	R	Biopsy (1 trocar)	60	No	No	Yes (3)	4	No	
AL	F	2010	8.07	TC	Suspicion of renal carcinoma metastasis (not confirmed at histology)	Inferior lobe	L	Biopsy	105	No	No	No	14	No	
BA	M	2010	3.94	TC	Nephroblastoma metastasis	Inferior lobe	L	Mass excision (atypical pulmonary excision)	155	No	No	No	2	No	
ML (1)	M	2010	18.16	TC	Casteman's disease	Anterior mediastinum	R	Biopsy	75	No	No	No	1	No	
PC	F	2010	4.79	TC	Ganglioneuroma metastasis	Costophrenic recess	L	Mass excision	180	No	No	No	3	No	
ML (2)	M	2011	18,65	TC	Casteman's disease	Anterior mediastinum	R	Mass excision	330	No	No	No	2	No	
CA	F	2012	0.50	TC MRI	Neuroblastoma	Superior mediastinum	L	Biopsy	90	No	No	No	3	No	
CS	F	2010	14.11	TC	Diffuse large B-cell lymphoma	Antero-Superior mediastinum	R	Biopsy	80	No	No	No	–**	No	
HL	M	2012	16.53	TC	Neuroblastoma	Posterior mediastinum	R	Biopsy	60	No	No	No	3	No	
DM	M	2012	11.04	TC	Precursor T-cell lymphoblastic lymphoma	Retrosternal region	R	Biopsy	150	No	No	No	–**	No	
PG	M	2012	0.35	TC	Cystic lymphangioma	Superior mediastinum	R	Mass excision	165	No	No	Yes (4)	2	Yes	Diaphragmatic paralysis, need for laparoscopic diaphragmatic plication (IVa) 1 year later
BL	M	2014	6.00	TC	Classical Hodgkin's lymphoma	Anterior mediastinum	R	Biopsy	70	No	No	No	3	No	

(Continued)

TABLE 1 | Continued

ID*	Sex	Year	Age (y)	Pre-op Imaging	Diagnosis	Localization	Side	Intervention	Operative Time (min)	Peri-op compli-cations	Conversion	Drain (days)	LHS (days)	Post-op complications	Type of complication (Clavien Dindo Classification)
BR	F	2014	10.00	MRI	Ganglioneuroblastoma	Posterior mediastinum	L	Mass excision	120	No	No	Yes (3)	5	No	
SR	F	2019	1.25	MRI	Lipoblastoma (recidive)	Lateral chest wall, medullar invasion	R	Mass excision	240	No	No	Yes (7)	–**	No	
FE (1)	F	2014	1.19	TC	Neuroblastoma	Antero-Superior mediastinum	R	Biopsy	180	No	No	No	5	No	
FE (2)	F	2014	1.84	TC MRI	Neuroblastoma	Antero-superior mediastinum	R	Biopsy	90	No	No	No	2	No	
GD	M	2014	13.61	TC	Osteosarcoma metastasis	Inferior lobe	L	Mass excision	90	No	No	No	2	No	
PI	F	2014	10.00	TC MRI	Ganglioneuroblastoma	Posterior mediastinum	L	Mass excision	120	No	No	Yes (3)	18	Yes	Pleural effusion after drain removal, need for thoracic drain re-insertion for 7 days (IIIb)
RG	F	2014	11.96	TC MRI	Myofibroblastic inflammatory tumor	Pulmonary hilum	R	Biopsy	250	No	No	Yes (4)	7	No	
VA	M	2014	16.13	TC	Germ cell tumor	Costophrenic recess	R	Biopsy	115	No	No	No	11	Yes	Post-op pneumonia (II)
AA (1)	F	2015	7.67	TC	Suspicion of neoplastic mass (not confirmed at histology)	Middle mediastinum	R	Biopsy	95	No	No	No	5	No	
AA (2)	F	2015	7.72	TC	Suspicion of neoplastic mass (not confirmed at histology)	Middle mediastinum	R	Biopsy	105	No	No	No	2	No	
AA (3)	F	2015	8.18	TC	Suspicion of neoplastic mass (not confirmed at histology)	Middle mediastinum	R	Biopsy + Culture test	110	No	No	No	3	No	
LAn	M	2015	15.77	TC	Classical Hodgkin's lymphoma	Costophrenic recess	L	Biopsy	160	No	No	No	2	No	
PB	M	2015	5.44	TC	Nephroblastoma metastasis	Superior lobe	R	Mass excision (atypical pulmonary excision)	350	Yes (bleeding)	Yes	Yes (4)	7	No	
RA	F	2015	10.00	MRI	Thymic teratoma	Anterior mediastinum	L	Mass excision (thymectomy)	200	No	No	Yes (5)	7	No	
ZS	M	2015	7.00	MRI	Thymic teratoma	Anterior mediastinum	R	Mass excision (thymectomy)	195	No	No	Yes (4)	6	No	
TM	F	2016	11.00	MRI	Thymoma	Anterior mediastinum	R	Mass excision (thymectomy)	220	No	No	Yes (5)	7	No	

(Continued)

TABLE 1 | Continued

ID*	Sex	Year	Age (y)	Pre-op Imaging	Diagnosis	Localization	Side	Intervention	Operative Time (min)	Peri-op compli-cations	Conversion	Drain (days)	LHS (days)	Post-op complications	Type of complication (Clavien Dindo Classification)
TL	F	2017	16.47	TC MRI	Pleomorphic liposarcoma	Costophrenic recess	R	Biopsy	110	No	No	No	3	No	
BB	F	2018	7.00	TC MRI	Neuroblastoma	Posterior mediastinum	L	Mass excision	190	No	No	Yes (3)	5	No	
BF	M	2018	12.00	MRI	Lipoblastoma	Lateral chest wall	R	Mass excision	180	No	No	Yes (5)	7	No	
EZ	F	2018	6.00	TC MRI	Myofibroblastic inflammatory tumor	Superior and medium lobe, trachea and heart invasion	R	Biopsy (1 trocar)	60	No	No	No	3	No	
LAr	M	2018	2.00	TC MRI	Neuroblastoma	Posterior mediastinum	L	Mass excision	119	No	No	Yes (4)	6	No	
LM	M	2018	7.00	TC MRI	Cystic lesions after pleuropulmonary blastoma excision	Superior, medium, and inferior lobe (3 different lesions)	R	Masses excision (atypical pulmonary excision)	190	No	No	Yes (2)	7	No	
LN	F	2018	7.00	TC MRI	Myoepithelial carcinoma	Superior and inferior lobe, heart invasion	L	Biopsy (with associated bronchoscopic biopsy)	80	No	No	No	7	No	
BG	F	2019	5.00	MRI	Lipoblastoma	Posterior mediastinum	L	Mass excision	150	No	No	Yes (4)	6	No	
BM	F	2020	13.28	TC MRI	Lipoblastoma	Superior mediastinum	R	Mass excision	305	No	No	Yes (7)	6	No	
FE (3)	F	2020	7.59	MRI	Ganglioneuroblastoma intermixed	Anterior mediastinum	R	Robot-Assisted mass excision	290	No	No	Yes (6)	7	No	
PD	M	2020	14.80	TC	Classical Hodgkin's lymphoma	Anterior mediastinum	R	Mass excision (thymectomy)	285	No	No	Yes (3)	5	No	
SL	F	2020	7.00	TC MRI	Immature teratoma metastases	Superior, medium and inferior lobe (6 different lesions)	R	Mass excision (multiple lesions)	420	No	No	Yes (7)	8	No	

**If in the same patient, a different number of procedures is specified within brackets.*

***LHS was not considered as they started further therapy during the same hospitalization.*

TABLE 2 | Review of the most recent literature.

References	Year	Study	Number	Indication*	Median age (y)	Types tumor*	LHS (days)	Conversion	Complications**	Port-Site metastases	Intraoperative rupture
Lautz et al. (9)	2021	Retrospective	48	AS	13.9 ± 4.5	Metastatic osteosarcoma	2	0%	2.1% SSI; 2.1%; DVT or PE 6.3%	0	0
Abdelhafeez et al. (10)	2019	Retrospective	179	B (81.6%) AS (18.5%)	NA	B: 113 Pulmonary lesions, 30 Mediastinal tumors, 3 Pleural lesions; AS: 21 Pulmonary metastases, 7 Neurogenic tumors, Other: 5	NA	15.1%	7.8% (B: 10 PNX, AS: 3 PNX, 2 bleeding, 1 SSI, 1 other)	0	0
Da et al. (12)	2019	Retrospective	43	AS	3.7 ± 2.9	13 Neurogenic tumors, 5 Cystic Teratoma, 4 Lymphangioma, Other: 21	10.0 ± 5.5	0%	4.7% (not precisely specified)	0	0
McDaniel et al. (15)	2018	Retrospective	35	AS	11.25 (0.67–23.50)	6 Osteosarcoma, 5 Ewing sarcoma, 5 Hepatoblastoma, 3 Rhabdomyosarcoma, 3 Synovial cell Sarcoma, Other: 13	NA	0%	17.0% (6 PNX)	0	0
Acker et al. (13)	2015	Retrospective	77	B (72.3%) AS (27.7%)	10.7 ± 6.3	B: Lymphoma 21, Metastases 29, Other: 6 AS: Neuroblastoma 11, Metastatic disease 9, schwannoma 1	5.9 (±8.1)	5.2%	11.0% (not precisely specified)	0	0
Sato et al. (11)	2016	Retrospective	21	AS	6.9 ± 4.6	11 Neurogenic tumors, 6 Germ Cell Tumors, Other: 4	8.0 ± 3.7	0%	20% (1 brachial plexus palsy, 1 Horner's syndrome, 1 atelectasis, 1 palsy of upper limb)	0	0
Irtan et al. (14)	2015	Retrospective	20	AS	3.3 (0.3–11.6)	Neuroblastic tumors	5.2 (2–10)	15%	20.0% (3 Chlyothorax, 1 Horner's syndrome)	0	0
Riccipetitoni et al. (2021)	2021	R	43	B (51.1%) AS (48.9%)	7.72 (0.35–18.6).	10 Neurogenic tumors, 9 Hematological diseases, 5 Metastases, 4 Lypoblastomas, 3 thymic pathologies, 3 germ-cell tumors, Other: 9 (see **Table 1**)	5 (1–18)	2.3%	7.0% (see **Table 1**)	0	0

**B, biopsy; AS, ablative surgery.*

***SSI, surgical site infection; DVT, deep venous thrombosis; PE, pulmonary embolism; PNX, pneumothorax.*

of exploring the entire surface of the lung and pleura, and performing multiple biopsies if required (e.g., germinal tumors). Morbidity, mortality, and length of hospitalization are lower when compared to open surgery (19). Success rate of thoracoscopic-assisted biopsies have been reported in literature ranging from 96.7 to 100% for both histological and/or bacteriological diagnosis (12, 19–28). Nonetheless, different techniques have been proposed to further enhance the accuracy of MIS, such as intraoperative ultrasound localization (both trans-pleural and endoscopic) (29), CT-guided needle localization with methylene blue staining, or micro-coil application (15, 30, 31).

Our experience confirms the feasibility of VATS for diagnostic procedures. Among our cases, we performed three one-trocar site procedures, without complications. Nevertheless, indication for this technique in pediatrics is limited to procedures with low risk of bleeding.

Thoracoscopic surgery has been largely applied to excise mediastinal malignancies, and its use has been extended in pediatrics as well. Although in our cohort we did not record conversion to open surgery, in the most recent literature, conversion rate has been reported in up to 15% of cases (10–14) (**Figure 1**).

When performing mediastinal mass excisions ($n = 14$), we positioned a chest drain in 85.7% of patients. Nonetheless, its use is not mandatory, and in literature, chest drainage is not performed in up to 35% of procedures (29–31). A recent review of 2021 by Yu-Wei Liu reported how eliminating chest drain placement after mediastinal tumor resection can decrease post-operative pain and hospital stay without increasing complications or compromising patient safety (32).

In pediatrics, the most common mediastinal neoplasms are neurogenic tumors (neuroblastoma, ganglioneuroblastoma, and ganglioneuroma). Surgical approach has been evolving, and their resection is now often performed thoracoscopically, guaranteeing the well-known advantages of MIS (30). Different studies have found similar oncological outcomes and comparable rates of complication between the MIS and open approaches (30, 31, 33). Nonetheless, at least one port-site dissemination has been described (34). To date, VATS for neurogenic tumors does not yet have specific guidelines, although there are no contraindications. Nonetheless, literature still reports the frequent use of open approach in case of a large mediastinal tumor (35). In our series, seven patients with neurogenic tumor underwent a total of 10 procedures (four biopsies and six mass excisions). Among the excision group, five patients were submitted to a thoracoscopic surgery and one patient to a robotics-assisted procedure. All children presented IDRF-negative tumors except the case treated by RATS.

Pre-operative diagnostic workup and identification of IDRFs obtained by computed tomography (CT) and/or magnetic resonance are essential to precisely localize the lesion and identify the extent of the disease. A recent systematic review conducted by the APSA Cancer Committee confirmed how a pre-operative objective assessment by IDRFs and size criteria are recommended to guide the approach, in order to follow oncologic principles of surgical resection of neuroblastic tumors with the least possible morbidity (36).

In recent years, 3D virtual reconstruction and printing technologies have been increasingly applied to further implement the possibility of a more precise surgical planning (37, 38). These technologies enable surgeons to simulate beforehand the surgical procedure, potentially reducing the risk of intraoperative complications and allowing a conservative surgery when indicated (39–41) (**Figures 2** and **3**). In our experience, these techniques were chosen in complex cases with multiple lesions and vessel encasement and allowed the formulation of a personalized surgical strategy.

VATS is largely used to perform segmentectomies and lobectomies for pulmonary lesions in oncological adult patients. A recent meta-analysis reviewed 34 studies (183,426 patients), comparing open-approach, VATS, and robotics-assisted surgery. Their results showed how MIS seemed safer compared to open surgery, with reduced 30-day mortality, pulmonary complications, and overall complications with equivalent oncologic outcomes and 5-year overall survival (42). Nevertheless, use of VATS in pediatric lung tumors is not yet validated, and only small case-series can be found.

As far as it concerns metastatic disease, osteosarcoma represents one of the most relevant causes of metastases in children. Surgical management of osteosarcoma is still strongly debated, knowing that the most important prognostic indicator for this disease is the complete resection of all lesions (43). One of the main disadvantages of VATS is the impossibility to perform digital palpation to detect possible lesions not identified at imaging. Compared to other neoplasia, the higher calcification of osteosarcoma metastases allows for manual palpation at sizes below the resolution of CT. Nonetheless, many centers have started using thoracoscopy for osteosarcoma metastases due to the acknowledged advantages of MIS compared to open thoracotomy. A recent collaborative study on 202 patients showed that, in patients with limited metastases, both mortality and risk of pulmonary recurrence were similar when comparing VATS and thoracotomy (44). The risk of possible port-site metastases should not be neglected, as it has already been reported in the case of an 18-year-old female who presented with port site metastases within 4 months of pulmonary metastasectomy for osteosarcoma (45).

In the last decades, robotics-assisted surgery (RAS) has been increasingly employed in several complex procedures, and its use is now standardized for many interventions. The known advantages are the 3D vision, seven degrees of freedom, tremor filtration, and precise camera control (46). In pediatrics, its usage has more limitations due to the mismatch between the robotic arms and trocar dimensions compared to small children, the absence of haptic feedback, and the potential risk of tumor rupture and spillage. No guidelines or recommendations have yet been proposed from the main association of pediatric surgery in this field (47). Despite this, RAS is starting to be implemented in this field as well. In a recent review of 2020 (48), a total of 13 thoracic oncological neoplasias were treated (thymoma, neuroblastoma, inflammatory myofibroblastic tumor, bronchial carcinoid tumor). No tumor recurrence or port-site metastases

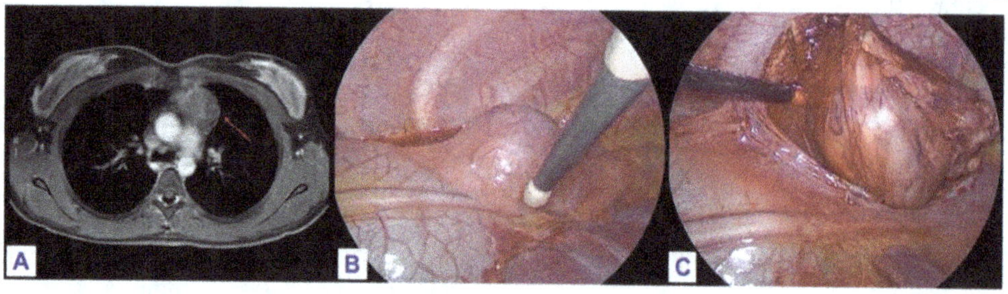

FIGURE 1 | Thymoma excision in an 11-year-old girl: **(A)** MRI pre-operative imaging. **(B)** Identification and preservation of the phrenic nerve. **(C)** Dissection of the thymus from the pericardium.

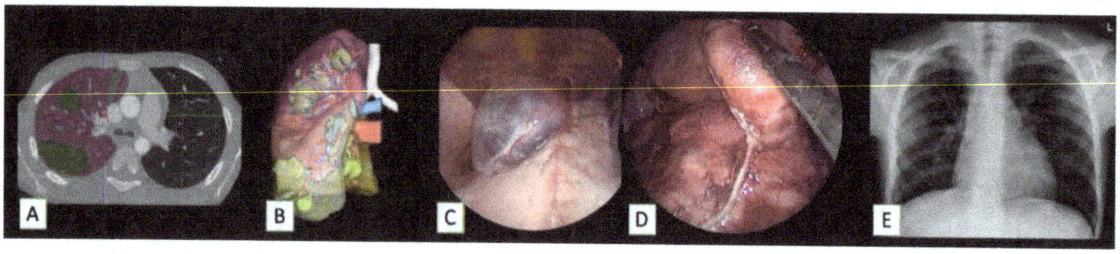

FIGURE 2 | Cystic lesions after surgery and chemotherapy for a pleuropulmonary blastoma in a 7-year-old boy, who then underwent MIS excision of multiple masses. **(A,B)** Reconstruction and 3D model of the lesions. **(C,D)** Intraoperative thoracoscopic view. **(E)** Post-operative X-ray.

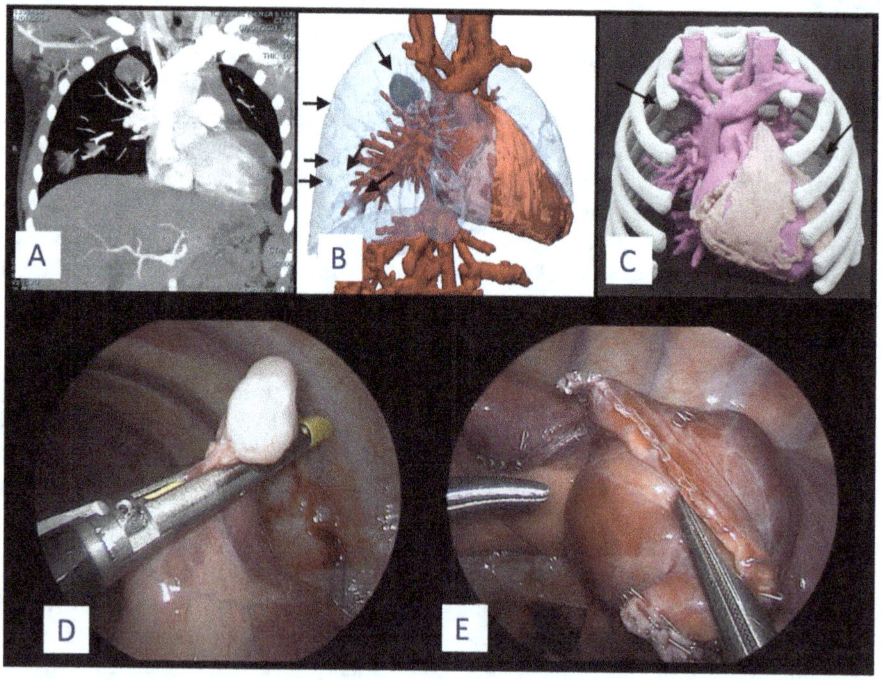

FIGURE 3 | Multiple metastases of immature teratoma in a 7-year-old girl. Left single metastasis was excised through an open procedure, due to dimension and site of the mass. The remaining lesions ($n = 6$, one solid, five cystic ones) on the right lobe were excised through VATS. **(A)** CT image. **(B)** 3D virtual reconstruction. **(C)** 3D printed model showing the two solid lesions (colored in gray). **(D,E)** Intraoperative view.

have been registered; two post-operative pneumothoraxes occurred, and one conversion due to difficult dissection of a neuroblastoma was recorded (48). In our single case, we did not observe any robot-related complications such as adjacent organ injury, positioning-related injury, or injury due to robotic arms. Despite some promising results of RAS reported in literature, its use should be reserved to highly selected cases and, due to lack of recommendations, surgical indication should be discussed by an expert multidisciplinary team (48–50).

LIMITATIONS OF THE STUDY

We should recognize some limitations of the study, related to the predictable low case-volume and heterogeneity of rare diseases that we treated. The analysis of the recent literature faces the same challenge. In addition, the comparison of MIS to open surgery may be problematic in ascertainment with observational studies due to potential unmeasured selection bias, difficulty of retrospective patient-level comparison, and lack of randomized trials (10, 51).

CONCLUSION

VATS has now become a standardized tool in pediatric surgery. From our experience, it may be applied effectively in thoracic pediatric oncology for both diagnostic and therapeutic purposes with low complication and conversion rate.

It is a challenging procedure that requires a dedicated multidisciplinary team with competencies in pediatric oncology, radiology, anesthesiology, and mini-invasive thoracic surgery.

Pre-operative patient selection requires a strict adherence to tumor protocols; IDRF evaluation; and assessment of biology, stage, and dimension of the tumor. Recent technologies such as 3D virtual reconstruction and 3D printing may optimize this selection and guarantee a safer and more targeted treatment. The role of robotics-assisted surgery needs to be defined.

ETHICS STATEMENT

Ethical review and approval was not required for the study on human participants in accordance with the local legislation and institutional requirements. Written informed consent to participate in this study was provided by the participants' legal guardian/next of kin. Written informed consent was obtained from the minor(s)' legal guardian/next of kin for the publication of any potentially identifiable images or data included in this article.

AUTHOR CONTRIBUTIONS

GR contributed to conception and design of the study. FV organized the database and performed the statistical analysis. FV, GR, and MB wrote the first draft of the manuscript. FV, MB, and GR wrote sections of the manuscript. MG and AR help the revision process and implemented sections of the manuscript. All authors contributed to manuscript revision, read, and approved the submitted version.

REFERENCES

1. Lacher M, Kuebler JF, Dingemann J, Ure BM. Minimal invasive surgery in the newborn: current status and evidence. *Semin Pediatr Surg.* (2014) 23:249–56. doi: 10.1053/j.sempedsurg.2014.09.004
2. Ponsky TA, Rothenberg SS. Minimally invasive surgery in infants less than 5 kg: experience of 649 cases. *Surg Endosc.* (2008) 22:2214–9. doi: 10.1007/s00464-008-0025-7
3. Ure BM, Schmidt AI, Jesch NK. Thoracoscopic surgery in infants and children. *Eur J Pediatr Surg.* (2005) 15:314–8. doi: 10.1055/s-2005-865793
4. Lawal TA, Gosemann JH, Kuebler JF, Glüer S, Ure BM. Thoracoscopy versus thoracotomy improves midterm musculoskeletal status and cosmesis in infants and children. *Ann Thorac Surg.* (2009) 87:224–8. doi: 10.1016/j.athoracsur.2008.08.069
5. Yang YF, Dong R, Zheng C, Jin Z, Chen G, Huang YL, et al. Outcomes of thoracoscopy versus thoracotomy for esophageal atresia with tracheoesophageal fistula repair. *Medicine.* (2016) 95:e4428. doi: 10.1097/MD.0000000000004428
6. Jaureguizar E, Vazquez J, Murcia J, Diez Pardo JA. Morbid musculoskeletal sequelae of thoracotomy for tracheoesophageal fistula. *J Pediatr Surg.* (1985) 20:511–4. doi: 10.1016/S0022-3468(85)80477-2
7. Korovessis P, Papanastasiou D, Dimas A, Karayannis A. Scoliosis by acquired rib fusion after thoracotomy in infancy. *Eur Spine J.* (1993) 2:53–5. doi: 10.1007/BF00301057
8. Durand M, Musleh L, Vatta F, Orofino G, Querciagrossa S, Jugie M, et al. Robotic lobectomy in children with severe bronchiectasis: a worthwhile new technology. *J Pediatr Surg.* (2021) 56:1606–10. doi: 10.1016/j.jpedsurg.2020.11.009
9. Lautz TB, Farooqui Z, Jenkins T, Heaton TE, Doski JJ, Cooke-Barber J, et al. Thoracoscopy vs thoracotomy for the management of metastatic osteosarcoma: a pediatric surgical oncology research collaborative study. *Int J Cancer.* (2021) 148:1164–71. doi: 10.1002/ijc.33264
10. Abdelhafeez A, Ortega-Laureano L, Murphy AJ, Davidoff AM, Fernandez-Pineda I, Sandoval JA. Minimally invasive surgery in pediatric surgical oncology: practice evolution at a contemporary single-center institution and a guideline proposal for a randomized controlled study. *J Laparoendosc Adv Surg Tech A.* (2019) 29:1046–51. doi: 10.1089/lap.2018.0467
11. Sato T, Kazama T, Fukuzawa T, Wada M, Sasaki H, Kudo H, et al. Mediastinal tumor resection via open or video-assisted surgery in 31 pediatric cases: experiences at a single institution. *J Pediatr Surg.* (2016) 51:530–3. doi: 10.1016/j.jpedsurg.2015.09.021
12. Da M, Peng W, Mo X, Fan M, Wu K, Sun J, et al. Comparison of efficacy between video-assisted thoracoscopic surgery and thoracotomy in children with mediastinal tumors: 6-year experience. *Ann Transl Med.* (2019) 7:653. doi: 10.21037/atm.2019.10.81
13. Acker SN, Bruny JL, Garrington TP, Partrick DA. Minimally invasive surgical techniques are safe in the diagnosis and treatment of pediatric malignancies. *Surg Endosc.* (2015) 29:1203–8. doi: 10.1007/s00464-014-3795-0
14. Irtan S, Brisse HJ, Minard-Colin V, Schleiermacher G, Canale S, Sarnacki S. Minimally invasive surgery of neuroblastic tumors in children: indications depend on anatomical location and image-defined risk factors. *Pediatr Blood Cancer.* (2015) 62:257–61. doi: 10.1002/pbc.25248
15. McDaniel JD, Racadio JM, Patel MN, Johnson ND, Kukreja K. CT-guided localization of pulmonary nodules in children prior to video-assisted thoracoscopic surgical resection utilizing a combination of two previously described techniques. *Pediatr Radiol.* (2018) 48:626–31. doi: 10.1007/s00247-018-4069-0
16. Smith TJ, Rothenberg SS, Brooks M, Bealer J, Chang J, Cook BA, et al. Thoracoscopic surgery in childhood cancer. *J Pediatr Hematol Oncol.* (2002) 24:429–35. doi: 10.1097/00043426-200208000-00004
17. Holcomb GW, Tomita SS, Haase GM, Dillon PW, Newman KD, Applebaum H, et al. Minimally invasive surgery in children with cancer. *Cancer.* (1995) 76:121–8.
18. Bassanezi BSB, Oliveira-Filho AG, Miranda ML, Soares L, Aguiar SS. Use of BiPAP for safe anesthesia in a child with a large anterior mediastinal mass. *Pediatr Anesth.* (2011) 21:985–7. doi: 10.1111/j.1460-9592.2011.03607.x
19. Rothenberg SS, Wagner JS, Chang JHT, Fan LL. The safety and efficacy of thoracoscopic lung biopsy for diagnosis and treatment in infants and children. *J Pediatr Surg.* (1996) 31:100–4. doi: 10.1016/S0022-3468(96)90328-0

20. Esposito C, Lima M, Mattioli G, Mastroianni L, Riccipetitoni G, Monguzzi G, et al. Thoracoscopic surgery in the management of pediatric malignancies: a multicentric survey of the Italian society of videosurgery in infancy. *Surg Endosc.* (2007) 21:1772–5. doi: 10.1007/s00464-007-9246-4
21. Sandoval C, Stringel G. Video-assisted thoracoscopy for the diagnosis of mediastinal masses in children. *JSLS.* (1997) 1:131–3.
22. Metzelder ML, Kuebler JF, Shimotakahara A, Glueer S, Grigull L, Ure BM. Role of diagnostic and ablative minimally invasive surgery for pediatric malignancies. *Cancer.* (2007) 109:2343–8. doi: 10.1002/cncr.22696
23. Spurbeck WW, Davidoff AM, Lobe TE, Rao BN, Schropp KP, Shochat SJ. Minimally invasive surgery in pediatric cancer patients. *Ann Surg Oncol.* (2004) 11:340–3. doi: 10.1245/ASO.2004.04.021
24. Iwanaka T, Arai M, Kawashima H, Kudou S, Fujishiro J, Imaizumi S, et al. Endosurgical procedures for pediatric solid tumors. *Pediatr Surg Int.* (2004) 20:39–42. doi: 10.1007/s00383-003-1078-2
25. Sailhamer E, Jackson CC, Vogel AM, Kang S, Wu Y, Chwals WJ, et al. Minimally invasive surgery for pediatric solid neoplasms. *Am Surg.* (2003) 69:566–8.
26. Holcomb GW. Minimally invasive surgery for solid tumors. *Semin Surg Oncol.* (1999) 16:184–92. doi: 10.3390/children5120158
27. Saenz NC, Conlon KC, Aronson DC, LaQuaglia MP. The application of minimal access procedures in infants, children, and young adults with pediatric malignancies. *J Laparoendosc Adv Surg Tech A.* (1997) 7:289–94. doi: 10.1089/lap.1997.7.289
28. Rodgers BM, Moazam F, Talbert JL. Thoracoscopy in children. *Ann Surg.* (1979) 189:176–80. doi: 10.1097/00000658-197902000-00008
29. Fraga JC, Aydogdu B, Aufieri R, Silva GVM, Schopf L, Takamatu E, et al. Surgical treatment for pediatric mediastinal neurogenic tumors. *Ann Thorac Surg.* (2010) 90:413–8. doi: 10.1016/j.athoracsur.2010.04.086
30. Fraga JC, Rothenberg S, Kiely E, Pierro A. Video-assisted thoracic surgery resection for pediatric mediastinal neurogenic tumors. *J Pediatr Surg.* (2012) 47:1349–53. doi: 10.1016/j.jpedsurg.2012.01.067
31. Malek MM, Mollen KP, Kane TD, Shah SR, Irwin C. Thoracic neuroblastoma: a retrospective review of our institutional experience with comparison of the thoracoscopic and open approaches to resection. *J Pediatr Surg.* (2010) 45:1622–6. doi: 10.1016/j.jpedsurg.2010.03.018
32. Liu YW, Chen HW, Lee JY, Chiang HH Li HP, Chang PC, et al. Is a chest tube necessary after video-assisted thoracoscopic mediastinal tumor resection? *Thorac Cardiovasc Surg.* (2019) 69:181–8. doi: 10.1055/s-0039-1683879
33. Malkan AD, Loh AHP, Fernandez-Pineda I, Sandoval JA. The role of thoracoscopic surgery in pediatric oncology. *J Laparoendosc Adv Surg Tech A.* (2014) 24:819–26. doi: 10.1089/lap.2014.0252
34. Pentek F, Schulte JH, Schweiger B, Metzelder M, Schündeln MM. Development of port-site metastases following thoracoscopic resection of a neuroblastoma. *Pediatr Blood Cancer.* (2015) 63:149–51. doi: 10.1002/pbc.25677
35. Christison-Lagay ER, Thomas D. Minimally invasive approaches to pediatric solid tumors. *Surg Oncol Clin N Am.* (2019) 28:129–46. doi: 10.1016/j.soc.2018.07.005
36. Gurria JP, Malek MM, Heaton TE, Gehred A, Lautz TB, Rhee DS, et al. Minimally invasive surgery for abdominal and thoracic neuroblastic tumors: a systematic review by the APSA cancer committee. *J Pediatr Surg.* (2020) 55:2260–72. doi: 10.1016/j.jpedsurg.2020.02.019
37. Sánchez-Sánchez Á, Girón-Vallejo Ó, Ruiz-Pruneda R, Fernandez-Ibieta M, García-Calderon D, Villamil V, et al. Three-Dimensional printed model and virtual reconstruction: an extra tool for pediatric solid tumors surgery. *European J Pediatr Surg Rep.* (2018) 06:e70–6. doi: 10.1055/s-0038-1672165
38. Smelt JLC, Suri T, Valencia O, Jahangiri M, Rhode K, Nair A, et al. Operative planning in thoracic surgery: a pilot study comparing imaging techniques and three-dimensional printing. *Ann Thorac Surg.* (2019) 107:401–6. doi: 10.1016/j.athoracsur.2018.08.052
39. Kiraly L, Tofeig M, Jha NK, Talo H. Three-dimensional printed prototypes refine the anatomy of post-modified Norwood-1 complex aortic arch obstruction and allow presurgical simulation of the repair. *Interact CardioVasc Thorac Surg.* (2015) 22:238–40. doi: 10.1093/icvts/ivv320
40. Barsness KA, Rooney DM, Davis LM. Collaboration in simulation: the development and initial validation of a novel thoracoscopic neonatal simulator. *J Pediatr Surg.* (2013) 48:1232–8. doi: 10.1016/j.jpedsurg.2013.03.015
41. Shiraishi I, Yamagishi M, Hamaoka K, Fukuzawa M, Yagihara, T. Simulative operation on congenital heart disease using rubber-like urethane stereolithographic biomodels based on 3D datasets of multislice computed tomography. *Eur J Cardiothorac Surg.* (2010) 37:302–6. doi: 10.1016/j.ejcts.2009.07.046
42. Aiolfi A, Nosotti M, Micheletto G, Khor D, Bonitta G, Perali C, et al. Pulmonary lobectomy for cancer: systematic review and network meta-analysis comparing open, video-assisted thoracic surgery, and robotic approach. *Surgery.* (2021) 169:436–46. doi: 10.1016/j.surg.2020.09.010
43. Tabone MD, Kalifa C, Rodary C, Raquin M, Valteau-Couanet D, Lemerle J. Osteosarcoma recurrences in pediatric patients previously treated with intensive chemotherapy. *J Clin Oncol.* (1994) 12:2614–20. doi: 10.1200/JCO.1994.12.12.2614
44. Lautz TB, Farooqui Z, Jenkins T, Heaton TE, Doski JJ, Cooke-Barber J, et al. Thoracoscopy vs thoracotomy for the management of metastatic osteosarcoma: a pediatric surgical oncology research collaborative study. *Int J Cancer.* (2020) 148:1164–71.
45. Sartorelli KH, Partrick D, Meagher DP Jr. Port-site recurrence after thoracoscopic resection of pulmonary metastasis owing to osteogenic sarcoma. *J Pediatr Surg.* (1996) 31:1443–4. doi: 10.1016/S0022-3468(96)90852-0
46. Meehan JJ. Robotic surgery for pediatric tumors. *Cancer.* (2013) 19:183–8. doi: 10.1097/PPO.0b013e318289486c
47. van Dalen EC, de Lijster MS, Leijssen LG, Michiels EM, Kremer LC, Caron HN, et al. Minimally invasive surgery versus open surgery for the treatment of solid abdominal and thoracic neoplasms in children. *Cochrane Database Syst Rev.* (2015) 1:CD008403. doi: 10.1002/14651858.CD008403.pub3
48. Blanc T, Meignan P, Vinit N, Ballouhey Q, Pio L, Capito C, et al. Robotic surgery in pediatric oncology: lessons learned from the first 100 tumours-A nationwide experience. *SSRN J [Preprint].* (2020). Available at: https://papers.ssrn.com/sol3/papers.cfm?abstract_id=3757404 (accessed September 5, 2021).
49. Blanc T, Pio L, Clermidi P, Muller C, Orbach D, Minard-Colin V, et al. Robotic-assisted laparoscopic management of renal tumors in children: preliminary results. *Pediatr Blood Cancer.* (2019) 66 (Suppl. 3):e28431. doi: 10.1002/pbc.27867
50. Mattioli G, Pini Prato A, Razore B, Leonelli L, Pio L, Avanzini S, et al. Da Vinci robotic surgery in a pediatric hospital. *J Laparoendosc Adv Surg Tech.* (2017) 27:539–45. doi: 10.1089/lap.2016.0390
51. Giordano SH, Kuo YF, Duan Z, Hortobagyi GN, Freeman J, Goodwin JS. Limits of observational data in determining outcomes from cancer therapy. *Cancer.* (2008) 112:2456–66. doi: 10.1002/cncr.23452

13

A Comprehensive Analysis of Robot-Assisted Surgery Uptake in the Pediatric Surgical Discipline

Nicolas Fernandez[1,2,3*] *and Walid A. Farhat*[1]

[1] *Division of Urology, Hospital for SickKids, University of Toronto, Toronto, ON, Canada,* [2] *Department of Urology, Fundación Santa Fe de Bogota, Bogota, Colombia,* [3] *Division of Urology, Hospital Universitario San Ignacio, Pontificia Universidad Javeriana, Bogota, Colombia*

***Correspondence:**
Nicolas Fernandez
nicolas.fernandez@sickkids.ca

Introduction: Robotic assisted surgery (RAS) is one of the most recent surgical approaches that has quickly been adopted by the pediatric urology community. Over the last decade, a vast amount of manuscripts has been published, supporting the safety and applicability of RAS in the pediatric population. The quality of published literature about this innovative technology remains supported by case-reports and retrospective case-series. Historical behavior of literature productivity and implementation of laparoscopy followed a similar trend. We present the historical publication uptake of RAS in pediatric urology and other surgical disciplines using a bibliometric comparison of the most cited manuscripts.

Materials and Methods: A systematic search and review of the literature was undertaken by the authors. Literature search was performed in OVID, PubMed, EMBASE, Scopus, Web of Science, and Google Scholar. The search period included all publications between 1985 and June 2018. All languages were included. Data analysis for graphical representation was performed using VOSviewer® version 1.6.8 and Impact Index Analysis was used to adjust the citations by the time since publication.

Results: A total of 1,014 titles were identified. After applying exclusion criteria, 200 papers were included for the RAS arm and 402 for the laparoscopic one. Case-series was the most common type of publication. Average citations for laparoscopic manuscripts was 23 ($SD \pm 31$) and for RAS was 20 ($SD \pm 31.5$). The impact index analysis showed an average of 95 ($SD \pm 167$) for laparoscopic manuscripts vs. 66 ($SD \pm 101$) for RAS. The laparoscopic manuscript with the highest citation count had 199 citations with an impact index of 12.1. And the RAS manuscript with the highest citation count had 280 citations and an impact index of 4.3.

Conclusion: Literature productivity in pediatric laparoscopic and RAS has quickly grown. Pediatric Urologists play a key role in the introduction of this innovative tool. Literature supporting its implementation and future consolidation requires to focus on increasing the level of evidence.

Keywords: robot-assisted surgery, laparoscopy, pediatrics, urology, minimally invasive surgery, bibliometric analysis

INTRODUCTION

Robotic surgery is one of the most recent surgical approaches that has quickly been adopted by the pediatric urology community. Since the first reported cases of laparoscopic surgery in the early 1990's and Peter's et al. first robot-assisted laparoscopic procedure on a pediatric patient in 2002, a vast amount of experience has been gained in the pediatric urological RAS field (1–3). By 2006, the application of RAS in children remained largely unexplored and the perspective of pediatric urologists was polarized (4, 5). Over the last decade, a vast amount of manuscripts have been published, supporting the safety and applicability of RAS in the pediatric population with an increase of 236.6% per year by 2016 (6).

Pediatric Urology has been the specialty that continue to lead this field with pyeloplasty being the most frequently performed procedure to date (7). More recent data support that more than 80% of pediatric urologists see a clear role for RAS in the pediatric population (5). The quick growth of RAS has been supported by the fact that surgeons can perform complex reconstructive procedures with much shorter learning curves compared to regular laparoscopy (8–10). In fact it has been seen that RAS-naïve surgeons who are performing suturing for the first time, they do it much faster than with laparoscopy (11). More recent studies are now supporting shorter lengths of stay and fewer complications for RAS cases compared to laparoscopic ones (12). Nonetheless, the quality of published literature about this innovative technology remains supported by case-reports and retrospective case-series. Historical behavior of literature productivity and implementation of laparoscopy followed a similar trend. Previous bibliometric analysis studies have shown how literature productivity and consumption (citations) cannot be interpreted the same way for all specialties in a universal way (13–15). For instance, topics like coronary artery disease, or cancer have more visibility and will be of more interest to more medical fields. This translates to higher citation counts for these publications, but specialties like pediatric RAS surgery where the amount of specialists interested in this field is smaller a proportional smaller citation count is seen. This proportion needs to be kept in mind when it comes to interpreting the citation counts based on the specialty "size".

Based on a Progressive Scholarly Acceptance analysis, RAS has not passed the transition point yet and remains un-accepted by the scientific community (16). Innovative technologies are rarely implemented universally and RAS is not the exception (6). Limitations for RAS and laparoscopy, as innovations, in the surgical field have gone through similar paths, both technologies have had to overcome critics and prove to be safe and replicable. We hypothesize that RAS has taken off in a much faster way compared to laparoscopy, considering that RAS enables surgeons the possibility of performing complex procedures with a shorter learning curve. For these reasons, we hereby present a mathematical analysis (need to consider statistical analysis) of a literature review to show the results of a historical bibliometric comparison of the most cited manuscripts since laparoscopy and RAS were implemented.

METHODS

A systematic search and review of the literature was undertaken by the authors following the PRISMA concepts. Literature search was performed in OVID, PubMed, EMBASE, Scopus, Web of Science, and Google Scholar. A comprehensive search included the MeSh terms: Pediatrics, minimally invasive surgical procedures, laparoscopy, urology, and robotics. The search period included all publications between 1985 and June 2018. Citation count per manuscript was taken from Scopus, Web of Science and Google Scholar. A secondary search was performed following the same methodology to include pediatric surgical procedures with the MeSh terms: Pediatric Surgery, robotics. No citation analysis was performed on this secondary analysis. Otolaryngologic and Neurosurgical publications were excluded. For manuscripts with different citation counts on each database, we used the highest citation count out of the three databases. Citation data extraction was performed in a 2-day period between June 20th and 21st of 2018. Impact index analysis (IIA) was initially developed as a way to adjust the citation count interpretation based on the time since publication. For this reason, we used the IIA in the present study to interpret our results. We followed the formula reported by Fernandez et al. considering influential manuscripts with low scores (13).

All extracted titles and abstracts were screened for relevance and disagreements were resolved by consensus. Duplicated titles and abstracts that did not disclose any information about pediatric urological robot-assisted or laparoscopic surgery were excluded. For manuscripts comparing regular laparoscopy with robot-assisted surgery, the title was included in the robot-assisted analysis. All languages were included. Data analysis for graphical representation was performed using VOSviewer® version 1.6.8 (http://www.vosviewer.com).

Comparisons of continuous variables was carried out with *t*-tests and ANOVA when more than two set of groups were compared. Statistical analyses were analyzed using SPSS v. 25.0 (SPSS 25.0—SPSS Inc., Chicago, Illinois). $P < 0.05$ were considered statistically significant.

RESULTS

A total of 1,014 titles were identified. After duplicated titles were excluded, 667 titles were screened and after applying exclusion criteria, 602 titles were included for analysis; 200 for the robot-assisted arm and 402 for the laparoscopic one. Case-series was the most common type of publication for both arms followed by review articles and case reports (**Figure 1**). There was only one experiment with an animal model and another with an inanimate one in the RAS analysis and 4 and 6, respectively, in the laparoscopic manuscripts. There are only 8 publications that were prospective studies. In the RAS analysis there were no randomized clinical trials as oppose to laparoscopic publications where we identified 4 manuscripts. There were more cost analysis studies in the RAS arm than laparoscopy. We looked for geographical distributions of the most cited manuscripts in order to compare centers' and their

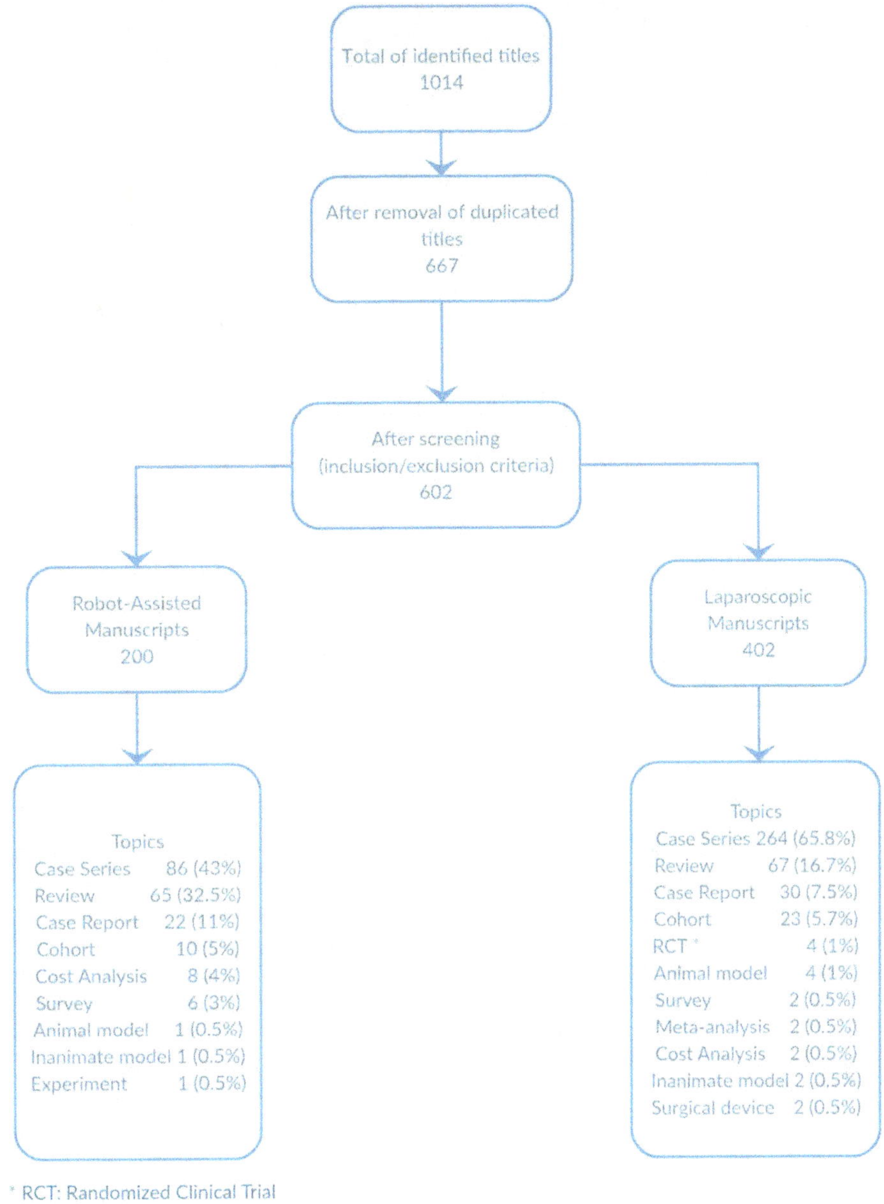

FIGURE 1 | Manuscript selection and distribution of types of studies.

citation counts and how they transitioned from laparoscopy into RAS. We found that the majority of authors and centers that were on the top ten positions of the most cited manuscripts were different for laparoscopy and RAS. The only author who remained at the top 10 for laparoscopy and RAS was Dr. Craig Peters.

When comparing the amount of publications per year between laparoscopic manuscripts and RAS, a higher and quicker proportional increase in the publication count for RAS manuscripts was noted (**Figure 2**). When comparing the amount of manuscripts published since 2,000 for pediatric urological laparoscopy, RAS urology and pediatric general surgery, the mean publication counts for this 18-year period was 20.78, 11.11, and 6.56, respectively ($p < 0.0000$) (**Figure 2**). When the same comparison is made for RAS in pediatric urology, pediatric general surgery and pediatric ENT there is a statistically significant difference favoring a higher productivity for pediatric urology ($p = 0.041$) (**Figure 2**).

In the first decade after either technique was introduced, there were less publications for laparoscopy (58 publications) than RAS (103 publications).

Average citations for laparoscopic manuscripts was 23 (*SD* ± 31) and for RAS was 20 (*SD* ± 31.5). The impact index analysis showed an average of 95 (*SD* ± 167) for laparoscopic manuscripts vs. 66 (*SD* ± 101) for RAS. When comparing average citation counts for publications before and after the year

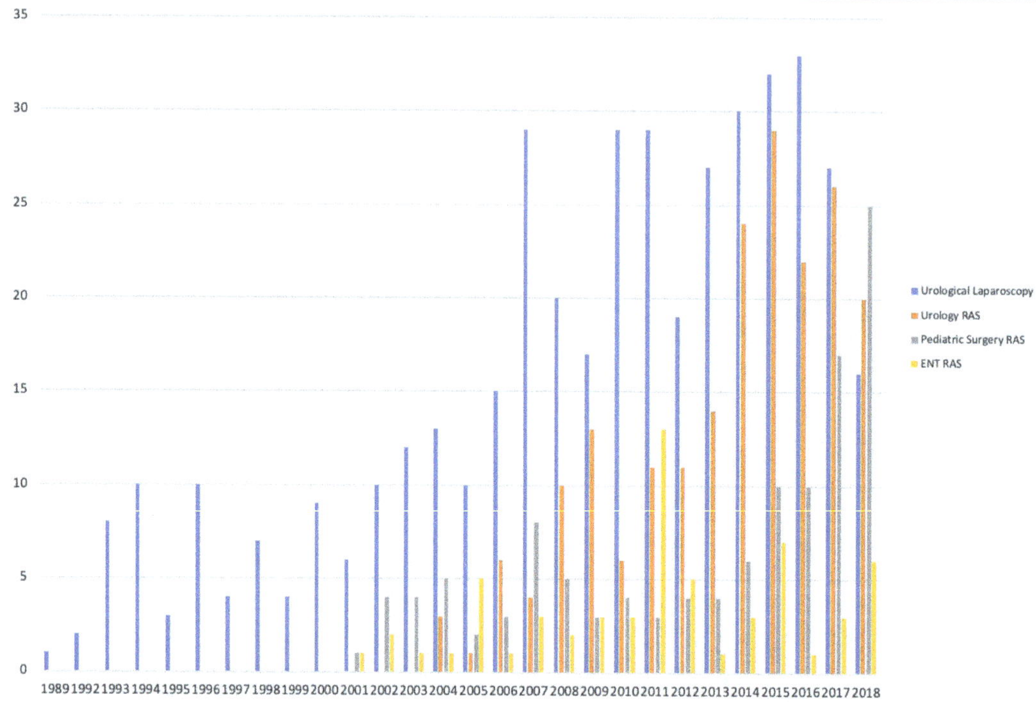

FIGURE 2 | Historical count of publications for laparoscopic and robot-assisted publications.

2000 for laparoscopic procedures, the average citation counts for publications after 2000 was 20 and before 47 (CI = 17.20–35.44) ($p < 0.0001$). We also did the same comparison using the impact index scores and found an average impact index of 86 for publications after the year 2000 and 157 for those published before ($p = 0.01$).

The laparoscopic manuscript with the highest citation count had 199 citations with an impact index of 12.1. And the RAS manuscript with the highest citation count had 280 citations and an impact index of 4.3.

Our impact index analysis showed low scores for landmark papers that have remained as highly influential since their publication time in the early 2000's. Historical impact index trends show that most recent papers have more impact (**Figures 4A,B**).

Almost all publications came from North-America (81%) followed by Europe (15%) and the remaining from Asian and Middle-East countries. The Journal where most of the RAS manuscripts were published was the Journal of Pediatric Urology with 26.5% of the publications followed by Journal of Urology with 10.5%. For regular laparoscopy, the journal with most manuscripts was Journal of Urology with 19.2% followed by Journal of Pediatric Urology with 13.6%. By the time laparoscopy was initially introduced, the Journal of Pediatric Urology was not yet indexed.

Secondary search identified a total of 118 publications in pediatric surgery. RAS and laparoscopy have steadily increased, but pediatric surgery has not had the same proportion of increase over time as in the pediatric urology subspecialty (**Figure 2**).

Most discussed topics were pyeloplasty followed by ureteral re-implantation (**Figure 3**). For Pediatric Surgery, the most common discussed topic was fundoplication. There has been a most recent increase in cost analysis publications over time for RAS. During the second decade after implementation of pediatric laparoscopy, a significant amount of manuscripts focused on the use of single port surgery. RAS literature was mainly about the presentation of applicability and safety of this technology. All publications were published exclusively in urology journals with Journal of Urology and Journal of Pediatric Urology being the ones with the most published and most cited manuscripts.

DISCUSSION

Minimally invasive surgery (MIS) has been a significant landmark in pediatric surgery discipline but robotic approach is evidently impacted pediatric urology evolution and practice far more than any other pediatric surgical disciplines. Our results show similar historical trends when comparing laparoscopy to RAS when looking at citation counts and level of evidence of supporting manuscripts. The main difference has been noticed on much quicker and higher manuscript productivity. Also, when adjusting by time since publication using our novel developed Impact index, we notice that RAS has had a better impact on the scientific community compared to laparoscopy. Implementation of innovative technologies depends on multiple factors and research with publications do enhance uptake of new technologies. RAS has had a quick take-off and one of the reasons for this trend is that literature acted as a catalyst for adopting it. At

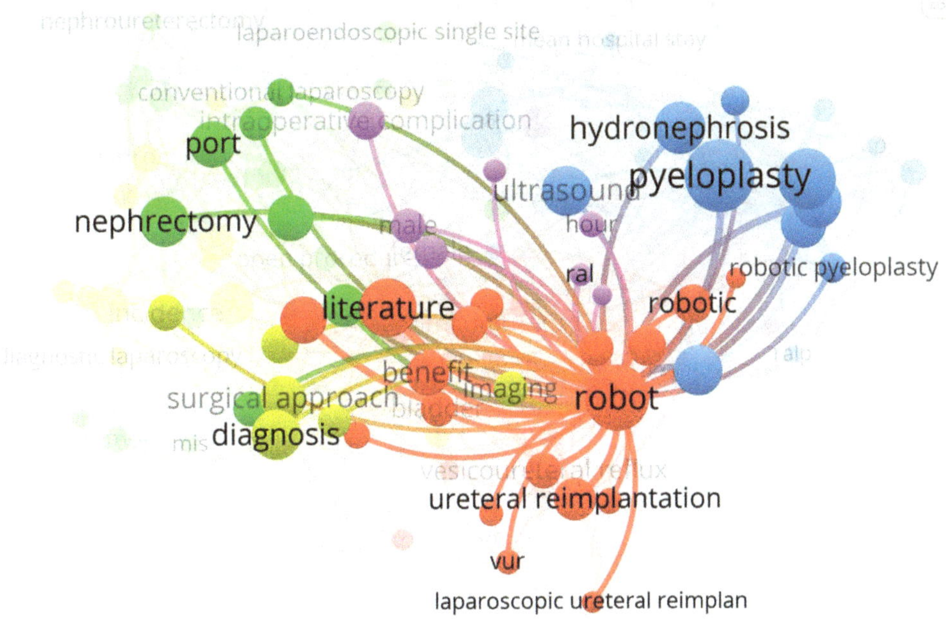

FIGURE 3 | Most discussed topics for manuscripts published in laparoscopy and robot-assisted pediatric urology.

some degree, this supports how new technologies are accepted by the surgical community. The urge to publicize and the pressure of community for recognition, may affect the quality of scientific productivity. Our results along with other authors like Cundy et al. show that 90% of published manuscripts in this topic are level IV (3, 17). Nevertheless, careful interpretation of literature is needed when new technologies are being implemented. (18, 19). Interestingly despite finding that there are 4 randomized studies and 2 meta-analysis in the laparoscopic literature, these have not been highly cited.

In the early 1990's, the implementation of laparoscopy as a novel technology, showed to be safe and reproducible when compared to open surgery for most of the procedures (20). The possibility of internet influencing the amount of citations is plausible when analyzing the impact index for publications before and after the year 2000. A similar trend has been seen for RAS. Nonetheless, none of either technology has enabled the creation of a novel surgical technique. Surgeons are the door of entrance for many innovative technologies. Our results support how such tool has evolved and is now broadly implemented (21).

Our results do not show the same evolution for pediatric surgery, similar to what has seen by other authors (3). Our results show that most publications focused on the applicability and safety of robotic surgery when compared to regular laparoscopy or open surgery. If considering open surgery as a "gold standard" the use of laparoscopy and RAS have shown to be comparable for procedures like pyeloplasty (22, 23). This explains why it is the most reported procedure in literature. For other procedures like nephrectomy, MIS has shown to be superior with less morbidity and shorter hospital stay (24). In the case of the management of vesicoureteral reflux, ureteral reimplantation performed laparoscopically and by RAS has now shown debatable results when compared to those of open surgery (25–27).

Bibliometrics and impact factor for published literature cannot be analyzed based only on the amount of citations. It is important to consider the specialty and discussed topic amongst other variables like time since publication at the moment of interpreting this data. Our results show how MIS in pediatric urology is a very specialized topic that is read and cited by a very selective group sub-specialists. This is proven by the fact that all manuscripts are published in urological journals for both, laparoscopy and RAS. The amount of literature produced per year has never been above 50 publications and average citation counts of 20 on our analysis compared to other topics. For instance vesicoureteral reflux, which is of more interest to other specialties besides pediatric urology, the average citation counts were 101, this confirms how selective this topic can be (13). Our impact index analysis also showed that despite having similar citation averages between laparoscopic surgery and RAS, the latter has had more impact in the community and is quickly growing with more publications in 2018 than regular laparoscopy. Trends for better impact index for more recent manuscripts might be due to the preference of readers for the most recent publications.

With the ongoing debate on the cost-effective of RAS in the pediatric population (28), we noted higher number of manuscripts that tackle this particular issue (cost analysis between RAS and regular laparoscopy). This reflects the common and significant need to justify and rationalize the use of such an expensive technology (7, 23, 25, 29).

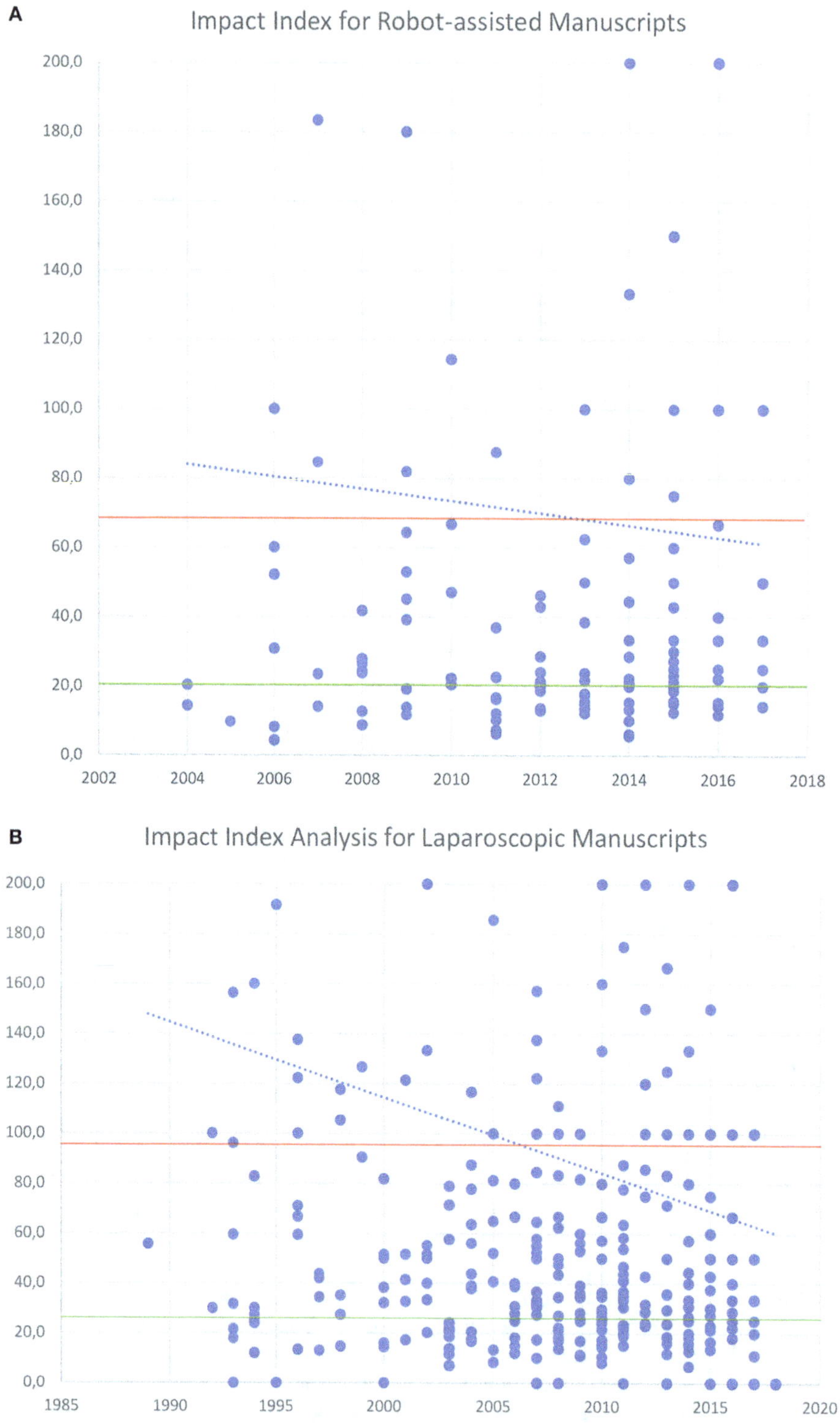

FIGURE 4 | (A) Impact Index analysis per manuscript over time for RAS. **(B)** Impact Index analysis per manuscript over time for Laparoscopy. In red average Impact Index and green average citations per manuscript. In blue the trend of Impact index over time.

Considering that MIS has been introduced as a new technology, its implementation was never supported by research based in basic science studies or experiments. Can we say that the implementation of novel technologies may not be necessarily supported by high quality type of studies to show its efficacy. It is our opinion that the adoption of new technology in surgery may not be because of the high quality studies *per se* but rather because it is doable and can be broadly adopted then some will adopt

Our results show that about 1% of the manuscripts describe results of experiments in animal or inanimate models. One reason for this might be the interest of authors to present information on how MIS can be clinically implemented. Nonetheless, the lack of this kind of experimental research misses the opportunity for innovation and probably for higher evidence-based literature that consolidates a safer path for the safe and efficient use of this novel tool. It is interesting to see that early adopters of RAS had the highest risk of litigation (30). But after the amount of procedures performed increased, the risks dropped. Most of the claims were due to surgical complications instead device failures from the DaVinci platform. This probably supports that novel technologies may not introduce a risk for legal actions if implemented and used in a responsible way. Good quality published literature may protect surgeons from legal actions against them.

Current efforts need to focus on the development of predictable inanimate models to help support the development of instruments that respond to the high technical demands of pediatric surgery. RAS instruments have been developed to be used on adults and pediatric surgeons have adopted these instruments into pediatric patients. The small working space is a challenge that few manuscripts have addressed and there is a need for scientific evidence to answer this question to help improve the usage of RAS in small patients (31). Literature productivity on this topic has tried to answer this question. The minimal effective volume that allows the performance of different surgical tasks without arm collision is between 125 and 130 cm^3 (31, 32). Abdominal characteristics for a suitable abdomen have been estimated to be a pubic-xyphoid length of 15 cm and an anterior superior iliac spine of 13 cm. Patient's weight has been defined as 10 kg. Considering all this variables, appropriate age range is around the 3 years of life. Considering this, many of upper tract reconstructive cases are performed earlier in life. For this reason, it is critical to focus our research on how to improve these technical limitations. Our group is currently working on developing a predictable 3-D inanimate model that simulates our results on small animal models reducing instrument collision and abdominal wall tension and traction (data presented at the NARUS conference 2018). This kind of results will allow the development of smaller instruments and improve the usage of current robot platforms in a better way.

CONCLUSIONS

Literature productivity in pediatric laparoscopic and robot-assisted surgery topic has quickly grown. Level of evidence literature productivity has been similar for both technologies with more impact for RAS in the community, exponentially growing at a faster pace than how laparoscopy was introduced. Current graduating generations have had a significant exposure to RAS during their adult training and for this reason we believe RAS has remained a leading topic in the pediatric urology specialty (33, 34). Future directives need to focus on increasing the level of evidence to support innovation and development of pediatric instruments.

AUTHOR CONTRIBUTIONS

NF proposed the idea of manuscript and did the data search and analysis. WF supervised the process of the entire manuscript and made the final corrections and elaborated the discussion.

REFERENCES

1. Koyle M, Woo H, Kavoussi L. Laparoscopic nephrectomy in the first year of life. *J Pediatr Sug.* (1993) 28:693e35.
2. Peters CA. Robotically assisted surgery in pediatric urology. *Urol Clin N Am.* (2004) 31:743–52. doi: 10.1016/j.ucl.2004.06.007
3. Cundy TP, Shetty K, Clark J, Chang TP, Sriskandarajah K, Gattas NE, et al. The first decade of robotic surgery in children. *J Pediatr Surg.* (2013) 48:858–65. doi: 10.1016/j.jpedsurg.2013.01.031
4. Lee RS, Retik AB, Borer JG, Peters CA. Pediatric robot assisted laparoscopic dismembered pyeloplasty: comparison with a cohort of open surgery. *J Urol.* (2006) 175:683–7. doi: 10.1016/S0022-5347(05)00183-7
5. Cundy TP, Marcus HJ, Hughes-Hallett A, Najmaldin AS, Yang GZ, Darzi A. International attitudes of early adopters to current and future robotic technologies in pediatric surgery. *J Pediatr Surg.* (2014) 49:1522–6. doi: 10.1016/j.jpedsurg.2014.05.017
6. Cundy TP, Harley SJD, Marcus HJ, Hughes-Hallett A, Khurana S. Global trends in paediatric robot-assisted urological surgery: a bibliometric and progressive scholarly acceptance analysis. *J Robot Surg.* (2018) 12:109–15. doi: 10.1007/s11701-017-0703-3
7. Bennett WE, Whittam BM, Szymanski KM, Rink RC, Cain MP, Carroll AE. Validated cost comparison of open vs. robotic pyeloplasty in American children's hospitals. *J Robot Surg.* (2017) 11:201–6. doi: 10.1007/s11701-016-0645-1
8. Nguyen HT, Passerotti CC, Penna FJ, Retik AB, Peters CA. Robotic assisted laparoscopic mitrofanoff appendicovesicostomy: preliminary experience in a pediatric population. *J Urol.* (2009) 182 (Suppl 4):1528–34. doi: 10.1016/j.juro.2009.06.055
9. Barashi NS, Rodriguez MV, Packiam VT, Gundeti MS. Bladder Reconstruction with bowel: robot-assisted laparoscopic ileocystoplasty with mitrofanoff appendicovesicostomy in pediatric patients. *J Endourol.* (2018) 32:119–26. doi: 10.1089/end.2017.0720
10. Passerotti C, Peters CA. Robotic-assisted laparoscopy applied to reconstructive surgeries in children. *World J Urol.* (2006) 24:193–7. doi: 10.1007/s00345-006-0084-0
11. Murthy PB, Schadler ED, Orvieto M, Zagaja G, Shalhav AL, Gundeti MS. Setting up a pediatric robotic urology program: a USA institution experience. *Int J Urol.* (2018) 25:86–93. doi: 10.1111/iju.13415
12. Silay M, Spinoit A, Undre S. Global minimally invasive pyeloplasty study in children: results from the pediatric urology expert group of the european association of urology young academic urologists working party. *J Pediatr Urol.* (2016) 12:229.e1-7. doi: 10.1016/j.jpurol.2016.04.007
13. Fernandez N, Puerto A, Azuero A, O'Kelly F, Hannick J, Rickard M, et al. Historical bibliometric analysis of the top cited articles on vesicoureteral reflux 1950-2016, and incorporation of a novel impact index. *J Pediatr Urol.* (2018) 14:446.e1-446.e9. doi: 10.1016/j.jpurol.2018.04.004
14. O'Kelly F, Nason GJ, McLoughlin LC, Flood HD, Thornhill JA. A comparative bibliometric analysis of the top 150 cited papers in hypospadiology (1945–2013). *J Pediatr Urol.* (2015) 11:85.e1-85.e11. doi: 10.1016/j.jpurol.2014.11.022

15. Rousseau R. Library science: forgotten founder of bibliometrics. *Nature.* (2014) 510:218. doi: 10.1038/510218e
16. Schnurman Z, Kondziolka D. Evaluating innovation. part 1: the concept of progressive scholarly acceptance. *J Neurosurg.* (2016) 124:207–11. doi: 10.3171/2015.1.JNS142661
17. Sackett D. Rules of evidence and clinical recommendations on the use of antithrombotic agents. *Chest.* (1989) 95:2s–4s. doi: 10.1378/chest.95.2_Supplement.2S
18. Jimbo M, Granberg CF, Osumah TS, Bandari J, Cannon GM, Routh JC, et al. Discrepancies in self-reported and actual conflicts of interest in pediatric urology robotic surgery. *J Urol.* (2018) 201:393–99. doi: 10.1016/j.juro.2018.07.043
19. Criss CN, Gadepalli SK. Sponsoring surgeons: an investigation on the influence of the da Vinci robot. *Am J Surg.* (2018) 216:84–7. doi: 10.1016/j.amjsurg.2017.08.017
20. Bansal D, Cost NG, Bean CM, Vanderbrink BA, Schulte M, Noh PH. Infant robot-assisted laparoscopic upper urinary tract reconstructive surgery. *J Pediatr Urol.* (2014) 10:869–74. doi: 10.1016/j.jpurol.2014.01.029
21. Senagore AJ. Adoption of laparoscopic colorectal surgery : it was quite a journey. *Clin Colon Rectal Surg.* (2015) 28:131–4. doi: 10.1055/s-0035-1560040
22. Varda BK, Johnson EK, Clark C, Chung BI, Nelson CP, Chang SL. National trends of perioperative outcomes and costs for open, laparoscopic and robotic pediatric pyeloplasty. *J Urol.* (2014) 191:1090–5. doi: 10.1016/j.juro.2013.10.077
23. Varda BK, Wang Y, Chung BI, Lee RS, Kurtz MP, Nelson CP, et al. Has the robot caught up? National trends in utilization, perioperative outcomes, and cost for open, laparoscopic, and robotic pediatric pyeloplasty in the United States from 2003 to 2015. *J Pediatr Urol.* (2018) 14:336.e1-336.e8. doi: 10.1016/j.jpurol.2017.12.010
24. Bowlin PR, Farhat WA. Laparoscopic nephrectomy and partial nephrectomy: intraperitoneal, retroperitoneal, single site. *Uro Clin North Am.* (2015) 42:31-42. doi: 10.1016/j.ucl.2014.09.012
25. Kurtz MP, Leow JJ, Varda BK, Logvinenko T, Yu RN, Nelson CP, et al. Robotic versus open pediatric ureteral reimplantation: costs and complications from a nationwide sample. *J Pediatr Urol.* (2016) 12:408.e1-408.e6. doi: 10.1016/j.jpurol.2016.06.016
26. De Lambert G, Fourcade L, Centi J, Fredon F, Braik K, Szwarc C, et al. How to successfully implement a robotic pediatric surgery program: Lessons learned after 96 procedures. *Surg Endosc Other Interv Tech.* (2013) 27:2137–44. doi: 10.1007/s00464-012-2729-y
27. Baek M, Koh CJ. Lessons learned over a decade of pediatric robotic ureteral reimplantation. *Investig Clin Urol.* (2017) 58:3–11. doi: 10.4111/icu.2017.58.1.3
28. Casella DP, Fox JA, Schneck FX, Cannon GM, Ost MC. Cost analysis of pediatric robot-assisted and laparoscopic pyeloplasty. *J Urol.* (2013) 189:1083–6. doi: 10.1016/j.juro.2012.08.259
29. Mahida JB, Cooper JN, Herz D, Diefenbach KA, Deans KJ, Minneci PC, et al. Utilization and costs associated with robotic surgery in children. *J Surg Res.* (2015) 199:169–76. doi: 10.1016/j.jss.2015.04.087
30. Nik-Ahd F, Souders CP, Zhao H, Houman J, McClelland L, Chughtai B, et al. Robotic urologic surgery: trends in litigation over the last decade. *J Robot Surg.* (2019). doi: 10.1007/s11701-018-00905-y
31. Thakre AA, Bailly Y, Sun LW, Van Meer F, Yeung CK. Is smaller workspace a limitation for robot performance in laparoscopy? *J Urol.* (2008) 179:1138–43. doi: 10.1016/j.juro.2007.10.091
32. Kutikov A, Guzzo TJ, Canter DJ, Casale P. Initial experience with laparoscopic transvesical ureteral reimplantation at the Children's Hospital of Philadelphia. *J Urol.* (2006) 176:2222–6. doi: 10.1016/j.juro.2006.07.082
33. Menhadji A, Abdelshehid C, Osann K, Alipanah R, Lusch A, Graversen J, et al. Tracking and assessment of technical skills acquisition among urology residents for open, laparoscopic, and robotic skills Over 4 years: is there a trend? *J Endourol.* (2013) 27:783–9. doi: 10.1089/end.2012.0633
34. Wang L, Diaz M, Stricker H, Peabody JO, Menon M, Rogers CG. Adding a newly trained surgeon into a high-volume robotic prostatectomy group: are outcomes compromised? *J Robot Surg.* (2017) 11:69–74. doi: 10.1007/s11701-016-0615-7

14

Resection of Giant Endotracheal Hamartoma by Electrosurgical Snaring via Fiberoptic Bronchoscopy in a 9-Year-Old Boy

Lei Wu [1,2†], *Wei Chen* [2,3†], *PengCheng Li* [2,4], *Shuxian Li* [1] *and Zhimin Chen* [1*]

[1] *Department of Pulmonology, The Children's Hospital, Zhejiang University School of Medicine, National Clinical Research Center for Child Health, Hangzhou, China,* [2] *Department of Endoscopy Center, The Children's Hospital, Zhejiang University School of Medicine, National Clinical Research Center for Child Health, Hangzhou, China,* [3] *Department of Pediatrics, The First Affiliated Hospital of USTC, Division of Life Sciences and Medicine, University of Science and Technology of China, Hefei, China,* [4] *Department of Pediatrics, Affiliated Hospital of Nantong University, Nantong, China*

***Correspondence:**
Zhimin Chen
zmchen@zju.edu.cn

† *These authors have contributed equally to this work*

Endotracheal hamartomas are rarely encountered in children. The symptoms of endotracheal hamartoma may include cough, dyspnea, hemoptysis, chest pain, purulent sputum, and fever. The non-specific symptoms often result in a delayed diagnosis. Among the various treatments of this rare disease, surgical resection seems to be the most widely used, while endoscopic treatment is rarely described. Herein, we describe the case of a 9-year-old boy with an endotracheal hamartoma that was successfully excised by electrosurgical snaring via fiberoptic bronchoscopy (FB). The resection of select benign endotracheal tumors in children can be conducted using electrocautery, which can be regarded as an alternative therapy to bronchotomy.

Keywords: endotracheal lesions, hamartoma, therapeutic bronchoscopy, airway tumors, case report

INTRODUCTION

Benign lung tumors represent <1% of all lung tumors; among these, hamartomas have an incidence of 0.025–0.32% in the adult population (1). Although still an uncommon occurrence, hamartoma is the most common type of benign pulmonary tumor, accounting for an estimated 77% of benign lung nodules and 8% of solitary lung lesions (2, 3). Most hamartomas occur in the peripheral parenchyma, but have in rare cases been present in the trachea or bronchi. A previous study reported that the hamartoma was in an endobronchial location in only 1.4% of 215 patients with hamartomas (4). Although hamartomas may be found at any age, the age at presentation is mostly between 40 and 60 years; primary pulmonary, tracheal, or bronchial hamartomas are significantly rarer in the pediatric population (2, 5). The most frequent clinical symptoms of tracheal or endobronchial hamartomas are fever, cough, hemoptysis, purulent sputum, dyspnea, and pain due to tracheal or bronchial obstruction. Tracheal or endobronchial hamartomas are traditionally treated by thoracotomy with bronchotomy or lung resection. At present, the first-line widely recommended approach in adults is endoscopic treatment; however, similar treatments have rarely been reported in children (6). We herein describe a case in which electrosurgical snaring via fiberoptic bronchoscopy (FB) was applied to successfully resect a rare tracheal hamartoma in a young boy, avoiding the need for bronchotomy.

CASE PRESENTATION

A 9-year-old boy was referred to our hospital with a 20-day history of cough, stridor, and shortness of breath. He had showed a poor clinical response to conventional therapy with antibiotics and systemic steroids at a local hospital. He was previously healthy with no relevant family history. A computed tomography (CT) scan performed at a local hospital revealed a homogeneous mass obstructing the trachea. During preparation for rigid bronchoscopy (RB) at the local hospital, he was found to be intolerant to general anesthesia and his dyspnea exacerbated. He was transferred to our hospital immediately. On admission to our hospital, the patient appeared dyspneic and had a characteristic biphasic stridor, with a percutaneous oxygen saturation of 93% under mask oxygen inhalation, body temperature of 37.7°C, pulse rate of 162 beats/min, respiration rate of 34 breaths/min, and blood pressure of 127/74 mmHg.

On day 2, contrast-enhanced multidetector CT revealed a mass lesion with a fat density that was nearly totally obstructing the tracheal lumen (**Figure 1**). The multidisciplinary consensus was to proceed with bronchoscopy to obtain a definitive diagnosis to guide management and determine the prognosis. After being fully informed about the surgical options and possible complications related to different surgical modalities, the patient's parents elected to have the mass removed by an electrocautery snare with FB. A rigid bronchoscope (Karl Storz, Germany), argon plasma coagulation (APC) (ERBE VIO200D+APC2), cryotherapy (ERBOKRYO CA), and Holmium: YAG laser (Dahua DHL-1, China) were available if necessary. The parents also agreed that if the treatment failed, surgical resection would be carried out immediately. Written informed consent for the interventional procedures was obtained from the patient's parents.

The mass resection was performed on day 3. Pulmonologists, otolaryngologists, thoracic surgeons, anesthesiologists, and pediatric intensive care unit doctors were all in the operating room to ensure the success of the treatment and the safety of the patient. General anesthesia was induced with 8% sevoflurane. After the intravenous administration of 2 mg of midazolam, a laryngeal mask airway (LMA) was inserted to maintain an open airway. Intraoperatively, anesthesia was maintained with 3% sevoflurane. Based on the depth of anesthesia, 10 mg of pentazocine and 50 mg of propofol were intravenously administered intraoperatively. A swivel adapter was used to connect the proximal end of the laryngeal mask to the T-piece anesthesia system. A flexible fiberoptic bronchoscope (Olympus 260; external diameter: 4.9 mm, working channel: 2 mm) operated by an experienced pulmonologist was inserted via the swivel adapter. A large mass covered by smooth mucosa with a stalk was obstructing approximately 85% of the trachea in the mid-tracheal region (**Figure 2A**). A flexible 1.9-mm electrocautery snare (Olympus CD-6C-1) was then introduced through the working channel of the bronchoscope. After placing the loop of the snare around the base of the mass (**Figure 2B**), the electrocautery snare was used in blend mode at 30 W to cut and coagulate the base of the mass (**Figure 2C**). The mass was resected without evidence of bleeding or perforation (**Figure 2D**). The inspired oxygen concentration was maintained at 25% to avoid potential combustion during the interventional procedure. Due to the broad base of the mass, part of the remaining tissue at the root was removed with biopsy forceps to reduce the amount of residual tissue. Postoperatively, the patient recovered completely and was discharged home on day 8. The pathologic examination suggested that the mass was a tracheal hamartoma predominantly constituted of mature fat cells (**Figure 3**). The patient's condition remained stable for 1 year following the interventional therapy. The patient returned to the hospital for repeat chest CT examination and bronchoscopy at 1 year postoperatively (**Figure 4**). There was a slight protrusion at the position of the incision (**Figure 2E**).

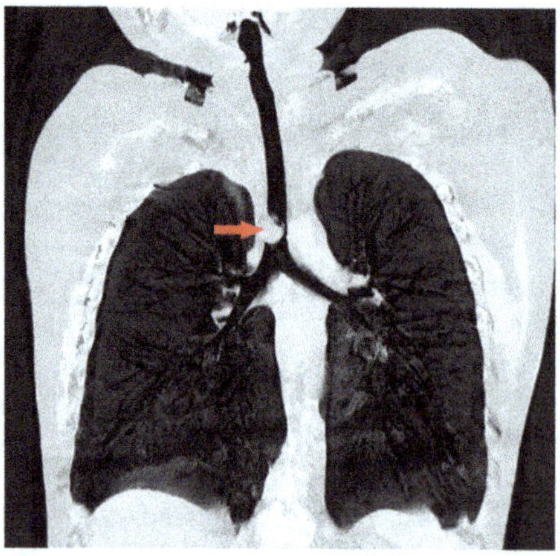

FIGURE 1 | Preoperative chest computed tomography reveals an endotracheal tumor nearly totally obstructing the tracheal lumen.

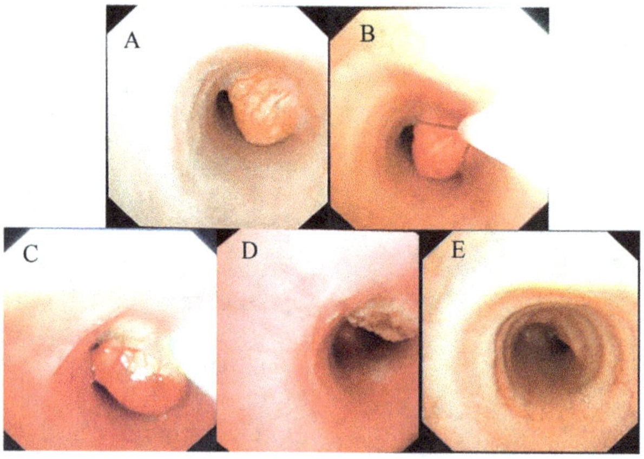

FIGURE 2 | (A) Fiberoptic bronchoscopy image of the large mass covered by smooth mucosa in the mid-tracheal region. **(B)** Placing the loop of the snare around the base of the mass. **(C)** The process of mass removal by electrocautery snare. **(D)** Most of the mass is removed by electrosurgical snaring under bronchoscopy. **(E)** Photograph showing a slight protrusion at the position of the incision at 1 year post-operatively.

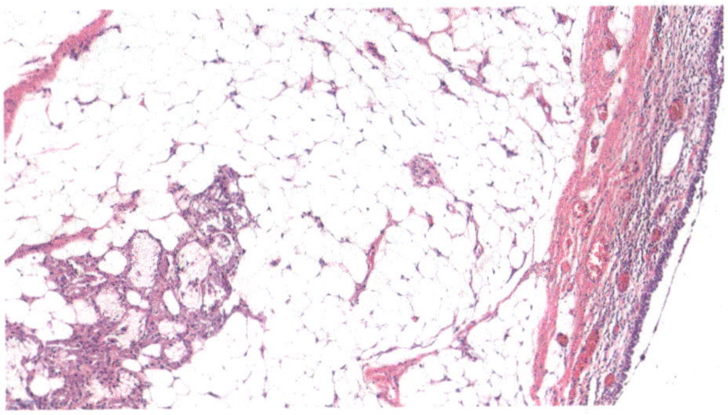

FIGURE 3 | The tumor was a hamartoma largely comprising mature fat cells.

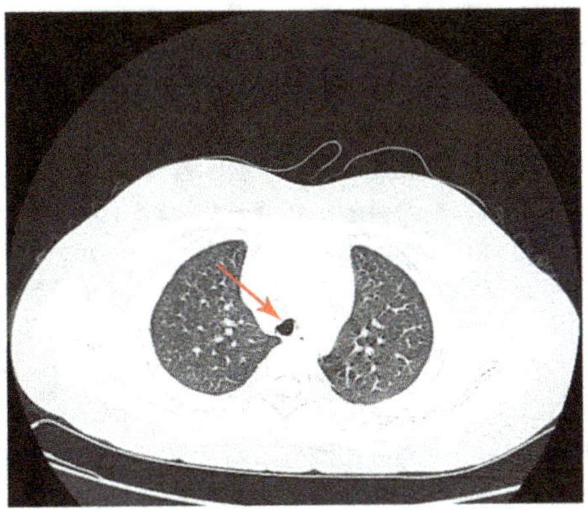

FIGURE 4 | Chest computed tomography at 1 year postoperatively shows that the anterior wall of the trachea has collapsed slightly.

DISCUSSION

Primary endobronchial and endotracheal tumors are uncommon in childhood. Of these, benign tumors consist of inflammatory pseudotumors (plasma cell granulomas), papillomas, hamartomas, mucus gland tumors, leiomyomas, and hemangiomas (7). Malignant tumors include mucoepidermoid carcinomas, carcinoids, adenoid cystic carcinomas, and bronchial adenomas (an obvious misnomer). The most common benign primary pulmonary tumors in children are inflammatory pseudotumors, followed by hamartomas (7).

Hamartomas in the lung are slow and abnormal growing neoplasms that are defined as a tumor-like malformation in which there is abnormal mixing of the normal components of the organ. In other words, a pulmonary hamartoma is a rare benign tumor that originates from the bronchial primitive mesenchymal tissue and can differentiate into various mature mesenchymal components (8). The histogenesis of hamartoma remains unclear. However, there are four etiologic theories: neoplasia, hyperplasia of a normal structure, congenital malformation, and response to inflammation. Both intraparenchymal and endobronchial hamartomas generally contain cartilage, bone, fat, and muscle tissue. Endobronchial hamartomas tend to have more fat than intraparenchymal hamartomas, which may be attributed to the relative abundance of fat in the tracheal walls as opposed to the lung parenchyma (9). This may partially explain why the mass in our patient was composed mainly of fatty tissue.

Patients with endotracheal hamartomas are generally asymptomatic, at least in the preocclusive early phase. The presenting symptoms including cough, dyspnea, hemoptysis, chest pain, purulent sputum, and fever are induced by tracheobronchial obstruction and can lead to recurrent pneumonia (10). As the clinical symptoms are not specific and depend on the size and localization of the tumor, endotracheal hamartomas are often misdiagnosed as more benign conditions, delaying definitive treatment (6, 11). Clinically, the differential diagnoses include aspirated foreign bodies, ectopic thyroid tissue, mucosal webs, cysts, as well as malignancies, including lipoma and lymphoma. With the popularization of CT and magnetic resonance imaging (MRI), it is often possible to determine a diagnosis or narrow the differential diagnosis list. Computed tomography (CT) is sensitive in diagnosing fat collections or calcifications. Fortunately, the hamartoma in our case mainly contained fat. In addition, the present patient was in a sitting breathing state because of airway obstruction caused by the hamartoma before surgery and could not tolerate lying flat for a long time for MRI examination. For these two reasons, we did not perform MRI. However, some hamartomas containing neither fat nor calcification are difficult to differentiate from malignant tumors. Magnetic resonance imaging is an excellent diagnostic tool for the evaluation of soft tissue tumors and has great diagnostic value for detecting the typical cleft-like structure in a pulmonary lesion when neither fat nor calcification is present on CT (12). Therefore, MRI may serve as an adjuvant or alternative diagnostic method to CT for thoracic lesions. However, the definitive diagnosis of hamartoma depends on the histological examination.

Surgical removal of the tumor in older patients should be done only when the tumor is symptomatic or if malignant transformation is suspected. In contrast to adults, peripheral and central hamartomas in children can cause marked symptoms and require prompt surgical removal. The traditional treatment is pneumonectomy or thoracotomy combined with bronchial resection in children (13). However, the first-line widely recommended therapy in adults is endoscopic treatment due to the benign nature of this disease with extremely rare malignant transformation and low recurrence rate (14). Our pediatric patient underwent successful airway recanalization via a flexible bronchoscope. However, due to the low incidence of this condition, experience with the endotracheal resection of hamartomas is relatively limited and there is no standard management for endotracheal hamartoma. Interventional bronchoscopic techniques utilized to manage airway lesions include electrosurgical snaring, APC, cryotherapy, and laser ablation. In the present case, the use of snare electrocautery minimized the bleeding risk by simultaneously cauterizing the base of the tumor during resection. Additionally, considering the unknown nature of the lesion at the time of presentation, we did not perform cryotherapy and APC to achieve hemostasis and destroy the residual tissue immediately after electrocautery. The bronchoscopic treatment options are dependent on the location and characteristics of the airway lesion, physician's preference, expertise, and device availability (6).

Rigid bronchoscopy is probably the best conduit for managing endotracheal lesions, although bronchoscopy via a LMA is a viable option. However, it is important to note that the parents of pediatric patients tend to choose FB. Because the patient could not tolerate anesthesia at the local hospital, he was unable to undergo RB there. Therefore, we chose to use bronchoscopy via a LMA rather than RB. The advantage of LMA general anesthesia is that it enables control of the patient's breathing and provides a large space for endoscopic operation. If it had been difficult to remove the tumor under FB, we would have attempted mechanical debulking under RB. If the patient had not been able to tolerate laryngeal mask anesthesia, we would have attempted to resect the mass via FB under tracheal intubation anesthesia. If we had been unable to remove the mass via FB under tracheal intubation anesthesia, the thoracic surgeon would have performed an open thoracotomy. The extracorporeal membrane oxygenation team was ready to provide emergency treatment if the vital signs became unstable. The management of pulmonary hamartoma might be highly center- and patient-dependent. There is no gold standard due to the rare nature of the lesion and lack of uniformity in expertise among centers in managing such cases. Therefore, a large prospective clinical trial is needed.

The electrocautery snare has the ability to sever a large mass quickly with concomitant hemostasis. The advantages of electrosurgery via FB are the provision of larger tissue specimens for more accurate histological diagnosis, recanalization of the involved airway, better assessment of the tumor base, more accurate surgical planning, stabilization of the patient to enable them to undergo surgery in a better general condition, and minimization of the bleeding risk by simultaneous cauterization of the base of the tumor during resection. Despite the partial residual tissue (**Figure 2D**), our patient's symptoms were relieved immediately after electrocautery, indicating that electrosurgical snaring is a potentially useful method with which to manage endotracheal hamartoma. Once the emergency situation was handled, the next step was to evaluate the need for further management depending on the histopathology. Although we advised further bronchoscopic debulking (e.g., cryotherapy and APC) of the residual mass (**Figure 2D**) based on the histopathologic result, the parents chose serial clinic visits, imaging, and airway inspections rather than bronchoscopic debulking. The patient remained recurrence- and symptom-free and the airway remained patent following bronchoscopic surveillance at the 1-year follow-up (**Figures 2E, 4**); this indicates that the outcome of electrosurgical snaring via FB for tracheal hamartoma appears to be satisfactory, although the long-term survival remains to be assessed. Hence, our experience suggests that bronchoscopic treatment can be considered as a bridging therapy to definitive treatment.

As hamartoma is a benign neoplasm, endoscopic treatment is now widely recommended as the first-line approach. Theoretically, hamartoma can be managed endoscopically in all age groups. However, the diameter of the electrosurgical snare and the working channel of the flexible bronchoscope limit the wide application of this technique. The diameter of the flexible electrocautery snare is 1.9 mm, which can pass through the working channel of the flexible bronchoscope BF-P260 (external diameter: 4.0 mm, working channel: 2.0 mm). As the smallest flexible bronchoscope with a 2.0-mm working channel, our experience suggests that the Olympus P260 can be used in children older than 2 years. Thus, electrosurgical snaring might be useful for endoscopically managing tumors in children $\geq$2 years.

The common complications of electrosurgical snaring include bleeding, perforation, and endotracheal burns (15). The main reason for bleeding during electrocautery snaring is that the snare shrinks too fast when cutting the tumor, which makes the electrical cut a simple mechanical cut, leading to tumor tearing and bleeding. The optimal strategy to prevent bleeding is to cut the mass slowly, so that there is enough time to cauterize the basal tissue while cutting the mass, and the basal tissue is coagulated and denatured. The main reason for airway wall perforation is that the direction of electric cutting deviates from the direction of the bronchus during the treatment process. Therefore, a good visual field should be maintained to avoid the cutting angle deviating from the direction of the bronchus. Using APC cauterization or cryotherapy at the mass root can reduce the risk of tumor recurrence. In the present case, we did not perform mass root interventional therapy because the airway obstruction was relieved after mass resection via the electrocautery snare, and the pathological diagnosis was not clear at that time. Although a small part of the tumor remained after resection, the patient had no symptoms, and the parents were not willing to consent to further thoracotomy. If the tumor continues to grow, thoracotomy is the best option.

Although interventional bronchoscopy is a mature technique in adults, it is seldom used in children. However, our case suggests that under careful preparation, interventional bronchoscopy can be safe and beneficial in pediatric patients.

CONCLUSION

Endotracheal hamartoma is a rare benign tumor, and bronchoscopic therapy is recommended as the first-line treatment, although surgical resection may be necessary under certain conditions. Clinicians should consider the presence of tracheal lesions such as hamartomas in pediatric patients who obtain no significant improvement of respiratory symptoms after conventional treatment.

AUTHOR CONTRIBUTIONS

ZC supervised research work. LW and SL participated in collecting information of this case and searched for literatures. All authors participated in the interpretation of the data, contributed to the article, and approved the submitted version.

ACKNOWLEDGMENTS

We thank Min Yang and Dongpi Wang for her assistance. We thank Liwen Bianji, Edanz Editing China (www.liwenbianji.cn/ac), for editing the English text of a draft of this manuscript.

REFERENCES

1. Murray J, Kielkowski D, Leiman G. The prevalence and age distribution of peripheral pulmonary hamartomas in adult males. An autopsy-based study. *S Afr Med J.* (1991) 79:247–9.
2. Ahmed S, Arshad A, Mador, MJ. Endobronchial hamartoma; a rare structural cause of chronic cough. *Respir Med Case Rep.* (2017) 22:224–7. doi: 10.1016/j.rmcr.2017.08.019
3. Lu Z, Qian F, Chen S, Yu G. Pulmonary hamartoma resembling multiple metastases: a case report. *Oncol Lett.* (2014) 7:1885–8. doi: 10.3892/ol.2014.2043
4. Gjevre JA, Myers JL, Prakash, UB. Pulmonary hamartomas. *Mayo Clin Proc.* (1996) 71:14–20. doi: 10.4065/71.1.14
5. Saadi MM, Barakeh DH, Husain S, Hajjar WM. Large multicystic pulmonary chondroid hamartoma in a child presenting as pneumothorax. *Saudi Med J.* (2015) 36:487–9. doi: 10.15537/smj.2015.4.10210
6. Pio L, Varela P, Eliott MJ, Couloigner V, Guillen Burrieza G, Paraboschi I, et al. Pediatric airway tumors: a report from the International Network of Pediatric Airway Teams (INPAT). *Laryngoscope.* (2019) 130:E243–51. doi: 10.1002/lary.28062
7. Jain V, Goel P, Kumar D, Seith A, Sarkar C, Kabra SK, et al. Endobronchial chondroid hamartoma in an infant. *J Pediatr Surg.* (2009) 44:e21–3. doi: 10.1016/j.jpedsurg.2009.06.011
8. Tomashefski JF. Benign endobronchial mesenchymal tumors: their relationship to parenchymal pulmonary hamartomas. *Am J Surg Pathol.* (1982) 6:531. doi: 10.1097/00000478-198209000-00005
9. Gaerte SC, Meyer CA, Winer-Muram HT, Tarver RD, Conces DJ Jr. Fat-containing lesions of the chest. *Radiographics.* (2002) 22:S61. doi: 10.1148/radiographics.22.suppl_1.g02oc08s61
10. Mondello B. Giant endobronchial hamartoma resected by fiberoptic bronchoscopy electrosurgical snaring. *J Cardiothorac Surg.* (2011) 6:97. doi: 10.1186/1749-8090-6-97
11. Varela P. Pio L, Torre M. Primary tracheobronchial tumors in children. *Semin Pediatr Surg.* (2016) 25:150–5. doi: 10.1053/j.sempedsurg.2016.02.013
12. Park KY, Kim SJ, Noh TW, Cho SH, Lee DY, Paik HC, et al. Diagnostic efficacy and characteristic feature of MRI in pulmonary hamartoma: comparison with CT, specimen MRI, and pathology. *J Comput Assist Tomogr.* (2008) 32:919–25. doi: 10.1097/RCT.0b013e31815abed4
13. Borro JM, Moya J, Botella JA, Padilla JD, Canto A, Paris F. Endobronchial hamartoma. Report of 7 cases. *Scand J Thorac Cardiovasc Surg.* (1989) 23:285–7. doi: 10.3109/14017438909106011
14. Sedat A, Levent D, Levent KC, Erdogan L, Sinem T, Nur S. Resection of giant endobronchial hamartoma by electrocautery and cryotherapy via flexible bronchoscopy. *Tüberk Toraks.* (2007) 55:390–4.
15. van Boxem TJ, Westerga J, Venmans BJ, Postmus PE, Sutedja, TG. Tissue effects of bronchoscopic electrocautery: bronchoscopic appearance and histologic changes of bronchial wall after electrocautery. *Chest.* (2000) 117:887–91. doi: 10.1378/chest.117.3.887

15

Thoracoscopy for Esophageal Diverticula After Esophageal Atresia with Tracheo-Esophageal Fistula

*Zhao Yong†, Wang Dingding†, Hua Kaiyun, Gu Yichao, Zhang Yanan, Liao Junmin, Yang Shen, Li Shuangshuang, Wang Peize and Huang Jinshi**

Department of Neonatal Surgery, Beijing Children's Hospital, National Center for Children's Health, Capital Medical University, Beijing, China

Correspondence:
Huang Jinshi
jsdr2002@126.com

Background: Esophageal diverticulum (ED) is an extremely rare complication of congenital esophageal atresia (EA) with or without tracheoesophageal fistula (TEF) surgery. We aimed to investigate feasible methods for the treatment of this rare complication.

Methods: We retrospectively reviewed all patients with EA/TEF at Beijing Children's Hospital from January 2015 to September 2019. The clinicopathological features of patients with ED after EA/TEF surgery were recorded. Follow-up was routinely performed after surgery until December 2020.

Results: Among 198 patients with EA/TEF, ED only occurred in four patients (2.02%; one male, three female). The four patients had varying complications after the initial operation, including anastomotic leakage (3/4), esophageal stenosis (3/4), and recurrence of TEF (1/4). The main clinical symptoms of ED included recurrent pneumonia (4/4), coughing (4/4), and dysphagia (3/4). All ED cases occurred near the esophageal anastomosis. Patients' age at the time of diverticulum repair was 6.6–16.8 months. All patients underwent thoracoscopic esophageal diverticulectomy (operation time: 1.5–3.5 h). Anastomotic leakage occurred in one patient and spontaneously healed after 2 weeks. The other three patients had no peri-operative complications. All patients were routinely followed up after surgery for 14–36 months. During the follow-up period, all patients could eat orally, had good growth and weight gain, and showed no ED recurrence or anastomotic leakage on esophagogram.

Conclusions: ED is a rare complication after EA/TEF surgery and is a clear indication for diverticulectomy. During the midterm follow-up, thoracoscopic esophageal diverticulectomy was safe and effective for ED after EA/TEF surgery.

Keywords: esophageal diverticulum, esophageal atresia, tracheoesophageal fistula, thoracoscopic, children

INTRODUCTION

Congenital esophageal atresia (EA) with or without tracheoesophageal fistula (TEF) is a serious digestive malformation with an incidence of ~1/2000–4500 (1). Esophageal diverticulum (ED) is a diverticulum of one or more layers of the esophageal wall. ED can be divided into two types; the true diverticulum includes the full layers of the esophageal wall, and the pseudo diverticulum only includes the mucosa and submucosa (2). ED is relatively rare in adults, with an incidence of ~0.06–4%, and mainly occurs in the elderly (3). Additionally, ED can occur as an extremely rare complication of EA/TEF surgery. Currently, only a few studies have reported the occurrence of ED after EA/TEF surgery. According to different reports, the incidence of ED is between 0.0% and 1.9% in patients who have undergone EA/TEF surgery (4–6). However, to the best of our knowledge, no reports have described the diagnosis and treatment of ED after EA/TEF surgery.

In this study, we retrospectively analyzed the diagnosis and treatment of patients with ED after EA/TEF surgery at our hospital. The objective of this study was to discuss feasible diagnostic and treatment methods for this rare complication after EA/TEF surgery.

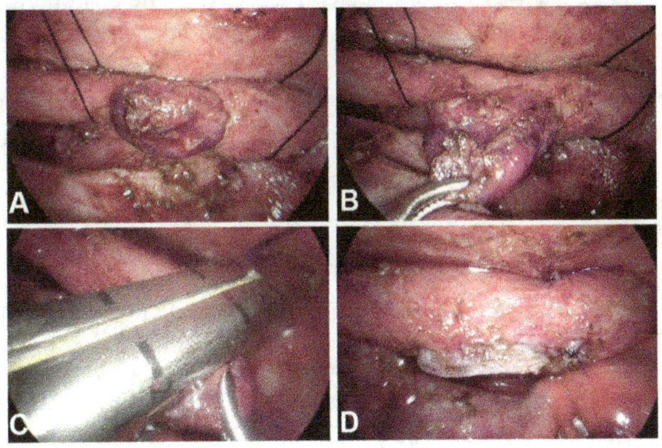

FIGURE 1 | (A,B) The neck of the esophageal diverticulum (ED) was fully exposed. **(C)** The linear cutter stapler was positioned at the neck of the ED and close to the esophagus. **(D)** The ED was excised by the stapler.

PATIENTS AND METHODS

Data Collection

We retrospectively reviewed all patients with EA/TEF at our institution between January 2015 and September 2019. Patients with ED after EA/TEF surgery were selected, and the clinicopathological features were recorded. Follow-up was routinely performed after surgery. This retrospective study was approved by the ethics committee of Beijing Children's Hospital (approval no. 2019-k-333), and the families of all patients provided written informed consent and agreed to participate in the study.

Diagnostic Method

Esophageal angiography was used to define the diagnosis of ED after EA/TEF and to evaluate the size and site of ED. Airway endoscopy, digestive endoscopy, and chest computed tomography (CT) were routinely performed to exclude other related diseases before diverticulectomy.

Surgical Method

Thoracoscopic esophageal diverticulectomy was routinely performed from the right side. A 5-mm thoracoscope was placed in the fifth intercostal space of the right infrascapular line. Two 3-mm trocars were placed in the second intercostal space in the mid axillary line and the fifth intercostal space in the posterior axillary line to establish operating channels. The intrathoracic pressure was maintained at 6–8 mmHg. The adhesion between the lung tissue and chest cavity was loosened, and the neck of the ED was fully exposed. The left-hand operating hole replaced with a 10-mm trocar, a surgical linear cutter stapler with a nail length of 30 mm, was inserted, and the diverticulum close to the esophagus was resected (**Figure 1**). The chest drainage tube was routinely indwelled. After the operation, patients were routinely transferred to the pediatric intensive care unit (PICU) under tracheal intubation.

Postoperative Follow-Up

Routine esophagogram was performed 7 and 14 days after the operation during hospitalization. Outpatient follow-up and esophagogram were routinely scheduled in the first month, third month and 6 month after surgery. Then outpatient follow-up was scheduled every 3 months during the first 1 year after surgery and every 6 months thereafter. If postoperative esophageal stenosis was found by esophagogram, endoscopy was used to detect and treat the stenosis with endoscopic balloon dilatation. All patients were followed up until the end of December 2020.

RESULTS

Among the 198 patients with EA/TEF at our institution between January 2015 and September 2019, ED only occurred in four patients (2.02%) during the follow-up period. Of these four patients, one was male, and three were female. EA repair surgery, including open or thoracoscopic ligation of the fistula and end-to-end anastomosis of esophageal segments, was performed in all patients 1 week after birth. The four patients had various complications after the initial operation, including anastomotic leakage (3/4), esophageal stenosis (3/4), and recurrence of TEF (1/4). Two patients also had malformations of other systems, including scoliosis (1/4) and vertebral deformities (2/4). The main clinical symptoms of ED included recurrent pneumonia (4/4), coughing (4/4), and dysphagia (3/4). All diverticula were located near the esophageal anastomosis, between T3 and T6, and all were therefore thoracic ED. Patient age at the time of diagnosing ED ranged from 2.5 to 9.3 months (median age: 6.2 months). The patient age of diverticulum repair was 6.6 to 16.8 months (median age: 9.5 months). By the time of diverticulectomy, the average long diameter of these EDs increased from 15.2 to 22.2 mm. Body weight at the time of operation was 6.5–9.5 kg (median weight: 7.3 kg). All four patients underwent a thoracoscopic esophageal diverticulectomy. Owing to recurrent TEF, patient 4 underwent thoracoscopic TEF resection at the same time. The operation time ranged from 1.5 to 3.5 h (average: 2.2 h). In all patients, intra-operative bleeding was <5 mL, and no blood transfusions were required during the operation. After the operation, patients were routinely transferred to the PICU. The postoperative time of invasive ventilator use was 1–7 days (average: 3 days). The postoperative hospital stay time was 10–20 days (average: 14 days). In patient 4, anastomotic leakage occurred 1 week after surgery, as observed by esophagogram. After enteral nutrition via a nasojejunal tube and conservative supportive treatment were performed, the anastomotic leakage healed after 2 weeks, as demonstrated by radiography. The other three patients had no peri-operative complications. Clinicopathological data for the four patients with ED after EA/TEF are shown in **Table 1**.

All patients were routinely followed up after surgery for 14–36 months. During the follow-up period, all patients were able to eat by mouth and had good growth and satisfactory weight gain, without coughing, pneumonia, or dysphagia. Additionally, esophagogram revealed no ED recurrence or anastomotic leakage.

Illustrative Cases

Patient 1 was a 6.6-month-old girl who was diagnosed with congenital EA type IIIa after birth. Five days after birth, the patient underwent thoracoscopic ligation of the fistula and end-to-end anastomosis of the esophageal segments. Esophagogram indicated leakage of esophageal anastomosis at 2 weeks after surgery, which healed after conservative treatment. At 2.5 months, the patient visited our outpatient clinic for choking and repeated pneumonia. Esophagogram revealed a 14.8 mm diverticulum at the right posterior edge of the esophagus. The symptoms were not significantly relieved by conservative treatment. The esophagus re-examination 6 months after birth showed that the long ED diameter increased to 25.5 mm, compared to its initial examination. Airway endoscopy and digestive endoscopy showed that the ED did not communicate with the trachea; chest CT was performed to exclude inflammatory consolidation of the lung. The patient underwent thoracoscopic esophageal diverticulectomy, and postoperative pathology revealed a pseudodiverticulum, which only contained mucosa and submucosa tissues without muscle tissue involvement. After the operation, the coughing and pneumonia symptoms disappeared, and the patient was gradually able to consume a normal diet. The patient was followed up for 23 months without symptoms.

Patient 2 was a 9.5-month-old girl diagnosed with congenital EA type IIIb and underwent thoracotomy ligation of the fistula and end-to-end anastomosis esophageal segments 5 days after birth. At 2 months, the patient had recurrent TEF. After conservative treatment and enteral nutrition for 2 months, she underwent thoracoscopic ligation of recurrent TEF 4 months after birth. In 6.2 months, the patient had dysphagia, and the esophagogram revealed esophageal stenosis and an ED at the upper edge of the esophageal stenosis. Then, she underwent endoscopic balloon dilatation three times, which was expanded to 10 mm. However, the patient still exhibited choking and repeated pneumonia. Esophagogram and endoscopy revealed that the ED increased from 15.7 mm to 22.1 mm. The patient underwent thoracoscopic esophageal diverticulectomy, and postoperative pathology revealed a true diverticulum, which contained a thickened muscle layer in the diverticula wall. After the operation, the symptoms of coughing and pneumonia

TABLE 1 | Clinicopathological features of patients with esophageal diverticulum after esophageal atresia/tracheoesophageal fistula surgery.

ID	Gender	Age of diagnosis (months)	Age of surgery (months)	Body Weight (kg)	Symptoms	Long diameter (mm)	Site	Complications after the initial surgery	Combined deformity	Operation time (h)	Tracheal intubation time (d)	Postoperative hospital stay	Postoperative complications	Postoperative pathology
1	Female	2.5	6.6	6.5	Coughing, recurrent pneumonia	25.5	T3-5	Anastomotic leakage	None	2	3	12	None	Pseudodiverticulum
2	Female	6.2	9.5	8.0	Dysphagia, Coughing, recurrent pneumonia	22.1	T4-5	Esophageal stricture	Scoliosis, vertebral deformities	1.5	1	10	None	True diverticulum
3	Female	6.8	13.1	9.5	Dysphagia, Coughing, recurrent pneumonia	24.6	T4-6	Anastomotic leakage, esophageal stricture	None	1.5	5	14	None	Pseudodiverticulum
4	Male	9.3	16.8	6.0	Dysphagia, Coughing, recurrent pneumonia	16.7	T4-5	Anastomotic leakage, esophageal stricture, recurrent TEF	Vertebral deformities	3.5	7	20	Anastomotic leakage, esophageal stricture	Pseudodiverticulum

ED, esophageal diverticulum; EA, esophageal atresia; TEF, tracheoesophageal fistula.

disappeared. The patient was followed up for 33 months without symptoms.

Patient 3 was a 13.1-month-old girl. Three days after birth, the patient underwent thoracotomy ligation of the fistula and end-to-end anastomosis of the esophageal segments due to congenital EA type IIIb. Anastomotic leakage occurred 2 weeks after surgery and healed after conservative treatment of 4 weeks. At 6.8 months of age, the patient exhibited repeated vomiting, choking, and pneumonia. Esophagogram showed gastroesophageal reflux and right-side ED at the T4–6 level (**Figure 2**). The 24-h pH test confirmed pathological reflux in the lower esophagus. At 8 months of age, she underwent laparoscopic fundoplication to improve gastroesophageal reflux. After the operation, coughing and repeated pneumonia symptoms were still observed, and endoscopic balloon dilatation of the esophageal stenosis was performed several times, gradually expanding to 12 mm. She still had repeated pneumonia and choking, and re-examination of esophagogram and endoscopy revealed that the ED increased from 17.1 mm to 24.6 mm. Thoracoscopic esophageal diverticulectomy was performed, and the pathological response showed no muscle layer in the diverticula wall, indicating the presence of pseudodiverticulum. After the operation, the patient's coughing symptoms improved, and she gradually returned to a normal diet. The patient was followed up for 36 months without symptoms.

Patient 4 was a 16.8-month-old boy with congenital EA type IIIb who underwent thoracotomy ligation of the fistula and end-to-end anastomosis of esophageal segments 3 days after birth. Postoperative esophageal anastomotic leakage occurred, and complication was alleviated after conservative treatment. Recurrent TEF was diagnosed 5 months after birth, and conservative treatment for pneumonia and enteral nutrition were performed. In 9.3 months, esophagogram and endoscopy revealed an ED on the right side of the esophagus, except for recurrent TEF and esophageal stenosis (**Figure 3**). Then, he underwent thoracoscopic ligation of recurrent TEF. However, he still had repeated pneumonia and choking after surgery. At 16 months after birth, esophagogram showed the ED increased from 13.0 mm to 16.7 mm and a novel recurrent TEF on the left side. Thoracoscopic ligation of the recurrent TEF and esophageal diverticulectomy were performed. Pathological examination showed no muscle layer in the diverticula wall, indicating pseudodiverticulum. One week after surgery, anastomotic leakage occurred by esophagogram, which healed spontaneously after conservative treatment for 1 week. Two months postoperatively, the patient underwent endoscopic balloon dilatation due to esophageal stenosis, which gradually expanded to 12 mm. He slowly returned to his normal diet after the operation and was followed up for 14 months without symptoms.

DISCUSSION

ED is an extremely rare complication of EA/TEF surgery. Myers et al. reported that among 498 patients with EA/TEF after surgery, the incidence of ED was only 0.2% (6). Taghavi et al. found that among 56 patients with H-type treated by surgery, the incidence of ED was 1.9% (5). Additionally, in a study evaluating the postoperative complications of 92 patients with EA/TEF, ED did not occur in any of the 92 patients after surgery (4). Among the 198 patients with EA/TEF at our institution, ED only occurred in four patients after surgery, with an incidence rate of 2.02%. This was consistent with the results of these previous studies, confirming that ED was a rare complication after EA/TEF surgery.

According to its pathogenesis, ED is divided into two types, i.e., pulsion diverticulum and traction diverticulum. Most ED cases are pulsion diverticulum, which is related to esophageal dysmotility, functional or mechanical obstruction, or weakness of the esophageal wall. The esophageal sphincter cannot relax normally, resulting in compression of the esophageal cavity and forcing the mucosa and submucosa to herniate through the esophageal muscles (pseudodiverticulum). Traction diverticulum is relatively rare. The inflammatory reaction around the esophagus causes scarring of the esophageal wall, and local traction of the esophageal wall leads to the formation of a diverticulum (true diverticulum). The primary pulsion diverticulum commonly occurs at the proximal and distal ends of the esophagus and includes Zenker diverticulum and epiphrenic diverticulum. In contrast, traction diverticulum, including thoracic ED, commonly occurs in the middle of the esophagus (2, 7, 8). In all four patients in our series, ED was considered thoracic ED; however, the pathogenesis of ED after EA/TEF surgery is different from that of the primary ED. Our four patients had various complications after the initial operation. For example, anastomotic leakage occurred in three patients after the initial surgery, and the pathological results of these three cases after diverticulectomy showed no muscle structures involved, suggestive of pseudodiverticulum. The formation mechanism in these cases may be related to continuous saliva and esophageal secretions through the anastomosis, resulting in persistent pleurisy and local inflammation around the esophagus and thereby causing the formation of cavities and local fibrosis. Moreover, the distal esophagus combined with stenosis resulted in increased pressure in the proximal esophagus, forcing the mucosa and submucosa to herniate via the anastomotic fistula to form the ED. The pathology results for patient 2 after diverticulectomy revealed the involvement of muscular structures, indicating true diverticulum. The patient did not experience anastomotic leakage after surgery; however, recurrent TEF occurred in the patient after 2 months. In the second surgery for recurrent TEF, the fistula was ligated close to the trachea, resulting in an excessively long esophageal fistula. Additionally, these features combined with anastomotic stricture of the esophagus led to increased pressure in the proximal esophageal cavity, and the stump of the esophageal fistula gradually expanded to form a diverticulum. Livaditis esophageal myotomy can lead to ED after EA/TEF surgery (9). None of the children in our study underwent Livaditis esophageal myotomy during the initial operation. The pathogenesis of ED after EA/TEF surgery was different from that of the primary ED and may be related to esophageal anastomosis leakage, anastomotic stricture or the long esophageal fistula stump, especially for patients with multiple

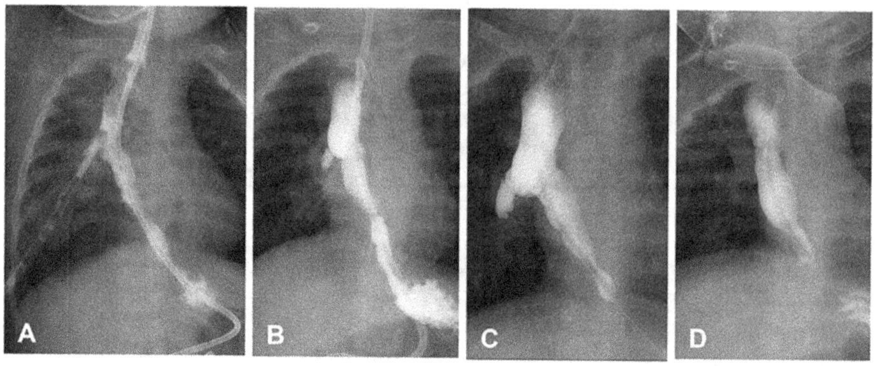

FIGURE 2 | Changes in the esophageal diverticulum (ED) of patient 3. **(A)** After esophageal atresia/tracheoesophageal fistula surgery, the contrast agent flowed into the chest drainage tube through the esophageal anastomosis leakage. **(B)** The thoracoscopic drainage tube was removed prematurely, and the ED appeared. **(C)** The ED was enlarged. **(D)** Two weeks after diverticulectomy, the esophagus was in good shape. In C and D, the patient underwent laparoscopic fundoplication, leading to postoperative distal esophageal stenosis.

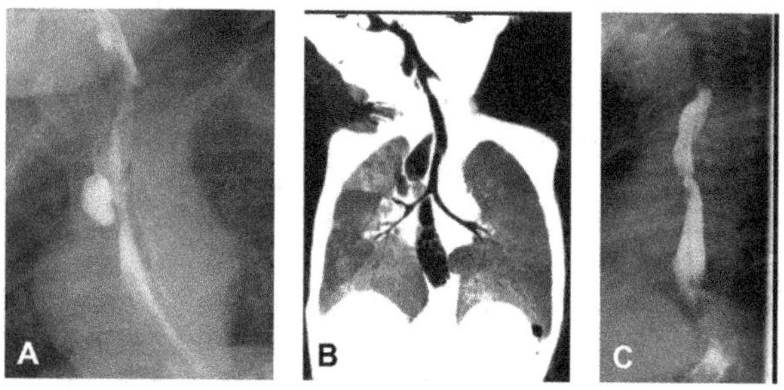

FIGURE 3 | The pre-operative and postoperative radiography of patient 4. **(A)** Esophagogram revealed esophageal diverticulum (ED) (on the right side of the esophagus) combined with recurrent tracheoesophageal fistula (on the left side of the esophagus). **(B)** ED on chest computed tomography. **(C)** Two weeks after diverticulectomy.

complications. For patients who had anastomosis leakage after surgery, early and aggressive endoscopic balloon dilatation for preventing anastomotic stricture might help in reducing the occurrence of ED. However, further studies are still needed to elucidate the detailed pathogenesis of this condition.

The common symptoms of thoracic ED in adults include dysphagia, gastroesophageal reflux, heartburn, aspiration pneumonia, and weight loss (10, 11). In our four patients, the main symptoms included recurrent pneumonia, dysphagia, coughing, and unsatisfactory weight gain. These symptoms were similar to the common symptoms of some complications after EA/TEF surgery, such as esophageal stenosis, gastroesophageal reflux, and recurrent TEF. Esophagogram is the preferred diagnostic method for ED; this approach can be used to confirm the diagnosis and evaluate the location and size of ED (12). Airway endoscopy, digestive endoscopy, and chest CT can be used to exclude other related diseases, such as recurrent TEF and inflammatory consolidation of the lung. Measurement of esophageal pressure is the gold standard for diagnosing esophageal dyskinesia. Studies have shown that more than 90% of ED patients may have abnormal esophageal motility; however, it is still unclear whether esophageal dyskinesia was the cause of ED or a symptom of ED (13). Some scholars have suggested that esophageal dyskinesia is always present in patients with ED, indicating that pressure measurement is not required (14). Gastroesophageal reflux is closely related to ED, and 24-h esophageal pH monitoring can confirm gastroesophageal reflux and guide surgical or drug treatment (12). All four patients underwent esophageal angiography to confirm the diagnosis of ED. All patients underwent airway endoscopy, digestive endoscopy, and chest CT, and recurrent TEF was diagnosed in patient 4. Moreover, 24-h esophageal pH monitoring was used to confirm the symptoms of gastroesophageal reflux in patient 3, which indicated pathological reflux, and laparoscopic fundoplication was performed. Esophagogram was a preferred diagnosis method for patients with ED after EA/TEF surgery. Moreover, airway endoscopy, digestive endoscopy, and chest CT should be performed to exclude surgical contraindications. Esophageal pH monitoring is a useful examination method for symptomatic patients. Comprehensive examination could contribute to the evaluation and provide direction for subsequent surgical approaches.

In adult thoracic ED, most surgeons agreed to surgical intervention in symptomatic patients; however, the treatment of patients with the mild or asymptomatic disease remains controversial (15-19). Altorki et al. reported that aspiration occurred in nine of 20 adult patients, and three experienced life-threatening complications (20). They strongly supported surgical intervention for all patients. Macke et al. summarized 15 years of experience in the treatment of thoracic ED in adults and concluded that surgical intervention should be carried out for patients with asymptomatic large diverticula or abnormal esophageal motility; additionally, asymptomatic patients, particularly those with a high risk of surgery, should be closely monitored (11). All four patients in this series had obvious clinical symptoms. Because infants and young children are more prone to aspiration, coughing, and other symptoms, we recommend that active surgical intervention be performed for mild or even asymptomatic ED after EA/TEF. Notably, anastomotic stricture should be treated aggressively before esophageal diverticulectomy, which might be the cause of ED.

The surgical treatment of thoracic ED mainly included open surgical approaches and minimally invasive approaches. With advancements in minimally invasive techniques, the surgical linear cutter stapler has become widely used in pediatric gastrointestinal surgery (20–22). All four patients in this group underwent thoracoscopic esophageal diverticulectomy, and we identified four technical details related to the surgery. First, it was necessary to fully expose the neck of the diverticulum during the separation of the diverticula. The surgical linear cutter stapler must be inserted close to the esophagus to avoid leaving a residual diverticulum. Second, placing a gastric tube could help stabilize the esophagus and prevent esophageal cavity stricture. Third, the muscles or pleura around the staple line of the esophagus should be freed to reduce the incidence of anastomotic leakage. Finally, three of the four patients in this series had pseudodiverticulum, and the diverticula wall had no muscle tissue. The cutter stapler might be useful to cut the pseudodiverticulum but not hand-tied ligature. Additionally, using a cutter stapler could reduce the operation time and the incidence of postoperative anastomotic leakage. None of the patients in the study underwent transit thoracotomy. Anastomotic leakage and esophageal stricture occurred in one patient 1 week after surgery; this symptom was alleviated by conservative treatment and balloon dilatation. The other three patients had no peri-operative complications. During the follow-up period, none of the patients had any other complications. Thoracoscopic esophageal diverticulectomy proved to be a reliable and effective treatment method for ED after EA/TEF, but must be performed by surgeons experienced in open and minimally invasive esophageal surgery.

Currently, the use of routine or selective esophageal Heller's myotomy during diverticulectomy for ED in adults is controversial. Studies have reported that the incidence of esophageal dyskinesia in adults with ED is 45–100% (23–27). Simple mechanical obstruction or combined functional obstruction could lead to increased pressure in the esophageal cavity and the formation of the ED. Therefore, some surgeons tend to routinely perform Heller's myotomy, regardless of the presence or absence of distal esophageal dyskinesia (25). In contrast, other researchers have been more inclined to perform Heller surgery when distal esophageal dyskinesia is clearly diagnosed before surgery (18). Because the pathogenesis of ED after EA/TEF is different from that of adult ED, the main factor resulting in increased pressure in the esophageal cavity was esophageal stenosis, which could be eliminated by endoscopic balloon dilation. Therefore, we recommend that ED after EA/TEF surgery may not require routine Heller surgery. None of the four patients in this study underwent Heller surgery. During the follow-up period, none of the patients had shown symptoms such as distal esophageal stenosis or recurrence of ED. However, long-term follow-up is still needed to assess this issue.

However, the study also has several limitations. Due to the rarity of this complication, the number of patients is small, which is not suitable for statistical analysis. The possible risk factors for ED after EA/TEF still need to be confirmed by larger samples. Additionally, the study is a single-center retrospective research, and more clinical prospective studies are required to confirm our results.

In summary, ED is a rare complication after EA/TEF surgery and is a clear indication for diverticulectomy. Our results showed that thoracoscopic esophageal diverticulectomy was safe and effective for ED after EA/TEF surgery during mid-term follow-up. Further follow-up is needed to assess the reliability of these results. Additionally, surgical treatment is suggested to be performed by surgeons with extensive thoracoscopic experience.

AUTHOR CONTRIBUTIONS

ZYo, WD, and HJ contributed to conception and design of the study. GY analyzed the data. HK and LJ processed the figures. ZYo and WD wrote the first draft of the manuscript. LS, WP, and ZYa wrote sections of the manuscript. All authors contributed to the article and approved the submitted version.

REFERENCES

1. Sfeir R, Michaud L, Salleron J, Gottrand F. Epidemiology of esophageal atresia. *Dis Esophagus.* (2013) 26:354–5. doi: 10.1111/dote.12051
2. Smith CD. Esophageal strictures and diverticula. *Surg Clin North Am.* (2015) 95:669–81. doi: 10.1016/j.suc.2015.02.017
3. Onwugbufor MT, Obirieze AC, Ortega G, Allen D, Cornwell EE, 3rd, Fullum TM. Surgical management of esophageal diverticulum: a review of the nationwide inpatient sample database. *J Surg Res.* (2013) 184:120–5. doi: 10.1016/j.jss.2013.05.036
4. Zhang J, Wu Q, Chen L, Wang Y, Cui X, Huang W, et al. Clinical analysis of surgery for type III esophageal atresia via thoracoscopy: a study of a Chinese single-center experience. *J Cardiothorac Surg.* (2020) 15:55. doi: 10.1186/s13019-020-01097-z
5. Taghavi K, Tan Tanny SP, Hawley A, Brooks JA, Hutson JM, Teague WJ, et al. H-type congenital tracheoesophageal fistula: insights from 70years of the royal children's hospital experience. *J Pediatr Surg.* (2020). doi: 10.1016/j.jpedsurg.2020.06.048. [Epub ahead of print].
6. Myers NA, Beasley SW, Auldist AW. Secondary esophageal surgery following repair of esophageal atresia with distal tracheoesophageal fistula. *J Pediatr Surg.* (1990) 25:773–7. doi: 10.1016/S0022-3468(05)80017-X
7. Steiner SJ, Cox EG, Gupta SK, Kleiman MB, Fitzgerald JF. Esophageal diverticulum: a complication of histoplasmosis in children. *J Pediatr.* (2005) 146:426–8. doi: 10.1016/j.jpeds.2004.10.020
8. Duda M, Sery Z, Vojacek K, Rocek V, Rehulka M. Etiopathogenesis and classification of esophageal diverticula. *Int Surg.* (1985) 70:291–5.
9. Bagolan P, Iacobelli Bd B, De Angelis P, di Abriola GF, Laviani R, Trucchi A, et al. Long gap esophageal atresia and esophageal replacement: moving toward a separation? *J Pediatr Surg.* (2004) 39:1084–90. doi: 10.1016/j.jpedsurg.2004.03.048
10. Rosati R, Fumagalli U, Elmore U, de Pascale S, Massaron S, Peracchia A. Long-term results of minimally invasive surgery

for symptomatic epiphrenic diverticulum. *Am J Surg.* (2011) 201:132–5. doi: 10.1016/j.amjsurg.2010.03.016

11. Macke RA, Luketich JD, Pennathur A, Bianco V, Awais O, Gooding WE, et al. Thoracic0. *Ann Thorac Surg.* (2015) 100:1795–802. doi: 10.1016/j.athoracsur.2015.04.122
12. Herbella FA, Patti MG. Modern pathophysiology and treatment of esophageal diverticula. *Langenbecks Arch Surg.* (2012) 397:29–35. doi: 10.1007/s00423-011-0843-2
13. Hoghooghi D, Coakley FV, Breiman RS, Qayyum A, Yeh BM. Frequency and etiology of midesophageal diverticula at barium esophagography. *Clin Imaging.* (2006) 30:245–7. doi: 10.1016/j.clinimag.2006.02.002
14. Soares R, Herbella FA, Prachand VN, Ferguson MK, Patti MG. Epiphrenic diverticulum of the esophagus. From pathophysiology to treatment. *J Gastrointest Surg.* (2010) 14:2009–15. doi: 10.1007/s11605-010-1216-9
15. Benacci JC, Deschamps C, Trastek VF, Allen MS, Daly RC, Pairolero PC. Epiphrenic diverticulum: results of surgical treatment. *Ann Thorac Surg.* (1993) 55:1109–13; discussion 14. doi: 10.1016/0003-4975(93)90016-B
16. Debas HT, Payne WS, Cameron AJ, Carlson HC. Physiopathology of lower esophageal diverticulum and its implications for treatment. *Surg Gynecol Obstet.* (1980) 151:593–600.
17. Streitz Jr JM, Glick ME, Ellis Jr FH. Selective use of myotomy for treatment of epiphrenic diverticula. Manometric and clinical analysis. *Arch Surg.* (1992) 127:585–7; discussion 7–8. doi: 10.1001/archsurg.1992.01420050109014
18. Castrucci G, Porziella V, Granone PL, Picciocchi A. Tailored surgery for esophageal body diverticula. *Eur J Cardiothorac Surg.* (1998) 14:380–7. doi: 10.1016/S1010-7940(98)00201-2
19. Altorki NK, Sunagawa M, Skinner DB. Thoracic esophageal diverticula. Why is operation necessary? *J Thorac Cardiovasc Surg.* (1993) 105:260–4. doi: 10.1016/S0022-5223(19)33810-3
20. Jackson HT, Kane TD. Advances in minimally invasive surgery in pediatric patients. *Adv Pediatr.* (2014) 61:149–95. doi: 10.1016/j.yapd.2014.03.011
21. Castro Salgado PC, Aragon Lopez SA, Garzon Gonzalez LN, Gutierrez I, Mateus LM, Molina Ramirez ID, et al. Characterization of patients with minimally invasive surgery converted in a pediatric hospital. *J Laparoendosc Adv Surg Tech A.* (2019) 29:1383–7. doi: 10.1089/lap.2019.0190
22. Blinman T, Ponsky T. Pediatric minimally invasive surgery: laparoscopy and thoracoscopy in infants and children. *Pediatrics.* (2012) 130:539–49. doi: 10.1542/peds.2011-2812
23. Vicentine FP, Herbella FA, Silva LC, Patti MG. High resolution manometry findings in patients with esophageal epiphrenic diverticula. *Am Surg.* (2011) 77:1661–4. doi: 10.1177/000313481107701239
24. Reznik SI, Rice TW, Murthy SC, Mason DP, Apperson-Hansen C, Blackstone EH. Assessment of a pathophysiology-directed treatment for symptomatic epiphrenic diverticulum. *Dis Esophagus.* (2007) 20:320–7. doi: 10.1111/j.1442-2050.2007.00716.x
25. Melman L, Quinlan J, Robertson B, Brunt LM, Halpin VJ, Eagon JC, et al. Esophageal manometric characteristics and outcomes for laparoscopic esophageal diverticulectomy, myotomy, and partial fundoplication for epiphrenic diverticula. *Surg Endosc.* (2009) 23:1337–41. doi: 10.1007/s00464-008-0165-9
26. D'Journo XB, Ferraro P, Martin J, Chen LQ, Duranceau A. Lower oesophageal sphincter dysfunction is part of the functional abnormality in epiphrenic diverticulum. *Br J Surg.* (2009) 96:892–900. doi: 10.1002/bjs.6652
27. Thomas ML, Anthony AA, Fosh BG, Finch JG, Maddern GJ. Oesophageal diverticula. *Br J Surg.* (2001) 88:629–42. doi: 10.1046/j.1365-2168.2001.01733.x

16

Robotic Ureteral Reconstruction in the Pediatric Population

Aylin N. Bilgutay[1*] *and Andrew J. Kirsch*[1,2]

[1] *Department of Pediatric Urology, Children's Healthcare of Atlanta, Atlanta, GA, United States,* [2] *Department of Urology, Emory University School of Medicine, Atlanta, GA, United States*

Correspondence:
Aylin N. Bilgutay
aylin.bilgutay@gmail.com

Robot-assisted laparoscopic (RAL) surgery is a safe, minimally invasive technique that has become more widely used in pediatric urology over recent decades. With several advantages over standard laparoscopy, robotic surgery is particularly well-suited to reconstructive surgery involving delicate structures like the ureter. A robotic approach provides excellent access to and visualization of the ureter at all levels. Common applications include upper ureteral reconstruction (e.g., pyeloplasty, ureteropelvic junction polypectomy, ureterocalicostomy, and high uretero-ureterostomy in duplex systems), mid-ureteral reconstruction (e.g., mid uretero-ureterostomy for stricture or polyp), and lower ureteral reconstruction (e.g., ureteral reimplantation and lower ureter-ureterostomy in duplex systems). Herein, we describe each of these robotic procedures in detail.

Keywords: robotic surgery, pediatric urology, pyeloplasty, ureteroureterostomy, vesicoureteral reflux, ureteropelvic junction obstruction, ureterovesical junction obstruction, megaureter

INTRODUCTION

Many considerations are involved in choosing surgical approach. Compared to open surgery, roboticsoffer several advantages including smaller incisions and more rapid convalescence. Robot-assisted laparoscopic (RAL) surgery may, however, be difficult or even impossible in very small patients, in whom pure laparoscopic intervention may be preferred. Pure laparoscopy allows for even smaller incisions than robotic surgery, with ports as small as 2–3 mm available. Another disadvantage of robotic surgery is increased cost compared to pure laparoscopic or open approaches. Benefits of robotic surgery include wristed movements and magnified vision, making it the ideal approach for delicate reconstructive procedures. Robotics continue to enjoy expanding applications and growing popularity among urologists and patient families alike.

UPPER URETERAL RECONSTRUCTION

Pyeloplasty

Pyeloplasty for ureteropelvic junction (UPJ) obstruction is the most common robotic surgery in pediatric urology (1). RAL retroperitoneoscopic pyeloplasty has been described in children (2); however, the transabdominal approach is more frequently utilized, providing a larger working space that facilitates dissection and anastomosis. Transabdominal robotic approach may involve transmesenteric UPJ exposure for left-sided cases to decrease operative time, as previously described for traditional laparoscopic pyeloplasty (3). However, reflecting the colon is usually rapid, and one should not risk limited exposure for potential time savings, particularly in complex cases.

Prior to positioning for the robotic portion of the case, we prefer starting with cystoscopy and retrograde pyelogram to delineate anatomy unless adequately assessed preoperatively with magnetic resonance urogram. A ureteral stent may be placed retrograde if desired. We prefer placing a ureteral stent antegrade during the robotic portion of the case.

Typical patient positioning for transabdominal robotic pyeloplasty is the modified flank/lateral decubitus position with affected side elevated ~45° over a roll, contralateral arm extended on an arm board, and ipsilateral arm straight against the patient's ipsilateral side or extended parallel to the contralateral arm using an elevated armrest or pillows. Alternatively, the patient may be positioned supine with table rotation to elevate the pathologic side (1). One must ensure that all pressure points are adequately padded and the patient is appropriately secured to the table.

The patient is flattened for port placement. The camera port is placed first, usually at the umbilicus, using either open Hasson or Veress needle technique. Some surgeons recommend against the use of Veress needle in children (4). However, we believe that this technique can be applied safely in pediatric cases and have successfully used it for several years at our high volume robotic institution with no complications. For the Si, we use the 8.5 mm robotic camera port. A 10 or 12 mm port (e.g., the Autosuture® balloon trocar) may also be used as the Si robot camera port (5). For the Xi, the camera and working ports are identical, allowing placement of the camera through any port. Robotic working ports are then placed under direct vision. For the Si, 8 and 5 mm robotic ports and instruments are available, while only 8 mm ports/instruments are available for the Xi. We prefer 8 mm robotic ports even with the Si because of the greater variety of instrumentation available. Another advantage of the 8 mm instruments is a shorter intracorporeal length of the wristed segment, with decreased required intracorporeal working distance (5).

For the Si, ideal port placement results in a triangular working field. One working port is placed cephalad to the camera port in the midline or midclavicular line, and the other is placed inferiorly at an ~30° angle rotated from midline toward the kidney of interest (**Figure 1A**). Ports are ideally spaced ~1 hand's breadth apart, but this may be impossible in smaller children and infants. All ports are instead placed in the midline to maximize the limited working space in infants, as close as 3 cm if necessary (5).

Optimal port placement for the Xi robot is in a line rather than triangulated. A third robotic port and/or assistant port(s) may be placed if desired. We usually do not find additional ports necessary. With our typical three-port setup, a robotic instrument must be removed to allow the assistant to suction or pass sutures. This positioning and port placement may be used for any renal or upper ureteral procedure.

The hidden incision endoscopic surgery (HIdES) port placement technique was developed to eliminate visible scarring (6). This involves placing the camera port and one robotic working port below the level of a Pfannenstiel incision and placing the second robotic working port infraumbilically (**Figure 1B**). Incisions are thus hidden beneath the underwear line, which has been shown to be preferable to patients and parents (6, 7).

After port placement, the next step is docking. The bed is rotated to raise the ipsilateral side, and the height of the bed is adjusted as desired. These changes must be made prior to robot docking unless using the Xi system with Trumpf Medical's TruSystem® 7000 dV OR table, which allows "integrated table motion" (OR table movement after docking). With the Si, docking is typically over the ispilateral shoulder at a slight angle or straight in from the side. Docking trajectory is more forgiving with the Xi system, as the robotic arms rotate on the boom into the optimal position when you perform anatomic targeting.

Next, the white line of Toldt is incised, and the colon is reflected medially to expose the retroperitoneum. One may alternatively utilize a transmesenteric approach for left-sided cases. The renal pelvis, UPJ, and ureter are then identified and dissected with limited, low-power cautery use. We routinely use a hitch stitch for traction to facilitate this dissection in the absence of an assistant port. We use a 4–0 Vicryl on an SH needle, which is manually straightened and passed directly through the abdominal wall by the assistant, through-and-through the renal pelvis, then back out the abdominal wall. The assistant may then adjust the tension as desired by the surgeon and snap the stitch in place at the level of the skin. A hitch stitch may not be necessary if the renal pelvis is not too floppy.

Dismemberment is the next step. Depending on UPJ configuration, one may choose an appropriate location and trajectory for renal pelvis transection in order to create an adequately wide pyelotomy for eventual anastomosis. If the UPJ insertion is high, an alternative is to ligate it, transect the proximal ureter, and create a new dependent pyelotomy for anastomosis. Non-dismembered techniques (e.g., Foley Y-V plasty or flap pyeloplasties) are preferred by some authors (8–10). Use of these methods has even been described in the setting of a crossing vessel, with concomitant cephalad translocation of the crossing vessel or Hellström technique (8, 9). Flaps can be particularly useful for long segments of UPJ/ureteral stricture, whereas a Heineke-Mikulicz type pelvotomy (Fenger-plasty) may be sufficient for short strictures (8, 11). We favor the classic Anderson-Hynes dismembered pyeloplasty technique in the majority of cases. Pelvic reduction may be performed if desired; however, this is rarely necessary in our experience.

The proximal ureter is then spatulated. Traditional descriptions favor spatulation along the lateral aspect because the proximal ureteral blood supply arises medially. Spatulation must be continued for an adequate length to ensure a wide anastomosis incorporating healthy ureter. A portion of the proximal ureter may ultimately be excised if it appears unsuitable for reconstruction; however, we recommend leaving such a segment attached for use as a handle until anastomosis is nearly complete. The anastomosis may be performed with running or interrupted fine absorbable suture. Typically, we perform half of the anastomosis with one running 5–0 Vicryl, then place a ureteral stent in antegrade fashion over a wire passed through an angiocatheter advanced directly through the abdominal wall. To confirm appropriate stent positioning, one may have the circulator instill dilute methylene blue solution into the bladder

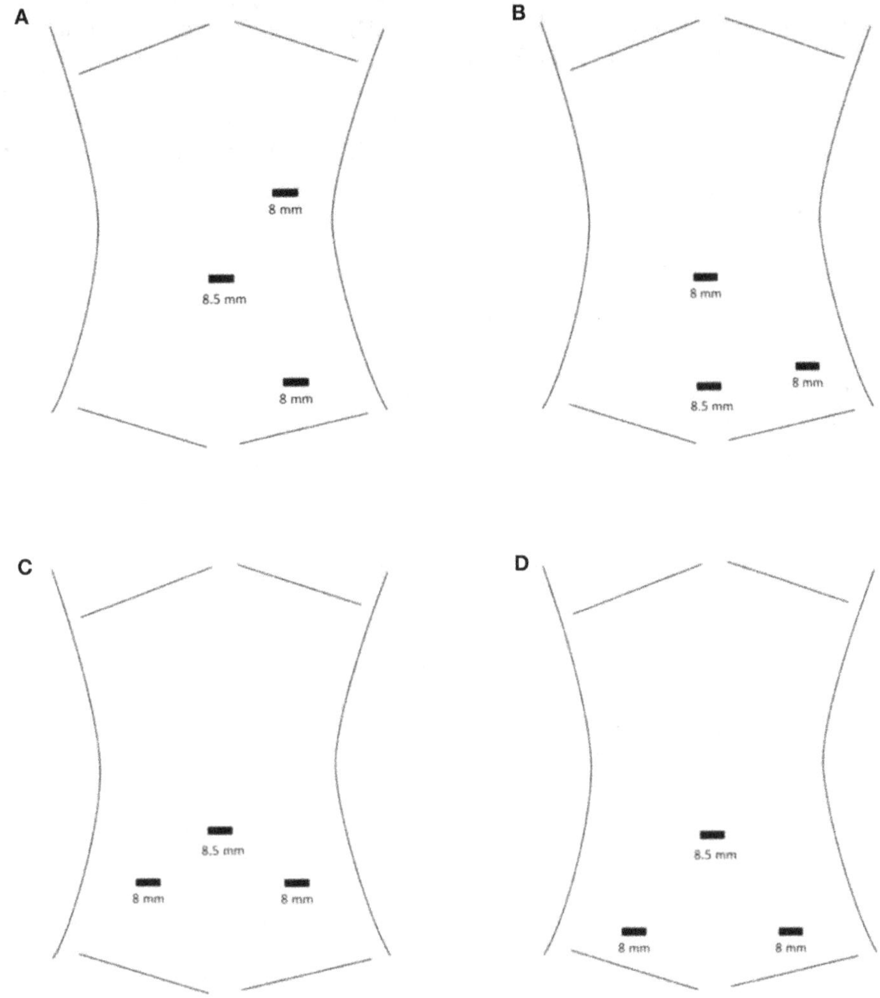

FIGURE 1 | (A) Standard port placement for RAL left pyeloplasty with the Si robot. The camera port is at the umbilicus. **(B)** HIdES port placement for RAL left pyeloplasty with the Si robot. The camera port is the inferior-most port. The camera port and one working port are hidden at or below the level of a Pfannenstiel incision, while the other working port is hidden in the umbilicus. **(C)** Standard port placement for RAL ureteral reimplantation with the Si robot. The camera port is at the umbilicus. **(D)** HIdES port placement for RAL ureteral reimplantation with the Si robot. The camera port is at the umbilicus. Skin incisions for the working ports are lower than in the standard port placement (at or below the level of a Pfannenstiel incision). Fascial entry sites for the working ports may be placed higher than the skin incisions in order to increase working space within the pelvis. This is achieved by applying cephalad traction during port placement.

through the Foley catheter, which should reflux up through the stent if the distal coil is in the bladder. The proximal stent coil is then placed within the pelvis, and the anastomosis is completed with a second running suture. Alternative approaches include placing a stent in retrograde fashion or leaving a percutaneous nephrostomy/nephroureterostomy tube or Penrose drain instead of an internal stent. Tubeless procedures have also been described with no short-term complications (12). Long-term success rates of tubeless robotic pyeloplasty have yet to be determined.

Robotic pyeloplasty is effective, with multiple series including ≥50 patients reporting success rates of 94–100% utilizing a transperitoneal or retroperitoneal approach (2, 13–20). A recent retrospective long-term study reported an 8-year failure-free rate of 91.5% after robotic pyeloplasty (21). A meta-analysis from 2014 showed comparable success and complication rates in pediatric patients after minimally invasive or open pyeloplasty (22). A recent retrospective cohort study using the national Premier database revealed that while the total number of pyeloplasties decreased by 7% annually between 2003 and 2015, robotic cases increased by 29% annually, accounting for 40% of all cases in 2015 (23). Increased robot utilization was greatest in the pediatric population. Complication rates were similarly low in open and robotic cases.

UPJ Reconstruction, Special/Complex Cases

Stones and/or UPJ polyps, if present, may be addressed concomitantly with retroperitoneoscopic or transperitoneal robotic pyeloplasty (24–27). Concurrent pyelolithotomy and pyeloplasty is safe and effective, with acceptable stone-free rates

(94, 83, and 72% at 1, 3, and 6 months, respectively) (25). Operative time was longer for pyeloplasty with pyelolithotomy (median 151 min) vs. pyeloplasty alone (120 min, $p < 0.0001$), with no difference in length of hospital stay.

Ureteral fibroepithelial polyps are an uncommon but important source of obstructive hydronephrosis in children and can be challenging to diagnose preoperatively (24). If a polyp is suspected, endoscopy may be the preferred approach. However, in cases of large or multifocal lesions, or if a concurrent UPJ stenosis is thought to be present, robotics provide superior definitive management (26).

Redo (salvage) pyeloplasties present a special challenge. Dense peripelvic fibrosis, longer strictures, and compromised vascularity may all contribute to the increased difficulty in such cases. One recent study looking at laparoscopic redo pyeloplasties found that operative times were longer compared to primary cases (191 vs. 145 min, $p = 0.0001$), but success rates were comparable at 93.3% (28). Other groups have reported success rates from 77.8 to 100% for small cohorts undergoing redo pyeloplasty (29–32). Use of buccal mucosal onlay grafts for robotic salvage pyeloplasty (33, 34) and complex ureteral stricture repairs (35–37) has been shown to be safe and effective with short-term follow up.

Ureterocalicostomy is an option for renal salvage in cases where pyeloplasty is not feasible. The open procedure was originally described by Neuwirt (38). Indications for ureterocalicostomy are relative and may include UPJ obstruction in with an intrarenal pelvis or recurrent UPJ obstruction with dense scarring making redo pyeloplasty difficult or impossible. It has been considered a last resort for kidney preservation, as an alternative to nephrectomy (39). Robotic ureterocalicostomy was first reported in the pediatric population by Casale et al. with steps based on the open procedure (40). These authors retrospectively studied 9 pediatric patients who underwent transperitoneal robotic ureterocalicostomy in the setting of recurrent UPJ obstruction or intrarenal UPJ. Two patients underwent concomitant ureteroscopic stone treatment. The hilum was mobilized to allow for rapid vascular control; however, hilar clamping was not required in any case. Diuretic renogram confirmed unobstructed systems in all patients 12 months postoperatively (40).

MID URETERAL RECONSTRUCTION

UU for mid Ureteral Stricture

RAL end-to-end UU may be indicated in the setting of mid ureteral stricture. Port placement for mid ureteral reconstruction can be achieved in a fashion similar to that described above for proximal ureteral reconstruction, with the ports shifted slightly inferiorly if needed. The diseased segment may be excised, and both ends spatulated at opposite aspects to achieve a wide anastomosis. For a relatively short stricture, a Heineke-Mikulicz repair may be adequate (41).

For long or multiple mid ureteral strictures, tension-free end-to-end anastomosis may not be possible. In such cases, the use of a graft may obviate the need for more morbid procedures such as ileal ureter, transureteroureterostomy, or autotransplantation. Buccal mucosal grafts may be used for complex pyeloplasties (33, 34) or complex ureteral stricture repairs (35–37). Use of the appendix as a ureteral substitute or as an onlay flap has also been described for complex right mid or upper ureteral stricture repair, initially in the open (42–44) or laparoscopic (45, 46) settings. Recently, Yarlagadda et al published a case report of robotic appendiceal interposition for right-sided ureteral stricture disease (47). In this case, a 5 cm obliterative ureteral stricture secondary to recurrent ureterolithiasis and pyelonephritis was repaired with interposition of the appendix between the proximal and distal healthy ureter. Resolution of hydronephrosis and flank pain was demonstrated at 10 months. Long-term results using this technique are needed.

LOWER URETERAL RECONSTRUCTION

Extravesical Reimplantation for VUR

The most common RAL distal ureteral surgery is extravesical ureteral reimplantation for VUR, following steps of the open Lich-Gregoir technique originally described in the 1960s (48, 49) VUR may also be treated endoscopically or with open or laparoscopic transvesical reimplantation. Open ureteral reimplantation has a reported success of 93.5–98% (50–52). Endoscopic VUR treatment is the least invasive option, but is associated with variable radiographic cure rates of 67–93% (53–57). Success is likely dependent on technique, surgeon experience, and patient factors. The hydrodistention implantation technique (HIT) provides better outcomes than the older subureteric transurethral injection (STING) procedure, and several authors have reported radiographic success rates ≥80% (58–60). The Double HIT has emerged as the most common injection technique in the United States (61), affording the highest endoscopic success rates (57, 62).

Patient positioning for RAL distal ureteral procedures is typically lithotomy for the Si, allowing for cystoscopy (if desired) and robotic surgery in a single prep and drape. The robot is docked between the legs in this scenario. Side-docking is also possible, especially with the Xi, allowing the patient to remain supine. Port placement at our institution involves an 8.5 mm Si robotic camera port at the umbilicus with open Hasson or Veress technique. One may also use a 10 or 12 mm port (e.g., the Autosuture® balloon trocar) for the Si robot (5). Xi camera and working ports are identical, allowing the camera to go through any of the ports.

After camera port placement, working ports are placed on either side of the umbilicus. These are placed inferiorly to the camera port to create a triangular working field for Si (**Figure 1C**), or in a line for the Xi. One may use 8 or 5 mm working ports for the Si, whereas only 8 mm instruments are available for the Xi. The HIdES port placement technique for lower urinary tract reconstruction involves placing the working ports at or below the level of a typical Pfannenstiel incision (**Figure 1D**) (6). Assistant port(s) and/or 3rd robotic port may be placed; however, we generally find this unnecessary. Unless the Xi and proprietary OR table are being used, one must adjust table height and position prior to docking.

Once docked, the first steps are opening the peritoneum (**Figure 2**) and mobilizing the ureter with judicious cautery use. The ureter is then followed distally to the ureterovesical junction (UVJ), taking care to preserve vas or uterine arteries in a boy or girl, respectively. A bladder hitch stitch may be utilized if the bladder is floppy and UVJ not clearly seen. A detrusor tunnel is created in the appropriate trajectory. The ideal location for detrusor tunnel may be more apparent in the absence of a hitch stitch, which may distort the anatomy. Ideal detrusor tunnel length has been described as 5:1 in comparison with the ureteral diameter (10). Flaps are developed on either side of the tunnel in order to prevent obstruction. Lastly, the tunnel is closed over the ureter. We use a running 3-0 V-loc for this, starting at the distal-most aspect and running proximally. Others may use different suture types, interrupted instead of running, and/or may start proximally, according to surgeon preference.

VUR resolution rates after extravesical RAL ureteral reimplantation (RALUR) reported in the literature range from 66.7 to 100% in multiple relatively small series (63–73). Overall success upon pooling these series is 91% (74). A multi-institutional retrospective study reported radiographic resolution in 87.9% of 280 ureters (75). More recently, a large prospective multi-institutional study reported 93.8% resolution in 199 ureters (76).

RALUR may be performed bilaterally; however, there is concern that bilateral dissection of the posterior bladder may disrupt the pelvic nerve plexus, resulting in higher rates of postoperative urinary retention. Nerve-sparing dissection has been proposed to reduce this complication (77). In 2008, Casale et al. reported a 97.6% success rate following bilateral nerve-sparing RALUR in 41 patients (65). There were no complications or instances of urinary retention. Herz et al. reported a 91.7% success rate for unilateral RALUR but a success rate of only 77.8% of ureters (72.2% of children) for bilateral cases (78). In this study, complication rates (including ureteral obstruction, readmission, and urinary retention) were higher for bilateral cases. A nerve-sparing technique was not utilized.

Peri-ureteral diverticula (if present) may be reduced/excised during reimplantation (79). In duplex systems, common sheath reimplantation with or without tapering has been described with good outcomes (80). Ureteral tapering may be performed while maintaining the native UVJ in the

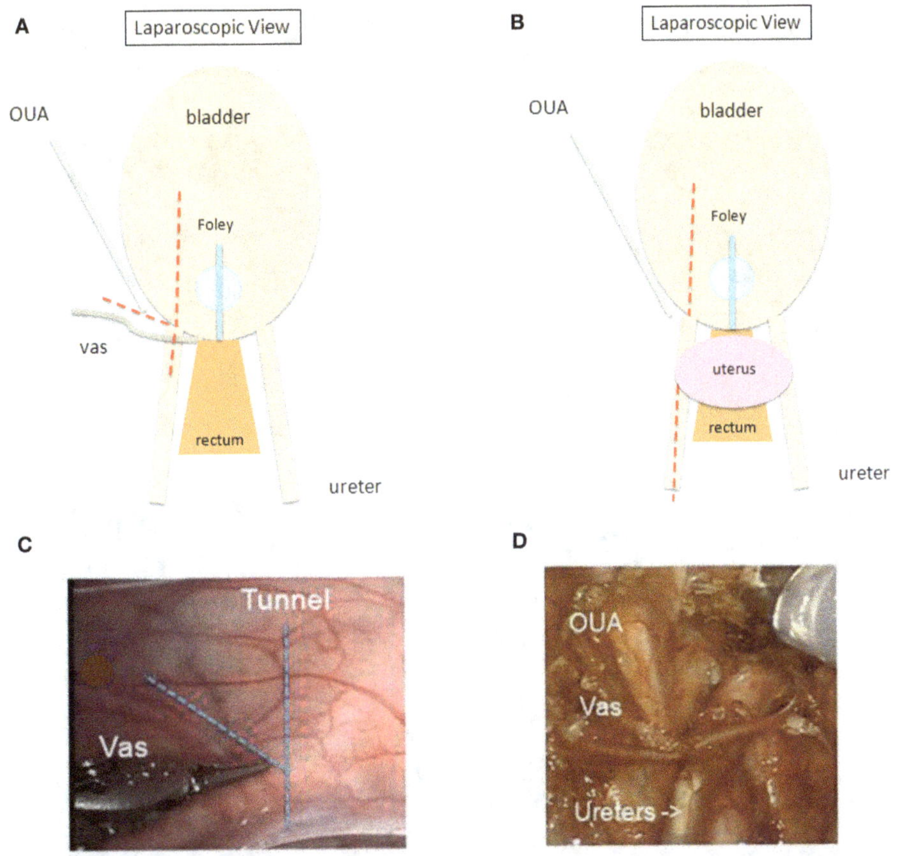

FIGURE 2 | (A,B) Schematic showing sites for opening peritoneum (- - -) during RAL ureteral reimplantation. Peritoneum may be opened in line with proposed detrusor tunnel or transversely for wider exposure. "V" flap **(A)** recommended for adequately exposing vas deferens in boys. One may open peritoneum further cephalad along the ureter to allow for additional ureteral mobilization **(B)**, especially in peri- or post-pubertal girls or in otherwise complex cases. OUA, obliterated umbilical artery. **(C,D)** Intraoperative view prior to **(C)** and after **(D)** opening peritoneum in a male patient. OUA, obliterated umbilical artery.

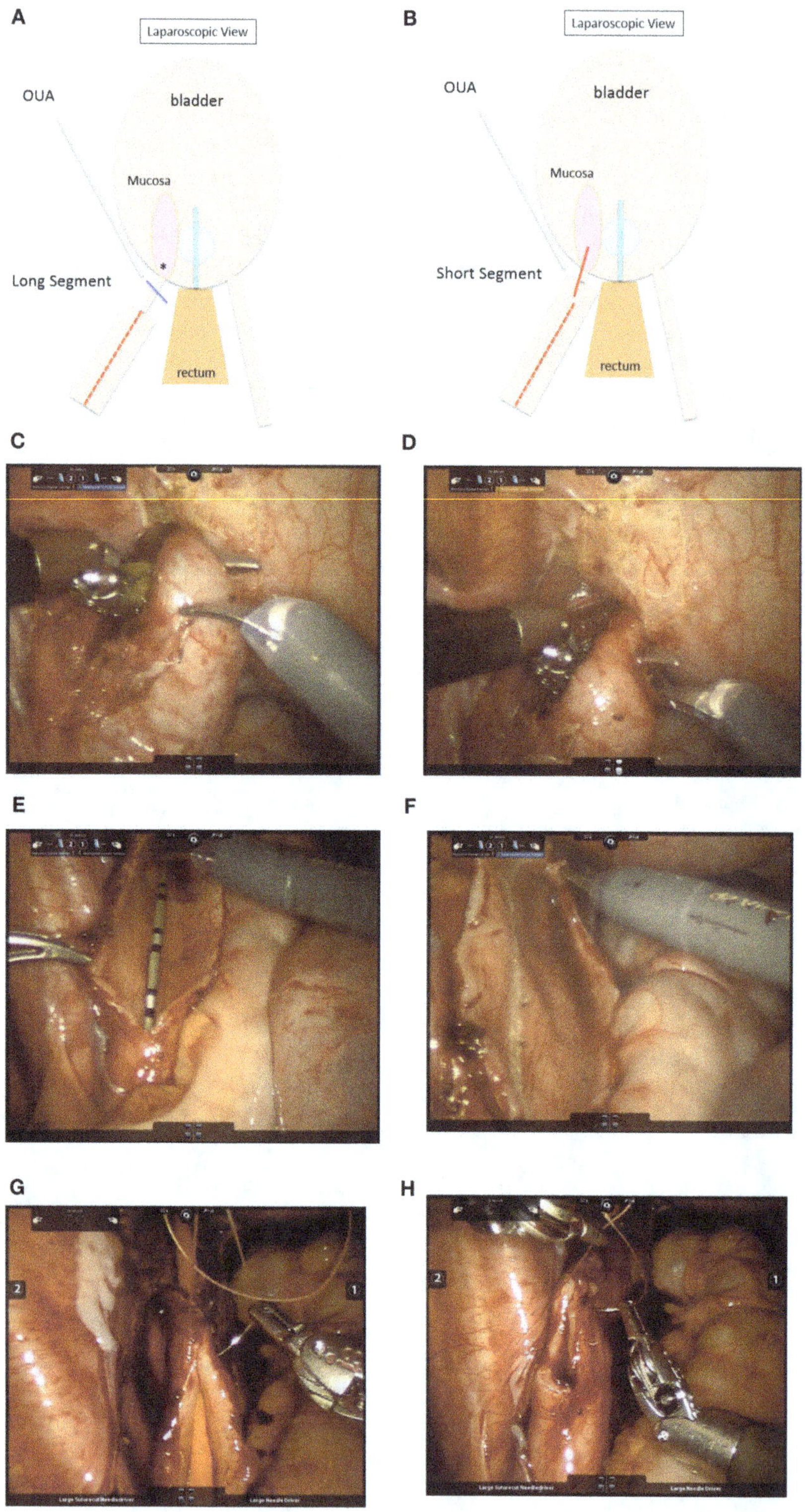

FIGURE 3 | (A) Schematic showing repair of obstructed megaureter with a long segment of stenotic UVJ. Steps: i. Keep ureter attached. ii. Taper megaureter (- - -) iii. Ligate UVJ (—). iv. Dismember ureter. v. Anastomosis at new site (*). Stent ± peritoneal closure. OUA, obliterated umbilical artery. **(B)** Repair of obstructed megaureter with a short stenotic UVJ segment. Steps: i. Keep ureter attached. ii. Taper megaureter (- - -) iii. Partially dismember (—). iv. *In situ* Heineke-Mikulicz anastomosis. Stent ± peritoneal closure. OUA, obliterated umbilical artery. **(C)** Intraoperative view during robotic repair of a left obstructed megaureter. The ureter has been mobilized circumferentially without devascularizing it. **(D)** The distally narrowed and obstructed segment is apparent in the view above. **(E)** A longitudinal

(Continued)

FIGURE 3 | ureterotomy has been created to allow for tapering. In this view, the ureter is still attached at the UVJ in order to maintain traction during tapering. **(F)** The ureter is scored to demarcate excess tissue for excisional tapering. **(G,H)** After excision of excess tissue, the ureter is closed/tapered using fine absorbable suture (5–0 Vicryl in the case above) over a 10 Fr catheter. The next steps include dismemberment at the UVJ, creation of ureteroneocystostomy, and creation of a detrusor tunnel to achieve a nonobstructed, nonrefluxing reimplantation.

setting of a non-obstructed, refluxing megaureter (81). For complex reimplants (i.e., those with history of prior anti-reflux surgery, requiring tapering and/or dismembering, or associated duplication or diverticulum), Arlen et al. found comparable success and complication rates for RAL vs. open cases, with shorter hospitalization in the RAL group (82). Older children were more likely to undergo RALUR.

Extravesical Reimplantation for UVJ Obstruction/Obstructed Megaureter

RAL dismembered extravesical ureteral reimplantation with or without tapering may be used for repair of obstructed megaureters (**Figures 3A,C–H**) (83, 84). The obstructed UVJ is divided, and a new ureteroneocystostomy anastomosis is created. A non-refluxing detrusor tunnel is created as described above. When tapering, we prefer to leave the ureter connected to the bladder during this process to provide retraction. Dismemberment is then performed after tapering is complete, similar to the process described by Khan et al. (85). A non-dismembered technique may also be used to repair obstructed megaureters, using the Heineke-Mikulicz principle (**Figure 3B**) (86).

UU in Duplex Systems

In appropriate duplex systems, end-to-side ureteroureterostomy (UU) can be performed proximally or distally depending on surgeon preference. We favor a distal approach, eliminating risk of hilar vessel injury, and allowing for intraoperative decision-making regarding performance of UU vs. ureteral reimplantation (vs. both concurrently in select settings). In some cases, it may be safer and more efficacious to perform UU in the mid ureter, thus avoiding both pelvic structures and renal hilar anatomy. Upper-to-lower UU may be performed for obstructed and/or ectopic upper moiety when there is no vesicoureteral reflux (VUR) into the lower moiety. Lower-to-upper UU may be performed in the setting of lower moiety VUR and unobstructed non-ectopic upper moiety (80).

Robot-assisted UU is a safe and effective alternative to open UU in children, with similar operative times and complication rates, and slightly shorter hospitalizations (87). UU has been shown to be safe and effective even in the setting of a minimally functioning/non-functioning moiety (as an alternative to upper moiety heminephrectomy) and irrespective of ureteral size difference (88).

When performing RAL UU, it is imperative to correctly identify each ureter. This can be facilitated with cystourethroscopy and passage of a temporary ureteral stent into one of the ureters. It is our practice to leave a double-J ureteral stent across the anastomosis, which is removed 4–6 weeks postoperatively. A renal-bladder ultrasound is performed ~4 weeks after stent removal, with additional imaging as clinically indicated.

CONCLUSION

RAL surgery is a safe, minimally invasive technique with various applications in pediatric ureteric reconstruction. A robotic approach allows access to the ureter at all levels. Multiple aspects of robotic surgery, including magnified three-dimensional view and wristed movements with multiple degrees of freedom, are particularly well-suited to these delicate reconstructive procedures. Robotic surgery continues to enjoy growing popularity among urologists and patient families alike.

AUTHOR CONTRIBUTIONS

AB and AK both contributed to deciding the structure, content of the manuscript and to writing, editing the manuscript.

REFERENCES

1. Van Batavia JP, Casale P. Robotic surgery in pediatric urology. *Curr Urol Rep.* (2014) 15:402. doi: 10.1007/s11934-014-0402-9
2. Olsen LH, Rawashdeh YF, Jorgensen TM. Pediatric robot assisted retroperitoneoscopic pyeloplasty: a 5-year experience. *J Urol.* (2007) 178:2137–2141. Discussion 2141. doi: 10.1016/j.juro.2007.07.057
3. Romero FR, Wagner AA, Trapp C, Permpongkosol S, Muntener M, Link RE, et al. Transmesenteric laparoscopic pyeloplasty. *J Urol.* (2006) 176(6 Pt 1):2526–9. doi: 10.1016/j.juro.2006.07.155
4. Spinoit AF, Nguyen H, Subramaniam R. Role of robotics in children: a brave New World! *Eur Urol Focus.* (2017) 3:172–80. doi: 10.1016/j.euf.2017.08.011
5. Chang C, Steinberg Z, Shah A, Gundeti MS. Patient positioning and port placement for robot-assisted surgery. *J Endourol.* (2014) 28:631–8. doi: 10.1089/end.2013.0733
6. Gargollo PC. Hidden incision endoscopic surgery: description of technique, parental satisfaction and applications. *J Urol.* (2011) 185:1425–31. doi: 10.1016/j.juro.2010.11.054
7. Garcia-Roig ML, Travers C, McCracken C, Cerwinka W, Kirsch JM, Kirsch AJ. Surgical scar location preference for pediatric kidney and pelvic surgery: a crowdsourced survey. *J Urol.* (2017) 197(3 Pt 2):911–9. doi: 10.1016/j.juro.2016.11.033
8. Amon Sesmero JH, Delgado MC, de la Cruz Martin B, Serrano MR, Mainez Rodriguez JA, Tapia Herrero AM. Laparoscopic pyeloplasty: always dismembered? *J Endourol.* (2016) 30:778–82. doi: 10.1089/end.2015.0800
9. Szydelko T, Apoznanski W, Koleda P, Rusiecki L, Janczak D. Laparoscopic pyeloplasty with cephalad translocation of the crossing vessel-a new approach to the Hellstrom technique. *Wideochir Inne Tech Maloinwazyjne.* (2015) 10:25–9. doi: 10.5114/wiitm.2015.48695
10. Wein AJ, Kavoussi LR, Campbell MF. Chapter 41: Management of upper urinary tract obstruction. In: Wein AJ, Kavoussi LR, et al, editors. *Campbell-Walsh Urology.* 10th ed. Philadelphia, PA: Elsevier Saunders (2012). p. 1122–68.

11. Janetschek G, Peschel R, Bartsch G. Laparoscopic fenger plasty. *J Endourol.* (2000) 14:889–93. doi: 10.1089/end.2000.14.889
12. Fichtenbaum EJ, Strine AC, Concodora CW, Schulte M, Noh PH. Tubeless outpatient robotic upper urinary tract reconstruction in the pediatric population: short-term assessment of safety. *J Robot Surg.* (2018) 12:257–60. doi: 10.1007/s11701-017-0722-0
13. Minnillo BJ, Cruz JA, Sayao RH, Passerotti CC, Houck CS, Meier PM, et al. Long-term experience and outcomes of robotic assisted laparoscopic pyeloplasty in children and young adults. *J Urol.* (2011) 185:1455–60. doi: 10.1016/j.juro.2010.11.056
14. Mufarrij PW, Woods M, Shah OD, Palese MA, Berger AD, Thomas R, et al. Robotic dismembered pyeloplasty: a 6-year, multi-institutional experience. *J Urol.* (2008) 180:1391–6. doi: 10.1016/j.juro.2008.06.024
15. Singh P, Dogra PN, Kumar R, Gupta NP, Nayak B, Seth A. Outcomes of robot-assisted laparoscopic pyeloplasty in children: a single center experience. *J Endourol.* (2012) 26:249–53. doi: 10.1089/end.201 1.0350
16. Patel V. Robotic-assisted laparoscopic dismembered pyeloplasty. *Urology.* (2005) 66:45–9. doi: 10.1016/j.urology.2005.01.053
17. Schwentner C, Pelzer A, Neururer R, Springer B, Horninger W, Bartsch G, et al. Robotic Anderson-Hynes pyeloplasty: 5-year experience of one centre. *BJU Int.* (2007) 100:880–5. doi: 10.1111/j.1464-410X.2007. 07032.x
18. Gupta NP, Nayyar R, Hemal AK, Mukherjee S, Kumar R, Dogra PN. Outcome analysis of robotic pyeloplasty: a large single-centre experience. *BJU Int.* (2010) 105:980–3. doi: 10.1111/j.1464-410X.2009.08983.x
19. Cestari A, Buffi NM, Lista G, Sangalli M, Scapaticci E, Fabbri F, et al. Retroperitoneal and transperitoneal robot-assisted pyeloplasty in adults: techniques and results. *Eur Urol.* (2010) 58:711–8. doi: 10.1016/j.eururo.2010.07.020
20. Sivaraman A, Leveillee RJ, Patel MB, Chauhan S, Bracho JE II, Moore CR, et al. Robot-assisted laparoscopic dismembered pyeloplasty for ureteropelvic junction obstruction: a multi-institutional experience. *Urology.* (2012) 79:351–5. doi: 10.1016/j.urology.2011.10.019
21. Hopf HL, Bahler CD, Sundaram CP. Long-term outcomes of robot-assisted laparoscopic pyeloplasty for ureteropelvic junction obstruction. *Urology.* (2016) 90:106–10. doi: 10.1016/j.urology.2015.12.050
22. Autorino R, Eden C, El-Ghoneimi A, Guazzoni G, Buffi N, Peters CA, et al. Robot-assisted and laparoscopic repair of ureteropelvic junction obstruction: a systematic review and meta-analysis. *Eur Urol.* (2014) 65:430–52. doi: 10.1016/j.eururo.2013.06.053
23. Varda BK, Wang Y, Chung BI, Lee RS, Kurtz MP, Nelson CP, et al. Has the robot caught up? National trends in utilization, perioperative outcomes, and cost for open, laparoscopic, and robotic pediatric pyeloplasty in the United States from 2003 to 2015. *J Pediatr Urol.* (2018) 14:336.e1–8. doi: 10.1016/j.jpurol.2017.12.010
24. Dai LN, Chen CD, Lin XK, Wang YB, Xia LG, Liu, Pet al. Retroperitoneal laparoscopy management for ureteral fibroepithelial polyps causing hydronephrosis in children: a report of five cases. *J Pediatr Urol.* (2015) 11:257 e251–5. doi: 10.1016/j.jpurol.2015.02.019
25. Jensen PH, Berg KD, Azawi NH. Robot-assisted pyeloplasty and pyelolithotomy in patients with ureteropelvic junction stenosis. *Scand J Urol.* (2017) 51:323–8. doi: 10.1080/21681805.2017.1 300188
26. Osbun N, Ellison JS, Lendvay TS. Robot-Assisted Laparoscopic Excision of ureteral and ureteropelvic junction fibroepithelial polyps in children. *J Endourol.* (2016) 30:896–900. doi: 10.1089/end.2016.0006
27. Skolarikos A, Dellis A, Knoll T. Ureteropelvic obstruction and renal stones: etiology and treatment. *Urolithiasis.* (2015) 43:5–12. doi: 10.1007/s00240-014-0736-2
28. Abraham GP, Siddaiah AT, Ramaswami K, George D, Das K. Laparoscopic management of recurrent ureteropelvic junction obstruction following pyeloplasty. *Urol Ann.* (2015) 7:183–7. doi: 10.4103/0974-7796.1 50489
29. Powell C, Gatti JM, Juang D, Murphy JP. Laparoscopic pyeloplasty for ureteropelvic junction obstruction following open pyeloplasty in children. *J Laparoendosc Adv Surg Tech A.* (2015) 25:858–63. doi: 10.1089/lap.20 15.0074
30. Basiri A, Behjati S, Zand S, Moghaddam SM. Laparoscopic pyeloplasty in secondary ureteropelvic junction obstruction after failed open surgery. *J Endourol.* (2007) 21:1045–51. Discussion 1051. doi: 10.1089/end.2006.0414
31. Braga LH, Lorenzo AJ, Skeldon S, Dave S, Bagli DJ, Khoury AE, et al. Failed pyeloplasty in children: comparative analysis of retrograde endopyelotomy versus redo pyeloplasty. *J Urol.* (2007) 178:2571–5. Discussion 2575. doi: 10.1016/j.juro.2007.08.050
32. Thomas JC, DeMarco RT, Donohoe JM, Adams MC, Pope JCt, Brock JW III. Management of the failed pyeloplasty: a contemporary review. *J Urol.* (2005) 174:2363–6. doi: 10.1097/01.ju.0000180420.11915.31
33. Zampini AM, Nelson R, Zhang JJH, Reese J, Angermeier KW, Haber GP. Robotic salvage pyeloplasty with buccal mucosal onlay graft: video demonstration of technique and outcomes. *Urology.* (2017) 110:253–6. doi: 10.1016/j.urology.2017.07.023
34. Ahn JJ, Shapiro ME, Ellison JS, Lendvay TS. Pediatric robot-assisted redo pyeloplasty with buccal mucosa graft: a novel technique. *Urology.* (2017) 101:56–9. doi: 10.1016/j.urology.2016.12.036
35. Arora S, Campbell L, Tourojman M, Pucheril D, Jones LR, Rogers C. Robotic buccal mucosal graft ureteroplasty for complex ureteral stricture. *Urology.* (2017) 110:257–8. doi: 10.1016/j.urology.2017.06.037
36. Lee Z, Waldorf BT, Cho EY, Liu JC, Metro MJ, Eun DD. Robotic ureteroplasty with buccal mucosa graft for the management of complex ureteral strictures. *J Urol.* (2017) 198:1430–5. doi: 10.1016/j.juro.2017.06.097
37. Zhao LC, Yamaguchi Y, Bryk DJ, Adelstein SA, Stifelman MD. Robot-assisted ureteral reconstruction using buccal mucosa. *Urology.* (2015) 86:634–8. doi: 10.1016/j.urology.2015.06.006
38. Neuwirt K. Implantation of the ureter into the lower calyx of the renal pelvis. *Urol Cutaneous Rev.* (1948) 52:351.
39. Gite VA, Siddiqui AK, Bote SM, Patil SR, Kandi AJ, Nikose JV. Ureterocalycostomy - final resort in the management of secondary pelvi-ureteric junction obstruction: our experience. *Int Braz J Urol.* (2016) 42:501–6. doi: 10.1590/S1677-5538.IBJU.2015.0368
40. Casale P, Mucksavage P, Resnick M, Kim SS. Robotic ureterocalicostomy in the pediatric population. *J Urol.* (2008) 180:2643–8. doi: 10.1016/j.juro.2008.08.052
41. Goel A, Singh D, Sengottayan VK, Sankhwar S. Nondismembered ureteroplasty for congenital midureteral stenosis: a new application of an old technique. *Urology.* (2010) 76:1004–6. doi: 10.1016/j.urology.2010. 03.093
42. Adani GL, Pravisani R, Baccarani U, Bolgeri M, Lorenzin D, Terrosu G, et al. Extended ureteral stricture corrected with appendiceal replacement in a kidney transplant recipient. *Urology.* (2015) 86:840–3. doi: 10.1016/j.urology.2015.06.010
43. Murai R, Ushida H, Osafune T, Johnin K, Kageyama S, Okada Y. [Repair of right ureteral stenosis by traumatic injury with appendiceal interposition: a case report]. *Nihon Hinyokika Gakkai Zasshi.* (2013) 104:667–70. doi: 10.5980/jpnjurol.104.667
44. Dagash H, Sen S, Chacko J, Karl S, Ghosh D, Parag P, et al. The appendix as ureteral substitute: a report of 10 cases. *J Pediatr Urol.* (2008) 4:14–9. doi: 10.1016/j.jpurol.2007.08.004
45. Duty BD, Kreshover JE, Richstone L, Kavoussi LR. Review of appendiceal onlay flap in the management of complex ureteric strictures in six patients. *BJU Int.* (2015) 115:282–7. doi: 10.1111/bju.12651
46. Reggio E, Richstone L, Okeke Z, Kavoussi LR. Laparoscopic ureteroplasty using on-lay appendix graft. *Urology.* (2009) 73:928 e927–10. doi: 10.1016/j.urology.2008.06.034
47. Yarlagadda VK, Nix JW, Benson DG, Selph JP. Feasibility of intracorporeal robotic-assisted laparoscopic appendiceal interposition for ureteral stricture disease: a case report. *Urology.* (2017) 109:201–5. . doi: 10.1016/j.urology.2017.08.017
48. Gregoir W. [The Surgical Treatment of Congenital Vesico-Ureteral Reflux]. *Acta Chir Belg.* (1964) 63:431–9.
49. Robert Lich Jr., Lonnie WH, and Lawrence AD. Recurrent urosepsis in children. *J Urol.* (1961) 86:554–8. doi: 10.1016/S0022-5347(17)65219-4
50. Nelson CP, Hubert KC, Kokorowski PJ, Huang L, Prasad MM, Rosoklija I, et al. Long-term incidence of urinary tract infection after ureteral reimplantation for primary vesicoureteral reflux. *J Pediatr Urol.* (2013) 9:92–8. doi: 10.1016/j.jpurol.2011.12.009

51. Elder JS, Peters CA, Arant BS Jr, Ewalt DH, Hawtrey CE, Hurwitz RS, et al. Pediatric Vesicoureteral Reflux Guidelines Panel summary report on the management of primary vesicoureteral reflux in children. *J Urol.* (1997) 157:1846–51. doi: 10.1016/S0022-5347(01)64882-1
52. Barrieras D, Lapointe S, Reddy PP, Williot P, McLorie GA, Bigli D, et al. Are postoperative studies justified after extravescial ureteral reimplantation? *J Urol.* (2000) 164(3 Pt 2):1064–6. doi: 10.1016/S0022-5347(05)67251-5
53. Hacker FM, Frech-Dorfler M, von Rotz M, Rudin C. Endoscopic hyaluronic acid/dextranomer gel implantation is effective as first-line treatment of vesicoureteral reflux (VUR) in children: a single centre experience. *Eur J Pediatr Surg.* (2011) 21:299–303. doi: 10.1055/s-0031-1279700
54. Elder JS, Diaz M, Caldamone AA, Cendron M, Greenfield S, Hurwitz R, et al. Endoscopic therapy for vesicoureteral reflux: a meta-analysis. I. Reflux resolution and urinary tract infection. *J Urol.* (2006) 175:716–22. doi: 10.1016/S0022-5347(05)00210-7
55. Friedmacher F, Colhoun E, Puri P. Endoscopic injection of dextranomer/hyaluronic acid as first line treatment in 851 consecutive children with high grade vesicoureteral reflux: efficacy and long-term results. *J Urol.* (2018) 200:650–5. doi: 10.1016/j.juro.2018.03.074
56. Kaye JD, Srinivasan AK, Delaney C, Cerwinka WH, Elmore JM, Scherz HC, et al. Clinical and radiographic results of endoscopic injection for vesicoureteral reflux: defining measures of success. *J Pediatr Urol.* (2012) 8:297–303. doi: 10.1016/j.jpurol.2011.02.006
57. Kalisvaart JF, Scherz HC, Cuda S, Kaye JD, Kirsch AJ. Intermediate to long-term follow-up indicates low risk of recurrence after Double HIT endoscopic treatment for primary vesico-ureteral reflux. *J Pediatr Urol.* (2012) 8:359–65. doi: 10.1016/j.jpurol.2011.07.006
58. Lee EK, Gatti JM, Demarco RT, Murphy JP. Long-term followup of dextranomer/hyaluronic acid injection for vesicoureteral reflux: late failure warrants continued followup. *J Urol.* (2009) 181:1869–74. Discussion 1874–65. doi: 10.1016/j.juro.2008.12.005
59. Gupta A, Snodgrass W. Intra-orifice versus hydrodistention implantation technique in dextranomer/hyaluronic acid injection for vesicoureteral reflux. *J Urol.* (2008) 180(4 Suppl.):1589–92. Discussion 1592–83. doi: 10.1016/j.juro.2008.04.073
60. Shim JS, Kim JW, Oh MM, Moon du G. Efficacy of hydrodistention implantation technique in treating high-grade vesicoureteral reflux. *Korean J Urol.* (2012) 53:194–9. doi: 10.4111/kju.2012.53.3.194
61. Kirsch AJ, Arlen AM, Lackgren G. Current trends in dextranomer hyaluronic acid copolymer (Deflux) injection technique for endoscopic treatment of vesicoureteral reflux. *Urology.* (2014) 84:462–8. doi: 10.1016/j.urology.2014.04.032
62. Molitierno JA, Scherz HC, Kirsch AJ. Endoscopic treatment of vesicoureteral reflux using dextranomer hyaluronic acid copolymer. *J Pediatr Urol.* (2008) 4:221–8. doi: 10.1016/j.jpurol.2007.11.015
63. Chan KW, Lee KH, Tam YH, Sihoe JD. Early experience of robotic-assisted reconstructive operations in pediatric urology. *J Laparoendosc Adv Surg Tech A.* (2010) 20:379–82. doi: 10.1089/lap.2009.0340
64. Lee RS, Sethi AS, Passerotti CC, Peters CA. Robot-assisted laparoscopic nephrectomy and contralateral ureteral reimplantation in children. *J Endourol.* (2010) 24:123–8. doi: 10.1089/end.2009.0271
65. Casale P, Patel RP, Kolon TF. Nerve sparing robotic extravesical ureteral reimplantation. *J Urol.* (2008) 179:1987–9. Discussion 1990. doi: 10.1016/j.juro.2008.01.062
66. Marchini GS, Hong YK, Minnillo BJ, Diamond DA, Houck CS, Meier PM, et al. Robotic assisted laparoscopic ureteral reimplantation in children: case matched comparative study with open surgical approach. *J Urol.* (2011) 185:1870–5. doi: 10.1016/j.juro.2010.12.069
67. Smith RP, Oliver JL, Peters CA. Pediatric robotic extravesical ureteral reimplantation: comparison with open surgery. *J Urol.* (2011) 185:1876–81. doi: 10.1016/j.juro.2010.12.072
68. Chalmers D, Herbst K, Kim C. Robotic-assisted laparoscopic extravesical ureteral reimplantation: an initial experience. *J Pediatr Urol.* (2012) 8:268–71. doi: 10.1016/j.jpurol.2011.04.006
69. Kasturi S, Sehgal SS, Christman MS, Lambert SM, Casale P. Prospective long-term analysis of nerve-sparing extravesical robotic-assisted laparoscopic ureteral reimplantation. *Urology.* (2012) 79:680–3. doi: 10.1016/j.urology.2011.10.052
70. Callewaert PR, Biallosterski BT, Rahnama'i MS, Van Kerrebroeck PE. Robotic extravesical anti-reflux operations in complex cases: technical considerations and preliminary results. *Urol Int.* (2012) 88:6–11. doi: 10.1159/000332953
71. Gundeti MS, Kojima Y, Haga N, Kiriluk K. Robotic-assisted laparoscopic reconstructive surgery in the lower urinary tract. *Curr Urol Rep.* (2013) 14:333–41. doi: 10.1007/s11934-013-0328-7
72. Schomburg JL, Haberman K, Willihnganz-Lawson KH, Shukla AR. Robot-assisted laparoscopic ureteral reimplantation: a single surgeon comparison to open surgery. *J Pediatr Urol.* (2014) 10:875–9. doi: 10.1016/j.jpurol.2014.02.013
73. Akhavan A, Avery D, Lendvay TS. Robot-assisted extravesical ureteral reimplantation: outcomes and conclusions from 78 ureters. *J Pediatr Urol.* (2014) 10:864–8. doi: 10.1016/j.jpurol.2014.01.028
74. Grimsby GM, Dwyer ME, Jacobs MA, Ost MC, Schneck FX, Cannon GM, et al. Multi-institutional review of outcomes of robot-assisted laparoscopic extravesical ureteral reimplantation. *J Urol.* (2015) 193(5 Suppl.):1791–5. doi: 10.1016/j.juro.2014.07.128
75. Boysen WR, Ellison JS, Kim C, Koh CJ, Noh P, Whittam B, et al. Multi-institutional review of outcomes and complications of robot-assisted laparoscopic extravesical ureteral reimplantation for treatment of primary vesicoureteral reflux in children. *J Urol.* (2017) 197:1555–61. doi: 10.1016/j.juro.2017.01.062
76. Boysen WR, Akhavan A, Ko J, Ellison JS, Lendvay TS, Huang J, et al. Prospective multicenter study on robot-assisted laparoscopic extravesical ureteral reimplantation (RALUR-EV): Outcomes and complications. *J Pediatr Urol.* (2018) 14:262 e261–6. doi: 10.1016/j.jpurol.2018.01.020
77. David S, Kelly C, Poppas DP. Nerve sparing extravesical repair of bilateral vesicoureteral reflux: description of technique and evaluation of urinary retention. *J Urol.* (2004) 172(4 Pt 2):1617–20. Discussion 1620. doi: 10.1097/01.ju.0000139951.37492.91
78. Herz D, Fuchs M, Todd A, McLeod D, Smith J. Robot-assisted laparoscopic extravesical ureteral reimplant: a critical look at surgical outcomes. *J Pediatr Urol.* (2016) 12:402 e401–9. doi: 10.1016/j.jpurol.2016.05.042
79. Noh PH, Bansal D. Pediatric robotic assisted laparoscopy for paraureteral bladder diverticulum excision with ureteral reimplantation. *J Pediatr Urol.* (2013) 9:e28–30. doi: 10.1016/j.jpurol.2012.06.011
80. Herz D, Smith J, McLeod D, Schober M, Preece J, Merguerian P. Robot-assisted laparoscopic management of duplex renal anomaly: comparison of surgical outcomes to traditional pure laparoscopic and open surgery. *J Pediatr Urol.* (2016) 12:44 e41–7. doi: 10.1016/j.jpurol.2015.04.046
81. Faasse MA, Lindgren BW, Gong EM. Robot-assisted laparoscopic ureteral reimplantation with excisional tailoring for refluxing megaureter. *J Pediatr Urol.* (2014) 10:773 e771–2. doi: 10.1016/j.jpurol.2014.01.023
82. Arlen AM, Broderick KM, Travers C, Smith EA, Elmore JM, Kirsch AJ. Outcomes of complex robot-assisted extravesical ureteral reimplantation in the pediatric population. *J Pediatr Urol.* (2016) 12:169 e161–6. doi: 10.1016/j.jpurol.2015.11.007
83. Fu W, Zhang X, Zhang X, Zhang P, Gao J, Dong J, et al. Pure laparoscopic and robot-assisted laparoscopic reconstructive surgery in congenital megaureter: a single institution experience. *PLoS ONE.* (2014) 9:e99777. doi: 10.1371/journal.pone.0099777
84. Hemal AK, Nayyar R, Rao R. Robotic repair of primary symptomatic obstructive megaureter with intracorporeal or extracorporeal ureteric tapering and ureteroneocystostomy. *J Endourol.* (2009) 23:2041–6. doi: 10.1089/end.2009.0103
85. Khan A, Rahiman M, Verma A, Bhargava R. Novel technique of laparoscopic extravesical ureteric reimplantation in primary obstructive megaureter. *Urol Ann.* (2017) 9:150–2. doi: 10.4103/0974-7796.204182
86. Landa-Juarez S, Guerra-Rivas A, Salgado-Sangri R, Castillo-Fernandez AM, de la Cruz-Yanez H, Garcia-Hernandez C. [Laparoscopic

ureterovesical repair for megaureter treatment]. *Cir Cir.* (2017) 85:196–200. doi: 10.1016/j.circir.2016.08.003

87. Lee NG, Corbett ST, Cobb K, Bailey GC, Burns AS, Peters CA. Bi-institutional comparison of robot-assisted laparoscopic versus open ureteroureterostomy in the pediatric population. *J Endourol.* (2015) 29:1237–41. doi: 10.1089/end.2015.0223
88. McLeod DJ, Alpert SA, Ural Z, Jayanthi VR. Ureteroureterostomy irrespective of ureteral size or upper pole function: a single center experience. *J Pediatr Urol.* (2014) 10:616–9. doi: 10.1016/j.jpurol.2014.05.003

17

Surgical Options for Pediatric Bilateral Vocal Cord Palsy: State of the Art

Marilena Trozzi, Duino Meucci, Antonio Salvati, Maria Luisa Tropiano and Sergio Bottero*

Airway Surgery Unit, Pediatric Surgery Department, Bambino Gesù Children's Hospital, Rome, Italy

***Correspondence:**
Duino Meucci
duino.meucci@opbg.net

Management of pediatric bilateral vocal cord palsy (BVCP) is a controversial and challenging topic. It may represent a severe obstructive condition usually associated with respiratory distress, and, in such condition, tracheostomy has been considered the gold standard for a long time. Many surgical options have been described and used to increase the glottic space in BVCP (1), with ongoing research of less invasive techniques. The challenge and current trend in our department and in many major pediatric centers is to avoid tracheotomy through an early treatment. Many techniques introduced in the last decade reduced the number of tracheotomies and increased the decannulation rate. Furthermore, we observed a recent increase in attention to preserve the quality of the voice with new techniques, such as endoscopic arytenoid abduction lateropexy which is in our opinion an important innovation to improve glottic space with satisfactory voice results. We present a review of the literature about the evolution of the treatment options for pediatric BVCP during the years.

Keywords: bilateral vocal cord palsy, pediatric, surgical options, voice quality, airway surgery

INTRODUCTION

Vocal cord paralysis (VCP) is the second most common congenital laryngeal anomaly in pediatric age (10–15%) (2).

Unilateral VCP and bilateral VCP differ in clinical presentation, etiology, and treatment. Bilateral vocal cord paralysis (BVCP) can be characterized by stridor, respiratory distress, suprasternal, and chest retractions, sleep apneas, and failure to thrive, and it represents up to 62% of all pediatric VCPs (3). Instead mild stridor, aspiration, and hoarse and breathy voice are generally suggestive of unilateral vocal cord paralysis (UVCP).

VCP results from laryngeal innervation disorders, posterior glottic stenosis, or cricoarytenoid joint's (CAj's) fixation. All the motility anomalies of the larynx are described with the term "laryngeal immobility."

An awake laryngeal endoscopy is the essential test for diagnosis of the paralysis, and a complete airway endoscopy under general anesthesia is always recommended to exclude other airway-associated pathologies and to differentiate the paralysis from vocal cord fixation (cricoarytenoid joint ankylosis, posterior glottic stenosis). About 45% of the cases of congenital BVCP have other airway diseases, and the most common are laryngomalacia, subglottic stenosis, and tracheomalacia (4).

In infants and children, VCP has mainly neurological, traumatic (birth trauma), and iatrogenic (post-surgical complications) (4–8) etiology. An MRI is often required to evaluate the central nervous system. In about one-third of the neurological cases, Arnold–Chiari II malformation is present with concomitant hydrocephalus and myelomeningocele. Furthermore, a large number of BVCPs are idiopathic (4, 5) and according to the literature, spontaneous recovery of vocal cord motility is possible within 1 or 2 years over the two-thirds of patients (3, 9, 10).

The treatment's choice has many variables; in particular, urgent intubation may be required in case of severe respiratory distress to ensure a safe airway. Placement of a tracheostomy can be required (11) in order to wait for a spontaneous recovery or the therapeutic choice.

In the last decade, the possibility of an early treatment avoiding tracheotomy has been considered, in particular with the proposal of minimally invasive treatments with preservation of the vocal folds, such as endoscopic arytenoid abduction lateropexy (1) or anterior–posterior cricoid split (12).

The best timing of surgical intervention is not standardized, and it is generally discussed case-by-case. Investigating the etiology of paralysis is crucial to predicting the possibilities of recovery and the timing of treatment. Other important prognostic variables are presence of comorbidities, associated airway diseases, age of the patients, and severity of the clinical condition.

Several surgical procedures to improve the glottic respiratory space have been proposed over the years, both endoscopic and open surgery, but a standard treatment has not been established.

The aim of this paper is a review of the literature on the treatment's options on pediatric bilateral vocal cord paralysis, focusing on the most recent techniques and the most promising and conservative approach currently available in this delicate field.

SURGICAL OPTIONS

Many surgical options have been described and used to increase the glottic space in BVCP (13), with continuous research of less invasive techniques. In 1946, Woodman (14) published a series of patients treated by arytenoidectomy and suture lateralization of the vocal process performed with the external posterolateral approach. This technique was reported with good results also by Cohen in 1973 (15) and Narcy in 1990 (16).

Other authors described partial and total arytenoidectomy with lateralization of the vocal process through the laryngofissure approach, making a midline incision of the thyroid cartilage (3, 17).

Thornell was one of the firsts to promote endoscopic procedures; he performed endoscopic arytenoidectomy using electrocautery (18). The development of the CO_2 laser gave new possibilities, ensuring greater precision, so in 1984 Ossoff et al. (19) described endoscopic CO_2 laser posterior cordotomy and in 1989 Dennis and Kashim (20) endoscopic laser CO2 arytenoidectomy (**Figure 1**).

In 1993, Crumley (21) proposed a variation of this procedure: endoscopic laser medial arytenoidectomy, preserving part of the cartilage including the vocal process, to reduce the consequences on the voice function. Bad voice quality is the main adverse effect of the surgery for BVCP, in particular after aritenoidectomy and posterior cordotomy (22, 23).

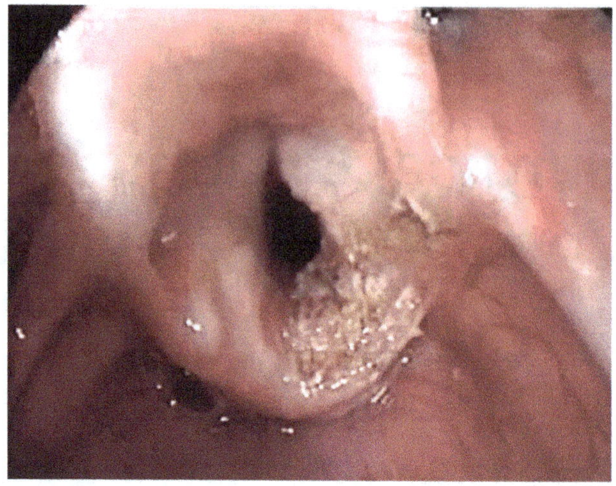

FIGURE 1 | CO_2 Laser right partial arytenoidectomy.

Most of the literature about the treatment of BVCP is referred to adult patients. One of the few describing a series of pediatric patients compared results of endoscopic vs. open arytenoidectomy [1994, Bower et al. (24)]. The series of 30 patients underwent endoscopic or external arytenoidectomy and lateralization, resulting in a higher decannulation rate for open arytenoidectomy (84%) than the endoscopic arytenoidectomy one (56%).

In 1989, Dennis and Kashima (20) introduced laser partial cordotomy (**Figure 2**) as a new endoscopic technique, which consisted of a triangular excision of the posterior true vocal fold and false vocal fold to improve the glottic respiratory space. In 2001, Friedman et al. (25) reported a series of pediatric patients all decannulated after posterior cordotomy. A combined endoscopic use of the two methods may be indicated (26).

A surgical revision may be often necessary both post arytenoidectomy than post posterior cordotomy for the presence of scar tissue or granulations, but the decannulation rate is high (27–29).

The use of new technologies has recently increased, with functional improvement and lower risk of thermal damage to the surrounding tissues: in 2015, Googe et al. (30) presented 14 cases of arytenoidectomy by coblator, and in 2018 Basterra et al. (31) described posterior cordotomy in bilateral vocal cord paralysis using monopolar microelectrodes and radiofrequency in 18 patients.

Ozturk et al. (32) compared laser cordotomy and diathermy-assisted cordotomy. Both the techniques gave a sufficient increase in respiratory space, stable over time, confirmed by respiratory functional test results. However, they showed a deterioration in terms of voice quality without significant differences between the two procedures.

Another procedure to improve the laryngeal respiratory space is the posterior cricoid split with rib grafting. This surgery,

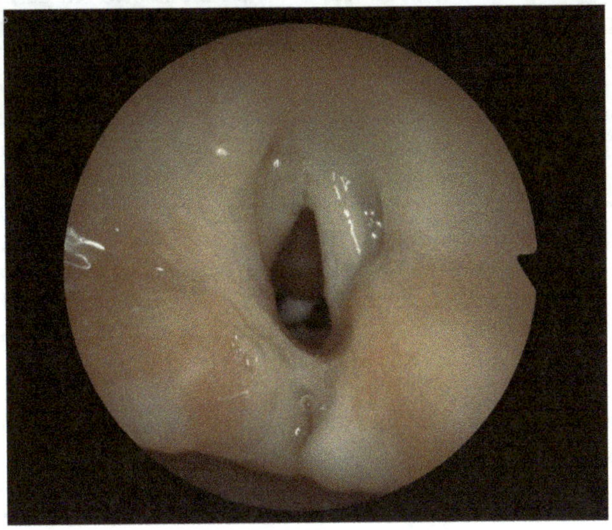

FIGURE 2 | Result after CO_2 laser left posterior cordotomy.

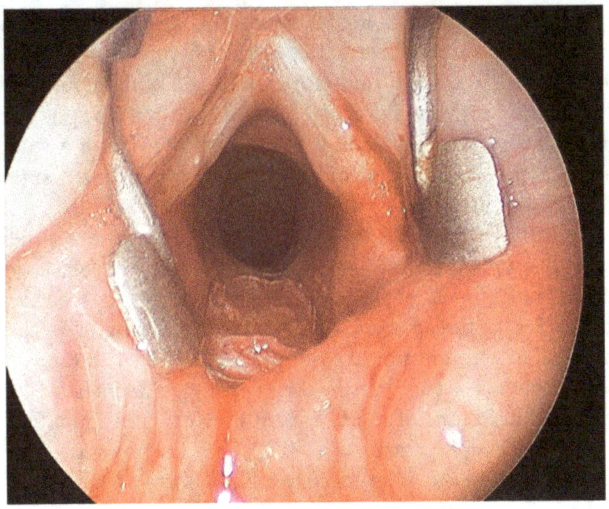

FIGURE 3 | Endoscopic posterior cricoid split with rib grafting.

mainly indicated for the treatment of glottic–subglottic stenosis and posterior glottic stenosis (33, 34), consists of a posterior enlargement of the interarytenoid space by splitting the cricoid plate and placing a rib cartilage graft, through laryngofissure (35) or using an endoscopic approach (12) (**Figure 3**). In 1994, Gray et al. (35) described the treatment of three cases of BVFP using this surgical procedure, with good outcomes in terms of decannulation (each patient was decannulated), and in 2003, Inglis et al. (12) published the results obtained in a series of 10 patients who underwent this surgery through endoscopic technique. For the latter, an excellent laryngeal and subglottic space exposure is crucial to performing midline posterior cricoid incision by CO_2 laser and splitting and where to put the cartilage rib graft opportunely shaped without appose sutures [no cases of graft dislodgment were described by Inglis in his paper (12)]. Recently, on 2017 again Inglis et al. (36) published a review of their experience about endoscopic posterior cricoid split during the last fifteen years. They described a series of 33 patients (32 had tracheostomy) with different pathologies (subglottic stenosis, posterior glottic stenosis, and bilateral vocal cord immobility) and a rate of decannulation after this surgery of 65.6% (only 28.6% for bilateral vocal fold immobility). This endoscopic procedure has the advantage of preserving the anatomy of the vocal folds and, theoretically, does not cause problems in case of spontaneous recovery of the motility and does not preclude the possibility of other surgeries, but its success was different for the pathologies treated, with worse results in subglottic stenosis combined with vocal cord paralysis. Furthermore, this surgery can be complicated by dysphagia and tracheotomy was considered before or during the endoscopic posterior cricoid split to prevent the risk of respiratory complications in case of dislodgment of the graft (36).

In 2018, Rutter et al. (37) proposed their results with the use of anterior–posterior cricoid split in a series of children in order to avoid tracheotomy. It consists in opening both sides of the cricoid cartilage endoscopically and dilating with an overestimate ETT for about a week. Between 2010 and 2016, they treated 19 patients with this technique and 14 (74%) avoided tracheostomy, demonstrating the effectiveness of the treatment under correct circumstances and so the opportunity to continue with further studies.

In 1922, Rethi (38) described the possibility of glottic enlargement with a lateralization of the vocal cord performed through a laryngofissure. Over the years, this technique has been resumed and perfected with the endoscopic approach as reported by Kirchner et al. in 1979 (39) and Ejnell et al. (40, 41). The laterofixation of the vocal cord is performed, after removal of the thyro-arytenoid muscle, by placing two sutures at the posterior third of the glottis, for each passing the thread above and below the vocal fold and pushing it out through the larynx, up to the skin where they are fixed in a little subcutaneous pouch over the muscle level.

Lichtenberger described the endoscopic vocal cord lateralization (42, 43) performed by using the Lichtenberger needle carrier (44), which more easily allows to pass the thread below and above the vocal fold through the thyroid cartilage, from the endolaryngeal lumen up to the skin. This procedure has been considered reversible from the authors; in case of recovery of vocal cord motility, the suture can be removed and a success rate up to 98% is described in literature (42, 43). Several variations of this technique have been proposed. Mathur et al. (45) tried to simplify the procedure using different instruments to reduce manipulation of the needle and thread inside the larynx and so the risks during the surgery. They performed lateralization of the vocal fold in a series of 10 pediatric patients by a set of spinal needles and a 2–0 stitch-passed extra laryngeal under endoscopic guidance, with a decannulation rate of 100% in the ten patients (45).

Woodson et al. (46, 47) described a very interesting alternative to laterofixation: arytenoid abduction. This technique simulates the natural contraction of posterior cricoarytenoid muscle and abduction of the vocal fold (**Figures 4A,B**). With a transverse skin incision at the midlevel of the thyroid cartilage, the posterior border of the thyroid cartilage is exposed to perform a suture laterofixation of the arytenoid cartilage by a permanent suture placed through the vocal process of the arytenoid and tied.

In 2010, Rovò et al. (48) proposed a new instrument for endoscopic arytenoid lateropexy, a modified endolaryngeal thread guide instrument (ETGI) based on a movable curved blade that guides the thread in and out from the endolaryngeal space up to the skin, with the aim to easily form a loop around the vocal process of the arytenoid cartilage and getting its abduction. They reported the results of the treatment of vocal cord immobility, including 22 adult patients with BVCP, showing how endoscopic arytenoid lateropexy is an effective solution for it (48).

In 2017, Madani et al. (1) described the possibility of using endoscopic arytenoid abduction lateropexy in 4 newborns by a new miniaturized ETGI, with good respiratory outcomes, no dyspnea, or swallowing disorder and satisfactory results about voice quality. Recently, the same Hungarian group (49) evaluated long-term results on the same patients after 3 years from endoscopic arytenoid abduction lateropexy. In terms of breathing, voice, and swallowing, every patient had durable resolution of dyspnea, a normal per os diet, an appropriate growth and development, and a normal voice in 2 cases and slightly impaired voice in 1 case.

Szakács et al. (50) published a comparison of the effects of different endoscopic glottis-widening procedures on cadaver; endoscopic arytenoid abduction lateropexy was the most effective and least destructive on phonation structures, providing with a physiological adduction movement the best phonation closure especially if recovery of adductor function occurs. Furthermore, the authors describe the reversibility of this technique without permanent damage to the vocal folds (49).

None of the surgical techniques above described can restore the normal laryngeal physiological movement of adduction and abduction.

With this purpose, laryngeal reinnervation techniques have been proposed.

In 1974, Miehlike (51) studied on animal model the anastomosis of the distal posterior branch of the laryngeal nerve (innervating the posterior crico-arytenoid muscle) with the main funiculus of the recurrent laryngeal nerve dissected out of the vagus. In 1975, Tucker (52) described a reinnervation procedure in adults consisting in dissecting a branch of the ansa hypoglossi joined to the corresponding area of omohyoid muscle to suture it at the level of the posterior cricoarytenoid muscle. In his series, three of five patients were decannulated with the increased glottic airway in over 80% of patients, but his results have never been reproducible in subsequent studies.

More recently, the use of foreign nerves has been deepened for the laryngeal reinnervation surgery in the treatment of bilateral paralysis. As described by Marina et al. (53) in 2011 and Li et al. (54) in 2013, the phrenic nerve can be used with good results to obtain a branch as a nerve substitute because it has a homogeneous composition of motoneurons involved during inspiration, with improvement of the movements in BVCP up to 93% (54).

Usually in BVFP, obstructive respiratory symptoms are predominant suggesting that adducting movement is partially preserved, so restoring the abduction function is the main purpose of these techniques with the possibility also of transecting the anterior laryngeal nerve branch to reduce the activity of the adductor muscles (53).

Recently, the rerouting of the thyrohyoid nerve for laryngeal reinnervation has been considered (55, 56) to reduce the length of the nerve graft and to find a reasonable alternative when ansa cervicalis is not available as a donor nerve, with good functional results and vocal outcomes (lower GIRBAS scores, higher maximal phonation time, stable, or improved postoperatively voice quality) (56).

Laryngeal reinnervation is a promising technique for BVCP, but the studies are still limited to adults with very limited experience in children (57) and in many cases, they refer to the treatment of unilateral vocal cord paralysis.

Alternative therapies have been investigated in recent years too, such as stem cell implant and gene therapy. Stem cell therapy for tissue regeneration in vocal cord paralysis may be applied by the use of autologous muscle-derived stem cells as Halum et al. (58) proposed in 2007 obtaining in rats the attenuation of muscle atrophy.

In 2016, Dirja et al. (59) tried the use of induced pluripotent stem cells with evidence of good differentiation in muscle cells *in vitro* and 2 weeks of survival in thyroarytenoid muscle of rats. Further papers show that adipose-derived stem cells (60) and olfactory ectomesenchymal stem cells (61) represent an interesting choice for this therapy; in particular, the latter have a high neuroregenerative potential in animal models. Always with the aim of promoting laryngeal nerve regeneration and muscle trophism, the idea of gene therapy has been proposed in several studies. It provides to use genes that encode neurotrophic factors for neuronal regeneration and growth factors for muscle cell proliferation and differentiation (62). These genes are linked to vectors that are injected into the laryngeal nerve and muscles (63, 64).

In 1998, Shiotani et al. studied the effect of insulin-like growth factor I gene in rats' denervated larynges (65), reporting an improvement of the size of muscle fibers and the number of axon terminals in the thyroarytenoid muscle, and in 2007 the effect of an adenoviral vector-encoding glial cell line-derived neurotrophic factor (GDNF) on the nucleus ambiguus of rats with vagus nerve injury (66), showing a lower loss of motoneurons after this treatment.

Both gene therapy and stem cell therapy are still experimental with *in vitro* and animal studies, therefore requiring further research and finding the solution to some problems such as ineffectiveness in preventing synkinesis, the risk of damage by viral vectors, and poor cell culture survival (51, 67).

Currently, functional electrical stimulation is another approach in progress for BVCP treatment. In 2016, Mueller et al. (68, 69) described the results of laryngeal pacing implant in 9 patients with evidence of spirometric parameter improvement,

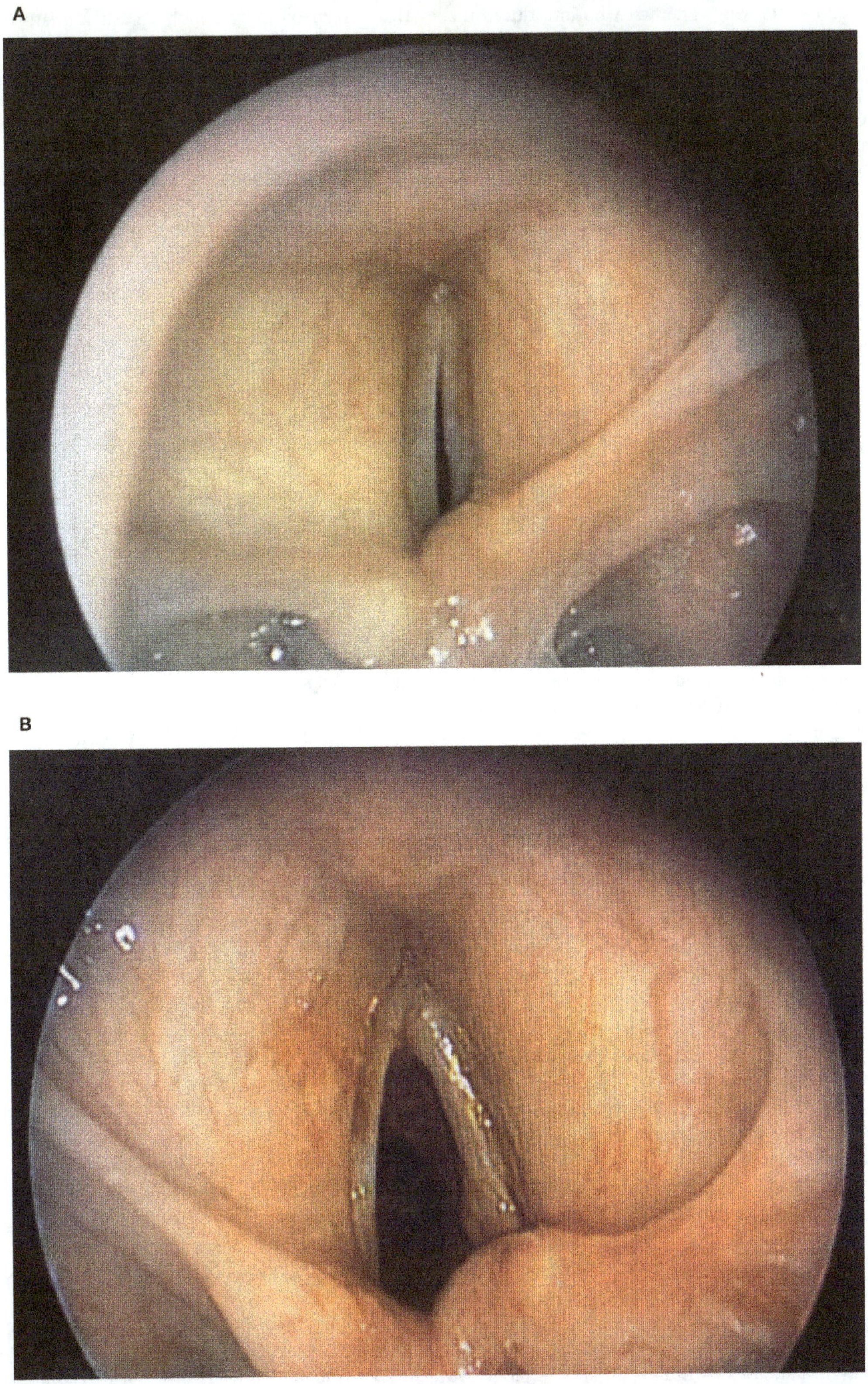

FIGURE 4 | (A) Endoscopic arytenoid lateropexy (before surgery). **(B)** Endoscopic arytenoid lateropexy (after surgery).

in particular of peak expiratory flow, without negative effects on the voice quality and swallowing. The first who introduced the functional electrical stimulation were Zealear and Dedo in 1977 (70), acting on unilaterally paralyzed cricothyroid muscle of the canine. In the following years, other authors reported the results about the stimulation of paralyzed posterior cricoarytenoid muscles, always in the canine model (71–73). Then in 1996, Zealear et al. (74) described the possibility of laryngeal pacing in humans, presenting in 2003 the results of unilateral laryngeal pacing in 7 patients with BVCP using an external device (75). In 2019, Muller and Pototschnig (76) showed their technique of electrical stimulation of the recurrent laryngeal nerve: one of the pacer electrodes is inserted into the PCA muscle, and the pacer is placed in a subcutaneous pocket over the sternum with another electrode on the lateral chest. Furthermore, they underline the importance of selection of patients who could have benefits from this procedure, as, for example, the presence of aberrant or synkinesis reinnervation is essential to ensuring good clinical performance of laryngeal pacemakers, although it is commonly considered an unfavorable condition for recovery of vocal cord movement (76). This technique has a high potentiality, ensuring a ventilatory improvement without compromising voice and swallowing (67). It could overcome the other surgical approach (76), and it has been described as superior to posterior cordotomy in ventilation and voice outcomes by Li et al. (77). However, it is still a complicated experimental procedure, more expensive than other surgeries considering also that the device must be replaced at least every 10 years (66), and so far there is no pediatric experience.

The comparisons of the different techniques do not show significant differences in literature, as reported by Gupta et al. (78), who found similar results in the decannulation rate between laser cordectomy, arytenoidectomy with fold lateralization, and endoscopic fold lateralization in a series of 61 patients (adults and children).

Partial arytenoidectomy and posterior cordotomy give an immediate respiratory space enlargement as well as vocal cord laterofixation, but the latter is certainly more conservative for laryngeal anatomy.

Laterofixation can be considered for its minimal invasiveness and reversibility (67, 79), ensuring minor impairment of voice. In particular, endoscopic arytenoid abduction lateropexy, characterized by an arytenoid abducted movement that preserves the vocal cordal anatomy and therefore the integrity of the mucosal wave, is a valid approach to obtain good respiratory outcomes preserving a good voice quality. During the last 2 years, at our Airway Surgery Unit, we focused the attention on this technique with excellent results that we are analyzing for an upcoming publication, characterized by significant improvement of the respiratory space and high decannulation rate maintaining a good quality of voice.

After diagnosis of BVCP, time of observation may be indicated especially in patients in whom spontaneous recovery can be expected (79), but the challenge and current trend in our department and in many major pediatric center is to avoid tracheotomy through an early treatment (67, 79). Our opinion, supported by literature (48), is that the endoscopic arytenoid abduction lateropexy is a good approach for an early treatment also in infants considering its characteristics of preservation of the vocal cord anatomy and reversibility in case of spontaneous recovery.

Exactly to evaluate the possibility of spontaneous recovery, laryngeal electromyography could have an important prognostic role identifying the candidates for early intervention, as described in several studies (80–84). Laryngeal electromyography shows the motor unit potentials, through hooked wire electrodes inserted into the thyro-arytenoid muscle and the posterior cricoarytenoid muscle, and it can be used to differentiate between mechanical (i.e., cricoarytenoid joint fixation) and neurological impairment of vocal fold and to localize the neuromuscular lesion.

As reported in a recent paper by Giotakis and Pototschnig (85), the presence of volitional activity in the multiple LEMG findings indicates the possibility of a full late recovery of laryngeal motility, allowing to select the cases for a wait-and-see strategy or a reversible approach, rather than a permanent laryngeal surgery. However, in the literature the opinion about the predictive value of this test is under debate, with data ranging from 13 to 96% (80, 81, 86).

SUMMARY

Identifying the best surgical approach for BVCP in pediatric patients is not easy, considering also that the experiences reported by many authors concern adult patients with very few and small series in children and that the comparisons of the different techniques do not show significant differences in literature.

Most studies report the results in terms of respiratory improvement and decannulation rate, with less attention to voice quality evaluation or assessing swallowing, even if common side effects of the BVCP surgery are dysphonia, dysphagia, and aspiration, but comparing with previous reviews in pediatrics' BVCP treatments, in addition to the global trend to reduce invasiveness, we observed a recent increasing in attention to preserve the quality of the voice.

The new techniques and therapies described above still require further studies and trials but are promising for the future in order to overcome more destructive surgical techniques and giving a potential dynamic functional recovery of the larynx.

AUTHOR CONTRIBUTIONS

MT, DM, AS, MLT, and SB contributed conception and design of the study. MT, DM, and AS wrote the manuscript. All authors contributed to manuscript revision, read and approved the submitted version.

REFERENCES

1. Madani S, Bach Á, Matievics V, Erdélyi E, Sztanó B, Szegesdi I, et al. A new solution for neonatal bilateral vocal cord paralysis: endoscopic arytenoid abduction lateropexy. *Laryngoscope.* (2017) 127:1608–14. doi: 10.1002/lary.26366
2. Holinger LD, Holinger PC, Holinger PH. Etiology of bilateral abductor vocal cord paralysis: a review of 389 cases. *Ann Otol Rhinol Laryngol.* (1976) 85(4Pt 1):428–36. doi: 10.1177/000348947608500402
3. Brigger MT, Hartnick CJ. Surgery for pediatric vocal cord paralysis: a meta-analysis. *Otolaryngol Head Neck Surg.* (2002) 126:349–55. doi: 10.1067/mhn.2002.124185
4. Daya H, Hosni A, Bejar-Solar I, Evans JN, Bailey CM. Pediatric vocal fold paralysis: a long-term retrospective study. *Arch Otolaryngol Head Neck Surg.* (2000) 126:21-25. doi: 10.1001/archotol.126.1.21
5. Rosin DF, Handler SD, Potsic WP, et al. Vocal cord paralysis in children. *Laryngoscope.* (1990) 100:1174–9. doi: 10.1288/00005537-199011000-00008
6. Miyamoto RC, Parikh SR, Gellad W, Licameli GR. Bilateral congenital vocal cord paralysis: a 16-year institutional review. *Otolaryngol Head Neck Surg.* (2005) 133:241–5. doi: 10.1016/j.otohns.2005.02.019
7. Zbar RI, Smith RJ. Vocal fold paralysis in infants twelve months of age and younger. *Otolaryngol. Head Neck Surg.* (1996) 114:18–21. doi: 10.1016/S0194-5998(96)70277-2
8. Kovesi T, Porcaro F, Petreschi F, Trozzi M, Bottero S, Cutrera R. Vocal cord paralysis appears to be an acquired lesion in children with repaired esophageal atresia/tracheoesophageal fistula. *Int J Pediatr Otorhinolaryngol.* (2018) 112:45–7. doi: 10.1016/j.ijporl.2018.06.031
9. Takamatsu I. Bilateral vocal cord paralysis in children. *Nihon Jibiinkoka Gakkai Kaiho.* (1996) 99:91–102. doi: 10.3950/jibiinkoka.99.91
10. Jomah M, Jeffery C, Campbell S, Krajacic A, El-Hakim H. Spontaneous recovery of bilateral congenital idiopathic laryngeal paralysis: systemat- ic non-meta-analytical review. *Int J Pediatr Otorhinolaryngol.* (2015) 79:202–9. doi: 10.1016/j.ijporl.2014.12.007
11. Smith ME. Vocal fold paralysis in children. In: Sulica L, Blitzer A, editors. *Vocal Fold Paralysis.* Berlin/Heidelberg: Springer (2006). p. 225–35. doi: 10.1007/3-540-32504-2_24
12. Inglis AF Jr, Perkins JA, Manning SC, Mouzakes J. Endoscopic posterior cricoid split and rib grafting in 10 children. *Laryngoscope.* (2003) 113:2004–9. doi: 10.1097/00005537-200311000-00028
13. Messner A. Congenital disorders of the larynx. In: Cummings C, editor. *Cummings Otolaryngology- Head And Neck Surgery. 4th edition.* Philadelphia: Mosby, Inc. (2005). p. 4226-7.
14. Woodman DG, Pennington CL. Bilateral abductor paralysis: 30 years experience with arytenoidectomy. *Ann Otol Rhinol Laryngol.* (1976) 85(4 Pt 1):437–9. doi: 10.1177/000348947608500403
15. Cohen SR. Arytenoidectomy in children. *Laryngoscope.* (1973) 83:1293–99. doi: 10.1288/00005537-197308000-00013
16. Narcy P, Contencin P, Viala P. Surgical treatment for laryngeal paralysis in infants and children. *Ann Otol Rhinol Laryngol.* (1990) 99:124–8. doi: 10.1177/000348949009900209
17. Hartnick CJ, Brigger MT, Willging JP, Cotton RT, Myer CM. Surgery for pediatric vocal cord paralysis: a retrospective review. *Ann Otol Rhinol Laryngol.* (2003) 112:1–6. doi: 10.1177/000348940311200101
18. Thornell WC. Intralaryngeal arytenoidectomy for bilateral abductor vocal cord paralysis. *Ann Otol Rhinol Laryngol.* (1952) 61:601–8.
19. Ossoff RH, Sisson GA, Duncavage JA, Moselle HI, Andrews PE, Mc Millan WG. Endoscopic laser arytenoidectomy for the treatment of bilateral vocal cord paralysis. *Laryngoscope.* (1984) 94:1293–7. doi: 10.1288/00005537-198410000-00006
20. Dennis DP, Kashima H. Carbon dioxide laser posterior cordectomy for treatment of bilateral vocal cord paralysis. *Ann Otol Rhinol Laryngol.* (1989) 98(12 Pt 1):930–4. doi: 10.1177/000348948909801203
21. Crumley RL. Endoscopic laser medial arytenoidectomy for airway management in bilateral laryngeal paralysis. *Ann Otol Rhinol Laryngol.* (1993) 102:81–4. doi: 10.1177/000348949310200201
22. Maurizi M, Paludetti G, Galli J, Cosenza A, Di Girolamo S, Ottavi- ani F. CO2 laser subtotal arytenoidectomy and posterior true and false cordotomy in the treatment of post-thyroidectomy bilateral laryngeal fixation in adduction. *Eur Arch Otorhinolaryngol.* (1999) 256:291–5. doi: 10.1007/s004050050248
23. Hillel AT, Giraldez L, Samad I, Gross J, Klein AM, Johns MM. Voice outcomes following posterior cordotomy with medial aryte- noidectomy in patients with bilateral vocal fold immobility. *JAMA Otolaryngol Head Neck Surg.* (2015) 141:728–32. doi: 10.1001/jamaoto.2015.1136
24. Bower CM, Choi SS, Cotton RT. Arytenoidectomy in children. *Ann Otol Rhinol Laryngol.* (1994) 103(4 Pt 1):271–8. doi: 10.1177/0003489494103 00403
25. Friedman EM, de Jong AL, Sulek M. Pediatric bilateral vocal fold immobility: the role of carbon dioxide laser posterior transverse partial cordectomy. *Ann Otol Rhinol Laryngol.* (2001) 110:723–8. doi: 10.1177/0003489401110 00805
26. Bizakis JG, Papadakis CE, Karatzanis AD, et al. The combined endoscopic CO(2) laser posterior cordectomy and total arytenoidectomy for treatment of bilateral vocal cord paralysis. *Clin Otolaryngol Allied Sci.* (2004) 29:51–4. doi: 10.1111/j.1365-2273.2004.00779.x
27. Yilmaz T, Suslu N, Atay G, Ozer S, Gunaydin RO, Bajin MD. Com- parison of voice and swallowing parameters after endoscopic total and partial arytenoidectomy for bilateral abductor vocal fold pa- ralysis: a randomized trial. *JAMA Otolaryngol Head Neck Surg.* (2013) 139:712–8. doi: 10.1001/jamaoto.2013.3395
28. Yilmaz T, Altuntas OM, Suslu N, Atay G, Ozer S, Kuscu O, et al. To- tal and partial laser arytenoidectomy for bilateral vocal fold paral- ysis. *Biomed Res Int.* (2016) 2016:3601612. doi: 10.1155/2016/3601612
29. Rashid M, Ayaz SB, Saleem H, Hussain R, Zaman S. Results of carbon dioxide laser-assisted posterior cordotomy in cases of bilateral vocal cord paralysis: An analysis of 34 casest. *J Pak Med Assoc.* (2019) 69:1539–42. doi: 10.5455/JPMA.302642798
30. Googe B, Nida A, Schweinfurth J. Coblator arytenoidectomy in the treatment of bilateral vocal cord paralysis. *Case Rep Otolaryngol.* (2015) 2015:487280. doi: 10.1155/2015/487280
31. Basterra J, Castillo-Lopez Y, Reboll R, Zapater E, Olavarria C, Krause F, et al. Posterior cordotomy in bilateral vocal cord paralysis using monopolar microelectrodes and radiofrequency in 18 patient. *Clin Otolaryngol.* (2018) 43:340–3. doi: 10.1111/coa.12940
32. Ozturk K, Turhal G, Kaya I, Aysel A, Benzer M, Korkmaz Ekren P, et al. A comparison of two endoscopic posterior cordotomy techniques: laser cordotomy vs diathermy-assisted cordotomy. *Clin Otolaryngol.* (2018) 43:256–60. doi: 10.1111/coa.12953
33. Zalzal GH. Posterior glottic stenosis. *Int J Pediatr Otorhinolaryngol.* (1999) 49(Suppl 1):S279–82. doi: 10.1016/S0165-5876(99)00173-1
34. Rutter MJ, Cotton RT. The use of posterior cricoid grafting in managing isolated posterior glottic stenosis in children. *Arch Otolaryngol Head Neck Surg.* (2004) 130:737–9. doi: 10.1001/archotol.130.6.737
35. Gray SD, Kelly SM, Dove H. Arytenoid separation for impaired pediatric vocal fold mobility. *Ann Otol Rhinol Laryngol.* (1994) 103:510–5. doi: 10.1177/000348949410300702
36. Dahl JP, Purcell PL, Parikh SR, Inglis AF Jr. Endoscopic posterior cricoid split with costal cartilage graft: a fifteen-year experience. *Laryngoscope.* (2017) 127:252–7. doi: 10.1002/lary.26200
37. Rutter MJ, Hart CK, Alarcon A, Daniel SJ, Parikh SR, Balakrishnan K, et al. Endoscopic anterior-posterior cricoid split for pediatric bilateral vocal fold paralysis. *Laryngoscope.* (2018) 128:257–63. doi: 10.1002/lary. 26547
38. Rethi A. Die operative lösung der bei der beiderseitigen postikuslähmung bestehenden medianlage. *Mschr Ohr Laryngorhinol.* (1922) 56:200–4.
39. Kirchner FR. Endoscopic lateralization of the vocal cord in abductor paralysis of the larynx. *Laryngoscope.* (1979) 89:1779–83. doi: 10.1288/00005537-197911000-00010
40. Ejnell H, Bake B, Hallen O, Lindstrom J, Maringnsson I, Stenborg R. A new simple method of laterofixation and its effects on orolaryngeal airway resistance and fonation. *Acta Otolaryngol.* (1982) 93(suppl 386):196–7. doi: 10.3109/00016488209108517
41. Ejnell H, Mansson I, Hallen O, Bake B, Stenborg R, Lindstrom J. A simple operation for bilateral vocal cord paralysis. *Laryngoscope.* (1984) 94:954–8. doi: 10.1288/00005537-198407000-00018

42. Lichtenberger G. Reversible immediate and definitive lateralization of paralyzed vocal cords. *Eur Arch Otorhinolaryngol.* (1999) 256:407–11. doi: 10.1007/s004050050176
43. Lichtenberger G. Reversible lateralization of the paralyzed vocal cord without tracheostomy. *Ann Otol Rhinol Laryngol.* (2002) 111:21–26. doi: 10.1177/000348940211100104
44. Lichtenberger G, Toohill RJ. The endo-extralaryngeal needle carrier. *Otolaryngol Head Neck Surg.* (1991) 105:755–56. doi: 10.1177/01945998911 0500522
45. Mathur NN, Kumar S, Bothra R. Simple method of vocal cord lateralization in bilateral abductor cord paralysis in pediatric patients. *Int J Pediatr Otorhinolaryngol.* (2004) 68:15–20. doi: 10.1016/j.ijporl.2003.08.050
46. Woodson G, Weiss T. Arytenoid abduction for dynamic rehabilitation of bilateral laryngeal paralysis. *Ann Otol Rhinol Laryngol.* (2007) 116:483–90. doi: 10.1177/000348940711600702
47. Woodson G. Arytenoid abduction for bilateral vocal fold immobility. *Curr Opin Otolaryngol Head Neck Surg.* (2011) 19:428–33. doi: 10.1097/MOO. 0b013e32834cd564
48. Rovó L, Madani S, Sztanó B, Majoros V, Smehák G, Szakács L, et al. A new thread guide instrument for endoscopic arytenoid lateropexy. *Laryngoscope.* (2010) 120:2002–7. doi: 10.1002/lary.21055
49. Sztanó B, Bach Á, Matievics V, Erdélyi E, Szegesdi I, Wootten CT, et al. Endoscopic arytenoid abduction lateropexy for the treatment of neonatal bilateral vocal cord paralysis - long-term results. *Int J Pediatr Otorhinolaryngol.* (2019) 119:147–50. doi: 10.1016/j.ijporl.2019.01.032
50. Szakács L, Sztanó B, Matievics V, Bere Z, Bach A, Castellanos PF, et al. A comparison between transoral glottis-widening techniques for bilateral vocal fold immobility. *Laryngoscope.* (2015) 125:2522–9. doi: 10.1002/lary.25401
51. Miehlike A. Rehabilitation of vocal cord paralysis: studies using the vagus recurrent bypass anastomosis, type ramus posterior shunt. *Arch Otolaryngol.* (1974) 100:431–41. doi: 10.1001/archotol.1974.00780040445005
52. Tucker HM. Human laryngeal reinnervation. *Laryngoscope.* (1976) 86:769–79. doi: 10.1288/00005537-197606000-00004
53. Marina MB, Marie JP, Birchall MA. Laryngeal reinnervation for bilateral vocal fold paralysis. *Curr Opin Otolaryngol Head Neck Surg.* (2011) 19:434–8. doi: 10.1097/MOO.0b013e32834c7d30
54. Li M, Chen S, Zheng H, Chen D, Zhu M, Wang W, et al. Reinnervation of bilateral posterior cricoarytenoid muscles using the left phrenic nerve in patients with bilateral vocal fold paralysis. *PLoS ONE.* (2013) 8:e77233. doi: 10.1371/journal.pone.0077233
55. Crampon F, Duparc F, Trost O, Marie JP. Selective laryngeal reinnervation: can rerouting of the thyrohyoid nerve simplify the procedure by avoiding the use of a nerve graft? *Surg Radiol Anat.* (2019) 41:145–50. doi: 10.1007/s00276-018-2117-y
56. Graham ME, Smith ME. The nerve to thyrohyoid muscle as a novel donor nerve for laryngeal reinnervation. *Ann Otol Rhinol Laryngol.* (2019) 18:3489419888956. doi: 10.1177/0003489419888956
57. Lee JW, Bon-Mardion N, Smith ME, Marie JP. Bilateral selective laryngeal reinnervation for bilateral vocal fold paralysis in children. *AMA Otolaryngol Head Neck Surg.* (2020) 146:401–7. doi: 10.1001/jamaoto.2019.4863
58. Halum SL, Naidu M, Delo DM, Atala A, Hingtgen CM. Injection of autologous muscle stem cells (myoblasts) for the treatment of vocal fold paralysis: a pilot study. *Laryngoscope.* (2007) 117:917–22. doi: 10.1097/MLG.0b013e31803 e8c8d
59. Dirja BT, Yoshie S, Ikeda M, Imaizumi M, Nakamura R, Otsuki K, et al. Potential of laryngeal muscle regeneration using induced pluripotent stem cell-derived skeletal muscle cells. *Acta Otolaryngol.* (2016) 136:391–6. doi: 10.3109/00016489.2015.1126351
60. Nishio N, Fujimoto Y, Suga K, Iwata Y, Toriyama K, Takanari K, et al. Autologous fat injection therapy including a high concentration of adipose-derived regenerative cells in a vocal fold paralysis model: animal pilot study. *J Laryngol Otol.* (2016) 130:914–22. doi: 10.1017/S00222151160 08707
61. Saïd Z, Pauline C, Claire B, Celia D, Jean-Paul M, Nicolas BM. Olfactory ecto-mesenchymal stem cells in laryngeal nerve regeneration in rats. *J Voice.* (2019). doi: 10.1016/j.jvoice.2019.10.012. [Epub ahead of print].
62. Bijangi-Vishehsaraei K, Blum K, Zhang H, Safa AR, Halum SL. Microarray analysis gene expression profiles in laryngeal muscle after recurrent laryngeal nerve injury. *Ann Otol Rhinol Laryngol.* (2016) 125:247–56. doi: 10.1177/0003489415608866
63. Rubin A, Mobley B, Hogikyan N, Bell K, Sullivan K, Boulis N, et al. Delivery of an adenoviral vector to the crushed recurrent laryngeal nerve. *Laryngoscope.* (2003) 113:985–9. doi: 10.1097/00005537-200306000-00013
64. Heavner SB, Rubin AD, Fung K, Old M, Hogikyan ND, Feldman EL. Dysfunction of the recurrent laryngeal nerve and the potential of gene therapy. *Ann Otol Rhinol Laryngol.* (2007) 116:441–8. doi: 10.1177/0003489407116 00609
65. Shiotani A, O'Malley BW Jr, Coleman ME, Alila HW, Flint PW. Reinnervation of motor endplates and increased muscle fiber size after human insulin-like growth factor I gene transfer into the paralyzed larynx. *Hum Gene Ther.* (1998) 9:2039–47. doi: 10.1089/hum.1998.9.14-2039
66. Shiotani A, Saito K, Araki K, Moro K, Watabe K. Gene therapy for laryngeal paralysis. *Ann Otol Rhinol Laryngol.* (2007) 116:115–22. doi: 10.1177/000348940711600207
67. Li Y, Garrett G, Zealear D. Current treatment options for bilateral vocal fold paralysis: a state-of-the-art review. *Clin Exp Otorhinolaryngol.* (2017) 10:203–12. doi: 10.21053/ceo.2017.00199
68. Mueller AH, Hagen R, Pototschnig C, Foerster G, Grossmann W, Baumbusch K, et al. Laryngeal pacing for bilateral vocal fold paralysis: voice and respiratory aspects. *Laryngoscope.* (2016) 2016:10. doi: 10.1002/lary.26428
69. Mueller AH, Hagen R, Foerster G, Grossmann W, Baumbusch K, Pototschnig C. Laryngeal pacing via an implantable stimulator for the rehabilitation of subjects suffering from bilateral vocal fold paralysis: a prospective first-in-human study. *Laryngoscope.* (2016) 126:1810–6. doi: 10.1002/lary.25792
70. Zealear DL, Dedo HH. Control of paralyzed axial muscles by electrical stimulation. *Trans Sect Otolaryngol Am Acad Ophthalmol Otolaryngol.* (1977) 84:310.
71. Obert PM, Young KA, Tobey DN. Use of direct posterior cricoarytenoid stimulation in laryngeal paralysis. *Arch Otolaryngol.* (1984) 110:88–92. doi: 10.1001/archotol.1984.00800280022007
72. Broniatowski M, Kaneko S, Jacobs G, Nose Y, Tucker HM. Laryngeal pacemaker: II. electronic pacing of reinnervated posterior cricoarytenoid muscles in the canine. *Laryngoscope.* (1985) 95:1194–8. doi: 10.1288/000 05537-198510000-00008
73. Herzon GD, Zealear DL. Use of an electronic laryngeal implant to restore glottic function in patients with bilateral vocal cord paralysis. *Cancer Focus.* (1986) 8:45–8.
74. Zealear DL, Rainey CL, Herzon GD, Netterville JL, Ossoff RH. Electrical pacing of the paralyzed human larynx. *Ann Otol Rhinol Laryngol.* (1996) 105:689–93. doi: 10.1177/000348949610500904
75. Zealear DL, Billante CR, Courey MS, Netterville JL, Paniello RC, Sanders I, et al. Reanimation of the paralyzed human larynx with an implantable electrical stimulation device. *Laryngoscope.* (2003) 113:1149–56. doi: 10.1097/00005537-200307000-00010
76. Mueller AH, Pototschnig C. Recurrent laryngeal nerve stimulator. *Otolaryngol Clin North Am.* (2020) 53:145–56. doi: 10.1016/j.otc.2019.09.009
77. Li Y, Pearce EC, Mainthia R, Athavale SM, Dang J, Ashmead DH, et al. Comparison of ventilation and voice outcomes between unilateral laryngeal pacing and unilateral cordotomy for the treatment of bilateral vocal fold paralysis. *ORL J Otorhinolaryngol Relat Spec.* (2013) 75:68–73. doi: 10.1159/000345501
78. Gupta AK, Mann SB, Nagarkar N. Surgical management of bilateral immobile vocal folds and long-term follow-up. *J Laryngol Otol.* (1997) 111:474–7. doi: 10.1017/S0022215100137685
79. Chen EY, Inglis AF. Bilateral vocal cord paralysis in children. *Otolaryngol Clin N Am.* (2008) 41:889–901. doi: 10.1016/j.otc.2008.04.003
80. Munin MC, Rosen CA, Zullo T. Utility of laryngeal electromyography in predicting recovery after vocal fold paralysis. *Arch Phys Med Rehabil.* (2003) 84:1150–3. doi: 10.1016/S0003-9993(03)00146-1
81. Grosheva M, Wittekindt C, Pototschnig C, Lindenthaler W, Guntinas-Lichius O. Evaluation of peripheral vocal cord paralysis by electromyogrphy. *Laryngoscope.* (2008) 118:987–90. doi: 10.1097/MLG.0b013e3181671b2d
82. Wang CC, Chang MH, De Virgilio A, Jiang RS, Lai HC, Wang CP, et al. Laryngeal electromyography and prognosis of unilateral vocal fold paralysis-a long-term prospective study. *Laryngoscope.* (2015) 125:898–903. doi: 10.1002/lary.24980

83. Munin MC, Heman-Ackah YD, Rosen CA, Sulica L, Maronian N, Mandel S, et al. Consensus statement: using laryngeal electromyography for the diagnosis and treatment of vocal cord paralysis. *Muscle Nerve.* (2016) 53:850–5. doi: 10.1002/mus.25090
84. Smith LJ, Rosen CA, Munin MC. Vocal fold motion outcome based on excellent prognosis with laryngeal electromyography. *Laryngoscope.* (2016) 126:2310–4. doi: 10.1002/lary.25910
85. Giotakis AI, Pototschnig C. Prognosis of congenital idiopathic abductor laryngeal paralysis with laryngeal electromyography. *Laryngoscope.* (2020) 130:E252–E7. doi: 10.1002/lary.28079
86. Sittel C, Stennert E, Thumfart WF, Dapunt U, Eckel HE. Prognostic value of laryngeal electromyography in vocal fold paralysis. *Arch Otolaryngology Head Neck Surg.* (2001) 127:155–60. doi: 10.1001/archotol.127.2.155

18

Reconstruction of Chest Wall by Cryopreserved Sternum Allograft After Resection of Sternal Hemangioma

Farahnaz Sadegh Beigee[1], *Ali Sheikhy*[2,3] *and Kambiz Sheikhy*[1*]

[1] *Department of Thoracic Surgery, Lung Transplantation Research Center, National Research Institute of Tuberculosis and Lung Diseases, Masih Daneshvari Hospital, Shahid Beheshti University of Medical Sciences, Tehran, Iran,* [2] *Research Department, Tehran Heart Center, Tehran University of Medical Sciences, Tehran, Iran,* [3] *Non-communicable Disease Research Center, Endocrinology and Metabolism Population Sciences Institute, Tehran University of Medical Sciences, Tehran, Iran*

Correspondence:
Kambiz Sheikhy
ksheikhy@sbmu.ac.ir

A 5-year-old girl was referred to our department for a mass of sternum that was previously biopsied and diagnosed as hemangioma. Chest X-ray and CT scan confirmed a large sternal mass. We resected the sternum completely and reconstructed a large anterior chest wall defect by a cryopreserved sternal allograft. In the follow-up of the patient, there was no instability of the chest wall and acceptable cosmetic results.

Keywords: sternal tumor, hemangioma, sternal allograft, cryopreserved bone allograft, case report

INTRODUCTION

Radical resection of the sternum is indicated in different situations, such as tumors, infection, radionecrosis, and trauma. In addition, it may be considered as an alternative surgical treatment in chest wall deformity (1). Sternum hemangioma is a rare benign bone tumor, and, to the best of our knowledge, about five cases have been reported in the literature, including adult and pediatric; meanwhile, any of them did not include pectus carinatum deformity coexisting with hemangioma of the sternum (2–5). In the case of sternal resection, reconstruction of the sternum is mandatory to prevent flail chest and ventilation impairment; besides, cosmetic consequences must also be considered. Due to mentioned difficulties, this procedure is challenging for most thoracic and reconstructive surgeons (6, 7).

Various techniques have been described previously, but there is no gold standard procedure for managing these defects (8). There is limited experience with a new method for the reconstruction of the sternum by utilizing cryopreserved sternal allograft; furthermore, no previous study was conducted in the pediatric group.

In this case report, we described a 5-year-old girl with the sternum hemangioma and pectus carinatum deformity, on whom reconstruction of the chest wall with a cryopreserved sternal allograft was conducted after complete surgical resection of the tumor (sternectomy).

CASE REPORT

A 5-year-old girl was referred to our thoracic surgery unit following diagnosis of hemangioma of the sternum (**Figure 1**). When she was 3 years old, following an attack of seizure, her brain MRI revealed a calcified hemangioma in addition to pectus carinatum deformity and thrombocytopenia (platelet count = 15,000/μL) in her primary evaluations. A chest CT scan was performed, which

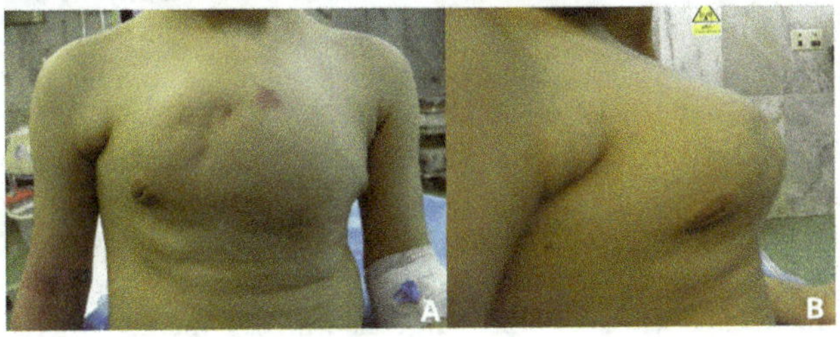

FIGURE 1 | Preoperative anterior **(A)** and lateral **(B)** view pictures showing a deformity and large mass.

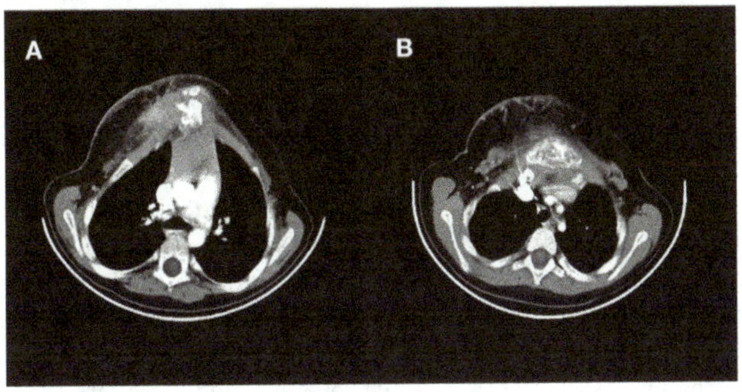

FIGURE 2 | Preoperative CT scan showing a large sternum mass. **(A)** Uppers segments, **(B)** lower segments.

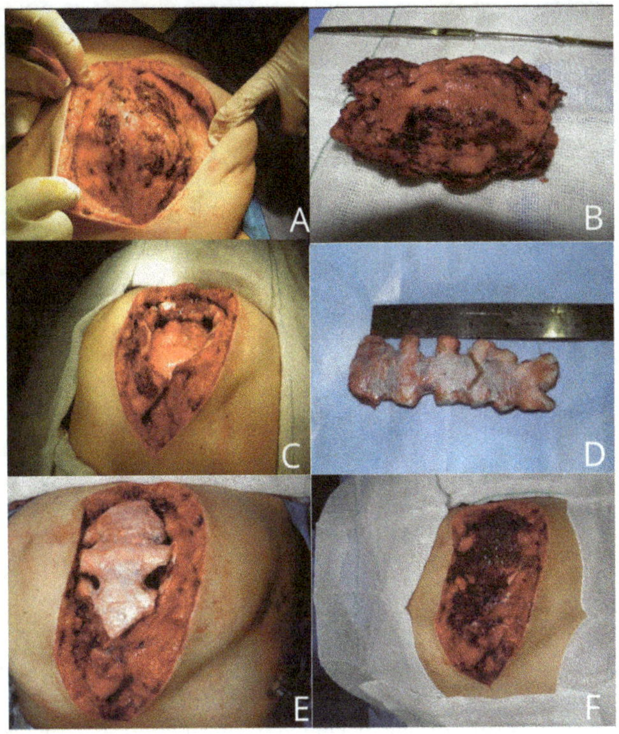

FIGURE 3 | An intraoperative picture of sternal mass **(A)**. Resected hemangioma with an acceptable margin **(B)**. Large chest wall defect **(C)**. Cryopreserved sternal allograft **(D)**. Covering of chest wall defect with graft **(E,F)**.

demonstrated a sternal expansile mass (**Figure 2**). Incisional biopsy of the mass was performed, and pathologic finding was compatible with hemangioma. Considering her thrombocytopenia, she underwent corticosteroid therapy. She experienced recurrent thrombocytopenia after corticosteroids withdrawal; therefore, she was referred for resection of sternal hemangioma as a potential genesis of thrombocytopenia. At the time of admission, she had a platelet count of 20,000/μL eventually; corticosteroid therapy was established before resection to normalize the platelet count.

According to CT findings, near-complete resection of the sternum was arranged. Based on predicted sternum size, measured according to anthropometric parameters and the resected area of the chest wall, a cryopreserved sternum was ordered from the tissue bank center. At the time of the surgery, a longitudinally elliptical midline incision was performed, which included a previous biopsy site. There was no infiltration or adhesion of mass to skin and subcutaneous tissue except the biopsied area, and a well-defined, capsulated but vascular mass was dissected from surrounding tissues. Due to the large dimension of the tumor, pectoralis major muscles were pushed laterally to nearly midclavicular lines (**Figures 3A,B**). The upper border of the manubrium seemed to be normal and preserved. The thoracic cavity was entered on the left side, and near-total sternectomy, including tumor and most parts of deformed cartilages, was achieved. Eventually, there was a 15 × 12-cm defect in the anterior chest wall. The previously preserved cryopreserved sternum allograft was prepared for the reconstruction (**Figures 3C,D**). The graft was dampened by 40°C normal salines, tailored gradually, fixed to the patient's ribs by titanium plates and screws, and fixed to remained manubrium (**Figures 3E,F**). Subsequently, the graft was covered by pectoralis muscles and after insertion of a bilateral chest tube and subcutaneous right side vacuum suction drainage; the skin was closed in the midline. The patient was extubated in the operation room. After surgery, the chest wall was completely stable, and there was no need for ventilator support. Chest tubes were removed on the 3rd day after the operation, and there was no evidence of wound infection. The patient was discharged after 7 days. In the 1st month after surgery, the defect was stable with no complications. The final pathologic finding was compatible with hemangioma (**Supplementary Figure 1**). Sixteen months after the operation, there was a minimal deformity in the anterior chest wall without any evidence of chest wall instability (**Figure 4**).

DISCUSSION

Hemangioma of the sternum is an extremely rare benign sternal tumor. To the best of our knowledge, <5 cases have been reported previously (2–5), and simultaneous occurrence of pectus carinatum and sternum hemangioma is a novel condition, although this type of anterior chest wall deformity

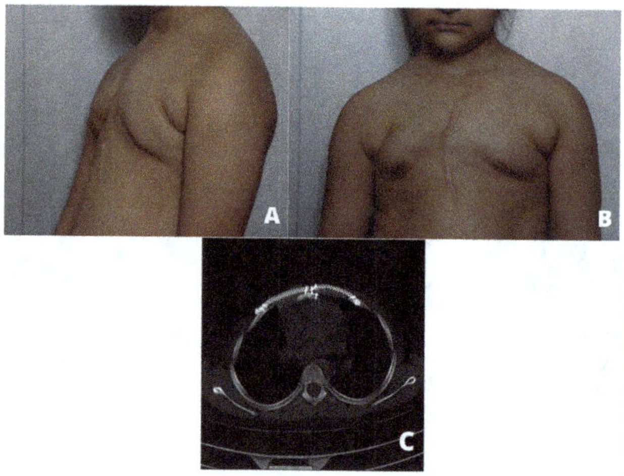

FIGURE 4 | An anterior, lateral photograph **(A,B)** and CT scan **(C)** 16 months after the operation.

may be acquired and secondary to abnormal overgrowth of the sternum (9). On the other hand, resection of sternum and repair strategies of the remained defect after resection based on different pathologies is challenging, especially in the pediatric. The most challenging part of the operation is the best reconstructive strategy selection for the reconstruction of the anterior chest wall. Reconstruction of soft tissue defects with various types of flaps is less challenging. The ongoing growth of a child and adverse effects of growth restriction following resection and reconstruction is the most important challenging points of pediatrics in contrast to adults.

Methyl methacrylate meshes and sandwiches, polytetrafluoroethylene (PTFE), and polypropylene patches are routinely used in thoracic surgery for reconstruction. The disadvantages of these prosthetic materials are the risk of infection, dislodgement, and long-term complications, including changes in thoracic morphology and function in pediatric patients (10). Metallic materials, such as titanium clips, plates, and moldable multi-hole plates, have been used for the stabilization of the chest wall (11, 12) and may have the same complications as other prosthetic materials. Turna et al. (13) described reconstruction of anterior chest wall defect after wide resection of this part with a well-designed patient-specific titanium implant. In addition, a hydroxyapatite tricalcium-phosphate compound (ceramic) that can be shaped has been introduced for reconstruction (11).

Due to complications related to using prosthetic material, such as infection, rigidity, and probable growth restriction in children, bone grafts have gained considerable attention in the reconstruction of the chest wall (14). Ribs can be harvested as autografts from the opposite surgical site or can be used as allografts. In extensive chest wall defects, as in sternum tumor resection, bone autograft harvest may lead to significant morbidity (15). A potentially inexhaustible source of bone for the reconstruction of chest wall defects in the human cadaver. The main advantage of bone grafts is their capability of integration with host tissue and chest wall stability without rejection, infection, and migration. Bone graft also acts as a scaffold for osteoprogenitor cells, which migrate within the graft, consequently, new bone will be formed (15). Some authors reported cryopreserved sternum allograft for a limited number of patients after sternum resection (15–18). Dell'Amore described this method and his experiences in fourteen patients, which is the largest group of patients (19). He has also described more limited experiences of other surgeons with this method in other centers (20). In all of these reports, no allograft complications have been reported.

Sternum allograft fixation by Titanium bridges and screws may result in a thoracic cage deformity in long term in a growing child; therefore, studies with longer follow-ups are mandatory to clarify this hypothesis.

Using an autologous flap in chest wall reconstruction is an option that is a complex but safe procedure; nevertheless, it may lead to inadequate functional and cosmetic results, especially in mid- and long-term follow-up. On the other hand, some surgeons have reported prosthetic material for reconstruction of the chest wall in this group of patients with acceptable results, but mid- and long-term results are not available and prosthetic material may interfere with the normal growth of the child (21); therefore, using bone allografts may be more beneficial for children.

In conclusion, in this case, we have reported three rare events occurring simultaneously. First, the rare occurrence of sternal hemangioma; second, the occurrence of sternum hemangioma with a pectus carinatum deformity (that most probably is acquired), and the last one is the use of a novel substitute for sternum reconstruction. Using cryopreserved sternum allograft for the reconstruction of the anterior chest wall after sternum resection is a simple and reproducible method.

To the best of our knowledge, this is the first report of chest wall reconstruction by utilizing cryopreserved sternum in children. The most important consideration in this reconstruction method is the restrictive effects on the sternum. Another question is why we did not try to repair pectus carinatum deformity completely? If we tried to resect more adjacent ribs and cartilages for cosmetic results, remained defect might have been as big as which could force us to use longer titanium bridges for sternum allograft fixation on the remained ribs. Still, we could repair the patient's carinatum deformity in the future to achieve more cosmetic results. Although, 16 months after the surgery, there was a minimal chest wall deformity in comparison with preoperative images. More studies with a larger sample size and longer follow up are mandatory to determine the long-term outcome of this type of transplantation, especially in children.

AUTHOR CONTRIBUTIONS

FS contributed in data gathering and drafting. AS contributed in revision and drafting. KS contributed in data gathering and final revision. All authors contributed to the article and approved the submitted version.

REFERENCES

1. Koppert LB, van Geel AN, Lans TE, van der Pol C, van Coevorden F, Wouter MW. Sternal resection for sarcoma, recurrent breast cancer, and radiation-induced necrosis. *Ann Thorac Surg.* (2010) 90:1102–8 e2. doi: 10.1016/j.athoracsur.2010.06.044
2. Boker SM, Cullen GM, Swank M, Just JF. Case report 593: Hemangioma of sternum. *Skeletal Radiol.* (1990) 19:77–8. doi: 10.1007/BF00197937
3. Medalion B, Bar I, Neuman R, Shargal Y, Merin G. Sternal hemangioma: a rare tumor. *J Thorac Cardiovasc Surg.* (1996) 112:1402–3. doi: 10.1016/S0022-5223(96)70165-4
4. Huang TW, Lee SC, Chen JC, Hsu HH, Cheng YL. Cavernous hemangioma of the sternum. *Thorac Cardiovasc Surg.* (2008) 56:500–1. doi: 10.1055/s-2007-989397
5. Onat S, Ulku R, Avci A, Mizrak B, Ozcelik C. Hemangioma of the sternum. *Ann Thorac Surg.* (2008) 86:1974–6. doi: 10.1016/j.athoracsur.2008.04.109
6. Chapelier AR, Missana MC, Couturaud B, Fadel E, Fabre D, Mussot S, et al. Sternal resection and reconstruction for primary malignant tumors. *Ann Thorac Surg.* (2004) 77:1001–7. doi: 10.1016/j.athoracsur.2003.08.053
7. Sheikhy K, Abbasi Dezfouli A, Sadegh Beigee F. Reconstruction of chest wall by cryopreserved sternal allograft after resection of aneurysmal bone cyst of sternum. *Case Rep Surg.* (2017) 2017:913565–7. doi: 10.1155/2017/91 35657
8. Chapelier A. Resection and reconstruction for primary sternal tumors. *Thorac Surg Clin.* (2010) 20:529–34. doi: 10.1016/j.thorsurg.2010.06.002
9. Fokin AA, Robicsek F. Acquired deformities of the anterior chest wall. *Thorac Cardiovasc Surg.* (2006) 54:57–61. doi: 10.1055/s-2005-865840
10. Marulli G, De Iaco G, Ferrigno P, De Palma A, Quercia R, Brascia D, et al. Sternochondral replacement: use of cadaveric allograft for the reconstruction of anterior chest wall. *J Thorac Dis.* (2020) 12:3–9. doi: 10.21037/jtd.201 9.07.82
11. Rocco G. Overview on current and future materials for chest wall reconstruction. *Thorac Surg Clin.* (2010) 20:559–62. doi: 10.1016/j.thorsurg.2010.06.005
12. De Palma A, Sollitto F, Loizzi D, Di Gennaro F, Scarascia D, Carlucci A, et al. Chest wall stabilization and reconstruction: short and long-term results 5 years after the introduction of a new titanium plates system. *J Thorac Dis.* (2016) 8:490–8. doi: 10.21037/jtd.2016.02.64
13. Turna A, Kavakli K, Sapmaz E, Arslan H, Caylak H, Gokce HS, et al. Reconstruction with patient-specific titanium implant after a wide anterior chest wall resection. *Interact Cardiovasc Thorac Surg.* (2014) 18:234–6. doi: 10.1093/icvts/ivt408
14. Arando JL, Varela G, Benito P, Juan A. Donor cryopreserved rib allograft for chest wall reconstruction. *Interact Cardiovasc Thorac Surg.* (2008) 7:858–60. doi: 10.1510/icvts.2008.183905
15. Dell' Amore A, Casanelli N, Dolci G, Stella F. An alternative technique for anterior chest wall reconstruction: the sternal allograft transplantation. *Interact Cardiovasc Thorac Surg.* (2012) 15:944–7. doi: 10.1093/icvts/ivs411
16. Nosotti M, Rosso L, Mendogni P, Tosi D, Palleschi A, Parafioriti A, et al. Sternal reconstruction for unusual chondrosarcoma: innovative technique. *J Cardiothorac Surg.* (2012) 7:40. doi: 10.1186/1749-8090-7-40
17. Stella F, Dell'Amore A, Dolci G, Cassanelli N, Caroli G, Zamagni C, et al. Allogenic sternal transplant after sternectomy for metastasis of ovarian carcinoma. *Ann Thorac Surg.* (2012) 93:e71–2. doi: 10.1016/j.athoracsur.2011.10.004
18. Kālab M, Karkoška J, Kamínek M, Šatavý P. Successful three- years outcome in a patients with allogenous sternal bone graft in the treatment of massive post-sternotomy defects. *Int J Surg Case.* (2015) 7:6–9. doi: 10.1016/j.ijscr.2014.12.027
19. Dell'Amore A, Ferrigno P, PangoniA, Natale G, Faccioli E, Schiavon M, et al. The biological approach for sternal replacement: sternochondral allograft transplantation. *Curr Chall Thorac Surg.* (2019) 1:9. doi: 10.21037/ccts.2019.08.02
20. Dell'Amore A, Kalab M, Miller AS 3rd, Dolci G, Liparulo V, Beigee FS, et al. Indications and results of sternal allograft transplantation: learning from a worldwide experience. *Ann Thorac Surg.* (2021) 112:238–47. doi: 10.1016/j.athoracsur.2020.08.032
21. Guillén G, García L, Marhuenda C, Pellisé F, Molino JA, Fontecha CG, et al. Thoracic wall reconstruction with bioabsorbable plates in pediatric malignant thoracic wall tumors. *J Pediatric Surg.* (2017) 52:377–81. doi: 10.1016/j.jpedsurg.2016.08.018

19

Robotic-Assisted Urologic Surgery in Infants: Positioning, Trocar Placement and Physiological Considerations

Soo Jeong Kim [1], *John S. Barlog* [2] *and Ardavan Akhavan* [1*]

[1] *Institute for Pediatric Urology, Komansky Children's Hospital, New York Presbyterian-Weill Cornell, New York, NY, United States,* [2] *SUNY Downstate Medical Center, Brooklyn, NY, United States*

Correspondence:
Ardavan Akhavan
apa9010@med.cornell.edu

Pediatric robotic-assisted laparoscopic procedures are becoming increasingly common. They have been shown to be safe in younger patients, including infants. Successful adoption of robotic-assisted surgery in infants requires an understanding of the technical factors unique to this patient population. This review will delineate the specific considerations to safely perform robotic-assisted laparoscopic procedures in infants, including physiological changes associated with pneumoperitoneum in infants, positioning, trocar placement, and docking.

Keywords: robotic-assisted laparoscopic surgery, surgery in infants, positioning and orientation, trocar placement, robotic-assisted laparoscopic pyeloplasty, robotic-assisted laparoscopic reimplant, robotic-assisted laparoscopic nephrectomy

INTRODUCTION

Since the introduction of laparoscopy in children (1), indications have expanded from simple diagnostic procedures to complex, reconstructive surgeries. While the most commonly performed pediatric robotic-assisted laparoscopic procedures are pyeloplasty, ureteral reimplantation, nephrectomy, and heminephrectomy (2), more complex procedures like appendicovesicostomy, bladder neck reconstruction, and augmentation cystoplasty are being performed by early adopters. Robotic surgical assistance has potentiated this adoption by adding high definition three-dimensional (stereoscopic) visualization as well as superior articulation, thereby allowing for more accurate movements and improved ergonomics (3). In addition, the magnified image can be combined with tremor filtration and motion scaling, allowing for delicate motions in small areas, which is particularly beneficial in pediatric cases. These benefits have propelled the adoption of robotically-assisted cases by 17.4% per year ($P < 0.0001$) between 2008 and 2013 (2). Furthermore, as experience has grown, the lower age of patients suitable for robotic surgery has declined, and several studies have demonstrated the safety of using robotic-assisted surgery in infants (4, 5).

Successful adoption of robotic-assisted surgery in infants requires understanding of the technical factors unique to this patient population. This review focuses on both the physiological changes associated with pneumoperitoneum in infants, as well as the positioning, trocar placement, and docking considerations that must be addressed in order to successfully execute robotic surgery in the youngest patients.

PHYSIOLOGICAL CONSIDERATIONS

Robotic-assisted laparoscopic surgery requires distension of the peritoneal cavity, and given the infant anatomy, there are several physiological factors to consider during robotic-assisted laparoscopic surgery in infants.

Respiratory

Increased intra-abdominal pressurefrom pneumoperitoneum can exert pressure on the lungs by cephalad displacement of the diaphragm, which decreases total lung capacity, and increases the peak inspiratory pressure, further decreasing the functional residual capacity. The Trendelenberg position can exacerbate these changes. Using CO_2 to maintain pneumoperitoneum also leads to direct increases in CO_2 absorption. These changes lead to acidosis, which is pressure-dependent. An increase in ventilatory minute volume is necessary to limit the respiratory perturbations following insufflation (6). This increase in CO_2 has been shown to be inversely correlated with age, possibly because the peritoneum of infants is relatively larger, and better perfused (7). Also, unlike adults, where the level of CO_2 tends to plateau during surgery, in infants the level of CO_2 continues to rise with the duration of surgery (6).

Cardiovascular

Pneumoperitoneum also exerts cardiovascular effects due to an increase in intraabdominal pressure, peritoneal absorption of CO_2, and stimulation of the neurohumoral vasoactive system. In young children aged 6–36 months, an intraabdominal pressure of 10 mmHg or greater (i.e., higher than the right atrial pressure) causes a decrease in venous return, right ventricular cardiac output, and left ventricular preload and cardiac output (8). In addition, increased intraabdominal pressure may cause a catecholamine release which could contribute to increased mean arterial pressure and systemic vascular resistance (9). Pediatric patients can also develop bradycardia due to a robust vagal reflex induced by pneumoperitoneum, which may require emergent desufflation (10, 11). In a prospective study evaluating 33 pediatric patients aged 1–14 years (median 5 years) undergoing laparoscopic surgery, no significant cardiovascular changes occurred during CO_2 insufflation if the intraabdominal pressure was maintained lower than 10 mmHg (12).

Positioning for robotic surgery can also affect cardiovascular status. The Trendelenberg position, for instance, can increase venous return to the heart and therefore cardiac filling pressure, while reverse-Trendelenberg reduces the two (13).

Renal

In adults, pneumoperitoneum is associated with a pressure-dependent, reversible decrease in renal blood flow, glomerular filtration, and resultant urinary output (14). When 8 patients aged 0–12 months with normal baseline renal function underwent laparoscopy with intraabdominal pressure maintained at 8 mmHg, 88% developed anuria (15). The anuria was reversible, however, with urine output significantly increased postoperatively, and maximum values were evident at 5 h after desufflation (15).

Pneumoperitoneum causes renal changes via stimulation of the renin-angiotensin-aldosterone system (increase in renin and subsequent aldosterone secretion) and excretion of anti-diuretic hormone. These hormonal changes contribute to salt and water retention with oliguria (16).

Insufflation

In addition to the physiologic changes as outlined above, mean postoperative pain score and requirement for analgesia have been shown to be positively correlated with pneumoperitoneal pressure during laparoscopic renal surgery in infants (17). Therefore, we recommend that the lowest possible insufflation pressure be used in infants [8–12 mmHg]. For infants and young children, we recommend beginning the insufflation with the lowest possible flow rate, in order to allow for any adverse physiological changes to be identified and immediately reversed, if necessary. Once the target pressure has been reached, the flow may be increased for the remainder of the case.

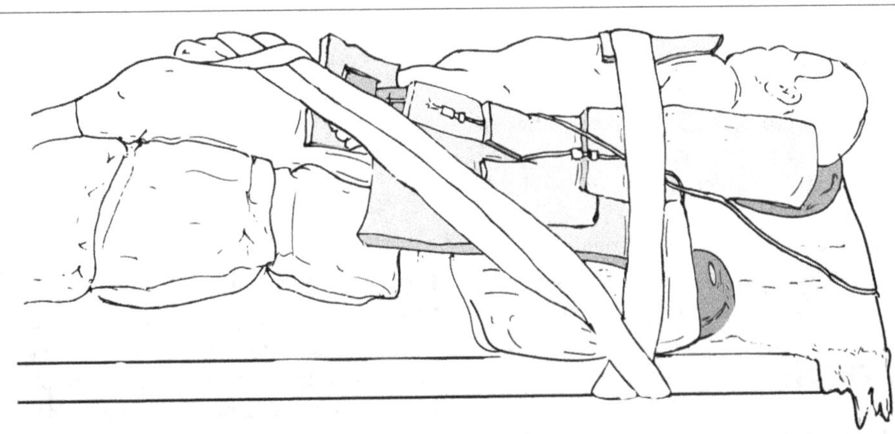

FIGURE 1 | Pad all pressure points and areas around tubing, wires, and nails.

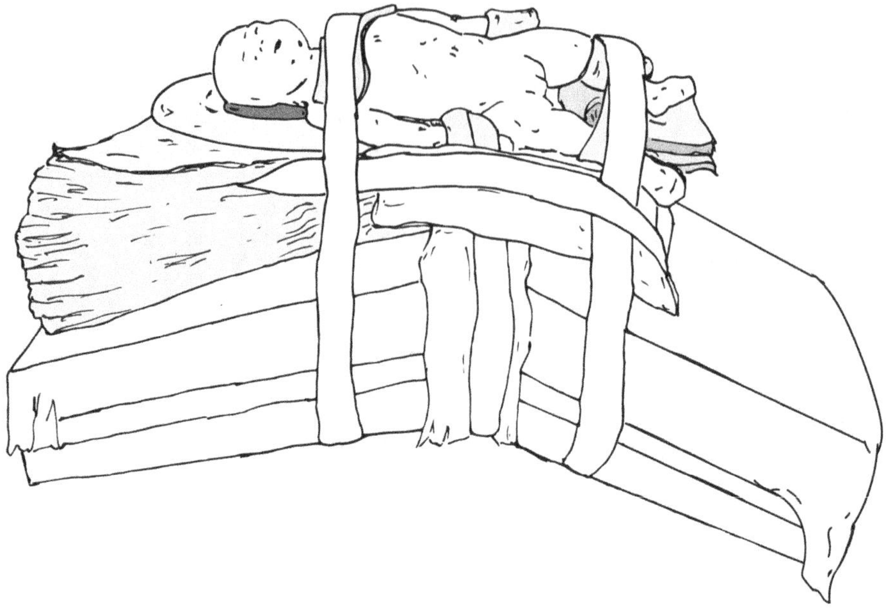

FIGURE 2 | Foam pads are used to elevate small infants (weight <10 kg) ~10 cm above the operating table to prevent the robot arms from hitting the table.

Other Anesthetic Concerns

There are several additional anesthesia-related considerations. First, no nitric oxide should be used in infants during robotic surgery as nitric oxide can lead to bowel distension, obscuring the surgical field. Second, intubation with an endotracheal tube is recommended as laryngeal mask airways will leak at a pressure less than required for robotic surgery. Third, patients should be paralyzed to allow for increased intraabdominal distension. Fourth, the robot is cumbersome and positioning for robotic surgery frequently requires the head of the patient to be far from the anesthesiologist. Anesthesiologists should know how to access the patient in case of emergency, and a plan should be in place to quickly undock if necessary. Lastly, aerosolized bupivacaine can be used to decrease the length of hospitalization, postoperative, and total postoperative narcotic requirements (18).

Physiologic Conclusions

Given the increased time-dependent physiological effects of pneumoperitoneum in infants, providers should take an honest assessment of their operative times and limit patient selection to older children until they are experienced enough to reliably execute procedures within a reasonable length of console time. Furthermore, surgeons should be quick to recognize failure to progress and have a set threshold to convert to an open procedure, should the surgery take longer than is reasonable.

PATIENT POSITIONING

Pediatric patients, particularly infants, are susceptible to crush injuries, and positional injuries. Proper positioning and padding are of paramount importance.

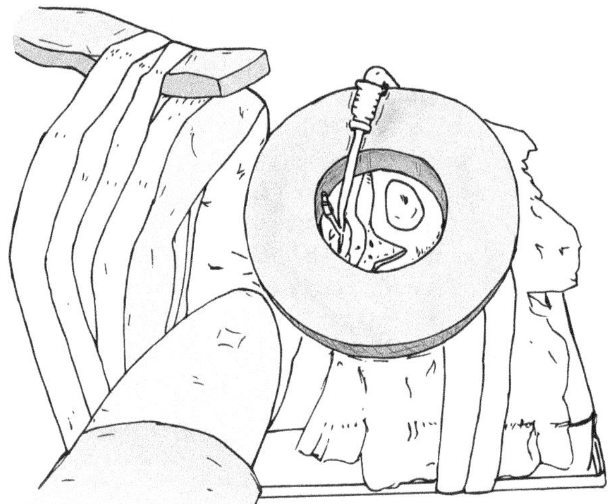

FIGURE 3 | Protect the face with foam to prevent injury or inadvertent manipulation of the endotracheal tube.

General Principles

The main goals of patient positioning and port placement are to avoid injuries to the patient and to allow maximum mobility of the robotic arms (3). All pressure points and areas around tubing, wires, and nails should be padded (**Figure 1**). We prefer to use cloth or silk tape and foam. Tape should not be applied directly to exposed skin. Small infants who weigh <10 kg should be elevated ~10 cm above the operating table using a foam pad to prevent the robot arms from hitting the table (**Figure 2**). The face should also be protected with foam to prevent injury to the eyes or inadvertent manipulation of the endotracheal tube (**Figure 3**). Prior to draping the patient, the table should be provoked to the most extreme position expected during the case in order to confirm that the patient is secure, no body part or tubing shifts or kinks, and that there are no anesthetic concerns.

Upper Urinary Tract Positioning

When preparing patients for renal and upper tract surgery, we prefer modified flank positioning over lateral decubitus positioning, as the former allows for port placement in a near-supine position, as well as bowel displacement and renal access via a table tilt (**Figures 4, 5**). For a modified flank position, arms can be placed on an arm board across the body or alongside the patient, depending on surgeon preferences. **Figure 6** illustrates the former. While there are many ways to secure the patient, we prefer placing a tape across the forehead in front of the face-foam, across the nipple-line of the chest, as well as diagonally from the arms across the legs on both sides (**Figure 5**). Egg crates, pillows, and/or an infant-sized bean bag may be used to help support the patient in position.

Lower Urinary Tract Positioning

When positioning a patient for lower urinary tract surgery, the patient may be placed in either lithotomy (**Figure 7A**), frog-leg position (**Figure 7B**), or supine (**Figure 7C**). If cystoscopy is necessary during the procedure, lithotomy is preferred.

TROCAR PLACEMENT

Trocar placement is a crucial step in robotic-assisted surgery in order to minimize instrument collision and operative time. A recent study demonstrated that collisions are minimized if the distance between both anterior superior iliac spines is >13 cm, or if the puboxyphoid distance is >15 cm (19).

Initial Access

Passerotti et al. published the outcomes of 806 laparoscopic procedures (conventional and robot assisted) and reported a 2% complication rate, 75% of which were access related (20). This finding is likely due to the fact that pediatric abdomens are more compliant than adult abdomens, and the pressure necessary to penetrate the pediatric peritoneum can easily cause injury. Therefore, we gain initial access using the open Hassan technique

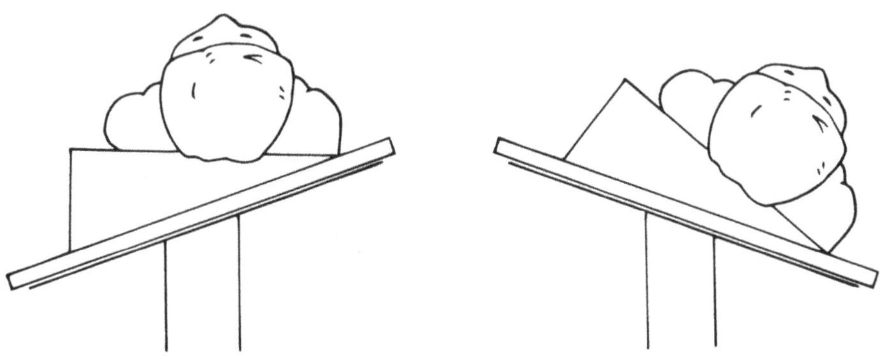

FIGURE 4 | Modified flank positioning used for upper tract surgery, which allows for port placement in a near-supine position (left), and subsequent bowel displacement and renal access via a table tilt (right).

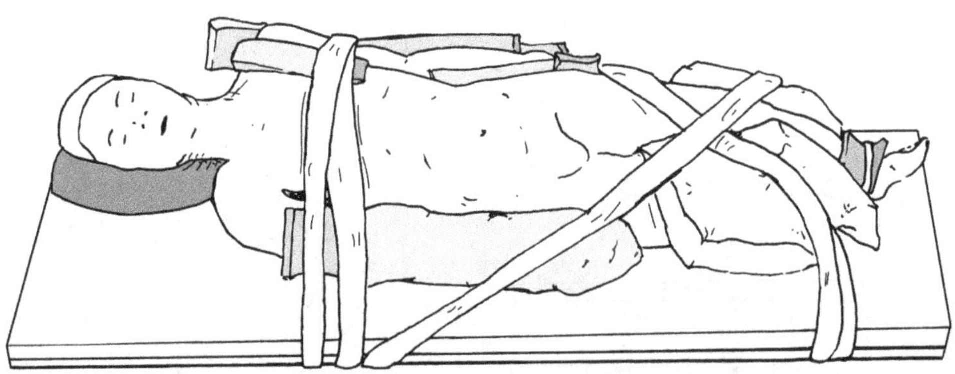

FIGURE 5 | Modified flank positioning used for upper tract surgery, with proper padding, and tape securing the patient to the operating table.

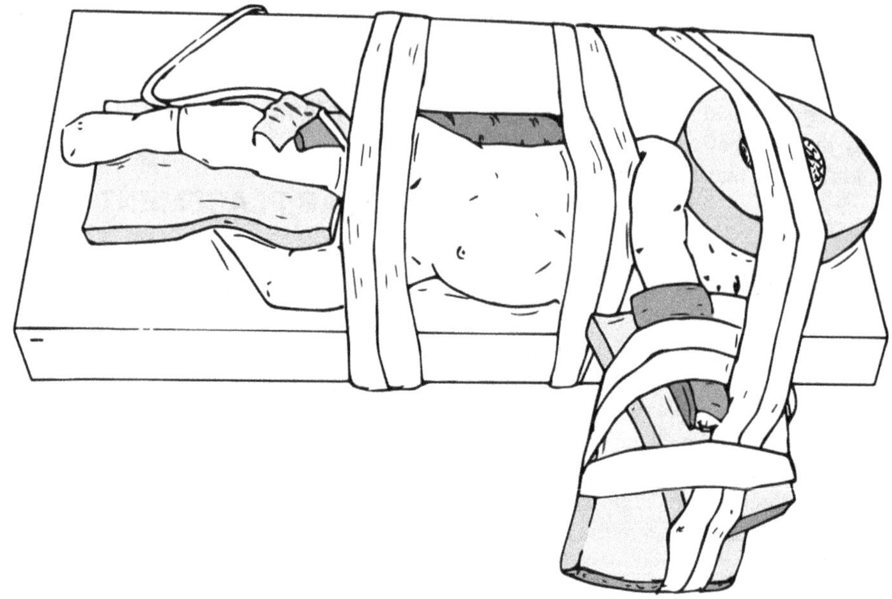

FIGURE 6 | Modified flank positioning with arms placed on an arm board across the body.

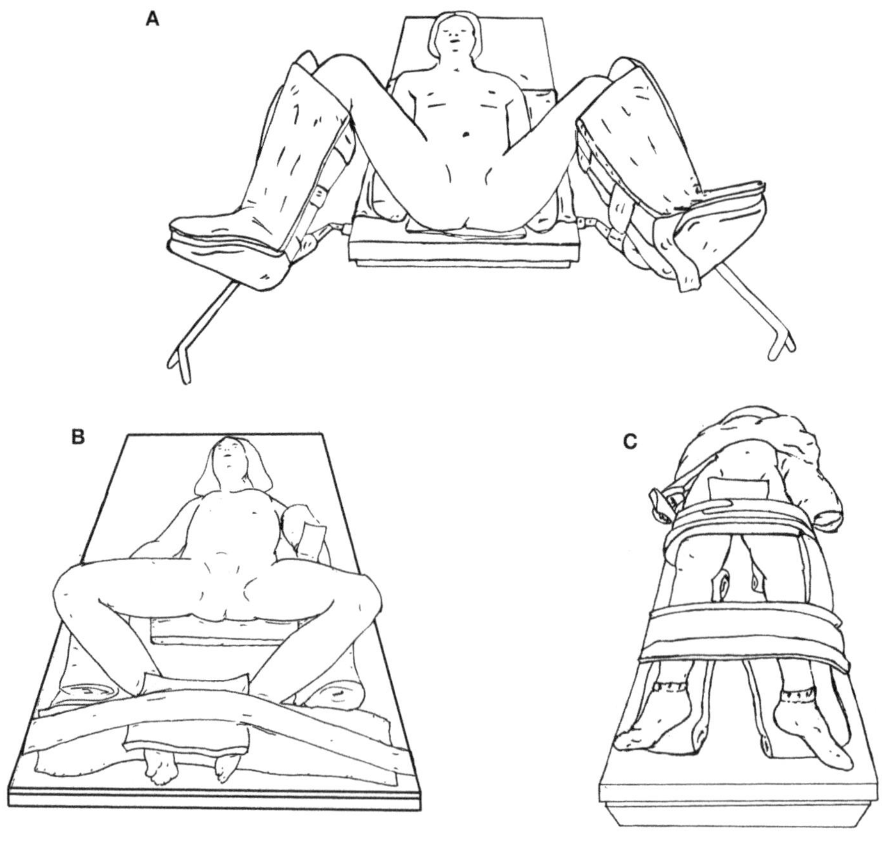

FIGURE 7 | Lower urinary tract surgery positioning options, including lithotomy **(A)**, frog-leg **(B)**, or supine **(C)**.

to place the 8.5 mm camera port, always using a blunt black obturator in order to minimize the risk of injury.

Instrument Ports

Under direct visualization, we employ sharp dissection through the peritoneum with an 11 blade, after injection of 0.25% bupivacaine. Once the port site is dilated with a mosquito clamp, the trocar is advanced with a blunt obturator. While the port is designed to be inserted at the level of the thick black line, in young infants, the port may often only be able to be placed a few mm into the peritoneum.

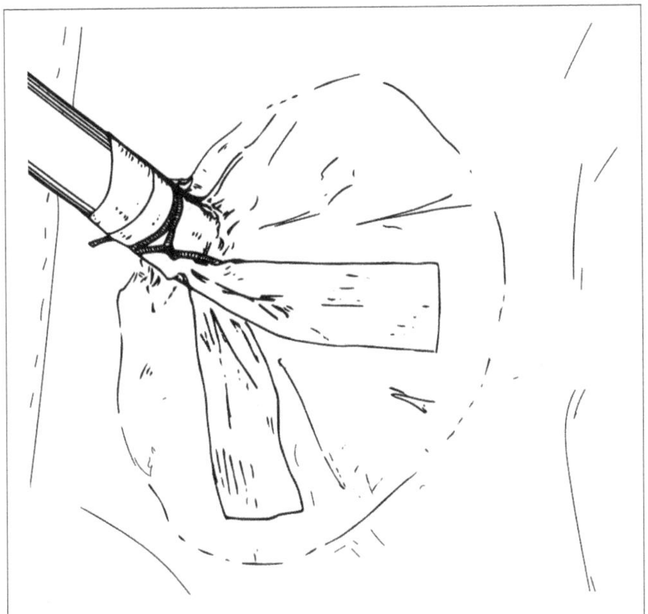

FIGURE 8 | Trocar secured to the skin using sutures, steri-strips, and Tegaderms.

When using an Si system, there is a longstanding debate regarding the preferred sizes of instrument ports in pediatric patients, as there is a pediatric option with an 8.5 mm camera and 5 mm instruments, compared with the standard option of a 12 mm camera and 8 mm instruments. Although the 5 mm ports require a slightly smaller incision, the 5 mm instruments paradoxically require an additional 2 cm intracorporeal working space due to the design of the instrument arms, as the articulating joints are further back on the 5 mm instruments than they are on the 8 mm instruments (3). In addition, the variety of instruments available in the 5 mm size is greatly limited compared to the 8 mm size, many of which are particularly useful during pediatric reconstruction cases, including Black diamond microforceps, and Potts scissors. We prefer to use a hybrid set with an 8.5 mm pediatric camera as well as the 8 mm instruments. On the Xi system, currently only 8-mm instruments are available.

While a 3–5 cm distance between ports is ideal, in infants, this distance is not always possible, so the trocars are just placed as far apart as possible. More distance will be evident after abdominal distension from the pneumoinsufflation. Furthermore, "burping" the ports out 1–2 cm after docking will tent the abdominal wall and also create some extra room. In order to prevent the trocars from falling out, in infants we advocate that they be secured to the skin using a combination of sutures, steri-strips, and Tegaderms (**Figure 8**). At the conclusion of the case, all ports are closed under direction vision.

14-Guage Angiocatheter Assist

A 14-guage angiocatheter in conjunction with cystoscopic tools can be used as an assistant port in order to avoid an additional port placement.

Trocar Positioning

Upper Urinary Tract Trocar Positioning

When performing upper urinary tract surgery such as pyeloplasty or nephrectomy in an infant, in order to prevent robotic

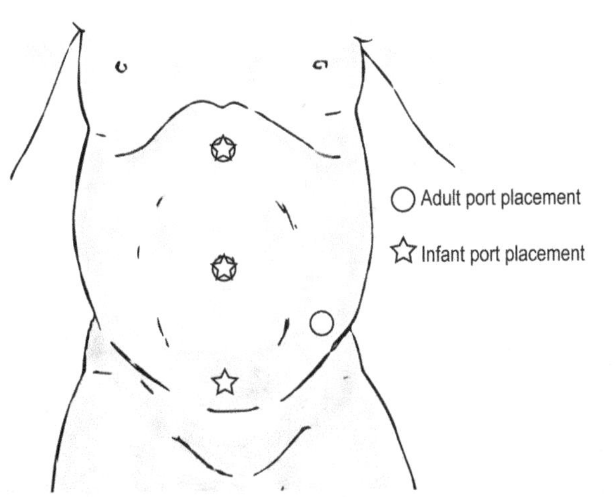

FIGURE 9 | Trocar positioning for upper urinary tract surgery in infants (☆) compared to that for adults (○).

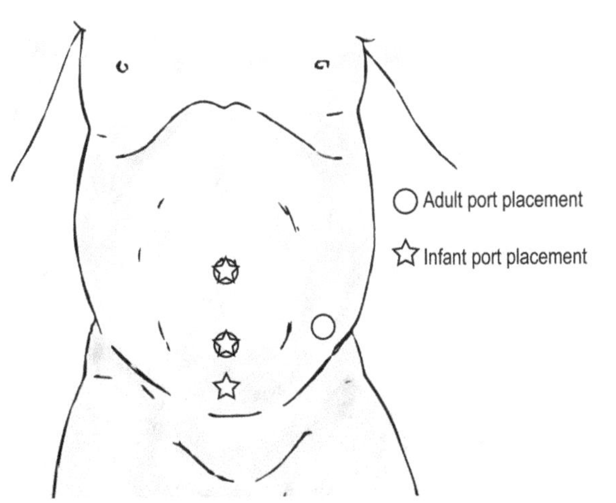

FIGURE 10 | Trocar positioning for upper urinary tract hidden incision endoscopic surgery (HIdES) in infants (☆) compared to that for adults (○).

arms from clashing, the most inferior port site can be moved medially (**Figure 9**). This adjustment is also useful when performing a pyeloplasty because a distended ureteropelvic junction can often be found in the lower abdomen in younger children. Of note, with the adjusted location of the most inferior port site, care must be taken to avoid injury to the bladder.

Upper Urinary Tract Hidden Incision Endoscopic Surgery (HIdES) Trocar Positioning

Hidden incision endoscopic surgery has been previously described for pediatric upper urinary tract surgery (21). The HIdES technique aims to eliminate visible scarring, and the robotic working port and camera port are placed below the line of a Pfannenstiel incision. A second working port is placed infraumbilically. Similar to standard upper urinary tract trocar positioning, the most inferior port can be moved medially in order to increase working room in an infant (**Figure 10**). Again, care must be taken to avoid injury to the bladder with this adjustment.

Extravesical Reimplant

When performing extravesical reimplant surgery with robotic assistance, the port site positioning will depend on the

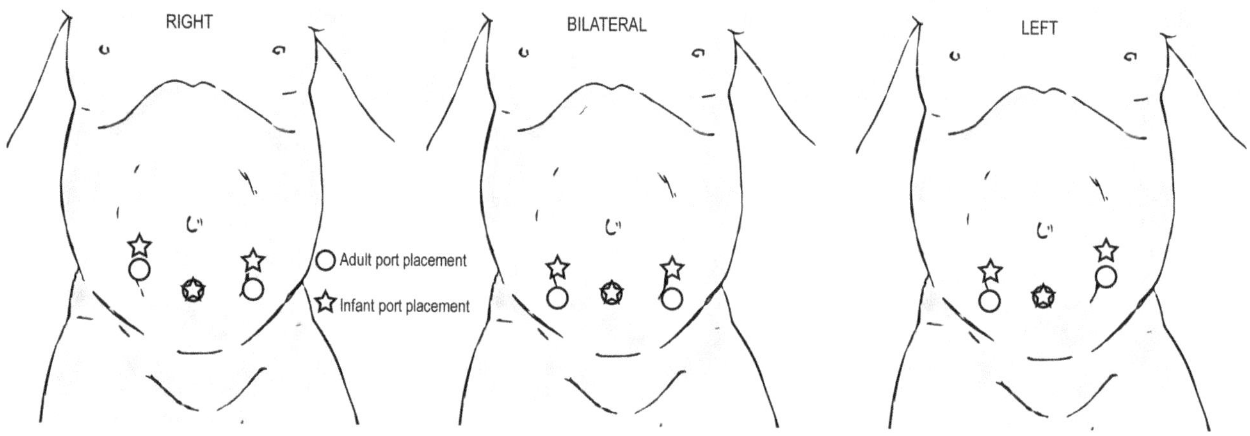

FIGURE 11 | Trocar positioning for extravesical reimplant surgery in infants (☆) compared to that for adults (○) based on laterality of procedure.

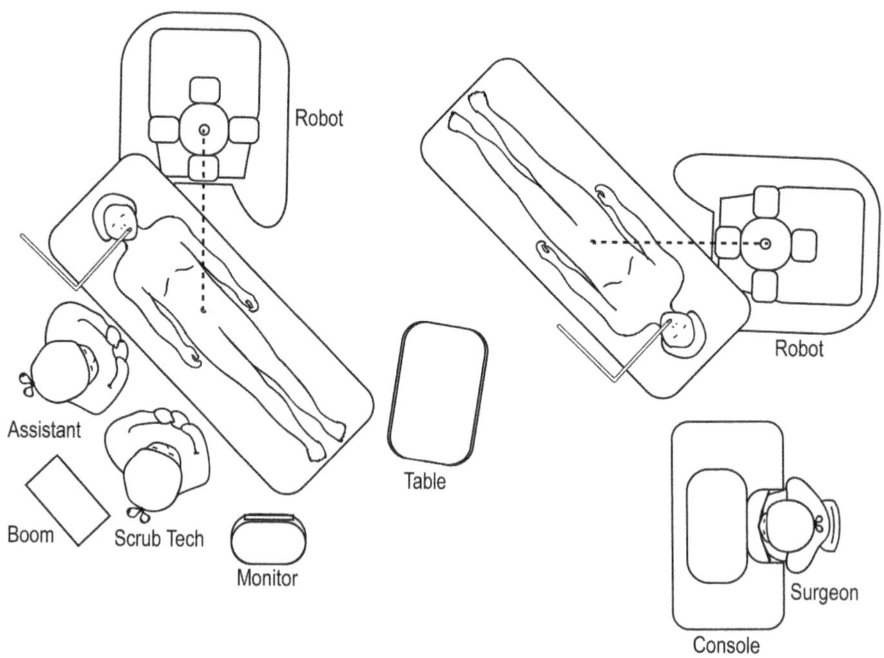

FIGURE 12 | Overhead view of room set-up for upper urinary tract surgery, with robot docked at ipsilateral shoulder.

laterality of the procedure. If bilateral, the port sites will be in a straight line. For infants, all port sites should be 2 cm above the umbilicus to ensure sufficient working room (**Figure 11**).

DOCKING/ROOM SET-UP

A standardized room set-up, including positioning of the robot, robotic console, scrub table, anesthesia machines, and surgical assistant, is important to maximize the utility of the robot while maintaining a safe and effective working environment. If using an Si system, we recommend maintaining the robot at one established location in the room and then moving/rotating the operating room table in position in order to minimize robotic manipulation. Communication with anesthesia is paramount, as extension tubing may be necessary. If using an Xi system, the robot arms can be rotated to the desired configuration without manipulating the operating room table.

Upper Urinary Tract Room Set-Up

The robot should be docked at a point that forms a straight line with the patient's umbilicus and the target location of the surgery (**Figure 12**), identified through either a preoperative retrograde pyelogram (if performing a pyeloplasty) or through direct gross inspection after the initial laparoscopy. The assistant and surgical technician stand on the contralateral side with an accessible table and Mayo stand.

Upper Urinary Tract Hidden Incision Endoscopic Surgery (HIdES) Room Set-Up

The room set-up for robotic-assisted upper urinary tract HIdES surgery is similar to that of standard upper urinary tract surgery, except that the robot is docked by coming in from above the ipsilateral shoulder. The feet of the robot should straddle the base of the operating room table (**Figure 13**).

Lower Urinary Tract Surgery

For robotic-assisted lower urinary tract surgery performed with the patient in the lithotomy or frog-leg supine position, the robot is docked at the patient's 6 o'clock position (**Figure 14**). The surgical tech, Mayo stand, and scrub table remain on one side of the patient, while the assistant stands at the other. For robotic-assisted lower urinary tract surgery performed with the patient in the supine position, the robot is docked laterally (**Figure 15**), with the feet of the Si system straddling the base of the table. The assistant and surgical technician remain on the contralateral side of the robot. If using an Xi system, the positioning of the robot is versatile as the arms can be rotated to the appropriate configuration.

TEAM CONSIDERATIONS

Robotic surgery is a team effort. A successful program requires dedicated support from the hospital as well as an established nursing team. While infant robotic cases are rarely performed daily, preoperative huddles, and standardized algorithms can be invaluable in helping establish a protocol for staff to

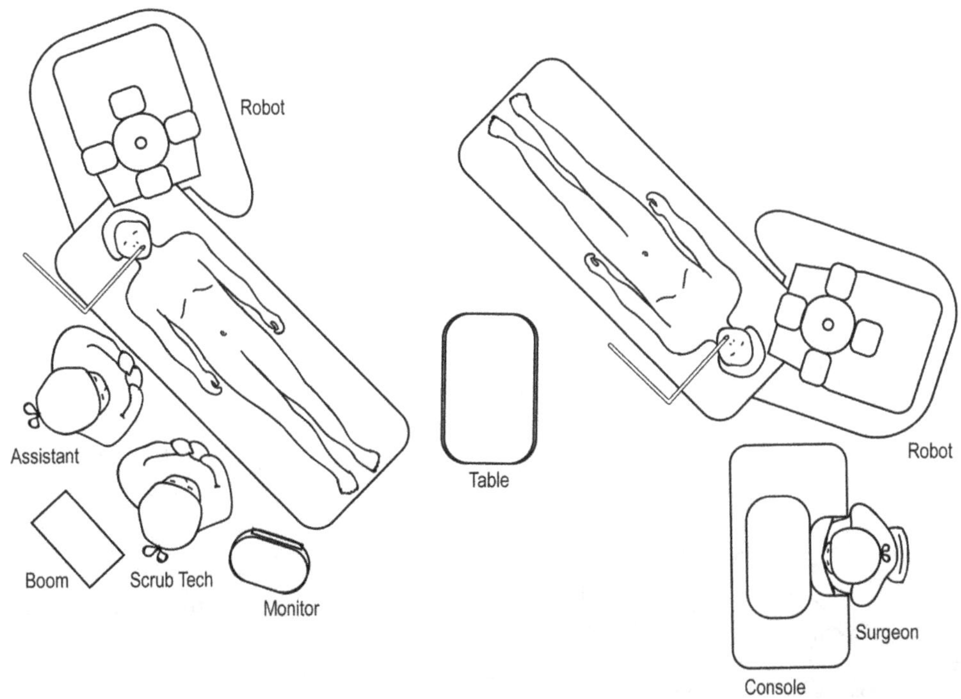

FIGURE 13 | Overhead view of room set-up for upper urinary tract hidden incision endoscopic surgery (HIdES), with robot docked at ipsilateral shoulder.

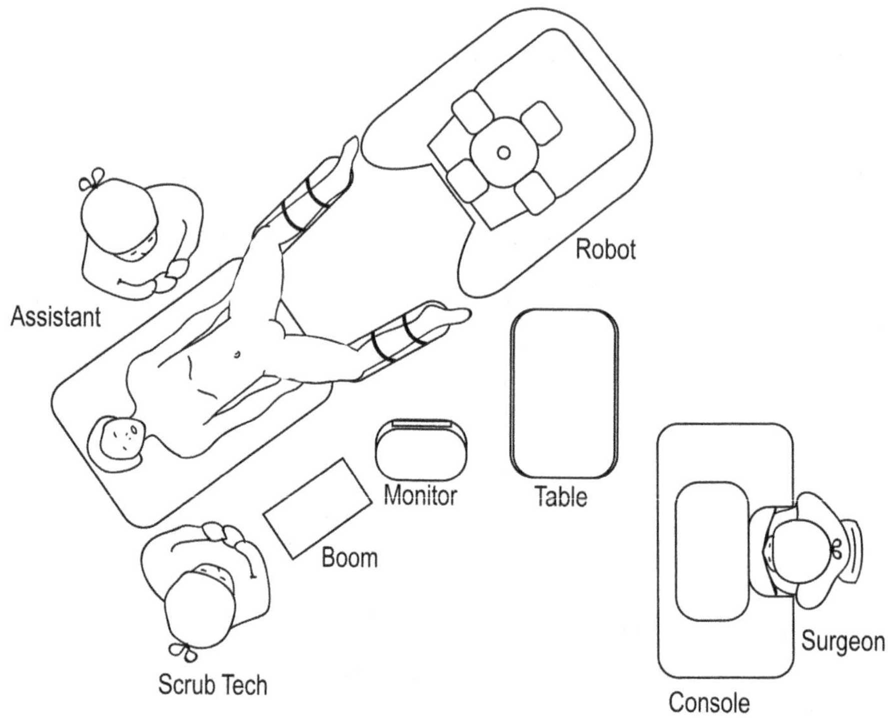

FIGURE 14 | Overhead view of room set-up for lower urinary tract surgery in the lithotomy or frog-leg supine positions.

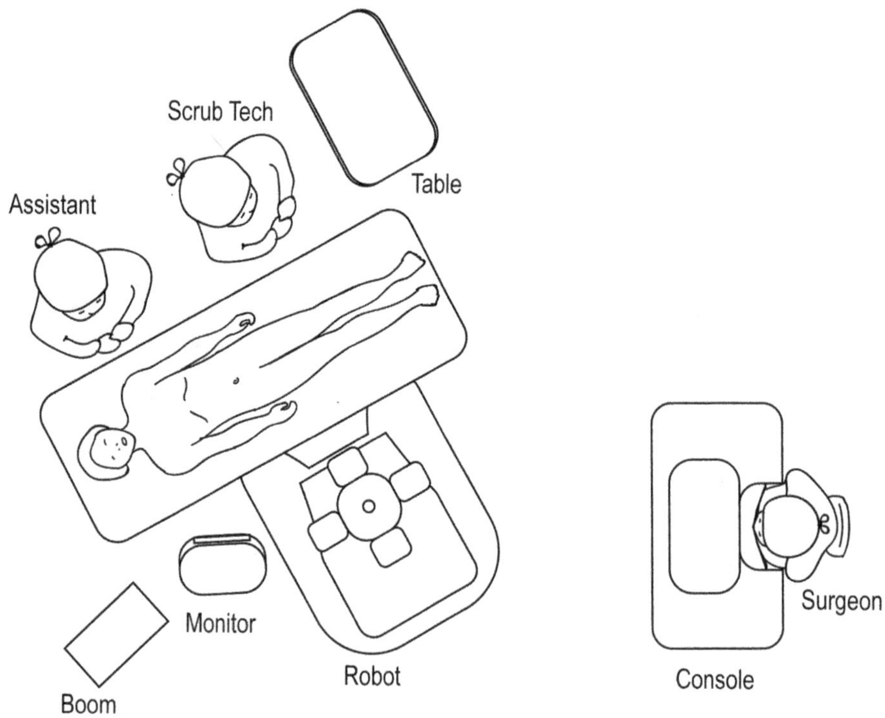

FIGURE 15 | Overhead view of room set-up for lower urinary tract surgery in the supine position.

follow, minimizing confusion, and variations in practice. Additionally, we recommend contingency plans for potential robotic emergencies. These include bleeding, loss of airway, equipment malfunction, and lost needle. Specific step-by-step plans and allocation of responsibilities should be established and practiced with the team in order to minimize reaction times.

CONCLUSION

Young infants warrant special consideration when considering robotic surgery. Their unique anatomy makes them particularly susceptible to the physiologic effects of pneumoperitoneum. When undertaking these cases, surgeons should strive to limit insufflation time and minimize the insufflation pressure to the lowest possible level in order to accomplish the surgery. Furthermore, while the DaVinci robotic system was designed to be used in adult patients, the machine can be used in young children, as long as the specific considerations outlined here are taken into account during positioning, port placement, and docking.

AUTHOR CONTRIBUTIONS

SK authored and edited the manuscript. JB edited the manuscript and contributed original illustrations. AA conceived focus of review and edited the manuscript.

REFERENCES

1. Cortesi N, Ferrari P, Zambarda E, Manenti A, Baldini A, Morano FP. Diagnosis of bilateral abdominal cryptorchidism by laparoscopy. *Endoscopy* (1976) 8:33–4. doi: 10.1055/s-0028-1098372
2. Mahida JB, Cooper JN, Herz D, Diefenbach KA, Deans KJ, Minneci PC, et al. Utilization and costs associated with robotic surgery in children. *J Surg Res.* (2015) 169–76. doi: 10.1016/j.jss.2015.04.087
3. Chang C, Steinberg Z, Shah A, Gundeti MS. Patient positioning and port placement for robot-assisted surgery. *J Endourol.* (2014) 28:631–8. doi: 10.1089/end.2013.0733
4. Avery DI, Herbst KW, Lendvay TS, Noh PH, Dangle P, Gundeti MS, et al. Robot-assisted laparoscopic pyeloplasty: multi-institutional experience in infants. *J Pediatr Urol.* (2015) 11:139.e1–5. doi: 10.1016/j.jpurol.2014.11.025
5. Kawal T, Srinivasan AK, Shrivastava D, Chu DI, Van Batavia J, Weiss D, et al. Pediatric robotic-assisted laparoscopic pyeloplasty: does age matter? *J Pediatr Urol.* S1477-5131:30215–8. doi: 10.1016/j.jpurol.2018.04.023
6. Kalfa N, Allal H, Raux O, Lopez M, Forgues D, Guibal MP, et al. Tolerance of laparoscopy and thoracoscopy in neonates. *Pediatrics* (2005) 116:e785–91. doi: 10.1542/peds.2005-0650
7. McHoney M, Corizia L, Eaton S, Kiely EM, Drake DP, Tan HL, et al. Carbon dioxide elimination during laparoscopy in children is age dependent. *J Pediatr Surg.* (2003) 38:105–10. doi: 10.1053/jpsu.2003.50021
8. De Waal EEC, Kalkman CJ. Haemodynamic changes during low-pressure carbon dioxide pneumoperitoneum in young children. *Pediatr Anesth.* (2003) 13:18–25. doi: 10.1046/j.1460-9592.2003.00973.x
9. Myre K, Rostrup M, Buanes T, Stokland O. Plasma catecholamines and haemodynamic changes during pneumoperitoneum. *Acta Anaesthesiol Scand.* (1998) 42:343–7. doi: 10.1111/j.1399-6576.1998.tb04927.x
10. Brady M, Kinn S, Ness V, O'Rourke K, Randhawa N, Stuart P. Preoperative fasting for preventing perioperative complications in children. *Cochrane Database Syst Rev.* 7:CD005285. doi: 10.1002/14651858.CD005285.pub2
11. Terrier G. Anaesthesia for laparoscopic procedures in infants and children: indications, intra- and post-operative management, prevention and treatment of complications. *Curr Opin Anaesthesiol.* (1999) 12:311–4. doi: 10.1097/00001503-199906000-00009
12. Mattioli G, Montobbio G, Pini Prato A, Repetto P, Carlini C, Gentilino V, et al. Anesthesiologic aspects of laparoscopic fundoplication for gastroesophageal reflux in children with chronic respiratory and gastroenterological symptoms. *Surg Endosc.* (2003) 17:559–66. doi: 10.1007/s00464-002-9077-2
13. Spinelli G, Vargas M, Aprea G, Cortese G, Servillo G. Pediatric anesthesia for minimally invasive surgery in pediatric urology. *Transl Pediatr.* (2016) 5:214–21. doi: 10.21037/tp.2016.09.02
14. Wever KE, Bruintjes MHD, Warlé MC, Hooijmans CR. Renal perfusion and function during pneumoperitoneum: a systematic review and meta-analysis of animal studies. *PLoS ONE* (2016) 11:e0163419. doi: 10.1371/journal.pone.0163419
15. Gómez Dammeier BH, Karanik E, Glüer S, Jesch NK, Kübler J, Latta K, et al. Anuria during pneumoperitoneum in infants and children: a prospective study. *J Pediatr Surg.* (2005) 40:1454–8. doi: 10.1016/j.jpedsurg.2005.05.044
16. Sodha S, Nazarian S, Adshead JM, Vasdev N, Mohan-S G. Effect of pneumoperitoneum on renal function and physiology in patients undergoing robotic renal surgery. *Curr Urol.* (2016) 9:1–4. doi: 10.1159/000442842
17. Sureka SK, Patidar N, Mittal V, Kapoor R, Srivastava A, Kishore K, et al. Safe and optimal pneumoperitoneal pressure for transperitoneal laparoscopic renal surgery in infant less than 10 kg, looked beyond intraoperative period: a prospective randomized study. *J Pediatr Urol.* (2016) 13:236. doi: 10.1016/j.jpurol.2017.01.003
18. Freilich DA, Houck CS, Meier PM, Passerotti CC, Retik AB, Nguyen HT. The effectiveness of aerosolized intraperitoneal bupivacaine in reducing postoperative pain in children undergoing robotic-assisted laparoscopic pyeloplasty. *J Pediatr Urol.* (2008) 4:337–40. doi: 10.1016/j.jpurol.2008.04.006
19. Finkelstein JB, Levy AC, Silva MV, Murray L, Delaney C, Casale P. How to decide which infant can have robotic surgery? Just do the math. *J Pediatr Urol.* (2015) 11:170.e1–4. doi: 10.1016/j.jpurol.2014.11.020
20. Passerotti CC, Nguyen HT, Retik AB, Peters CA. Patterns and predictors of laparoscopic complications in pediatric urology: the role of ongoing surgical volume and access techniques. *J Urol.* (2008) 180:681–5. doi: 10.1016/j.juro.2008.04.042
21. Gargollo PC. Hidden incision endoscopic surgery: description of technique, parental satisfaction and applications. *J Urol.* (2011) 185:1425–31. doi: 10.1016/j.juro.2010.11.054

20

Endoscopic Preoperative Assessment, Classification of Stenosis and Decision-Making

Marta Filauro[1,2†], *Francesco Mazzola*[1,2†], *Francesco Missale*[1,2,3*‡], *Frank Rikki Canevari*[1,2] *and Giorgio Peretti*[1,2]

[1] IRCCS Ospedale Policlinico San Martino, Genoa, Italy, [2] Unit of Otorhinolaryngology—Head and Neck Surgery, University of Genoa, Genoa, Italy, [3] Department of Molecular and Translational Medicine, University of Brescia, Brescia, Italy

***Correspondence:**
Francesco Missale
missale.francesco@gmail.com

Pediatric Laryngo-Tracheal Stenosis (LTS) comprises different conditions that require precise preoperative assessment and classification. According to the guidelines, the optimal diagnostic work-up of LTS patients relies both on a comprehensive anamnesis and on endoscopic and radiological assessments. All the causes of LTS result in an impairment in airflow, mucociliary clearance, phonation, and sometimes in swallowing disorders. The main goals of treatment are to maintain an adequate respiratory space and restore the Upper Aero-Digestive Tract (UADT) physiology. The first step when dealing with LTS patients is to properly assess their medical history. The main causes of pediatric LTS can be divided into two groups, i.e., congenital and acquired. The most common causes of congenital LTS are: laryngomalacia (60%), vocal fold paralysis (15–20%), subglottic stenosis (SGS) (10–15%), laryngeal webs and atresia (5%), subglottic hemangioma (1.5–3%), and others. On the other hand, 90% of acquired pediatric LTS cases are subsequent to post-intubation injuries. Other less frequent causes are: iatrogenic complications from endoscopic laryngeal interventions, benign tumors, caustic or thermal injuries, external blunt force injury or trauma, chronic inflammatory disorders, or idiopathic causes. Diagnostic work-up consists in a step-by-step investigation: awake and asleep transnasal fiberoptic laryngoscopy (TNFL), direct laryngoscopy with 0° and angled telescopes to investigate the type of stenosis (arytenoid mobility, craniocaudal extension, involved anatomical sites, and active or mature scar tissue), and broncho-esophagoscopy to rule out associated mediastinal malformations. To date there are several available classifications for each of the involved sites: Cohen's classification for anterior glottic stenosis, Bogdasarian's for posterior glottic stenosis (PGS) and Myer-Cotton's for subglottic stenosis, even though others are used in daily practice (Lano-Netterville, FLECS, etc.). The European Laryngological Society recently proposed a new classification which is applicable in all LTS cases. In this chapter we deal with preoperative assessment and staging, reviewing the most relevant classifications applicable in patients affected by LTS, *conditio sine qua non* in order to tailor the best treatment modality to each subject. We'll also detail the comprehensive radiological, endoscopic and functional assessment for the correct use of each staging classification.

Keywords: classification, laryngotracheal stenosis, decision-making, pediatric airway, European laryngological society

INTRODUCTION

Pediatric laryngotracheal stenosis (LTS) comprises a wide number of conditions that require precise pre- and intraoperative assessment.

The main causes of pediatric LTS can be divided into two groups, i.e., congenital and acquired. The most common causes of congenital LTS include laryngomalacia (60%), vocal fold paralysis (15–20%), subglottic stenosis (SGS) (10–15%), laryngeal webs and atresia (5%), subglottic hemangioma (1.5–3%), and others (1). On the other hand, 90% of acquired pediatric LTSs occur after post-intubation injuries. Other less frequent causes include iatrogenic complications from endoscopic laryngeal interventions, benign tumors, caustic or thermal injuries, external blunt force injury or trauma, chronic inflammatory disorders or idiopathic causes (2).

The aims of the initial assessment are to establish or confirm the diagnosis, to identify disease-specific risk factors and prognostic variables, to set goals with the patient and his/her parents and to establish an initial management plan (3).

Accurate preoperative and intraoperative diagnostic work-up is of paramount importance to obtain crucial information which could impact on the postoperative outcome. Information that must be collected includes vocal fold mobility, the presence of glottic and/or supraglottic scar tissue, crico-arytenoid joint(s) fixation, possible additional tracheal damage (stenosis, malacia) related to stoma or cannula, secondary airway lesions (i.e., granuloma, scar tissue), obstructive sleep apnea (OSA)-related obstructions, swallowing difficulties with/without chronic aspiration, severe gastroesophageal reflux (GOR), eosinophilic esophagitis, medical comorbidities, or congenital anomalies.

Any of the following scenarios may be encountered in a child with acquired LTS: (1) neonatal intubation for respiratory distress; (2) intubation for infection or traumatic injury later in life; (3) previous history of endotracheal intubation presenting as "idiopathic" LTS (4).

An important distinction that must be pointed out is between incipient and mature stenosis. Incipient LTS results from acute or subacute post-intubation airway narrowing (e.g., edema, ulcerations, granulation tissue), which is treated endoscopically or by a cricoid split procedure in newborns in an effort to prevent cicatricial stenosis. The final goal is to avoid tracheotomy or allow decannulation in already tracheostomized patients (2).

Mature cicatricial stenoses correspond to well-established airway narrowing that can pose a therapeutic challenge to the surgeon. It is thus of paramount importance to understand the individual characteristics of the stenosis and the clinical context of each patient (5).

In order to identify the best therapeutic option, an appropriate diagnostic work-up must include correct staging of the lesion and an endoscopic pre- and intraoperative assessment.

CLASSIFICATIONS OF LTS

In the last few decades, the broad variety of laryngotracheal stenosis presentations has been in great need of standardized definitions. In an attempt to fill this gap, laryngotracheal stenosis classifications have proliferated in the literature due to the need to describe the complex anatomy of this district, the varied clinical presentations and the treatment possibilities. The most relevant classifications are reported in this chapter.

Myer-Cotton

This classification was proposed by Myer et al. (3), taking cues from a previous version published by Cotton (4). The Myer-Cotton classification was intended for firm, mature subglottis stenoses, thus excluding any other lumen narrowing conditions (e.g., trachea- and/or laryngomalacia, vocal cord paralysis, immature stenosis, tracheal stenosis, suprastomal collapse, supraglottic collapse and suprastomal granulation tissue). While it was initially used to predict lumen surface reduction in case of endotracheal tube application, it was then extended to describe both pediatric and adult subglottic and/or tracheal stenosis. It consists of IV grades: Grade I—0 to 50% decrease in lumen surface; Grade II—51 to 70% decrease; Grade III—71 to 99% decrease, and Grade IV–no evidence of detectable lumen (**Figure 1**). Healthy and stenotic lumen surfaces can be accurately calculated and compared by radiological imaging or intra-operative investigation using the formula $A = \pi r^2$ to obtain circle area values.

McCaffrey

In 1992, McCaffrey proposed a classification to describe the extension of the stenosis among the most commonly involved subsites: glottis, subglottis and trachea (6). This system was initially validated on an adult population but was later extended to pediatric patients. This classification was conceived after both univariate and multivariate analyses showed that the involved site had the most consistent significant predictive value for determining time to decannulation. Stage I is located in the subglottis or trachea, with a craniocaudal extension of <1 cm. Stage II stenosis is limited to the subglottis and has a craniocaudal extension of more than 1 cm. Stage III stenosis involves both the subglottis and trachea, while Stage IV stenosis extends to the glottis with fixation or paralysis of at least one vocal cord (**Figure 2**).

Lano-Netterville

In 1998, Lano et al. (7) proposed a simpler staging system based on anatomical subsite involvement. The authors described three stages according to the number of involved subsites: Stage I in case of single subsite involvement, stage II for two involved subsites and stage III in case of glottic-tracheal involvement (**Table 1**). The Authors recommended the use of this classification in order to have a good correlation between surgical success and stage categories, which in their retrospective population resulted 94, 78, and 20% for Stage I, II, and III, respectively.

Cohen

A new classification proposed by Cohen (8) attempted to describe anterior glottic webs occurring at the time of glottic lumen formation during laryngeal embryological development (1985). The four types of anterior glottic web correlate with the severity of symptoms. Type 1 is an anterior web involving 35% or less of the glottic lumen. Type 2 ranges between 35 and 50%, Type 3

Classification	From	To	Endoscopic appearance
Grade I	No Obstruction	50% Obstruction	
Grade II	51%	70%	
Grade III	71%	99%	
Grade IV	No detectable lumen		

FIGURE 1 | Myer-Cotton classification, adapted from Myer et al. (3) with unpublished clinical pictures.

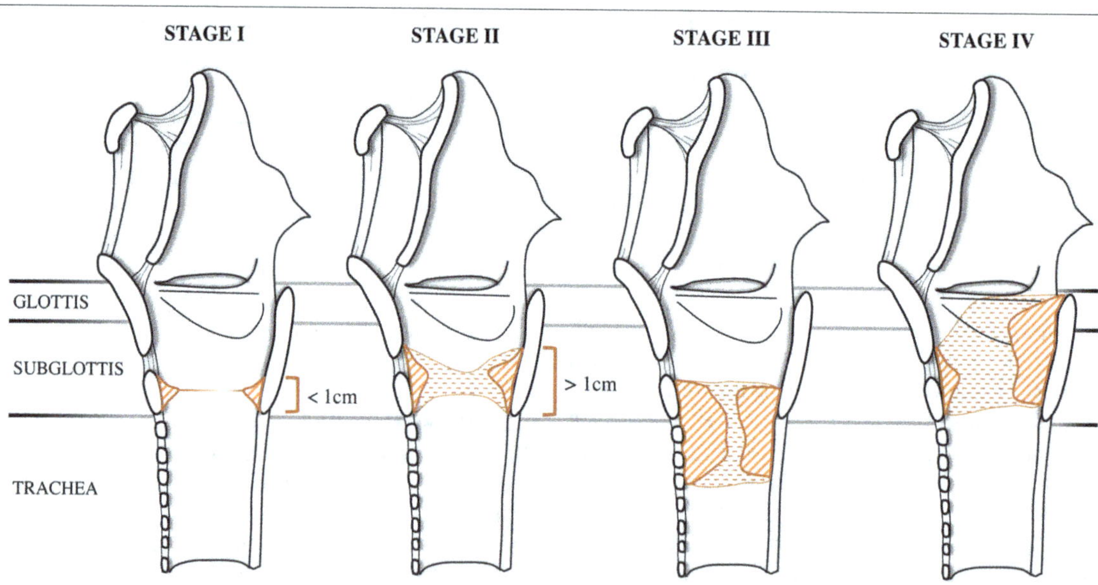

FIGURE 2 | McCaffrey Classification. The stenosis can be located in the subglottis or in the trachea in stage I and in stage II, adapted from McCaffrey (6) with unpublished draws.

between 51 and 75% while Type 4 involves 76% or more of the glottic lumen (**Figure 3**).

Other Classifications

As previously mentioned, other classifications have been proposed, and while each of them describes stenotic lesions differently, they have limited relevance in clinical practice.

Laccourrey et al. (9) proposed a detailed staging system taking into account larynx fixation, subsites, and laryngeal joint involvement.

Bogdasarian et al. (10) published a new classification to describe post-intubation posterior glottic stenosis (PGS) in the pediatric population. Moreover, the FLECS staging system (11) was proposed by the American Society of Pediatric Otolaryngology (ASPO) to encompass a detailed description of the Function, Lumen, Diameter, Extent and Site of stenosis. Although this classification was probably the most complete, it was abandoned because it was considered too confusing.

With regard to laryngomalacia, the most widely used classification was proposed by Olney et al. (12). Type 1 corresponds to a prolapse of the mucosa overlying the arytenoid cartilage, type 2 to foreshortened aryepiglottic folds and type 3 to posterior displacement of the epiglottis.

ELS Classification

In 2015, the European Laryngological Society (ELS) published a consensus paper (5) presenting a five-step endoscopic airway assessment and a reporting system. The authors attempted to standardize the pre- and intraoperative assessment techniques in order to fully investigate the lesion in all its aspects (type of stenosis, involved subsites, extension, laryngeal motility, and airway lumen). Furthermore, other conditions describing airway pathological status or concurrent comorbidities were integrated to help provide a more comprehensive evaluation of the patient.

TABLE 1 | Lano-Netterville classification Lano et al. (7).

	N. of involved subsites	Subsites
Stage I	1	Glottis or sub-glottis or trachea
Stage II	2	Glottis and sub-glottis or sub-glottis and trachea
Stage III	3	Glottis and sub-glottis and trachea

All these data are enclosed in a practical checklist which generates a final score.

The ELS classifications has been applied to large retrospective cohorts from the centers that contributed to its developing and it was confirmed to be as accurate for the prediction of both peri-operative outcome, i.e., complication rate or need for further treatments as long as for long-term outcomes, i.e., decannulation rate, both in pediatric (13) and adult groups (14) affected by laryngotracheal stenosis, and treated by tracheal or crico-tracheal resection and anastomosis. Its value for the prediction of the outcomes of patients submitted to endoscopic treatments has not been assessed yet.

The endoscopic work-up for LTS according to the ELS consists of five key-point procedures:

1. Awake indirect laryngoscopy or transnasal fiberoptic laryngoscopy (TNFL);
2. Asleep TNFL;
3. Direct transoral laryngotracheoscopy with a bare zero-degree rod-lens telescope;
4. Suspension microlaryngoscopy;
5. Bronchoesophagoscopy;

See the next paragraph for a detailed description of each step (5).

Radiological Assessment

Unlike indications for radiological evaluation in adult patients, those for pediatric stenosis are still under debate. CT scan can be helpful for studying craniocaudal extension and severity of the obstruction, capable to provide also 3D reconstruction of the airways (15, 16), especially when awake TNFL is unable

Classification	From	To	Endoscopic appearance
Grade I	No Obstruction	35% Obstruction	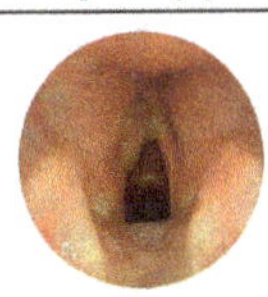
Grade II	35%	50%	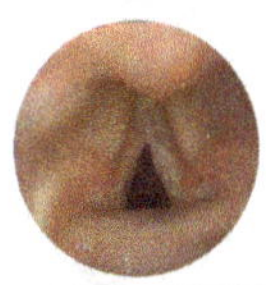
Grade III	51%	75%	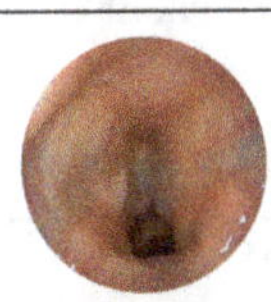
Grade IV	76%	100%	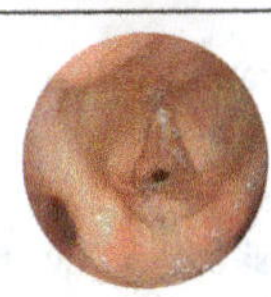

FIGURE 3 | Cohen Classification, adapted from Monnier et al. (5) with unpublished clinical pictures.

to show a clear view of them. Indeed, before performing any procedure under sedation or general anesthesia, radiological investigation is always mandatory in patients with Cotton-Meyer grade III or IV stenosis, except for subjects requiring immediate tracheotomy. Good quality imaging can be obtained without sedation using a CT scan with ultrafast acquisition frames. Otherwise, radiological imaging is indicated to study neck masses or abnormal mediastinal vessels (17). If the child can be safely sedated, standard CT or MRI scans can be performed in the presence of an anesthetist. MRI provides high resolution images allowing the assessment of airway compression secondary to mediastinal malformations (5).

Functional Assessment

Voice evaluation and respiratory function assessment should be obtained before carrying out any conservative or open neck procedures in order to establish the baseline condition. Documentation regarding stridor at-rest or during exercise, and physical activity and pulmonary function tests, such as spirometry, must be reported (18). Moreover, voice evaluation should be performed using the GRBAS-scale, including voice range profile and maximum phonation time for the vowels/e/and/a/. In case of infant patients these clinical data are meaningless if the tests cannot be performed properly (5).

Assessment of the Patient's General Condition

A comprehensive assessment of concomitant comorbidities must be included in the work-up. Pulmonary and cardiac check-ups are required, together with a full neurological evaluation. In case of previous tracheostomy, the grade of stenosis can easily be tested by temporarily occluding the cannula. This test provides immediate feedback on pulmonary capacity and low-flow/high-pressure resistance of the stenotic area (5).

Final Scoring

ELS final scoring is obtained by combining the Myer-Cotton grading system, a revised version of the Lano-Netterville classification, and the presence of severe comorbidities. The Myer-Cotton score defines the degree of stenosis and, similarly to the original classification, assigns a value from I to IV.

Thereafter, a revised version of the Lano-Netterville classification, which includes the supraglottis as the fourth subsite, is applied: (a) establishes a single subsite involvement and so forth up to (d) for involvement of all subsites. Lastly, in case of severe comorbidity or congenital abnormalities, a (+) sign is added to the score (**Figures 4, 5**) (5).

Advantages and Limits of ELS Classification

The main advantage of ELS classification is its comprehensive value and its aid guiding the whole work-up for a patient affected by laryngotracheal stenosis; regarding the scoring system it introduces the three-dimensional view, taking into account together the cranio-caudal shape of the stenosis and its smaller area on the axial plane; furthermore, relevant comorbidities of the patient are included, as they are crucial for the correct decision-making process. Beyond all these favorable features of the ELS classification, it has some limits as it lacks specificity for some subsites of the airway, such as the different compartments of the glottis, for which the older Cohen's and Bogdasarian's classification still play a relevant role for the staging of anterior and posterior glottic stenosis, respectively. Secondary, the functional investigation, such as spirometry, is included in the suggested work-up but its specific parameters are not taken into consideration in detail; beneath this kind of test is mostly applicable in adults population, the results by the recent literature about the usefulness of such exam are rising the value of spirometry for an objective evaluation of patients both for the pre-treatment staging and for follow-up period (19, 20).

PREOPERATIVE ENDOSCOPIC ASSESSMENT

The endoscopic diagnostic work-up includes TNFL, asleep TNFL, direct transoral laryngoscopy with 0° and 70° telescope, suspension microlaryngoscopy (SML), and bronchoesophagoscopy. Upon completion of the endoscopic work-up, a radiological study with CT and/or MRI must be performed, as must an assessment of respiratory and voice function and of the patient's general conditions.

Transnasal Fiberoptic Laryngoscopy

TNFL is part of the in-office examination. Patency of the nasal cavities, choanae, nasopharynx, pharynx, and larynx should be carefully assessed.

Flexible nasoendoscopy is performed to detect any obstructive supraglottic lesions (e.g., laryngomalacia, lymphovascular malformations, and cysts), vocal fold movements, and any evidence of impaired swallowing such as hypopharyngeal pooling of secretions. If restricted abduction or true immobility is observed, then a complete examination under general anesthesia is warranted in order to distinguish neurogenic bilateral vocal cord paralysis from posterior glottic stenosis, especially if the patient has been subjective to an orotracheal intubation. TNFL always yields incomplete information as the subglottis and trachea cannot be properly visualized.

Not all patients need direct laryngoscopy, especially when a clear diagnosis of mild laryngomalacia is made following a comprehensive medical history and physical examination (21). However, in case of symptom worsening, associated abnormalities or atypical clinical presentations, a complete laryngotracheobronchoscopy and esophagoscopy must be performed under general anesthesia.

Asleep TNF

Clinical indicators such as feeding difficulties, growth slowdown, obstructive sleep apneas and pulmonary hypertension required further investigation. Moreover, inadequate patient compliance is an absolute indication for TNFL under general anesthesia but in spontaneous respiration. Anesthesia is maintained with sevoflurane or i.v propofol. Before starting the laryngoscopy, atropine is administered intravenously.

ENDOSCOPY • preoperative assessment ☐ yes ☐ no
• postoperative assessment ☐ yes ☐ no

Awake indirect laryngoscopy/Awake TNFL ☐ yes ☐ no

• **VF mobility**

normal bilaterally	☐ yes	☐ no	
restricted abduction	☐ left	☐ right	☐ bilateral
VF immobility	☐ left	☐ right	☐ bilateral

Asleep TNFL (under GA in spontaneous respiration) ☐ yes ☐ no

• **OSA-related narrowings** ☐ yes ☐ no
☐ nose ☐ nasopharynx ☐ oropharynx ☐ pharyngolarynx

description :..

• **VF mobility** (if awake TNFL was impossible) ☐ yes ☐ no (please report above)

• **Tracheomalacia** ☐ yes ☐ no ☐ diffuse ☐ localized

• **Secondary Airway Lesions** ☐ yes ☐ no

description :..

Direct laryngotracheoscopy +/- SML (under GA)

• **Congenital LTS** ☐ yes ☐ no

• **Acquired LTS**

fresh, incipient LTS	☐ yes	☐ no
mature cicatricial LTS	☐ yes	☐ no
mixed (acquired on congenital) LTS	☐ yes	☐ no

• **Grade of stenosis**	• **Cranio-caudal extent of stenosis**	
☐ I ≤ 50 %	≤ 5mm	☐
☐ II 51 to 70%	> 5mm ≤ 15 mm	☐
☐ III 71 to 99%	> 15mm ≤ 30mm	☐
☐ IV no lumen	> 30mm	☐

• **Site of stenosis** (more than one answer possible)

supraglottic	☐ yes	☐ no
glottic	☐ yes	☐ no
subglottic	☐ yes	☐ no
tracheal	☐ yes	☐ no

• **Abnormal VF mobility**

neurogenic VF paresis ☐, paralysis ☐	☐ unilateral	☐ bilateral
VF fixation	☐ partial unilat.	☐ partial bilat.
	☐ complete unilat.	☐ complete bilat.

• **Posterior glottic stenosis (PGS)** ☐ yes ☐ no
interarytenoid adhesion (cicatricial bridge) ☐
true PGS ☐ yes ☐ no
☐ without CAA ☐ with unilat. CAA ☐ with bilat. CAA

FIGURE 4 | ELS checklist for pre-operative assessment and decision making (1/2) Monnier et al. (5).

Inspection of the nasal cavities on both sides is mandatory to identify possible pathologies, such as vestibular stenosis, deviated septum, choanal atresia, adenoid hyperplasia, or tumor masses. In cases of obstructive sleep apnea, when patients undergo general anesthesia with spontaneous breathing, their muscle tone decreases and the level of obstruction can then

- **VF web, synechia** ☐ yes ☐ no
  ≤ 25% VF length ☐ 25% ≤ 50% VF length ☐ 50% ≤ 75% VF length ☐ > 75% VF length ☐

- **Trachea**
  Stenosis ☐ yes ☐ no
  Malacia ☐ yes ☐ no
  primary diffuse ☐ yes ☐ no
  localized post-tracheostomy ☐ yes ☐ no
  extrinsic vascular compression ☐ yes ☐ no
  Tracheostomy ☐ yes ☐ no
  location ☐ 1st 2nd rings ☐ 3rd 4th rings ☐ ≥ 5th rings
  additional distal tracheal stenosis ☐ yes ☐ no
  localized tracheostoma malacia ☐ yes ☐ no

- **Bronchial tree and esophagus**
  Bronchomalacia ☐ yes ☐ no Bacteriological aspirate ☐ yes ☐ no
  Extrinsic bronchial compression ☐ yes ☐ no Bronchoalveolar lavage ☐ yes ☐ no
  Gastroesophageal refux ☐ yes ☐ no Esophageal biopsies ☐ yes ☐ no
  Eosinophilic esophagitis ☐ yes ☐ no
  Other...

COMORBIDITIES ☐ yes ☐ no

- **Airway** ☐ yes ☐ no
  OSA-related narrowings ☐ yes ☐ no
  Secondary LTS/ malacia ☐ yes ☐ no
  description :...

- **Medical** ☐ yes ☐ no
  respiratory insufficiency (O_2 dependence) ☐ yes ☐ no
  Symptomatic cardiac/vascular disease ☐ yes ☐ no
  Neurologic sequelae/mental impairment ☐ yes ☐ no
  Swallowing disorder/aspiration ☐ yes ☐ no
  Symptomatic gastroesophageal reflux ☐ yes ☐ no
  Eosinophilic esophagitis ☐ yes ☐ no
  Syndromic/non-syndromic anomalies ☐ yes ☐ no
  Other : .... ☐ yes ☐ no

FINAL SCORING

☐ Ia	☐ Ib	☐ Ic	☐ Id
☐ IIa	☐ IIb	☐ IIc	☐ IId
☐ IIIa	☐ IIIb	☐ IIIc	☐ IIId
☐ IVa	☐ IVb	☐ IVc	☐ IVd

a = only one site involved (supraglottis/glottis/subglottis/trachea)
b = two sites involved } in any order
c = three sites involved }
\+ is added to any final score to indicate an additional severe comorbidity or congenital anomaly

TREATMENT PLAN **Primary surgery** ☐ **Salvage surgery** ☐: **1st** ☐ **2nd** ☐ **3rd** ☐ **>3rd** ☐

- **Description :** 1...
  2...
  3...
  4...

FIGURE 5 | ELS checklist for pre-operative assessment and decision making (2/2) Monnier et al. (5).

be identified. Various causes of dynamic obstruction that are detectable by fiberoptic endoscopy include retroposition of the soft palate, lingual tonsillar hypertrophy and epiglottic and supraglottic prolapse. This assessment is extremely relevant, especially in the preoperative evaluation of subglottic stenosis. A jaw lift is mandatory to raise the tongue base, allowing a better visualization of the pharyngolarynx. When the videobronchoscope reaches the laryngeal aditus, deeper anesthesia is needed in order to further advance into the lower airway tract without risking laryngospasm.

Passing behind the epiglottis and reaching the laryngeal inlet allows for a detailed and careful assessment of vocal cord mobility (22): it should be noted that large cuneiform cartilage and short aryepiglottic folds can obscure the laryngeal inlet and prevent a proper view of the vocal cords. Flexible laryngoscopy in the office setting might not be able to identify oropharyngolaryngeal obstructions that may be responsible for OSA.

Evaluation of the larynx during spontaneous breathing allows us to identify webs, posterior glottic stenosis, vocal fold palsy or paralysis.

Furthermore, dynamic examination of the trachea and bronchi is of paramount importance for the diagnosis of localized or diffuse tracheomalacia and anatomical narrowings of the lower airways. When vocal cord immobility is detected during TNFL, SML must be carried out.

In conclusion we can say that both awake and asleep TNFL are required in the evaluation of a compromised airway.

Direct Transoral Laryngoscopy With 0° and 70° Telescope

In order to better visualize and characterize a possible glottic, subglottic or tracheal stenosis the child must be deeply anesthetized and completely paralyzed. The larynx is visualized using a general-purpose Storz laryngoscope with the blade inserted at the level of the vallecula. A rigid 4 mm diameter magnifying telescope offers a clear view of the endolarynx, subglottis and trachea as far as the carena. In case of subglottic or tracheal stenosis, attention has to be paid not to damage the mucosa. Indeed, the slightest injury to a narrow airway could decompensate a stable obstructive dyspnea, thus requiring a tracheotomy. If the 4 mm diameter endoscope is too large, then a 2.7 mm or even a 1 mm diameter (sialendoscopy) scope should be used to assess the length of the stenosis and the integrity of the distal airway. The degree of SGS is calculated by passing telescopes or bougies of different sizes through the stenosis. The Myer–Cotton airway grading system is commonly utilized (3). Generally speaking, a tracheostomy caused by diagnostic upper airway endoscopy must be considered unacceptable.

Suspension Microlaryngoscopy

The Benjamin-Lindholm laryngoscope is preferable for visualizing the pharynx, larynx, and subglottis (23).

Specific tools are needed during the procedure: 0° and 70° telescopes, a Lindholm vocal cord retractor, angulated probes, and tapered bougies.

Telescopes are used to measure the craniocaudal extension of the stenosis. Bougies of given size are used to measure the degree of the stricture. Lastly, in order to distinguish between bilateral vocal cord paralysis (BVCP) and posterior glottic stenosis, Lindholm vocal cord retractor and angulated telescopes are used. To get the most precise measurement of the craniocaudal extension of the stenosis, the telescope is inserted through the laryngoscope and further advanced as far as the vocal cords, pointing the distance on the shaft of the telescope. Repeated measurements are taken at the upper and lower borders of the stenosis and tracheostoma, if present, and lastly at the level of the carina (**Figure 6**). In order to program the surgery correctly, especially in case of tracheal resection and anastomosis, such measurements are mandatory. With complete airway obstruction, CT scans with 3D reconstructions are very useful.

Once we had carefully assed the craniocaudal extension and the degree of the stenosis, differential diagnosis between BVCP and PGS is mandatory. Important information can be provided by the patient's medical history. Lindholm cord retractor and an angulated probe are used to precisely assess the posterior laryngeal commissure and cricoarytenoid joint function in all the patients who have previously undergone orotracheal intubation. The former is placed at the level of the vocal fold and is opened. In patients with neurogenic BVCP, the interarytenoid distance is restored to its normal size, while in patients with PGS it remains narrow, and a stretched band of scar tissue may be observed (**Figures 7A,B**).

By using the angulated probe, it thus becomes possible to precisely identify the different types of PGS according to Bogdasarian's classification (**Figure 8**) (10).

Bronchoesophagoscopy

The diagnostic work-up of children affected by SGS must be completed by the evaluation of lower airways and esophagus. In case of tracheostomized patients, rigid or flexible bronchoscope has to be introduced through the tracheostoma. If the distal end of the cannula has caused strictures of the lower trachea, the rigid bronchoscope is not advanced any further in order to avoid mucosal damages. In this case the use of a flexible bronchoscope is mandatory. If the tracheal wall has not been damaged by the cannula, then all of the rings can be identified. The linear measure between the lower border of the tracheostoma and the carina should be measured as described in the previous paragraph (**Figure 6**). When planning possible resection and anastomosis of the airway it is of paramount importance to count the number of residual normal tracheal rings. Further investigation down to the basal bronchi is performed on both sides.

Biopsies and bronchoalveolar lavage (BAL) should always be executed at the end of bronchoscopic evaluation, as bleeding might affect any further examination.

During the bronchoscopy we have to investigate the presence of congenital or acquired lesions such as tracheo-esophageal fistula, bronchus suis, localized or diffuse malacia, extrinsic compressions, anomalous distribution of the bronchial tree and lesions caused by local trauma induced by the tracheostomy cannula as well as from suction catheters at the level of the carina. The characteristics of bronchial secretions (serous, mucus, muco-purulent) and mucosa (inflammation and friability) must be documented. Precise assessment of their effects on the ventilation through the stenotic segmental bronchi is required. Bacteriological testing of the aspirate should be conducted systematically, while BAL is necessary to confirm the diagnosis of chronic aspiration when lipid-laden macrophages are seen on the smear examination. Missing the diagnose of infection of the

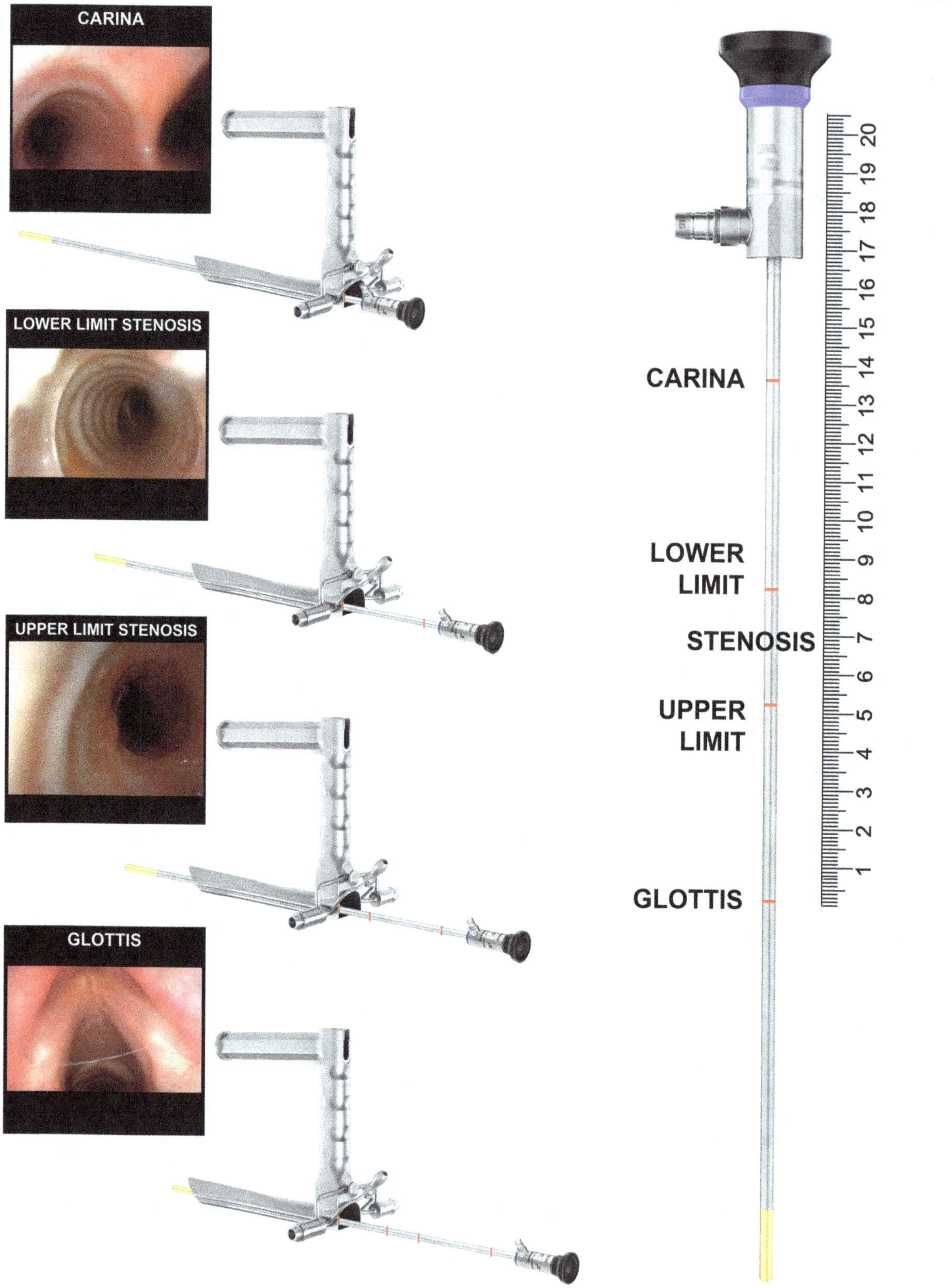

FIGURE 6 | Intraoperative measurement of a 3 cm tract of the tracheal stenosis during suspension microlaryngoscopy.

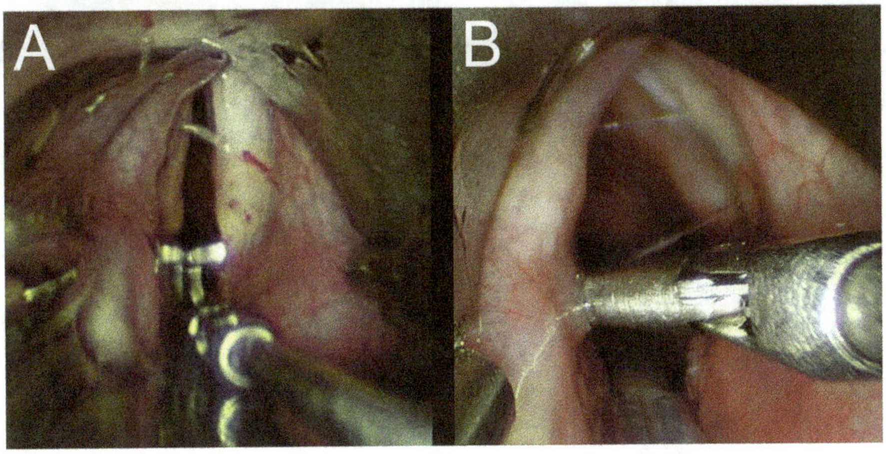

FIGURE 7 | (A,B) Lindholm cord retractor.

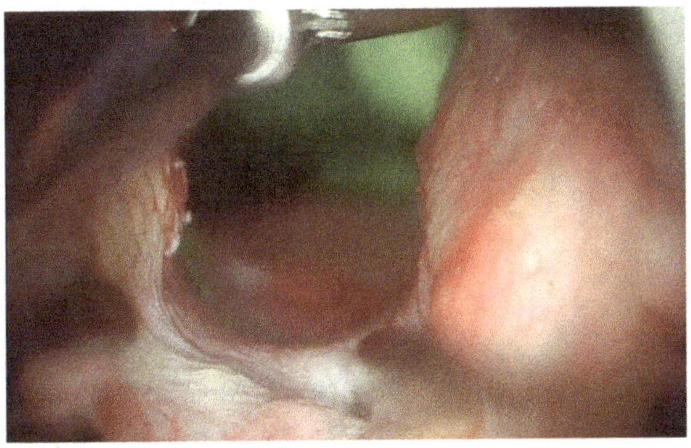

FIGURE 8 | Angulated probe to better visualize the posterior commissure.

lower airways could affect surgical outcome, leading to adverse complications such as anastomotic dehiscence, cartilage graft infection and secondary tracheostomy.

As well as bronchosocopy, esophagoscopy can be performed with flexible or rigid scopes. The use of rigid scope is easier in infants and children than in adults (24, 25).

Esophagoscopy must address the presence of gastroesophageal reflux and eosinophilic esophagitis.

GOR is best diagnosed using 24-h pH monitoring or impedancemetry, but endoscopy may reveal signs of erosive esophagitis (25). The absence of the angle of His, with the cardia opening located in a direct line to the gastric pouch, is an anatomical pattern that may cause chronic reflux.

Thickened or annulated mucosa may be indicative of eosinophilic esophagitis (26). Biopsies are necessary to confirm this diagnosis.

DECISION MAKING

Comprehensive pre-operative assessment is helpful for identifying which children affected by laryngotracheal stenosis would most benefit from surgery. It would also be useful to the multi-disciplinary laryngotracheal stenosis board team made up of ENT surgeons, pulmonologists, gastroenterologists, cardiologists, neurologists, neonatologists, and intensivists in making the best choices regarding type and timing of surgery (2). The goal of any laryngotracheal surgical procedure is to achieve decannulation and to re-establish an airway while preserving adequate laryngeal function for airway protection, swallowing, and voicing (27).

Tracheotomy

Patients affected by mild stenosis (grade I-II) are often kept under observation due to the lack of severe symptoms and pending airway growth that usually leads to widening of the free lumen. If the patient's respiratory condition starts deteriorating it is advisable to take airway reconstruction surgery into consideration to avoid a tracheotomy, the latter making further treatment more challenging and being a potential worsening factor for learning effective communication in a growing child.

In some cases, however, tracheotomy is unavoidable in order to safely secure a compromised laryngeal airway, especially in the presence of local or systemic medical conditions which are contraindicated in airway reconstruction surgery (28). It must be highlighted that the mortality rate of tracheostomized children with significant laryngeal obstruction has decreased from 24% in the 1970s to 2–3% by the year 2000 (2). When dealing with a laryngeal stenosis, the tracheotomy should be placed immediately below the cricoid to maximally preserve the normal trachea distally, or far below, sparing a sufficient amount of uninvolved tracheal rings between the stenosis and the tracheostomy. With this aim in mind, the best site to perform the procedure in patients with purely tracheal stenosis is through the stenotic site, maximally preserving the uninvolved tracheal rings.

Surgical Timing

The main factors affecting the choice to proceed to surgery primarily regard open neck laryngo-tracheal reconstruction procedures, meaning partial cricotracheal resection and

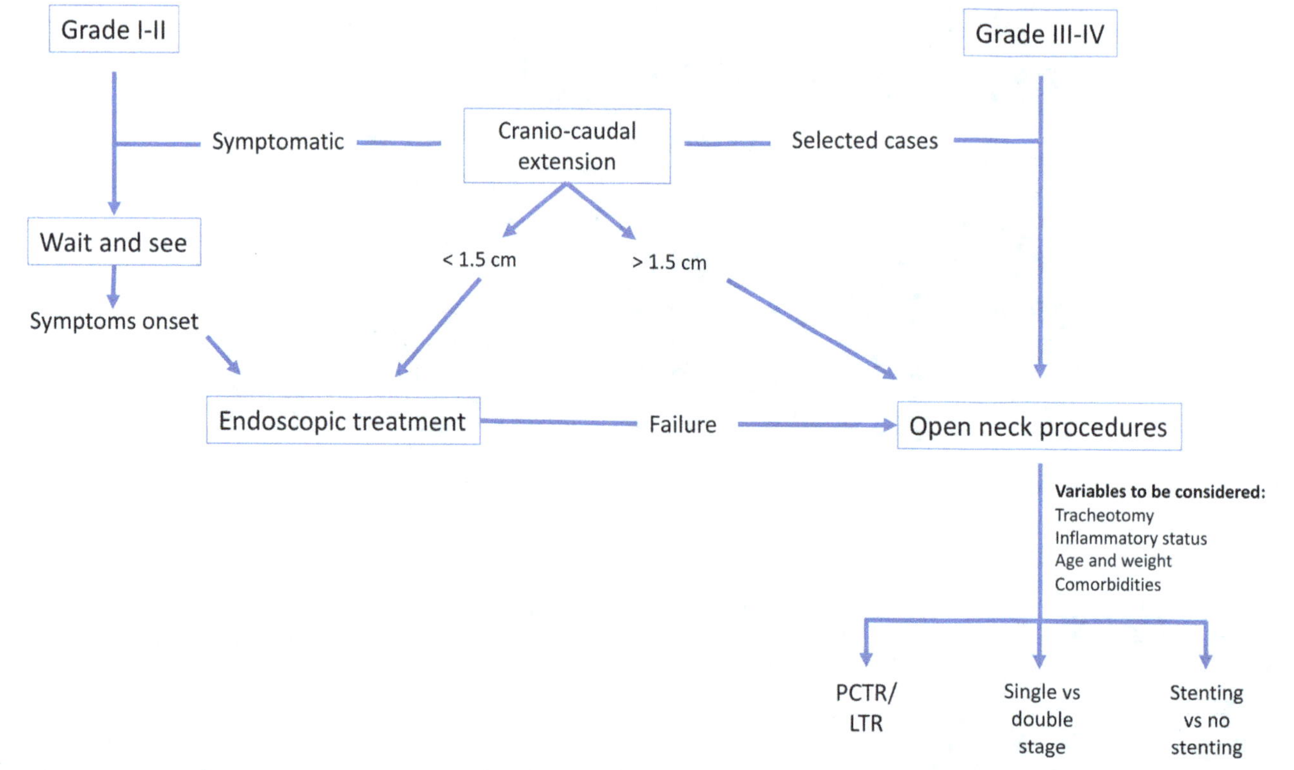

FIGURE 9 | Decision-making flow-chart.

anastomosis (PCTR) or laryngotracheal reconstruction (LTR), and can be summarized in three main items: grade of stenosis, inflammatory status of the stenosis and/or medical comorbidities, age and weight of the child.

1. Grade: for children affected by mild stenosis (Grade I-II) a wait and see policy can be chosen, especially facing with congenital, knowing that the airway is expected to become wider with growth. Endoscopic follow-up should be done every 6 months, until complete resolve of the symptoms. If a worsening of the respiratory condition is seen, an airway reconstruction surgery must be taken into account, to avoid emergency tracheostomy, potentially compromising further airway reconstructive procedures (2);
2. Inflammatory status and comorbidities: the presence of laryngeal or tracheal reactivity, as proven by the presence of erythematous mucosa or edema, is a contraindication for proceeding to open neck surgery; the same policy should be followed if the child is suffering from unresolved concomitant cardiopulmonary disease, neurological impairment associated with pharyngolaryngeal discoordination and/or aspiration or uncontrolled gastroesophageal reflux disease.
3. Age and weight of the child: when an infant has no significant comorbidities, early intervention during the first months of life is appropriate (2). Thanks to the established use of magnification devices and the experience that has been accrued in tertiary referral centers for the treatment of infants weighing <10 kg (29), the weight criterion no longer needs to be considered an absolute contraindication. As we are dealing with growing tracheostomized children, it must always be kept in mind that a delay would ultimately affect both communication learning (30) and the mortality rate associated with the tracheostomy tube.

Patient Management

Currently available treatments can be summarized as including endoscopic procedures, open neck laryngo-tracheal reconstruction (single stage/double stage PCTR/LTR) and the use of non-surgical devices, such as continuous positive airway pressure (C-PAP) therapy. Patients with mild stenosis (grade I-II) often have intermittent stridor associated with respiratory tract infection, but tracheostomy is not usually needed. In this scenario the airway is not severely compromised and in most cases no treatment is necessary, especially if the stenosis is congenital and therefore it is expected to enlarge as the child grows.

When dealing with a symptomatic child requiring treatment, once the whole diagnostic algorithm has been followed, the decision-making should be discussed among the multidisciplinary airway team in order to reach a consensus for the best timing and type of surgery.

Monnier proposed a list of queries that the laryngotracheal stenosis board team should address so as to make the best treatment choice (2):

1. What type of surgery should be appropriate?

   a. Endoscopic, LTR, PCTR or extended PCTR?
   b. Which type of grafting if needed?

2. Single-stage or double-stage surgery?
   a. With or without stenting?
   b. Need for intensive care unit?

3. What type and risk of complications to expect?
   a. PCTR: anastomotic dehiscence and/or RLN injury
   b. LTR: high recurrence rate for grade III-IV subglottic stenosis

4. Which kind of results can be predicted about airway, voice and deglutition?
5. Have all relevant comorbidities been studied?
   a. GOR disease?
   b. Neurologic, pulmonary and cardiac diseases?
   c. Nutritional status?
   d. Airway infection or contamination?

6. Is surgical timing appropriate?
   a. Maturity of the stenosis?
   b. Patient's age and comorbidities?

7. Does the theoretically best surgical procedure fit with the child's comorbidities or other airway abnormalities?

We propose our decision-making flow chart (**Figure 9**) since there is a broad number of treatment options and it is the task of the multidisciplinary team to establish which is the best for each individual patient while keeping in mind the aforementioned issues. Moreover, choosing the correct treatment modality at the very beginning is of paramount importance, otherwise the success of the entire treatment could be compromised.

AUTHOR CONTRIBUTIONS

Material preparation and literature search were performed by MF, FMa, and FMi. The first draft of the manuscript was written by MF, FMa, and FMi. GP and FC reviewed the manuscript. All authors contributed to the study conception and design, read, and approved the final manuscript.

REFERENCES

1. Clark CM, Kugler K, Carr MM. Common causes of congenital stridor in infants. *JAAPA*. (2018) 31:36–40. doi: 10.1097/01.JAA.0000546480.64441.af
2. Monnier P. *Pediatric Airway Surgery Management of Laryngotracheal Stenosis in Infants and Children*. Heidelberg: Springer (2011).
3. Myer CM, O'connor DM, Cotton RT. Proposed grading system for subglottic stenosis based on endotracheal tube sizes. *Ann Otol Rhinol Laryngol*. (1994) 103(4 Pt 1):319–23. doi: 10.1177/000348949410300410
4. Cotton RT. Pediatric laryngotracheal stenosis. *J Pediatr Surg*. (1984) 19:699–704. doi: 10.1016/S0022-3468(84)80355-3
5. Monnier P, Dikkers FG, Eckel H, Sittel C, Piazza C, Campos G, et al. Preoperative assessment and classification of benign laryngotracheal stenosis: a consensus paper of the European Laryngological Society. *Eur Arch Oto-Rhino-Laryngology*. (2015) 272:2885–96. doi: 10.1007/s00405-015-3635-4
6. McCaffrey T V. Classification of laryngotracheal stenosis. *Laryngoscope*. (1992) 102:1335–40. doi: 10.1288/00005537-199212000-00004
7. Lano CFJ, Duncavage JA, Reinisch L, Ossoff RH, Courey MS, Netterville JL. Laryngotracheal reconstruction in the adult: a ten year experience. *Ann Otol Rhinol Laryngol*. (1998) 107:92–7. doi: 10.1177/000348949810700202
8. Cohen S. Congenital glottic webs in children. A retrospective review of 51 patients. *Ann Otol Rhinol Laryngol Suppl*. (1985) 121:2–16. doi: 10.1177/00034894850940S601
9. Laccourreye H, Beutter P, Brasnu D. [Laryngeal and laryngotracheal stenoses. Classification and treatment (author's transl)]. *Ann Otolaryngol Chir Cervicofac*. (1981) 98:571–9.
10. Bogdasarian RS, Olson NR. Posterior glottic laryngeal stenosis. *Otolaryngol Head Neck Surg*. (1980) 88:765–72. doi: 10.1177/0194599880088 00625
11. Phillips JS, Erskine S. *Landmark Papers in Otolaryngology*. Oxford: Oxford University Press (2018). doi: 10.1093/med/9780198834281.001.0001
12. Olney DR, Greinwald JHJ, Smith RJ, Bauman NM. Laryngomalacia and its treatment. *Laryngoscope*. (1999) 109:1770–5. doi: 10.1097/00005537-199911000-00009
13. Fiz I, Monnier P, Koelmel JC, Di Dio D, Torre M, Fiz F, et al. Implementation of the European Laryngological Society classification for pediatric benign laryngotracheal stenosis: a multicentric study. *Eur Arch Oto Rhino Laryngol*. (2019) 276:785–92. doi: 10.1007/s00405-019-0 5353-4
14. Fiz I, Monnier P, Koelmel JC, Di Dio D, Fiz F, Missale F, et al. Multicentric study applying the european laryngological society classification of benign laryngotracheal stenosis in adults treated by tracheal or cricotracheal resection and anastomosis. *Laryngoscope*. (2019) doi: 10.1002/lary.28274. [Epub ahead of print].
15. Lambert V, Sigal-Cinqualbre A, Belli E, Planché C, Roussin R, Serraf A, et al. Preoperative and postoperative evaluation of airways compression in pediatric patients with 3-dimensional multislice computed tomographic scanning: effect on surgical management. *J Thorac Cardiovasc Surg*. (2005) 129: 1111–8. doi: 10.1016/j.jtcvs.2004.08.030
16. McDaniel LS, Poynot WJ, Gonthier KA, Dunham ME, Crosby TW. Image-Based 3-dimensional characterization of laryngotracheal stenosis in children. *OTO Open*. (2018) 2:2473974X17753583 doi: 10.1177/2473974X17753583
17. Singh C, Gupta M, Sharma S. Compression of trachea due to double aortic arch: demonstration by Multi-slice CT Scan (MSCT). *Hear Lung Circ*. (2006) 15: 332–33. doi: 10.1016/j.hlc.2006.02.006
18. Bogaard JM, Pauw KH, Versprille A, Stam H, Verbraak AFM, Maas AJJ. Maximal expiratory and inspiratory flow–volume curves in bilateral vocal–cord paralysis: changes after surgical treatment and comparison with glottic resistance characteristics. *ORL J Otorhinolaryngol Relat Spec*. (1987) 49:35–41. doi: 10.1159/000275904
19. Franco RA, Husain I, Reder L, Paddle P. Awake serial intralesional steroid injections without surgery as a novel targeted treatment for idiopathic subglottic stenosis. *Laryngoscope*. (2018) 128:610–7. doi: 10.1002/lary.26874
20. Abdullah A, Alrabiah A, Habib SS, Aljathlany Y, Aljasser A, Bukhari M, et al. The value of spirometry in subglottic stenosis. *Ear Nose Throat J*. (2019) 98:98–101. doi: 10.1177/0145561318823309
21. Stern, Y, Cotton R. Evaluation of the noisy infant. In: Cotton RT, Myer CM III, editors. *Practical Pediatric Otolaryngology*. Philadelphia, PA; New York, NY: Lippincott-Raven (1999) p. 471–476.
22. Chen EY, Inglis AF. Bilateral vocal cord paralysis in children. *Otolaryngol Clin North Am*. (2008) 41:889–901. doi: 10.1016/j.otc.2008.04.003
23. Benjamin B. Pediatric laryngoscopes: design and application. *Ann Otol Rhinol Laryngol*. (2001) 110:617–23. doi: 10.1177/000348940111000705
24. Green C, Holinger L, Gartlan M. Technique. In: Holinger ID, Lusk RP, Green CGM, editors. *Paediatric Laryngology and Bronchoesophagology*. Philadelphia; New York, NY: Lippincott-Raven (1997). p. 106–7.
25. Savary, M., Miller G. *The Esophagus: Handbook and Atlas of Endoscopy*. Solothurn: Verlag Gassmann AG (1978).
26. Shannon R. Eosinophilic esophagitis in children. *Gastroenterol Nurs*. (2009) 32:123–5. doi: 10.1097/SGA.0b013e31819f7a20
27. Baker S, Kelchner L, Weinrich B, Lee L, Willging P, Cotton R, et al. Pediatric laryngotracheal stenosis and airway reconstruction: a review of

voice outcomes, assessment, and treatment issues. *J Voice.* (2006) 20:631–41. doi: 10.1016/j.jvoice.2005.08.012

28. Meier JD, White DR. Multisystem disease and pediatric laryngotracheal reconstruction. *Otolaryngol Clin North Am.* (2012) 45:643–51, viii. doi: 10.1016/j.otc.2012.03.004
29. Garabedian E-N, Nicollas R, Roger G, Delattre J, Froehlich P, Triglia J-M. Cricotracheal resection in children weighing less than 10 kg. *Arch Otolaryngol Head Neck Surg.* (2005) 131:505–8. doi: 10.1001/archotol.131.6.505
30. Zalzal GH, Choi SS, Patel KM. Ideal timing of pediatric laryngotracheal reconstruction. *Arch Otolaryngol Head Neck Surg.* (1997) 123:206–8. doi: 10.1001/archotol.1997.01900020094014

21

Necessity of Prophylactic Extrapleural Chest Tube During Primary Surgical Repair of Esophageal Atresia

Martin Riis Ladefoged[1,2], Steven Kwasi Korang[1,3], Simone Engmann Hildorf[4], Jacob Oehlenschlæger[4], Susanne Poulsen[5], Magdalena Fossum[2,4,6] and Ulrik Lausten-Thomsen[5]*

[1] Copenhagen Trial Unit, Department 7812, Centre for Clinical Intervention Research, Copenhagen University Hospital Rigshospitalet, Copenhagen, Denmark, [2] Department of Clinical Medicine, University of Copenhagen, Copenhagen, Denmark, [3] Department of Anesthesiology Critical Care Medicine, Childrens Hospital Los Angeles, Los Angeles, CA, United States, [4] Department of Paediatric Surgery, Copenhagen University Hospital Rigshospitalet, Copenhagen, Denmark, [5] Department of Neonatology, Copenhagen University Hospital Rigshospitalet, Copenhagen, Denmark, [6] Department of Women's and Children's Health, Karolinska Institutet, Stockholm, Sweden

***Correspondence:**
Martin Riis Ladefoged
martin-riis@hotmail.com

Background: Esophageal atresia is corrected surgically by anastomosing and recreating esophageal continuity. To allow the removal of excess fluid and air from the anastomosis, a prophylactic and temporary intraoperative chest tube (IOCT) has traditionally been placed in this area during surgery. However, whether the potential benefits of this prophylactic IOCT overweigh the potential harms is unclear.

Objective: To assess the benefits and harms of using a prophylactic IOCT during primary surgical repair of esophageal atresia.

Data Sources: We conducted a systematic review with a meta-analysis. We searched Cochrane Central Register of Controlled Trials (2021, Issue 12), MEDLINE Ovid, Embase Ovid, CINAHL, and Science Citation Index Expanded and Conference Proceedings Citation Index—(Web of Science). Search was performed from inception until December 3rd, 2021.

Study Selection: Randomized clinical trials (RCT) assessing the effect of a prophylactic IOCT during primary surgical repair of esophageal atresia and observational studies identified during our searches for RCT.

Data Extraction and Synthesis: Two independent reviewers screened studies and performed data extraction. The certainty of the evidence was assessed by GRADE and ROBINS-I.

PROSPERO Registration: A protocol for this review has been registered on PROSPERO (CRD42021257834).

Results: We included three RCTs randomizing 162 neonates, all at overall "some risk of bias." The studies compared the placement of an IOCT vs. none. The meta-analysis did not identify any significant effect of profylacitic IOCT, as confidence intervals were compatible with no effect, but the analyses suggests that the placement of an IOCT might lead to an increase in all-cause mortality (RR 1.66, 95% CI 0.76–3.65; three trials), serious adverse events (RR 1.08, 95% CI 0.58–2.00; three trials), intervention-requiring pneumothorax (RR 1.65, 95% CI 0.28–9.50; two trials), and anastomosis leakage (RR 1.66, 95% CI 0.63–4.40). None of our included studies assessed esophageal stricture or pain. Certainty of evidence was very low for all outcomes.

Conclusions: Evidence from RCTs does not support the routine use of a prophylactic IOCT during primary surgical repair of esophageal atresia.

Keywords: chest tube, neonates, tracheoesophageal fistula, esophageal atresia, pediatric surgery

INTRODUCTION

Esophageal atresia refers to a group of congenital anomalies in which the continuity of the esophagus is interrupted (1). Tracheoesophageal anomalies are divided into subtypes depending on anatomy and the most prominent (85%) subtype has a tracheoesophageal fistula to the distal esophageal segment (1). The prevalence of esophageal atresia varies according to country and time period (2–8). Observational studies from 1981 to 2018 have estimated the prevalence to span from 0.88 to 4.55 per 10,000 births in China and in Germany, respectively. Recent European studies suggest that the prevalence is relatively stable over time (9–11) and that males are most affected with a male:female ratio of 1:0.74 (9).

At birth, the neonate presents with typical drooling of saliva, inability to swallow, choking, coughing, cyanotic attacks, and distended abdomen if the subtype involves a fistula to the trachea (11). The diagnosis is confirmed by the inability to pass a feeding tube into the stomach (11, 12) and a plain X-ray showing the non-progression of the feeding tube located in a blind-ending pouch (11, 12). Prenatal diagnostics having improved from 26 to 36% during the last 30 years (9). Postnatal diagnosis occurs on the first day after birth in 83% of cases, the remaining 15% of cases within the first week, and only in 1.2% after the first week (9).

Most cases seem to occur sporadically, therefore the etiology is likely to be multifactorial involving multiple genes and complex gene-environment interactions (13, 14). Despite observational studies suggesting various maternal risk factors (10, 13, 15), the exact etiology is still unclear (13, 14). Since esophageal atresia is an early organogenesis defect, associated anomalies are frequency found (9, 16–19). Isolated esophageal atresia occurs in ~45–53% of the cases, whereas 32–47% have multiple anomalies, and 24–25% have an association or a syndrome, the most common being VACTERL association occurring in ~10% (9, 16–21). Among the most common associated anomalies are congenital heart defects (23–29% of cases), other gastrointestinal anomalies (16–21%), urinary tract anomalies (15–16%), and limb anomalies (13–14%) (9, 16–19).

Left untreated, the condition is fatal due to starvation, infection, and respiratory complications and survival therefore relies on early surgical correction (1, 11). The surgery aims to reconstruct the continuity of the esophagus and eliminate any possible fistulae (11, 14), which can be done either as a transpleural thorascopical procedure, or as open surgery, most commonly extrapleural (11, 22).

The mortality rate in isolated esophageal atresia range from 4.3 to 8.1% (7, 8, 17, 23–25), but varies with the type of atresia (with higher mortality and morbidity in the long gap esophageal atresia presentation), and mortality increases furthermore in case of prematurity and/or low birth weight, and with the presence of associated abnormalities, notably major cardiac and chromosomal anomalies (2, 6, 9, 26, 27). Even after hospital discharge, the children have increased mortality with post-discharge mortality is primarily due to respiratory compromise, including sudden infant death, aspiration, tracheomalacia, and reactive airway disease (23, 28, 29).

The most common postoperative complications are anastomosis leakage, fistula recurrence, anastomotic strictures, respiratory complications, and infections (25, 30–40). Anastomotic leakage is one of the most common serious complications occurring in about 5–17% of cases (25, 34, 35). Leakage into the mediastinum result mainly from anastomotic tension (particularly in cases with increased gap length) leading to ischemia of the esophageal ends, particularly in the small, friable lower segment and sub-optimal surgical technique; sepsis and even use of prosthetic materials can contribute (36–38). Major leaks are uncommon and tend to present with acute deterioration associated with pneumothorax and sepsis, and may require emergency decompression with placement of a postoperative chest tube (35, 39, 40). Most leaks heal spontaneously given proper drainage and antibiotics and only few require surgical intervention (35, 39, 40).

Long-term complications include strictures of the anastomotic region [incidence 25–75% (25, 34, 41, 42)], gastroesophageal reflux [incidence 22–63% (43)], esophagitis, tracheomalacia, feeding difficulties [incidence up to 80% (30, 44)], pulmonary symptoms, and developmental challenges (30–33, 45). These long-term complications have an impact on quality of life (28) in both patients and parents, especially in the case of tracheal and esophageal complications (6, 31, 46–50).

During the esophageal repair a prophylactic intraoperative chest tube (IOCT) has traditionally been placed close to the anastomosis to drain access fluid and air through a one-way system (51, 52). The routine use of prophylactic IOCTs is now debated (11, 39, 40, 52) and at the European Reference Network for rare Inherited and Congenital Anomalies (ERNICA) consensus conference, no consensus was found with only 21.4% of the members voting for the use of IOCTs (22). However, IOCTs are still used and reported as common as in 54% of the cases in the UK (53), 57% in Belgium (54), and 69% in an international survey, respectively (55).

IOCTs are not without drawback as they can cause insertion site infection (56) and when improperly placed, the tube can cause disruption of the site of anastomosis or penetration of proximal myotomy (57). IOCTs may also cause considerable postoperative pain, which would decrease inspiratory effort tand need for administration of more opoids, both leading to secondary effects such as atelectasis and pneumonia (58). Importantly, in some cases, IOCTs are insufficient to drain major leaks, necessitating the placement of a new chest tube (39, 40).

Whether the potential benefits of the prophylactic IOCT overweigh the potential harms is therefore unclear (22). Accordingly, the objective of this study was to examine the benefits and harms of prophylactic IOCT during primary surgical repair of esophageal atresia.

METHODS

We conducted a systematic review of the existing literature according to the Preferred Reporting Items for Systematic Reviews and Meta-Analysis guidelines (PRISMA) and the Cochrane Handbook for Systematic Reviews of Intervention (59, 60). The predefined methodology, and method for this review in general, is described in our protocol, registered in June 2021 (61).

Eligibility Criteria

We searched for RCTs assessing the effect of a prophylactic IOCT during primary surgical repair of esophageal atresia and related observational studies identified during our searches for RCTs.

Search and Study Selection

We searched the Cochrane Central Register of Controlled Trials, MEDLINE Ovid, Embase Ovid, CINAHL, and Science Citation Index Expanded and Conference Proceedings Citation Index—(Web of Science). The search strategy was developed by an information specialist from the Cochrane Hepato-Biliary Group. The search strategy can be found in **Appendix 1**.

Studies were included irrespectively of publication type, publications status, and language. Two independent reviewers (MRL and SKK) screened and found relevant studies, performed data-extraction using an EXCEL data extraction sheet, and systematically checked risks of bias. We planned to contact trial authors if relevant data were unclear or missing. A description of the data collection process can be found in our protocol.

Risk of Bias Assessment

We followed the Cochrane Handbook for Systematic Reviews of Interventions to examine the risk of bias (62), including the ROBIN-I tool for non-randomized studies (63). Two authors, MRL and SKK, independently assessed the risk of bias in the included trials. In case of disagreements, a third author (ULT) would arbitrate.

Outcomes and Subgroup Analyses

The primary outcomes were: (1) all-cause mortality, (2) serious adverse events, and (3) pneumothorax - requiring intervention. Secondary outcomes were: (1) sepsis or mediastinitis, (2) anastomosis leakage, (3) esophageal stricture, and (4) pain (measured by any valid score). For every relevant outcome, the risk ratios (RRs) were calculated with a 95% confidence interval (CI).

Data Synthesis

We pooled the data from relevant studies that were estimated to be clinically homogeneous using the Review Manager 5.4.1 software. If more than one study provides usable data in any single comparison, we performed a meta-analysis. We used RR for dichotomous outcomes, and by utilizing the fixed-effect (Mantel-Haenszel model).

RESULTS

A systematic search done December 3rd, 2021, identified a total of 953 records from databases and registers. A total of 894 were excluded based on the title and abstract. We assessed 19 full-text original articles, of which following studies were included: three RCTs (64–66) and two case-control studies (51, 52) for narrative description in the discussion. See **Figure 1**: PRISMA flowchart and **Table 1**: Table of excluded studies regarding details on inclusion and exclusion of the studies.

Included Trials

We identified and included three RCTs randomizing a total of 162 neonates with esophageal atresia and distal tracheoesophageal fistula into intervention and control group. The trials compared mortality, serious adverse events, intervention-requiring pneumothorax, and anastomosis leakage (see **Table 2**: summary of findings). The risk of bias assessment is shown in **Figure 2**. All trials were assessed to be at overall "some concerns" for risk of bias. None of the trials adequately describe the randomization process or referred to a publish protocol.

Effects of Interventions

Primary Outcomes

All-Cause Mortality

A meta-analysis of three trials, randomizing 162 participants, showed that an IOCT might result in an increased risk of mortality compared to neonates undergoing surgery without an IOCT, but the confidence interval was compatible with no effect [RR 1.66, 95% CI 0.76–3.65; $P = 0.21$; 2.8% of optimal information size (OIS); very low certainty of evidence; **Figure 3**].

Proportion of Participants With One or More Serious Adverse Events

A meta-analysis of three trials, randomizing 162 participants, showed that an IOCT might result in an increased risk of having a serious adverse event compared with neonates with esophageal atresia undergoing surgery without an IOCT, but the confidence

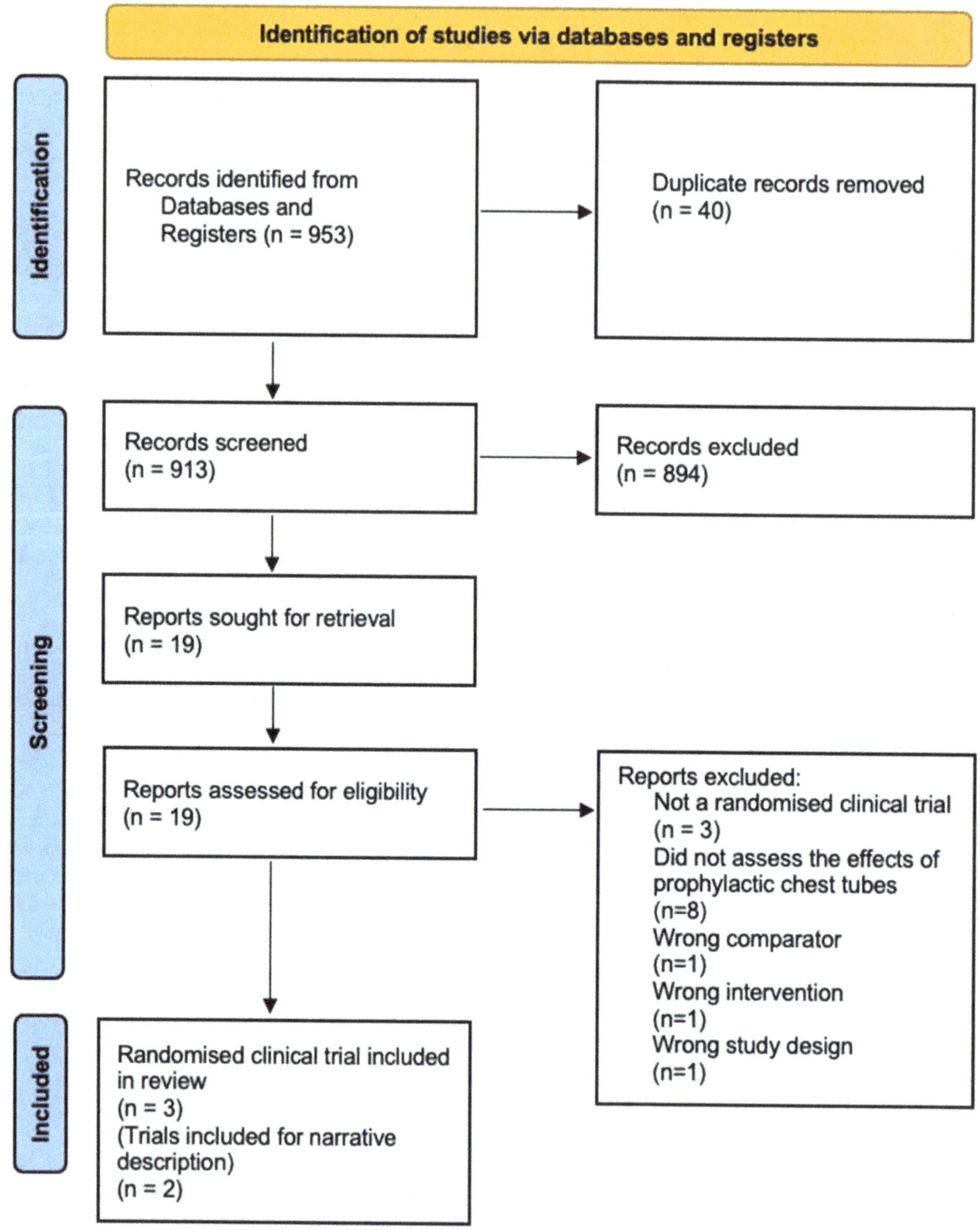

FIGURE 1 | PRISMA flowchart.

interval was compatible with no effect (RR 1.08, 95% CI 0.58–2.00; $P = 0.81$; 7.4% of OIS; very low certainty of evidence; **Figure 4**).

The serious adverse effects assessed in the trials were respiratory complications including respiratory distress, pneumonia, pneumothorax, lung collapse, and apnea as well as mortality.

Proportion of Participants With an Intervention-Requiring Pneumothorax

A meta-analysis of the two trials, randomizing 112 participants, showed that an IOCT might result in an increased risk of having an intervention-requiring pneumothorax compared with neonates with esophageal atresia undergoing surgery without an IOCT, but the confidence interval was compatible with no effect

TABLE 1 | Table of excluded studies.

Study id	Reason for exclusion	The authors's conclusion on IOCT (if any)
Brohi et al. (67)	Not a randomized clinical trial	NA
Castilloux et al. (68)	Did not assess the effects of prophylactic chest tubes	NA
Donoso et al. (69)	Did not assess the effects of prophylactic chest tubes	NA
Esteves et al. (70)	Did not assess the effects of prophylactic chest tubes	NA
Fasting and Winther (71)	Did not assess the effects of prophylactic chest tubes	NA
Grebe et al. (72)	Wrong intervention	NA
Johnson and Wright (57)	Wrong study design	An IOCT can perforate esophagus after primary repair.
Kay and Shaw (73)	Wrong comparator	An IOCT may not be necessary.
McCallion et al. (40)	Not a randomized clinical trial	IOCT unable to drain major leaks sufficiently, requiring placement of an additional drain.
Paramalingam et al. (74)	Not a randomized clinical trial	Drain appears not to be needed in all cases.
Vazquez et al. (75)	Did not assess the effects of prophylactic chest tubes	NA
Vercauteren et al. (76) Vol 8	Did not assess the effects of prophylactic chest tubes	NA
Zhang et al. (77)	Did not assess the effects of prophylactic chest tubes	NA
Zhang et al. (78)	Did not assess the effects of prophylactic chest tubes	NA

NA, not applicable.

(RR 1.65, 95% CI 0.28–9.50; $P = 0.58$; 0.46% of OIS; very low certainty of evidence; **Figure 5**).

Secondary Outcomes

Participants With Sepsis or Mediastinitis

One included trial (65), reporting sepsis, showed that an IOCT might result in an increased risk of having sepsis compared with neonates with esophageal atresia undergoing surgery without an IOCT, but the confidence interval was compatible with no effect (RR 3.00, 95% CI 0.14–64.26).

Participants With Anastomosis Leakage

Three trials, randomizing 162 participants, showed that an IOCT might result in an increased risk of anastomosis leakages compared with neonates with esophageal atresia undergoing surgery without an IOCT, but the confidence interval was compatible with no effect (RR 1.66, 95% CI 0.63–4.40; $P = 0.30$; 2.24 % of OIS; very low certainty of evidence; **Figure 6**).

Participants With Esophageal Stricture

None of the included trials reported on esophageal stricture.

Pain (Measured by Any Valid Score)

None of the included studies did a measurement of pain.

DISCUSSION

Summary of Main Findings

We identified and included three RCTs randomizing a total of 162 neonates with esophageal atresia and distal tracheoesophageal fistula into intervention and control group. The trials compared mortality, serious adverse events, intervention-requiring pneumothorax, and anastomosis leakage.

We found no evidence of a beneficial effect of placing a prophylactic IOCT during primary surgical repair from neither of the included studies. The evidence from RCTs shows potential harm when assessing all-cause mortality and serious adverse events, but the results were very uncertain. All studies were assessed to be at overall "some concerns" for risk of bias. The risk of bias assessment is shown in **Figure 2**. The statistical heterogeneity was low for all our meta-analyses. It was not possible to assess the preplanned subgroups regarding esophageal stricture and pain due to the lack of relevant data.

Two observational studies (51, 52) seem to support the overall results from the three RCTs in terms of mortality, serious adverse events, and anastomosis leakage that found no beneficial effect of placing a prophylactic IOCT. Furthermore, observational data from Nquyen et al. (51) suggest that the placement of a prophylactic IOCT may increase the risk of various complications such as an increase in the risk of developing esophageal stricture. These observational studies were assessed by ROBINS-I to be at overall serious (51) and critical risk of bias (52) and should therefore be interpreted with caution. Finally, we identified but excluded for various reasons (see **Table 1**) an additional 4 studies, no of which were in favor of routine ICOT (see **Table 1**).

Strengths and Limitations

This review draws strengths from the strict methodology, including following a protocol registered before the literature search began, systemically assessing for risk of bias, and adhering to all recommendations from the Cochrane Collaboration, including the use of ROBINS-I. The search strategy was developed by an information specialist from the Cochrane Hepato-Biliary Group. Our study also differs from a recent review by Anand et al. (79) on the topic by adding GRADE assessment of the included studies and abstaining from mixing RCTs with observational studies in the meta-analyses. In Anand et al., the meta-analysis included a mix of extrapleural and transpleural repair (51, 52) and an observation study, where some of the participants received IOCTs by a non-prophylactic indication (74). Although the overall conclusions in the present study are fairly similar to the study by Anand et al., inclusion of non-randomized studies with their inherently different study designs in a meta-analysis may severely compromise the validity of their results, as their lack of randomization makes them highly at risk for confounding bias resulting in an imbalance in prognostic factors associated with the outcome (80).

TABLE 2 | Summary of findings, randomized clinical trials.

Use of prophylactic chest tubes vs. control

Population: Neonates with esophageal atresia.
Intervention: Prophylactic chest tube in primary surgical repair.
Comparison: Control (no prophylactic chest tube).

Outcomes	Illustrative comparative risks* (95% CI)		Relative effect (95% CI)	No of participants (No of studies)	Quality of the evidence (GRADE)	Comments
	Assumed risk (controls)	Corresponding risk (chest tube)				
	Study population					
All-cause mortality						
Maximum follow-up	109 per 1,000	182 per 1,000 (83–398)	RR 1.66 (0.76, 3.65)	162 (3)	⊕⊖⊖⊖ **Very low**	OIS 5822 (alpha 5%, beta 20%, RR 0.8 and Pc 10.9%) Downgraded one level due to serious risk of bias and two levels due to very serious imprecision.
Serious adverse events						
Maximum follow-up	250 per 1,000	270 per 1,000 (145–500)	RR 1.08 (0.58, 2.00)	162 (3)	⊕⊖⊖⊖ **Very low**	OIS 2188 (alpha 5%, beta 20%, RR 0.8 and Pc 25%) The adverse events reported were respiratory complications. Downgraded one level due to serious risk of bias and two levels due to very serious imprecision.
Intervention-requiring pneumothorax						
Maximum follow-up	28 per 1,000	47 per 1,000 (8–271)	RR 1.65 (0.28, 9.50)	112 (2)	⊕⊖⊖⊖ **Very low**	OIS 24124 (alpha 5%, beta 20%, RR 0.8 and Pc 25%)
Sepsis or mediastinitis						
Maximum follow-up	NA	NA	RR 3.00 (0.14, 64.26)	16 (1)	⊕⊖⊖⊖ **Very low**	
Anastomosis leakage						
Maximum follow-up	89 per 1,000	148 per 1,000 (56–393)	RR 1.66 (0.63, 4.40)	162 (3)	⊕⊖⊖⊖ **Very low**	OIS 7240 (alpha 5%, beta 20%, RR 0.8 and Pc 8.9%) Downgraded one level due to serious risk of bias and two levels due to very serious imprecision.
Esophageal stricture						
Maximum follow-up	NA	NA				

**The basis for the assumed risk (e.g., the median control group risk across studies) is provided in footnotes. The corresponding risk (and its 95% confidence interval) is based on the assumed risk in the comparison group and the relative effect of the intervention (and its 95% CI).*
CI, Confidence interval; Pc, Proportion in control group with outcome; RR, Risk ratio; NA, Not applicable.
GRADE Working Group grades of evidence.
High quality: Further research is very unlikely to change our confidence in the estimate of effect.
Moderate quality: Further research is likely to have an important impact on our confidence in the estimate of effect and may change the estimate.
Low quality: Further research is very likely to have an important impact on our confidence in the estimate of effect and is likely to change the estimate.
Very low quality: We are very uncertain about the estimate.

We only identified three RCTs, systematically comparing the intervention with an IOCT to no IOCT in 162 neonates undergoing primary repair for esophageal atresia. None of our meta-analyses reached the optimal information size. In addition to evaluate overall improvement in treatment techniques and clinical outcomes, future trials should also assess pain and esophageal stricture as this would be an important outcome for the children and parents. Importantly, the associated malformations and genetic aberrations often found in esophageal atresia and the difference in exact anatomical presentation [with or without fistula(e)] make this a relatively heterogeneous pathology. The patients included in these RCTs all presented with distal tracheoesophageal fistula, but with various details on pre-surgical gap length and on associated malformations; further complicating the comparison between studies and the transferability of the conclusion to other patient subgroups.

Esophageal atresia is a relatively rare condition; particularly considering the numerous subtypes with various possible

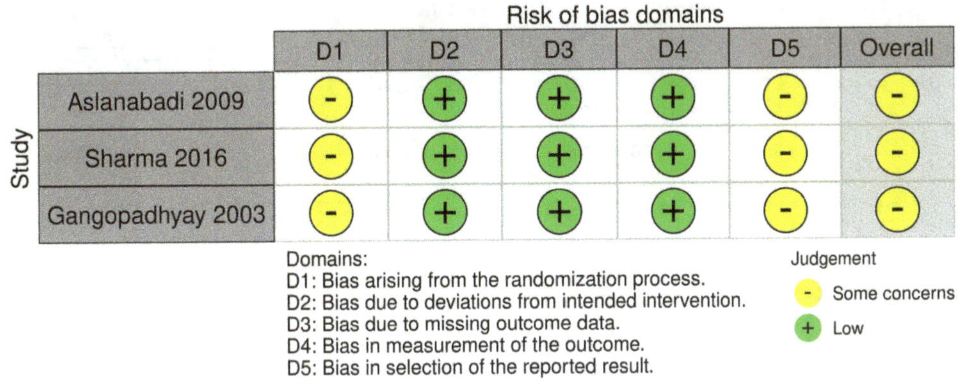

FIGURE 2 | Risk of bias assessment.

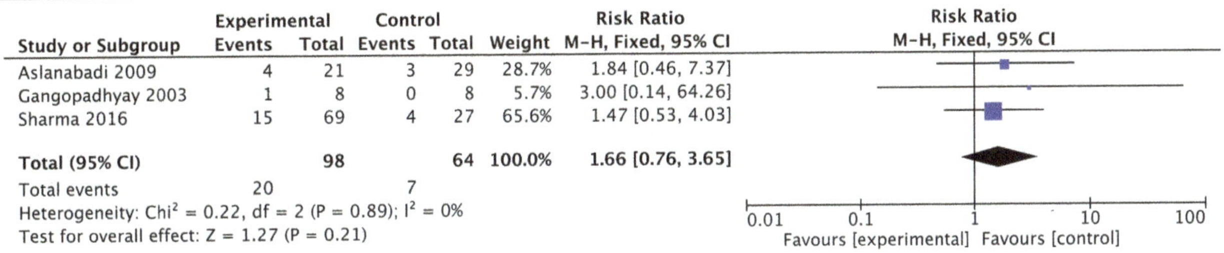

FIGURE 3 | Forest plot for all-cause mortality.

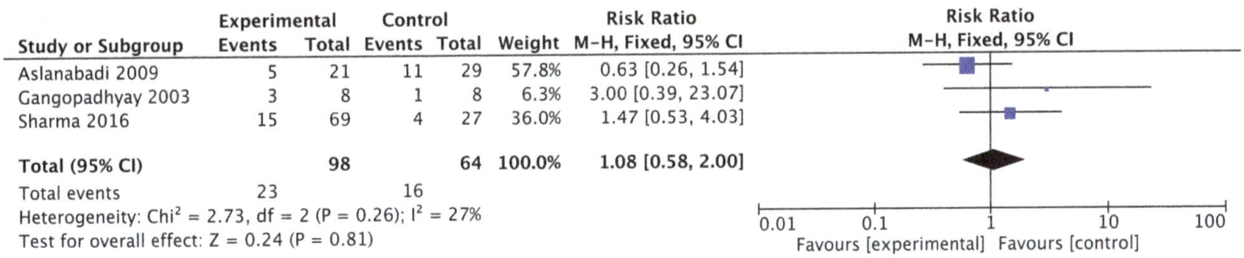

FIGURE 4 | Forest plot for serious adverse events.

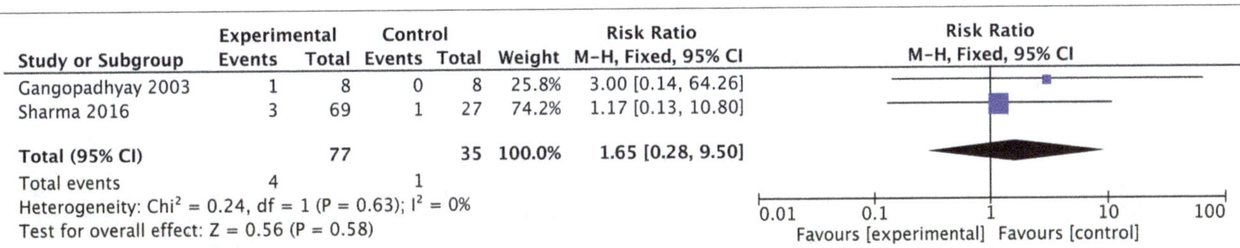

FIGURE 5 | Forest plot for intervention-requiring pneumothorax.

anatomical presentations and associated malformation. Rare diseases pose challenges to methodology when designing RCTs that are adequately powered to draw definitive conclusions, as small patient sample sizes are statistically vulnerable to small deviations in the observed number of outcomes (81). Innovative clinical trial methods minimizing sample size requirements

Study or Subgroup	Experimental Events	Experimental Total	Control Events	Control Total	Weight	Risk Ratio M-H, Fixed, 95% CI
Aslanabadi 2009	2	29	2	21	37.4%	0.72 [0.11, 4.74]
Gangopadhyay 2003	3	8	1	8	16.1%	3.00 [0.39, 23.07]
Sharma 2016	10	69	2	27	46.4%	1.96 [0.46, 8.35]
Total (95% CI)		**106**		**56**	**100.0%**	**1.66 [0.63, 4.40]**
Total events	15		5			

Heterogeneity: $Chi^2 = 1.12$, df = 2 (P = 0.57); $I^2 = 0\%$
Test for overall effect: Z = 1.03 (P = 0.30)

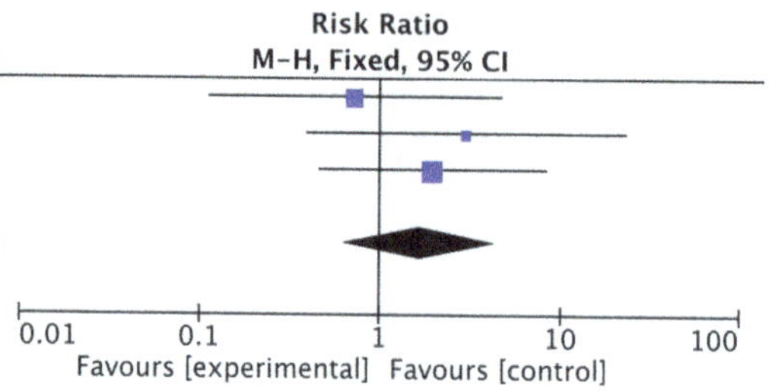

FIGURE 6 | Forest plot for anastomosis leakage.

(82) and optimal research infrastructure (83), possibly through international collaborations, may improve future productivity of robust research in esophageal atresia.

CONCLUSION

We did not identify any studies advocating for the use of prophylactic IOCTs. Based on the limited amount of research on this topic and results from the included studies, we did not find sufficient evidence to support or discontinue the routine use of prophylactic IOCTs for neonates undergoing surgical repair of esophageal atresia, as all confidence intervals were compatible with no effect. Further trials, ideally multicentric, are warranted to explore the effects of the prophylactic IOCT for neonates undergoing surgical repair of esophageal atresia. Importantly, future trials should adhere to SPIRIT guidelines (84).

AUTHOR CONTRIBUTIONS

ML drafted the protocol and review, extracted data, co-ordinated the review, analyzed the data, and revised the review. SK drafted and revised the protocol, extracted data, analyzed the data, interpreted the data, commented on, revised the review, interpreted the data, provided supervision, and provided a methodological and statistical expertise. SH revised and commented on the protocol and review and provided supervision. JO and MF revised and commented on the protocol and review and provided clinical expertise. SP revised and commented on the review. UL-T drafted the protocol, conceived and designed the review, revised the protocol, commented on, revised the review, provided supervision, and clinical expertise. All authors contributed to the article and approved the submitted version.

ACKNOWLEDGMENTS

The review author team would like to acknowledge the information specialist Sarah Klingenberg from the Cochrane Hepato-Biliary Group for the development of our search strategy.

REFERENCES

1. Spitz L. Oesophageal atresia. *Orphanet J Rare Dis.* (2007) 2:24. doi: 10.1186/1750-1172-2-24
2. Zhou Y, Mao X, Zhou H, Qin Z, Wang L, Cai Z et al. Epidemiology of birth defects based on a birth defect surveillance system in Southern Jiangsu, China, 2014–2018. *J Matern Fetal Neonatal Med.* (2020) 35:1–7. doi: 10.3389/fpubh.2020.00378
3. Sfeir R, Michaud L, Sharma D, Richard F, Gottrand F. National esophageal atresia register. *Eur J Pediatr Surg.* (2015) 25:497–9. doi: 10.1055/s-0035-1569466
4. Demikova NS, Vydrych YV, Podolnaya MA, Lapina AS, Asanov AY. Prevalence and descriptive epidemiology of esophageal atresia in the Russian Federation. *Birth Defects Res A Clin Mol Teratol.* (2016) 106:854–9. doi: 10.1002/bdra.23553
5. Lupo PJ, Isenburg JL, Salemi JL, Mai CT, Liberman RF, Canfield MA et al. Population-based birth defects data in the United States, 2010-2014: a focus on gastrointestinal defects. *Birth Defects Res.* (2017) 109:1504–14. doi: 10.1002/bdr2.1145
6. Wittekindt B, Schloesser R, Doberschuetz N, Salzmann-Manrique E, Grossmann J, Misselwitz B et al. Epidemiology and outcome of major congenital malformations in a large German county. *Eur J Pediatr Surg.* (2019) 29:282–9. doi: 10.1055/s-0038-1642630
7. Cassina M, Ruol M, Pertile R, Midrio P, Piffer S, Vicenzi V et al. Prevalence, characteristics, and survival of children with esophageal atresia: a 32-year population-based study including 1,417,724 consecutive newborns. *Birth Defects Res A Clin Mol Teratol.* (2016) 106:542–8. doi: 10.1002/bdra.23493
8. Schmedding A, Wittekindt B, Schloesser R, Hutter M, Rolle U. Outcome of esophageal atresia in Germany. *Dis Esophagus.* (2020) 34:doaa093. doi: 10.1093/dote/doaa093
9. Pedersen RN, Calzolari E, Husby S, Garne E, EUROCAT working group. Oesophageal atresia: prevalence, prenatal diagnosis and associated anomalies in 23 European regions. *Arch Dis Child.* (2012) 97:227–32. doi: 10.1136/archdischild-2011-300597
10. Oddsberg J, Lu Y, Lagergren J. Maternal diabetes and risk of esophageal atresia. *J Pediatr Surg.* (2010) 45:2004–8. doi: 10.1016/j.jpedsurg.2010.06.008
11. Höllwarth ME, Till H. Chapter 44. Esophageal atresi. In: Puri P, editor. *Pediatric Surgery: General Principles and Newborn Surgery.* Berlin; Heidelberg: Springer (2020). p. 661–80.
12. Morini F, Conforti A, Zani A, Sindjic-Antunovic S, Koivusalo A, Friedmacher F, et al. Diagnostic workup of neonates with esophageal atresia: results from the EUPSA esophageal atresia registry. *Front Pediatr.* (2020) 8:489. doi: 10.3389/fped.2020.00489

13. Felix JF, de Jong EM, Torfs CP, de Klein A, Rottier RJ, Tibboel D. Genetic and environmental factors in the etiology of esophageal atresia and/or tracheoesophageal fistula: an overview of the current concepts. *Birth Defects Res A Clin Mol Teratol.* (2009) 85:747–54. doi: 10.1002/bdra.20592
14. Harmon CM, Coran AG. Chapter 69. Congenital anomalies of the esophagus In: Coran AG, editor. *Pediatric Surgery.* 7th ed. Philadelphia, PA: Mosby (2012). p. 893–918. doi: 10.1016/B978-0-323-07255-7.00069-6
15. Källén B, Finnström O, Lindam A, Nilsson E, Nygren K-G, Otterblad PO. Congenital malformations in infants born after *in vitro* fertilization in Sweden. *Birth Defects Res A Clin Mol Teratol.* (2010) 88:137–43. doi: 10.1002/bdra.20645
16. Oddsberg J, Lu Y, Lagergren J. Aspects of esophageal atresia in a population-based setting: incidence, mortality, and cancer risk. *Pediatr Surg Int.* (2012) 28:249–57. doi: 10.1007/s00383-011-3014-1
17. Sfeir R, Michaud L, Salleron J, Gottrand F. Epidemiology of esophageal atresia. *Dis Esophagus.* (2013) 26:354–5. doi: 10.1111/dote.12051
18. Stoll C, Alembik Y, Dott B, Roth M-P. Associated malformations in patients with esophageal atresia. *Eur J Med Genet.* (2009) 52:287–90. doi: 10.1016/j.ejmg.2009.04.004
19. van Heurn LWE, Cheng W, de Vries B, Saing H, Jansen NJG, Kootstra G et al. Anomalies associated with oesophageal atresia in Asians and Europeans. *Pediatr Surg Int.* (2002) 18:241–3. doi: 10.1007/s003830100692
20. Stoll C, Alembik Y, Dott B, Roth M-P. Associated anomalies in cases with esophageal atresia. *Am J Med Genet A.* (2017) 173:2139–57. doi: 10.1002/ajmg.a.38303
21. Brosens E, Ploeg M, van Bever Y, Koopmans AE, IJsselstijn H, Rottier RJ et al. Clinical and etiological heterogeneity in patients with tracheo-esophageal malformations and associated anomalies. *Eur J Med Genet.* (2014) 57:440–52. doi: 10.1016/j.ejmg.2014.05.009
22. Dingemann C, Eaton S, Aksnes G, Bagolan P, Cross KM, De Coppi P et al. ERNICA consensus conference on the management of patients with esophageal atresia and tracheoesophageal fistula: diagnostics, preoperative, operative, and postoperative management. *Eur J Pediatr Surg.* (2020) 30:326–36. doi: 10.1055/s-0039-1693116
23. Choudhury SR, Ashcraft KW, Sharp RJ, Murphy JP, Snyder CL, Sigalet DL. Survival of patients with esophageal atresia: influence of birth weight, cardiac anomaly, and late respiratory complications. *J Pediatr Surg.* (1999) 34:70–3. doi: 10.1016/S0022-3468(99)90231-2
24. Lilja HE, Wester T. Outcome in neonates with esophageal atresia treated over the last 20 years. *Pediatr Surg Int.* (2008) 24:531–6. doi: 10.1007/s00383-008-2122-z
25. Zimmer J, Eaton S, Murchison LE, De Coppi P, Ure BM, Dingemann C. State of play: eight decades of surgery for esophageal atresia. *Eur J Pediatr Surg.* (2019) 29:39–48. doi: 10.1055/s-0038-1668150
26. Sfeir R, Rousseau V, Bonnard A, Gelas T, Aumar M, Panait N, et al. Risk factors of early mortality and morbidity in esophageal atresia with distal tracheoesophageal fistula: a population-based cohort study. *J Pediatr.* (2021) 234:99–105.e1. doi: 10.1016/j.jpeds.2021.02.064
27. Bairdain S, Zurakowski D, Vargas SO, Stenquist N, McDonald M, Towne MC, et al. Long-gap esophageal atresia is a unique entity within the esophageal atresia defect spectrum. *Neonatology.* (2017) 111:140–4. doi: 10.1159/000449241
28. Tan Tanny SP, Comella A, Hutson JM, Omari TI, Teague WJ, King SK. Quality of life assessment in esophageal atresia patients: a systematic review focusing on long-gap esophageal atresia. *J Pediatr Surg.* (2019) 54:2473–8. doi: 10.1016/j.jpedsurg.2019.08.040
29. Tan Tanny SP, Fearon E, Hawley A, Brooks J-A, Comella A, Hutson JM et al. Predictors of mortality after primary discharge from hospital in patients with esophageal atresia. *J Pediatr.* (2020) 219:70–5. doi: 10.1016/j.jpeds.2019.12.031
30. Acher CW, Ostlie DJ, Leys CM, Struckmeyer S, Parker M, Nichol PF. Long-term outcomes of patients with tracheoesophageal fistula/esophageal atresia: survey results from tracheoesophageal fistula/esophageal atresia online communities. *Eur J Pediatr Surg.* (2016) 26:476–80. doi: 10.1055/s-0035-1570103
31. Harmsen WJ, Aarsen FJ. van der Cammen-van Zijp MHM, van Rosmalen JM, Wijnen RMH, Tibboel D, et al. Developmental problems in patients with oesophageal atresia: a longitudinal follow-up study. *Arch Dis Child Fetal Neonatal Ed.* (2017) 102:F214–9. doi: 10.1136/archdischild-2015-309976
32. Nurminen P, Koivusalo A, Hukkinen M, Pakarinen M. Pneumonia after repair of esophageal atresia-incidence and main risk factors. *Eur J Pediatr Surg.* (2019) 29:504–9. doi: 10.1055/s-0038-1675775
33. Rayyan M, Allegaert K, Omari T, Rommel N. Dysphagia in children with esophageal atresia: current diagnostic options. *Eur J Pediatr Surg.* (2015) 25:326–32. doi: 10.1055/s-0035-1559818
34. Allin B, Knight M, Johnson P, Burge D, BAPS-CASS. Outcomes at one-year post anastomosis from a national cohort of infants with oesophageal atresia. *PLoS ONE.* (2014) 9:e106149. doi: 10.1371/journal.pone.0106149
35. Chittmittrapap S, Spitz L, Kiely EM, Brereton RJ. Anastomotic leakage following surgery for esophageal atresia. *J Pediatr Surg.* (1992) 27:29–32. doi: 10.1016/0022-3468(92)90098-R
36. Lal DR, Gadepalli SK, Downard CD, Ostlie DJ, Minneci PC, Swedler RM et al. Challenging surgical dogma in the management of proximal esophageal atresia with distal tracheoesophageal fistula: outcomes from the Midwest Pediatric Surgery Consortium. *J Pediatr Surg.* (2018) 53:1267–72. doi: 10.1016/j.jpedsurg.2017.05.024
37. Upadhyaya VD, Gangopadhyaya AN, Gopal SC, Upadhyaya A, Sharma SP, Gupta DK et al. Is ligation of azygos vein necessary in primary repair of tracheoesophageal fistula with esophageal atresia? *Eur J Pediatr Surg.* (2007) 17:236–40. doi: 10.1055/s-2007-965693
38. Teague WJ, Karpelowsky J. Surgical management of oesophageal atresia. *Paediatr Respir Rev.* (2016) 19:10–5. doi: 10.1016/j.prrv.2016.04.003
39. Spitz L. Esophageal atresia. Lessons I have learned in a 40-year experience. *J Pediatr Surg.* (2006) 41:1635–40. doi: 10.1016/j.jpedsurg.2006.07.004
40. McCallion WA, Hannon RJ, Boston VE. Prophylactic extrapleural chest drainage following repair of esophageal atresia: is it necessary? *J Pediatr Surg.* (1992) 27:561. doi: 10.1016/0022-3468(92)90446-E
41. Friedmacher F, Kroneis B, Huber-Zeyringer A, Schober P, Till H, Sauer H, et al. Postoperative complications and functional outcome after esophageal atresia repair: results from longitudinal single-center follow-up. *J Gastrointest Surg.* (2017) 21:927–35. doi: 10.1007/s11605-017-3423-0
42. Koivusalo AI, Pakarinen MP, Rintala RJ. Modern outcomes of oesophageal atresia: single centre experience over the last twenty years. *J Pediatr Surg.* (2013) 48:297–303. doi: 10.1016/j.jpedsurg.2012.11.007
43. Krishnan U, Mousa H. Dall'Oglio L, Homaira N, Rosen R, Faure C, et al. ESPGHAN-NASPGHAN guidelines for the evaluation and treatment of gastrointestinal and nutritional complications in children with esophageal atresia-tracheoesophageal fistula. *J Pediatr Gastroenterol Nutr.* (2016) 63:550–70. doi: 10.1097/MPG.0000000000001401
44. Gibreel W, Zendejas B, Antiel RM, Fasen G, Moir CR, Zarroug AE. Swallowing dysfunction and quality of life in adults with surgically corrected esophageal atresia/tracheoesophageal fistula as infants: forty years of follow-up. *Ann Surg.* (2017) 266:305–10. doi: 10.1097/SLA.0000000000001978
45. Morini F, Conforti A, Bagolan P. Perioperative complications of esophageal atresia. *Eur J Pediatr Surg.* (2018) 28:133–40. doi: 10.1055/s-0038-1636941
46. Legrand C, Michaud L, Salleron J, Neut D, Sfeir R, Thumerelle C, et al. Long-term outcome of children with oesophageal atresia type III. *Arch Dis Child.* (2012) 97:808–11. doi: 10.1136/archdischild-2012-301730
47. Rozensztrauch A, Smigiel R, Patkowski D. Congenital esophageal atresia-surgical treatment results in the context of quality of life. *Eur J Pediatr Surg.* (2019) 29:266–70. doi: 10.1055/s-0038-1641597
48. Sistonen SJ, Pakarinen MP, Rintala RJ. Long-term results of esophageal atresia: Helsinki experience and review of literature. *Pediatr Surg Int.* (2011) 27:1141–9. doi: 10.1007/s00383-011-2980-7
49. Witt S, Dellenmark-Blom M, Dingemann J, Dingemann C, Ure BM, Gomez B et al. Quality of life in parents of children born with esophageal atresia. *Eur J Pediatr Surg.* (2019) 29:371–7. doi: 10.1055/s-0038-1660867
50. Witt S, Dellenmark-Blom M, Flieder S, Dingemann J, Abrahamsson K, Jönsson L et al. Health-related quality of life experiences in children and adolescents born with esophageal atresia: a Swedish-German focus group study. *Child Care Health Dev.* (2019) 45:79–88. doi: 10.1111/cch.12619
51. Nguyen MVL, Delaplain PT, Lim JC, Golden JM, Gayer CP. The value of prophylactic chest tubes in tracheoesophageal fistula repair. *Pediatr Surg Int.* (2020) 36:687–96. doi: 10.1007/s00383-020-04664-6
52. Gawad N, Wayne C, Bass J, Nasr A. A chest tube may not be needed after surgical repair of esophageal atresia and tracheoesophageal fistula. *Pediatr Surg Int.* (2018) 34:967–70. doi: 10.1007/s00383-018-4307-4

53. Burge DM, Shah K, Spark P, Shenker N, Pierce M, Kurinczuk JJ, et al. Contemporary management and outcomes for infants born with oesophageal atresia. *Br J Surg.* (2013) 100:515–21. doi: 10.1002/bjs.9019
54. Reusens H, Matthyssens L, Vercauteren C, van Renterghem K, Belgian Association of Paediatric Surgery (BELAPS). Multicentre survey on the current surgical management of oesophageal atresia in Belgium and Luxembourg. *J Pediatr Surg.* (2017) 52:239–46. doi: 10.1016/j.jpedsurg.2016.11.010
55. Zani A, Eaton S, Hoellwarth ME, Puri P, Tovar J, Fasching G, et al. International survey on the management of esophageal atresia. *Eur J Pediatr Surg.* (2014) 24:3–8. doi: 10.1055/s-0033-1350058
56. Kwiatt M, Tarbox A, Seamon MJ, Swaroop M, Cipolla J, Allen C, et al. Thoracostomy tubes: A comprehensive review of complications and related topics. *Int J Crit Illn Inj Sci.* (2014) 4:143–55. doi: 10.4103/2229-5151.134182
57. Johnson JF, Wright DR. Chest tube perforation of esophagus following repair of esophageal atresia. *J Pediatr Surg.* (1990) 25:1227–30. doi: 10.1016/0022-3468(90)90511-7
58. Ponsky TA, Rothenberg SS, Tsao K, Ostlie DJ, St Peter SD, Holcomb GW. Thoracoscopy in children: is a chest tube necessary? *J Laparoendosc Adv Surg Tech A.* (2009) 19(Suppl 1):S23–25. doi: 10.1089/lap.2008.0090.supp
59. Lefebvre C, Glanville J, Briscoe S, Littlewood A, Marshall C, Metzendorf M-I, et al. Chapter 4 - Searching for and selecting studies. In: Higgins JPT, Thomas J, Chandler J, Cumpston M, Li T, Page MJ, Welch VA, editors. *Cochrane Handbook for Systematic Reviews of Interventions* Version 6.2 *(updated February 2021).* Cochrane (2021). Available online at: www.training.cochrane.org/handbook (accessed January 10, 2022).
60. Moher D, Liberati A, Tetzlaff J, Altman DG, PRISMA Group. Preferred reporting items for systematic reviews and meta-analyses: the PRISMA statement. *PLoS Med.* (2009) 6:e1000097. doi: 10.1371/journal.pmed.1000097
61. *Link to protocol registred on PROSPERO.* Available online at: https://www.crd.york.ac.uk/prospero/display_record.php?RecordID=257834 (accessed June 28, 2021).
62. Higgins JPT, Savović J, Page MJ, Elbers RG, Sterne JAC. Chapter 8 - Assessing risk of bias in a randomized trial. In: Higgins JPT, Thomas J, Chandler J, Cumpston M, Li T, Page MJ, Welch VA, editors. *Cochrane Handbook for Systematic Reviews of Interventions* version 6.2. Cochrane (2021). Available online at: www.training.cochrane.org/handbook (accessed January 10, 2022).
63. Sterne JA, Hernán MA, Reeves BC, Savović J, Berkman ND, Viswanathan M et al. ROBINS-I: a tool for assessing risk of bias in non-randomised studies of interventions. *BMJ.* (2016) 355:i4919. doi: 10.1136/bmj.i4919
64. Aslanabadi S, Jamshidi M, Tubbs RS, Shoja MM. The role of prophylactic chest drainage in the operative management of esophageal atresia with tracheoesophageal fistula. *Pediatr Surg Int.* (2009) 25:365–8. doi: 10.1007/s00383-009-2345-7
65. Gangopadhyaya A. Is retropleural drainage necessary after definitive repair of esophageal atresia and tracheoesophageal fistula? *J Indian Assoc Pediatr Surg.* (2003) 8:86–90.
66. Sharma S, Pathak S, Husain A, Pandey DC, Kunwer R, Chaturvedi J. Retropleural drainage: yes or no in primary repair of esophageal atresia with tracheoesophageal fistula. *Int J Contemp Med Res.* (2016) 3:3.
67. Brohi AR, Syal AA, Mengal N. Oesophageal atresia - Experience of 7 years with data evaluation. *Med Forum Monthly.* (2011) 22:3–7.
68. Castilloux J, Noble AJ, Faure C. Risk factors for short- and long-term morbidity in children with esophageal atresia. *J Pediatr.* (2010) 156:755–60. doi: 10.1016/j.jpeds.2009.11.038
69. Donoso F, Kassa A-M, Gustafson E, Meurling S, Lilja HE. Outcome and management in infants with esophageal atresia - a single centre observational study. *J Pediatr Surg.* (2016) 51:1421–5. doi: 10.1016/j.jpedsurg.2016.03.010
70. Esteves E, Pessoa C, Paguada-Ruiz LK, Castro KC. Thoracoscopic management of esophageal atresia and its related complications: lessons after the first 106 cases. In: *Proceedings of the 28th Annual Congress for Endosurgery in Children.* Santiago (2019). doi: 10.1089/lap.2019.29028.abstracts
71. Fasting H, Winther LK. Oesophageal atresia and tracheo-oesophageal fistula. Early and late results in 86 patients. *Scand J Thorac Cardiovasc Surg.* (1978) 12:147–51. doi: 10.3109/14017437809100366
72. Grebe S, Schnapka J, Menardi G. Esophageal atresia - analysis of the postoperative morbidity in 61 cases. *Zentralbl Chir.* (1999) 8:144–6.
73. Kay S, Shaw K. Revisiting the role of routine retropleural drainage after repair of esophageal atresia with distal tracheoesophageal fistula. *J Pediatr Surg.* (1999) 34:1082–5. doi: 10.1016/S0022-3468(99)90571-7
74. Paramalingam S, Burge DM, Stanton MP. Operative intercostal chest drain is not required following extrapleural or transpleural esophageal atresia repair. *Eur J Pediatr Surg.* (2013) 23:273–5. doi: 10.1055/s-0032-1330845
75. Vazquez AG, Novillo IC, Diaz ML, Sanchez RT, Carretero SF, Zegarra CM, et al. Technical modifications in thoracoscopic repair of esophageal atresia. Our experience. *J Laparoendosc Adv Surg Tech.* (2011) 21:A76. doi: 10.1089/lap.2011.9999
76. Vercauteren C, Reusens H, De Backer A, Tambucci R, Van Cauwenberge S, Leyman P, et al. Oesophageal atresia: a multicenter retrospective study on surgical treatment and 1-year follow-up. *ISDE.* (2019) 32(Supplement 1):30. doi: 10.1093/dote/doz047.92
77. Zhang J, Wu Q, Chen L, Wang Y, Cui X, Huang W, et al. Clinical analysis of surgery for type III esophageal atresia via thoracoscopy: a study of a Chinese single-center experience. *J Cardiothorac Surg.* (2020) 15:55. doi: 10.1186/s13019-020-01097-z
78. Zhang M, Lin Y, Xie W, Yu J, Huang Q, Li J, et al. The multidisciplinary management of recurrent tracheoesophageal fistula after esophageal atresia: Experience with 135 cases from a tertiary center. *J Pediatr Surg.* (2021) 56:1918–25. doi: 10.1016/j.jpedsurg.2020.12.019
79. Anand S, Singh A, Krishnan N, Yadav DK. Whether prophylactic intraoperative chest drain insertion in esophageal atresia-tracheoesophageal fistula is an evidence-based practice or just a prejudice: a systematic review and meta-analysis. *J Pediatr Surg.* (2021). doi: 10.1016/j.jpedsurg.2021.06.015. [Epub ahead of print].
80. Higgins JPT, Thomas J, Chandler J, Cumpston M, Li T, Page MJ, editors. *Cochrane Handbook for Systematic Reviews of Interventions version 6.2.* Cochrane (2021). Available online at: www.training.cochrane.org/handbook (accessed January 10, 2022).
81. Mitani AA, Haneuse S. Small data challenges of studying rare diseases. *JAMA Netw Open.* (2020) 3:e201965. doi: 10.1001/jamanetworkopen.2020.1965
82. Gagne JJ, Thompson L, O'Keefe K, Kesselheim AS. Innovative research methods for studying treatments for rare diseases: methodological review. *BMJ.* (2014) 349:g6802. doi: 10.1136/bmj.g6802
83. Whicher D, Philbin S, Aronson N. An overview of the impact of rare disease characteristics on research methodology. *Orphanet J Rare Dis.* (2018) 13:14. doi: 10.1186/s13023-017-0755-5
84. Chan A-W, Tetzlaff JM, Altman DG, Laupacis A, Gøtzsche PC, Krleža-Jerić K et al. SPIRIT 2013 statement: defining standard protocol items for clinical trials. *Ann Intern Med.* (2013) 158:200–7. doi: 10.7326/0003-4819-158-3-201302050-00583

APPENDIX 1

Search Strategies (search performed 3rd of December 2021)
Cochrane Central Register of Controlled Trials [*via* Ovid Evidence-Based Medicine Reviews Database (EBMR)]

#1	MeSH descriptor: [Esophageal Atresia] explode all trees
#2	MeSH descriptor: [Esophagus] explode all trees
#3	(esophag∗ or oesophag∗)
#4	(artresia∗ or atretic∗)
#5	#1 or [(#2 or #3) and #4]
#6	MeSH descriptor: [Chest Tubes] explode all trees
#7	(chest tube∗ or catheter∗ or drain∗ or intubat∗ or artificial respirat∗ or suction∗ or IOCT∗)
#8	#6 or #7
#9	#5 and #8

MEDLINE Ovid

1.	exp Esophageal Atresia/
2.	exp Esophagus/
3.	(esophag∗ or oesophag∗).tw,kw.
4.	(artresia∗ or atretic∗).tw,kw.
5.	1 or [(2 or 3) and 4]
6.	exp Chest Tubes/
7.	(chest tube∗ or catheter∗ or drain∗ or intubat∗ or artificial respirat∗ or suction∗ or IOCT∗).mp. [mp=title, abstract, original title, name of substance word, subject heading word, floating sub-heading word, keyword heading word, organism supplementary concept word, protocol supplementary concept word, rare disease supplementary concept word, unique identifier, synonyms]
8.	6 or 7
9.	5 and 8

Embase Ovid

1.	exp esophagus atresia/
2.	exp esophagus/
3.	(esophag∗ or oesophag∗).tw,kw.
4.	(artresia∗ or atretic∗).tw,kw.
5.	1 or [(2 or 3) and 4]
6.	exp chest tube/
7.	(chest tube∗ or catheter∗ or drain∗ or intubat∗ or artificial respirat∗ or suction∗ or IOCT∗).mp. [mp=title, abstract, heading word, drug trade name, original title, device manufacturer, drug manufacturer, device trade name, keyword, floating subheading word, candidate term word]
8.	6 or 7
9.	5 and 8

CINAHL

S9	S5 AND S8
S8	S6 OR S7
S7	TX (chest tube∗ or catheter∗ or drain∗ or intubat∗ or artificial respirat∗ or suction∗ or IOCT∗)
S6	MH chest tubes
S5	S1 or [(S2 or S3) and S4]
S4	TX (artresia∗ or atretic∗)
S3	TX (esophag∗ or oesophag∗)
S2	MH Esophagus
S1	MH Esophageal Atresia

Science Citation Index Expanded and Conference Proceedings Citation Index – (Web of Science)

#3	#2 AND #1
#2	TS = (chest tube∗ or catheter∗ or drain∗ or intubat∗ or artificial respirat∗ or suction∗ or IOCT∗)
#1	TS = [(esophag∗ or oesophag∗) and (artresia∗ or atretic∗)]

22

The Robot-Assisted Extravesical Anti-Reflux Surgery: How we Overcame the Learning Curve?

*Ravindra Sahadev, Katelyn Spencer, Arun K. Srinivasan, Christopher J. Long and Aseem Ravindra Shukla**

Division of Pediatric Urology, Children's Hospital of Philadelphia, Philadelphia, PA, United States

Correspondence:
Aseem Ravindra Shukla
shuklaa@email.chop.edu

Management of vesicoureteral reflux (VUR) has evolved over the past several decades, with a trend toward a decrease in surgical management. In spite of this, ureteral reimplantation remains a commonly performed procedure by pediatric urologists in selected cases. Although the basic tenets of the ureteral reimplant procedure remain the same, the extra- vs. intravesical approach, and the traditional open vs. minimally invasive approach remain the primary options to correct reflux. Considering the advantages conferred by the robotic surgery platform, many leading centers have preferentially adopted robot-assisted laparoscopic extravesical anti-reflux surgery, or in common surgical parlance, the robot-assisted laparoscopic ureteral reimplantation (RALUR), over pure laparoscopic or open approaches. Predicated on our experience of performing over 170 cases of RALUR, we have made technical modifications which we posit reduce the morbidity of the procedure while offering acceptable outcomes. This review highlights the evolution and establishment of RALUR as a standardization of care in the surgical management of VUR at our institution. In particular, we emphasize the technical nuances and specific challenges encountered through the learning curve in hopes of facilitating this process for others.

Keywords: robotic, ureteral reimplantation, RALUR, learning curve, extravesical approach

INTRODUCTION

Over the past two decades, both the evaluation and therapeutic interventions for vesicoureteral reflux (VUR) have undergone extensive evolutions, with a clear trend toward non-operative management and a focus on voiding dysfunction as the major risk factor for urinary tract infection (UTI) (1–3).

In spite of significant investigations aimed at identifying risk factors for the development of recurrent urinary tract infections and predicting the potential for VUR resolution and/or the development of renal scarring, our ability to do so remains limited. Still, when conservative management fails, and febrile UTIs or significant renal scarring occurs, children do require surgical management.

The surgical principles for the correction of VUR remain consistent, several years after its initial description (4). In order to prevent VUR the length of the anti-refluxing tunnel is extended, traditionally in a 5:1 ratio of tunnel length to width of the ureter. While the open ureteral reimplant has been the traditional gold standard repair for VUR, the minimally invasive approaches, such as sub-ureteral injections or laparoscopic and robotic assisted laparoscopic ureteral reimplant (RALUR), have been established as viable alternatives (3).

Although initial enthusiasm for RALUR has waned for some due to concerns about a steep learning curve which can potentially increase the risk of patient morbidity or persistent VUR (5, 6), the well-established benefits of the robotic approach encourage its use (7, 8). Benefits of the robotic vs. the open approach include an improved field of vision via magnification intraperitoneal visualization of the ureters and bladder, improved cosmesis for the patient, and a more rapid recovery in the immediate postoperative period due to an extravesical approach. In our experience several technical modifications mitigate the aforementioned risk of RALUR while maximizing patient outcomes.

In this review, we seek to explore the evolution of extravesical RALUR–as it is the most widely adapted robotic approach–and describe technical modifications that render this procedure reproducible across surgeons and lessen the learning curve trajectory.

EVOLUTION OF RALUR

Since its first description by Peters (9), the technical aspects of the RALUR have undergone several modifications. Along with the initial descriptions of robotic assisted pediatric urologic procedures, Peters highlighted the advantages of the robotic system, the need for evolution and evaluation (9). The surgical principles illustrated for both the robotic-assisted intravesical (RAIVUR) and extravesical techniques were adapted to the new platform while adhering to the principles of contemporary open surgical procedures. The intravesical techniques were favored in bilateral cases due the concerns of urinary retention with bilateral extravesical reimplantation (9).

Since then, while the RAIVUR confers advantages of decreased hematuria and bladder spasms compared to the open approach, it failed to gain widespread adaptation, largely due to technical challenges such as insufflation leaks through the larger trocar hiatus and limited working space of a small bladder (10, 11). Only three groups have reported their experience with RAIVUR, with modest success rates (83, 92, and 100% reflux resolution in 6, 19, and 3 patients, respectively) and highly variable complication rates (17, 52, and 0%) (10–12).

Meanwhile, the Lich-Gregoir technique has become popular for the robotic approach due to its ready adaptability to the technology. This trans-abdominal approach provides excellent visualization of the retrovesical space, particularly when compared to the open approach. The magnification of the robotic camera facilitates meticulous detrusor dissection, which combined with judicious use of energy devices limits the potential for collateral damage to the nerve bundles of the bladder (13).

As with other minimally invasive approaches, RALUR confers the significant benefits of minimally invasive surgery including a shorter convalescence, reduced hospital stay, and improved cosmesis. The realization of the potential improved experience for patients has led to more widespread acceptance for utilization of RALUR. This had led to more centers having a higher number of RALUR over open ureteral reimplants, including ours, and this is reflected in publication trends as well (**Figure 1**).

A negative postoperative voiding cystourethrogram (VCUG) remains the gold standard to declare surgical success after a ureteral reimplantation. But, traditionally high success rates of the open approach obviated a post-operative VCUG in practice. Similarly, with accumulating experience with the RALUR, and pilot studies have demonstrated that our technique delivers reliable VCUG proven success (14). Our institution now defines surgical success as a lack of postoperative febrile UTI and a negative VCUG, if obtained in the postoperative period (15). Potential short term complications reported after RALUR include minor self-limiting adverse events such as bladder spasms, hematuria, and GI disturbances. Other reported complications include urinary extravasation, UTIs, incisional hernia, ureteral obstruction resulting in anuria, and the rare complication of ureteral strictures.

Early reports for RALUR are typical for most new techniques: they are comprised of single institution experiences with small patient numbers. To compound this, there is a lack of uniformity in data reporting, including the age at the time of repair, the indication for ureteral reimplantation (VUR vs. obstruction), and the degree of reflux at the time of surgery. Bladder and bowel dysfunction has proven to be a significant risk factor for surgical failure yet remains under reported in the literature (16). Overview of the literature review (**Table 1**) suggests, in the first decade of utilization of RALUR, there were inconsistencies in reported success (66.7–100%) and complication (0–100%) rates (7–9, 11–15, 17–28). It is notable that higher Clavien grade complications occurred in reports following smaller patient cohorts. However, recent growing evidence in literature has been relatively consistent in proving the safety and efficacy of RALUR in prospective multi-institutional collaborative efforts (7, 8).

THE LEARNING CURVE

The learning curve refers to variations in the productivity of a new surgical procedure or surgeon over a specific time period that leads to achieving a consistent level of expertise to meet contemporary standards. Defining a learning curve is a challenging concept. Although some authors claim that proxies such as operative time, complication rates, and functional outcomes are inadequate measures to assess a true learning curve, most reports have defaulted to these as practical measures of surgical success (28, 29).

As outlined above, the heterogeneity of the published literature on RALUR on key variables such as patient demographics, grades of reflux, comorbidities, in addition to variable study catchment periods makes assessment of a true learning curve difficult.

In order to trace the influence of a learning curve to surgical parameters and outcomes for RALUR at our institution, we have compared the failure rates (need for secondary anti-reflux surgery), radiographic reflux resolution rate, operative time,

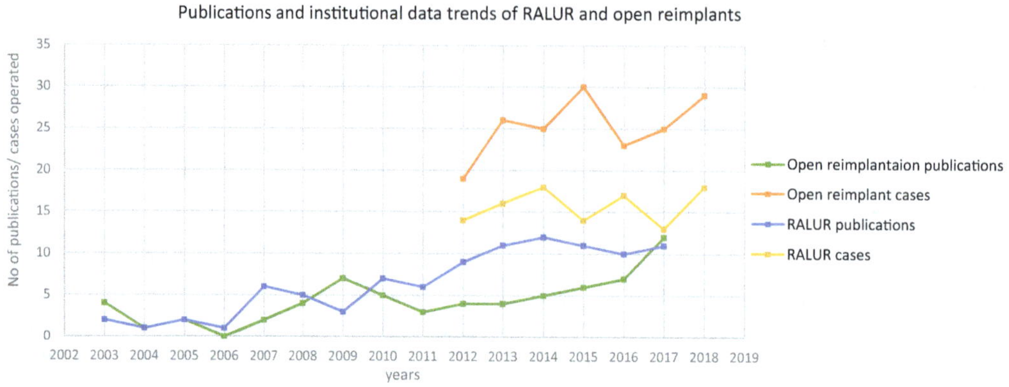

FIGURE 1 | Trends in publications and number of RALURs performed at our institute. Source: PubMed search report of terms "Open ureteral reimplantation" and "Robot-assisted ureteral reimplantation" as on 23 July 2018.

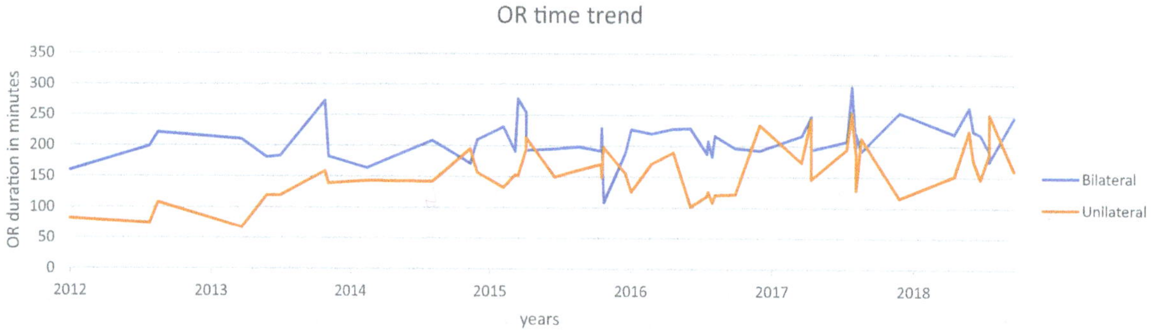

FIGURE 2 | Institutional- OR time trends over 2012 to 2018.

and/or complication rates over defined time frames (yearly trends) for a series of consecutive cases (**Table 2**). We feel as though a single institution center with a relatively high surgical volume as well as 5 different surgeons provides a unique opportunity to carry out this analysis.

A review of data from a prospectively maintained database from 2012 till October 2018, includes six surgeons performing RALUR on 170 patients, of which 60 were bilateral. One hundred twenty-seven were female patients. In our series, the average age at surgery was 5.9 years with a general trend toward higher age at surgery each year, contrary to the literature on national data (3). A Majority of RALUR were done for dilating VUR (Grade 3 or higher) with breakthrough UTIs or renal scarring (100 cases), 36 cases had a duplex anomaly, 23 obstructive megaureter and 10 bladder diverticula. Additionally, 18 cases had a prior history of failed sub-ureteric injection. Among VUR cases, 40% had high grade VUR (IV and V). The operative time varied depending on the number of ureters, need for cystoscopy, retrograde pyelography, placement of a suprapubic tube, and other concomitant procedures depending on the associated pathology (nephrectomy, heminephrectomy, etc.). For unilateral procedures without any concomitant procedure the mean operative time was 161 min (49 cases), and it was 208 min for bilateral cases (48 cases). Operative time includes time of first incision or procedure start, to procedure end time as recorded by the nursing staff. The operative time did not vary significantly between the first and last quarters of consecutive case series (**Figure 2**). Blood loss was minimal in most of the cases from the beginning.

Over the follow up period of 1 to 75 months (mean 23, median 20 months), six cases had transient urinary retention and four cases needed surgery for port site hernia (we now meticulously close fascia even for 5 mm port sites under direct vision). Four cases of ureteral obstruction were noted based on increased dilation of calyces on renal ultrasound with symptoms of flank pain with nausea; of which three cases resolved with cystoscopy and ureteral stenting for 6 weeks and, in another case, required open ureteral reimplantation. We previously reported our surgical outcomes on an initial cohort and found that postoperative febrile UTIs occurred in 15.8% of unilateral cases compared with 20% of bilateral cases ($p = 0.61$) (15). Surgical failure, denoted by postoperative febrile UTI and a positive VCUG was noted in five (8.7%) of the unilateral cases vs. three (8.6%) of the bilateral RALUR cases ($p = 0.98$). The updated demographic and clinical information is summarized in **Table 2**.

Although the intraoperative surgical time has remained consistent over the years, we note that the number and complexity of complications are decreasing over subsequent

TABLE 1 | A literature review of RALUR-EV.

References	Study year†	Baseline			Outcomes			
		No of patients	No of Ureters	OR time in min	Success rate#	Complications %*		
						Clavien grade 1	Clavien grade 2	Clavien grade 3
Peters (9)	2004	24	27	165	88		11	5
Chan et al. (12)	2005–2008	3	4	210	66.7	33	0	0
Boysen et al. (7)	2005–2014	260	363	177	87.9	5	1.9	2.7
Casale et al. (13)	2006–2007	41	82	139.8	97.6	0	4.87	0
Smith et al. (17)	2006–2009	25	33	185	95.6	16	0	4
Akhavan et al. (18)	2006–2013	50	78	–	92.3	4	14	4
Chalmers et al. (19)	2007–2010	16	22	152	90.9	0	0	0
Marchini et al. (11) (EV)	2007–2010	20	27	233.5	100	10	10	0
Schomburg et al. (14)	2008–2010	20	25	196	100	0	0	10
Gundeti et al. (20)	2008–2015	58	83	–	82	1.7	0	0
Silay et al. (21)	2008–2015	72	91	–	97.9	2.7	0	0
Katsturi et al. (22)	2009–2011	150	300	–	99.3	0	0.7	0
Dangle et al. (23)	2010–2013	29	40	–	80	–	–	–
Grimsby et al. (24)	2010–2013	61	93	–	72	1.6	1.6	8.2
Srinivasan et al. (15)	2012–2016	92	–	164	91.3	4.3	17	2.1
Hayashi et al. (25)	2013	9	15	268.78	93.3	100	0	0
Arlen et al. (26)	2013–2014	17	20	169.3	94.1	0	11.76	0
Herz et al. (27)	2013–2015	54	72	–	85.2	5.5	9.8	11
Boysen et al. (8)	2015–2017	143	199	194	93.8	4.9	0.7	5.6

† Approximate period.
 # Clinical or radiological success rates.
**Some reports did not report complications as per Clavien-Dindo grading directly; The reports were graded based on the description. Some authors included UTIs in the complications. There were no Grade-4 complications related to surgery reported in any of the studies. In many series, same patients have had complications of different grades, hence they cannot be summated.*

TABLE 2 | Summary of institutional RALUR data: patient characteristics and operative outcomes.

Year	No of pts.	Age in yrs.	No of renal units	VUR- I, II, III, IV, V, OMs	OR time in min	Need for subsequent anti-reflux surgery	Complications-Grade- 1, 2, 3,4	Mean follow up (months)
2012	15	4.53	18	0,3,3,7,1,1	132	1	3,1,1,0	23.36
2013	34	5.39	41	0,5,12,7,2,8	174	0	2,1,3,0	32.76
2014	25	5.18	30	3,2,9,5,3,3	165	1	0,1,1,0	33.43
2015	29	5.31	43	0,3,10,11,2,3	194	3	1,1,3,0	25.99
2016	24	7.62	38	0,4,8,7,2,3	206	0	1,0,1,0	20.35
2017	22	6.25	31	0,3,9,3,2,5	203	0	0,0,0,0	11.75
2018#	21	5.52	29	0,4,6,4,4,3	197	0	1,0,0,0	3.57

OM-Obstructive megaureter. # till October 2018.

years, concomitant to a reduced need for secondary interventions. Indeed, these results encouraged increasing use of RALUR at our institution with the increase in expertise and confidence level. Backed by comparable outcomes there has been an increase in the proportion of RALUR cases as compared to open ureteral reimplants (**Figure 1**). We expect, also, that being an academic teaching institute with many surgeons and trainees, inherent variations in the proficiency levels with atypical learning curve patterns would affect continued improvement in specific parameters.

TECHNICAL MODIFICATIONS TO ACHIEVE A SUCCESSFUL RALUR

Based on our experiences with RALUR, in addition to standard steps (**Table 3**), we have adopted several key technical modifications that we believe have improved our institutional outcomes (**Table 4**). Proper case selection is vital and must consider patient age, toilet training status, and the presence or absence of dysfunctional elimination. If there is a concern for secondary reflux due to a neurogenic bladder, this must be worked up prior to intervention. If significant bowel and/or bladder dysfunction persists in spite of adequate therapy, a suprapubic tube should be considered in order to ensure proper, low-pressure post-operative voiding prior to removing within a week.

In order to avoid collateral damage to the detrusor muscle and the nerve plexus, meticulous dissection and judicious use of electrocautery is vital (**Figure 3B**). We recommend that estimating tunnel length is inaccurate–and overestimated–when the bladder is even slightly distended, hence we now delineate the tunnel length–ensuring a measurement of tunnel length five times the diameter of the distal ureter–while the bladder is completely drained with a foley catheter (**Figure 3C**). We regularly utilize a hitch stitch not only to aid detrusor dissection but also to mark the direction of proposed tunnel (**Figure 3D**). We use only the tip of the hook to cauterize the identified bleeding spots and spread the muscles bluntly, rather than cutting those layers (**Figure 4B**).

Once the tunnel length of the detrusor is delineated, we begin dissecting the tunnel midway between the hitch stitch and ureterovesical junction until the bladder mucosal layer is defined (**Figure 4A**). Utilizing this window, we find that further progression proximally and distally proceeds more easily without the risk of inadvertent cystotomies (**Figure 4C**). We avoid medial and inferior dissection close to the VUJ, which poses damage to the nerve plexus and may increase the risk of detrusor injury and urinary retention. The ureters must be adequately mobilized in a cephalad direction in order to remove any proximal tension that may tease the ureter out of the tunnel.

Once the detrusorrhaphy begins, we prefer interrupted suturing with long term absorbable sutures (5–0 polydiaxone) in a "bottom up" approach, starting from uretero-vesical junction and then moving distally toward the hitch stitch (dome), as it allows for a tailored formation of the tunnel depending on the available ureter length and amount of tension. This technique can be confusing for the beginner and requires careful passing of suture underneath the ureter and back toward the initial bite

TABLE 3 | Standard steps of RALUR.

- Preoperative cystoscopy and retrograde pyelogram, if there is a suspicion of ectopic ureter, duplex systems, solitary system
- Patient position: Supine (younger patients) or modified lithotomy; Attention to pressure points and careful strapping to prevent shifting when patient put into lithotomy position.
- Port placement: 8.5 mm camera port at the umbilicus, 5 mm working instruments in midclavicular line on either side, or utilizing lower incisions with cephalad tunneling of the trocar.
- Cephalad ureteral mobilization to release tension
- Tunnel measurement and marking to achieve a 5:1 ratio
- Mild hydrodistension, hitch placement
- Detrusor tunnel creation
- Detrusorrhaphy-suturing
- Closure

TABLE 4 | Challenges and cautions/modifications.

Outcomes of concerns	Possible technical reasons	Modifications adopted
Urinary retention	Damage to nerve plexus	Precise dissection at VUJ between ureter and bladder, avoiding medial and caudal detrusor dissection (**Figure 4C**)
		Judicious use of electrocautery
Incomplete reflux resolution	Inadequate tunnel length	Standardized measurement of the tunnel length in the collapsed bladder (**Figure 3C**)
	Cephalad slippage of the ureter out of the tunnel	Including the ureter adventitia in the first few and last tunnel closure suture ("advancement stitches").
		Proximal ureteral mobilization to release tension on tunnel closure
	Incomplete detrusor separation for the tunnel creation	Use of hitch stitch for adequate traction and bladder distension to facilitate dissection (**Figure 3D**)
Ureteral obstruction	Ureteral injury	Avoiding pre-stenting unless absolutely necessary (e.g., Duplex system), avoiding excessive traction and direct cautery usage on the ureter
	Excessive ureteral mobilization	Ureteral mobilization to the required length with frequent assessments
	Tight tunnel	"Bottom-up" approach starting at the UVJ with careful and stepwise closure of tunnel, raising adequate detrusor flaps to have a spacious tunnel
	Acute angulation of the ureter	Studying the course of the ureter and its angulation prior to hitch stitch and marking the corresponding tunnel line (**Figure 3C**)
Urinary leak	Cystotomy	Careful identification and repair prior to closure of detrussorotomy
	Leak from ureteral suture-line	Maximize urinary drainage with bladder catheter and/or suprapubic tube, and place ureteral stent if necessary.
	Refluxing stumps in cases of ectopic ureteral insertion	Adequate exposure, resection of residual, and closure of the stump.
Multiple post site scars	Multiple port site scars	HidES (Hidden incision for endoscopic surgery) groin ports, hide umbilical camera port within umbilical crease; only two working 5 mm ports; no assist port.
Injury to vas and vessels	Poor field of vision	Preservation of uterine vessels; Under-vision dissection distal to the vas deferens. Starting the distal ureteral dissection with good hemostasis to maintain optimum visibility (**Figure 3A**).

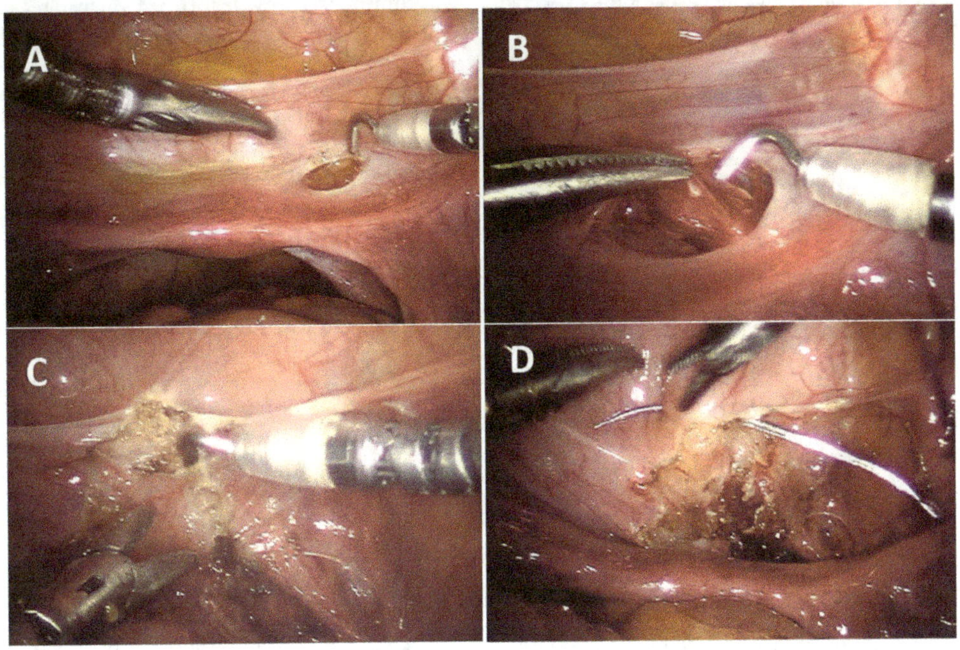

FIGURE 3 | Operative steps of RALUR. **(A)** Small window created in the broad ligament to access the ureter directly. **(B)** Ureteral mobilization: gentle handling by grasping only the ureteral adventitia. **(C)** Marking the detrusor tunnel in a collapsed bladder in line with the ureter. **(D)** Hitch stitch at the distal end of tunnel marking.

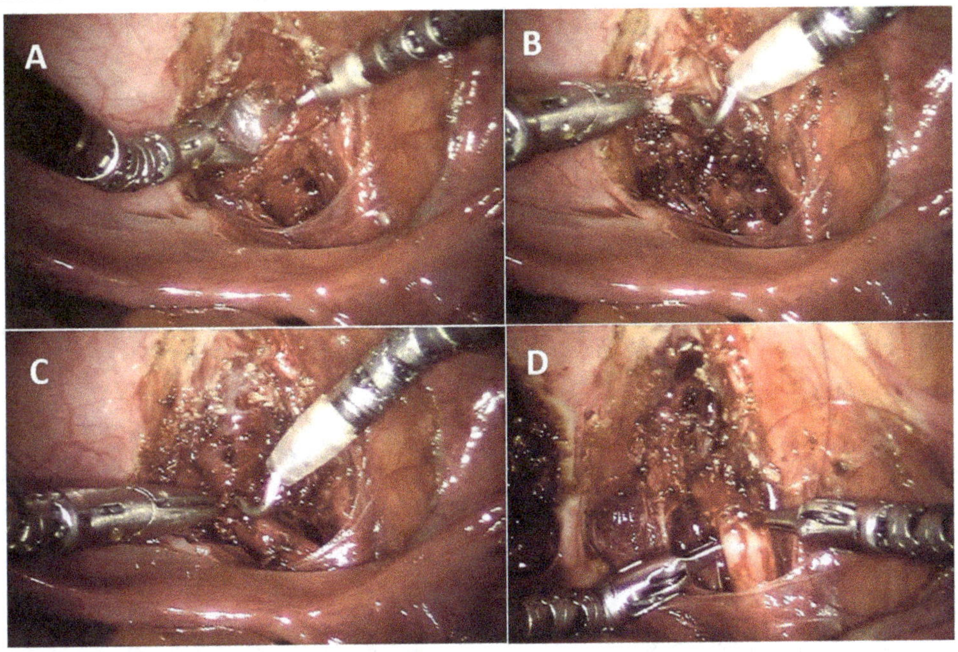

FIGURE 4 | Operative steps of RALUR. **(A)** Making a detrusor window till bluish bladder mucosa is delineated. **(B)** Detrusor muscle separated with direct pinpoint electrocautery tip combined with blunt spreading of the muscle fibers. **(C)** Detrusor tunnel opened proximally to ureterovesical junction. **(D)** Passing suture underneath the ureter to advance the ureter into the detrusor trough (left to right).

side (**Figure 4D**) to allow placement of the ureter deep in the tunnel with close approximation of the detrusor edges. It is important to include ureteral adventitia in the initial and ending detrusor closure stitch. In cases of dismembered reimplants, solitary kidney, tapered or complex reimplants we prefer to leave a double J stent, but we do not stent typical RALUR cases. We also do not routinely place a drain. We leave a urinary catheter overnight and discharge the patient once they are able to void, leaving residuals that are <25% of the expected bladder capacity.

Table 4 summarizes the common pitfalls and technical modification adopted to address those concerns.

CHALLENGES

In their recent review, Baek et al. analyzes the reasons for slower adoption of RALUR in comparison to the widespread and quickly adopted robotic prostatectomy among adult counterparts. The steeper learning curve and concerns about the efficacy compared to open reimplants were oft-cited reasons, and the authors suggested that the procedure be deferred to a later point in the robotic experience (30). However, from our learning curve experience, we deduce that careful adherence to outlined steps allows the RALUR to be safely and reproducibly performed. Standardization of salient steps with adequate training and judicious use of electrocautery will ensure the avoidance of common pitfalls.

Although there are debates regarding the efficacy of the RALUR in comparison to open ureteral reimplantation, we must be cautious while comparing the historical reports to the contemporary outcomes as the population characteristics (age group, voiding dysfunction, etc.) have been changing. Eventually, the trends suggest RALUR inexorably will be adopted more widely, and reports and ongoing multi-institutional consortiums will continue to provide further evidence regarding its safety and affirming its efficacy.

CONCLUSIONS

RALUR utilization has increased since its inception, but concerns over the procedure's technical difficulty, safety, risk of urinary retention and outcomes has limited its widespread use. Herein, we demonstrate that the learning curve of RALUR can be shortened with specific modifications predicated on experience, and that with technical adaptations, clinically significant improvements in surgical outcomes may be expected. In appropriately selected patients and with adequate preparation, we posit that the RALUR is a safe and effective technique that confers the well-described advantages of minimally invasive surgery to the treatment of VUR.

AUTHOR CONTRIBUTIONS

ARS conceived the idea, laid the platform for the review with substantial additions to the manuscript, along with proofreading. RS prepared the initial manuscript and collected the raw data. KS prepared the literature review and part of data abstraction. CL and AKS reviewed the manuscript and made significant corrections.

REFERENCES

1. Routh JC, Bogaert GA, Kaefer M, Manzoni G, Park JM, Retik AB, et al. Vesicoureteral reflux: current trends in diagnosis, screening, and treatment. *Eur Urol.* (2012) 61:773e82. doi: 10.1016/j.eururo.2012.01.002
2. Qureshi AH, Ajayi O, Schwaderer AL, Hains DS. Decreased Identification of vesicoureteral reflux: a cautionary tale. *Front Pediatr.* (2017) 5:175. doi: 10.3389/fped.2017.00175
3. Kurtz MP, Leow JJ, Varda BK, Logvinenko T, McQuaid JW, Yu RN, et al. The decline of the open ureteral reimplant in the United States: National data from 2003 to 2013. *Urology.* (2017) 100:193–7. doi: 10.1016/j.urology.2016.07.024
4. Paquin AJ. Ureterovesical anastomosis: the description and evaluation of a technique. *J Urol.* (1959) 82:573–83. doi: 10.1016/S0022-5347(17)65934-2
5. Cannon GM, Ost MC. Robot-assisted laparoscopic extravesical ureteral reimplantation for primary vesicoureteral reflux in children *J Urol.* (2017) 197:1379–81. doi: 10.1016/j.juro.2017.03.112
6. Gargollo PC. Editorial comment regarding: Prospective multicenter study on robot-assisted laparoscopic extravesical ureteral reimplantation (RALUR-EV): outcomes and complications. *J Ped Urol.* (2018) 14:263–4. doi: 10.1016/j.jpurol.2018.02.018
7. Boysen W, Ellison JS, Kim C, Koh CJ, Noh P, Whittam B, et al. Multi-institutional review of outcomes and complications of robot-assisted laparoscopic extravesical ureteral reimplantation for treatment of primary vesicoureteral reflux in children. *J Urol.* (2017) 197:1555–61. doi: 10.1016/j.juro.2017.01.062
8. Boysen WR, Akhavan A, Ko J, Ellison JS, Lendvay TS, Huang J, et al. Prospective multicenter study on robot-assisted laparoscopic extravesical ureteral reimplantation (RALUR-EV): Outcomes and complications. *J Pediatr Urol.* (2018) 14:262.e1–6. doi: 10.1016/j.jpurol.2018.01.020
9. Peters CA. Robotically assisted surgery in pediatric urology. *Urol Clin North Am.* (2004) 31:743–52. doi: 10.1016/j.ucl.2004.06.007
10. Peters CA, Woo R. Intravesical robotically assisted bilateral ureteral reimplantation. *J Endourol.* (2005) 19:618–21. doi: 10.1089/end.2005.19.618
11. Marchini GS, Hong YK, Minnillo BJ, Diamond DA, Houck CS, Meier PM, et al. Robotic assisted laparoscopic ureteral reimplantation in children: case matched comparative study with open surgical approach. *J Urol.* (2011) 185:1870–5. doi: 10.1016/j.juro.2010.12.069
12. Chan KW, Lee KH, Tam YH, Sihoe JD. Early experience in robotic-assisted laparoscopic bilateral intravesical ureteral reimplantation for vesicoureteral reflux in children. *J Robot Surg.* (2012) 6:259–62. doi: 10.1007/s11701-011-0288-1
13. Casale P, Patel RP, Kolon TF. Nerve sparing robotic extravesical ureteral reimplantation. *J Urol.* (2008) 179:1987–9; discussion 1990. doi: 10.1016/j.juro.2008.01.062
14. Schomburg JL, Haberman K, Willihnganz-Lawson KH, Shukla AR. Robot-assisted laparoscopic ureteral reimplantation: a single surgeon comparison to open surgery. *J Pediatr Urol.* (2014) 10:875–9. doi: 10.1016/j.jpurol.2014.02.013
15. Srinivasan AK, Maass D, Shrivastava D, Long CJ, Shukla AR. Is robot-assisted laparoscopic bilateral extravesical ureteral reimplantation associated with greater morbidity than unilateral surgery? A comparative analysis. *J Pediatr Urol.* (2017) 13:494.e1–7. doi: 10.1016/j.jpurol.2017.01.021
16. Sillén U. Bladder dysfunction and vesicoureteral reflux. *Adv Urol.* (2008) 8:815472. doi: 10.1155/2008/815472
17. Smith RP, Oliver JL, Peters CA. Pediatric robotic extravesical ureteral reimplantation: comparison with open surgery. *J Urol.* (2011) 185:1876–81. doi: 10.1016/j.juro.2010.12.072
18. Akhavan A, Avery D, Lendvay TS. Robot-assisted extravesical ureteral reimplantation: outcomes and conclusions from 78 ureters. *J Pediatr Urol.* (2014) 10:864–8. doi: 10.1016/j.jpurol.2014.01.028

19. Chalmers D, Herbst K, Kim C. Robotic-assisted laparoscopic extravesical ureteral reimplantation: an initial experience. *J Pediatr Urol.* (2012) 8:268–71. doi: 10.1016/j.jpurol.2011.04.006
20. Gundeti MS, Boysen WR, Shah A. Robot-assisted laparoscopic extravesical ureteral reimplantation: technique modifications contribute to optimized outcomes. *Eur Urol.* (2016) 70:818–23. doi: 10.1016/j.eururo.2016.02.065
21. Silay MS, Baek M, Koh CJ. Robot-assisted laparoscopic extravesical ureteral reimplantation in children: top-down suturing technique without stent placement. *J Endourol.* (2015) 29:864–6. doi: 10.1089/end.2014.0815
22. Kasturi S, Sehgal SS, Christman MS, Lambert SM, Casale P. Prospective long-term analysis of nerve-sparing extravesical robotic-assisted laparoscopic ureteral reimplantation. *Urology.* (2012) 79:680–3. doi: 10.1016/j.urology.2011.10.052
23. Dangle PP, Shah A, Gundeti MS. Robot-assisted laparoscopic ureteric reimplantation: extravesical technique. *BJU Int.* (2014) 114:630–2. doi: 10.1111/bju.12813
24. Grimsby GM, Dwyer ME, Jacobs MA, Ost MC, Schneck FX, Cannon GM, et al. Multi-institutional review of outcomes of robot-assisted laparoscopic extravesical ureteral reimplantation. *J Urol.* (2015) 193(5 Suppl.):1791–5. doi: 10.1016/j.juro.2014.07.128
25. Hayashi Y, Mizuno K, Kurokawa S, Nakane A, Kamisawa H, Nishio H, et al. Extravesical robot-assisted laparoscopic ureteral reimplantation for vesicoureteral reflux: initial experience in Japan with the ureteral advancement technique. *Int J Urol.* (2014) 21:1016–21. doi: 10.1111/iju.12483
26. Arlen AM, Broderick KM, Travers C, Smith EA, Elmore JM, Kirsch AJ. Outcomes of complex robot-assisted extravesical ureteral reimplantation in the pediatric population. *J Pediatr Urol.* (2016) 12:169.e1–6. doi: 10.1016/j.jpurol.2015.11.007
27. Herz D, Fuchs M, Todd A, McLeod D, Smith J. Robot-assisted laparoscopic extravesical ureteral reimplant: A critical look at surgical outcomes. *J Pediatr Urol.* (2016) 12:402.e1–402.e9. doi: 10.1016/j.jpurol.2016.05.042
28. Pruthi R, Smith A, Wallen E. Evaluating the learning curve for robot-assisted laparoscopic radical cystectomy. *J Endourol.* (2008) 22:2469–74. doi: 10.1089/end.2008.0320
29. Kaul S, Shah N, Menon M. Learning curve using robotic surgery. *Curr Urol Reports.* (2016) 7:125–29. doi: 10.1007/s11934-006-0071-4
30. Baek M, Koh CJ. Lessons learned over a decade of pediatric robotic ureteral reimplantation. *Investig Clin Urol.* (2017) 58:3–11. doi: 10.4111/icu.2017.58.1.3

23

Recurrent Wheezing in Pre-School Age: Not Only Airway Reactivity!

Marco Roversi[1], *Federica Porcaro*[2*], *Paola Francalanci*[3], *Adriano Carotti*[4] *and Renato Cutrera*[2]

[1] Academic Department, University of Rome Tor Vergata, Rome, Italy, [2] Paediatric Pulmonology and Respiratory Intermediate Care Unit, Sleep and Long-Term Ventilation Unit, Academic Department of Paediatrics, Research Institute, Bambino Gesù Children's Hospital, Rome, Italy, [3] Department of Pathology, Research Institute, Bambino Gesù Children's Hospital, Rome, Italy, [4] Unit of Pediatric Cardiac Surgery, Research Institute, Bambino Gesù Children's Hospital, Rome, Italy

***Correspondence:**
Federica Porcaro
federica.porcaro@opbg.net

Background: About a fifth of all mediastinal masses are primary cysts arising in the absence of other underlying pathology. Bronchogenic cysts, although rare, are the most frequent type responsible for lower airways compression as they often develop in the peripheral branches of the tracheobronchial tree.

Case presentation: We report the case of a 6-months-old child admitted for acute respiratory distress and wheezing not responsive to asthma treatment. Digestive and airway endoscopy proved a mild and a marked reduction of the esophageal and tracheal lumen, respectively. The nocturnal polygraphy showed an underlying obstructive disorder and the chest CT scan confirmed the presence of a wide mediastinal cyst compressing the trachea. The mass, later identified as a bronchogenic cyst, was surgically removed with complete resolution of the patient's respiratory symptoms.

Discussion: Our case shows that differential diagnosis of wheezing in pre-school aged children should encompass causes others than airway reactivity, thus prompting further evaluation and management.

Keywords: pediatrics, wheezing, asthmatic bronchitis, bronchogenic cyst, airways abnormalities

BACKGROUND

Despite being one of the most common finding in infants and children, wheezing never ceased to be an alarming symptom for both the parents and the physician. It consists of a continuous sound heard during normal expiration or inspiration when airways obstruction is severe (1). A wheezing sound is usually caused by turbulent airflow passing through a narrowed medium-sized airway. Particularly under pre-school age (<6 years), a heterogeneous group of diseases, ranging from a self-limited viral process to a life-threatening disease, can be responsible for this symptom (2, 3). Diagnosis and treatment of young children with wheezing can thus be challenging and assessment of any kind of wheezing should always include a careful examination and detailed medical history, comprising the time of onset and the concurrent clinical manifestations (**Figure 1**). A chronic wheezing unresponsive to any treatment should prompt further evaluation with advanced imaging as to exclude congenital anomalies of the tracheobronchial tree, comprising vascular rings and slings (4), or a mediastinal mass (**Table 1**). We discuss the case of an infant with persistent wheezing and acute respiratory failure due to a large mediastinal mass compressing the lower airways.

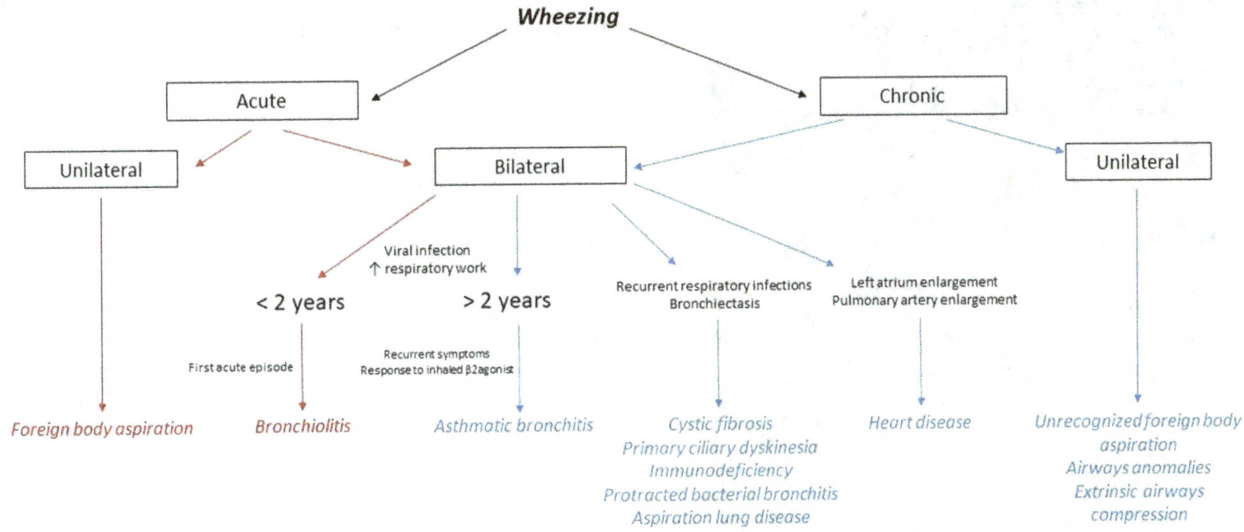

FIGURE 1 | Flow chart on differential diagnosis of wheezing in children. The main causes of acute wheezing are highlighted in red, whereas the conditions underlying a chronic wheezing are colored in blue.

TABLE 1 | Causes of recurrent/chronic wheezing in children.

Tracheo-bronchomalacia*
Vascular compression/rings*
Tracheal stenosis/web*
Extrinsic compression of trachea-bronchial tree (cyst or tumor, lymphadenopathy, cardiomegaly)
Asthma
Gastroesophageal reflux, aspiration
Not recognized foreign body
Bronchopulmonary dysplasia
Cystic fibrosis
Primary ciliary dyskinesia
Immunodeficiency
Bronchiolitis obliterans

*These alterations tend to be present in pre-school aged children.

CASE PRESENTATION

A 6-months-old child was admitted at our hospital for acute respiratory failure. Her family history was positive for atopy. She was born at term from a vaginal birth and an uncomplicated pregnancy. Weight at birth was 2,790 g and respiratory distress in the immediate perinatal period was not reported. Recurrent asthmatic bronchitis not responsive to short course of inhaler bronchodilator and corticosteroids and growth retardation without clear symptoms of dysphagia (inability to swallow, regurgitation, gagging, cough during feeding) had occurred in the previous months. The parents reported a progressive worsening of the respiratory load. Physical examination showed dyspnoea, polypnea, prolonged expiration and wheezing worsening while eating. Chest X-ray revealed a normal tracheal air column and main stem bronchi with diffuse thickening of the bronchial walls, as for a non-specific inflammation of the bronchi and their surroundings. Blood tests and microbiologic analysis on respiratory secretions were negative. The echocardiography was limited by a poor acoustic window (due to significant air trapping) and was inconclusive for vascular rings. Based on the history of recurrent symptoms partially responsive to inhaler short term β2 agonists, the patient underwent airway and digestive endoscopy, which revealed a severe tracheomalacia at the T2-T3 level. Antero-posterior compression with a 1:1 ratio between the cartilage rings and the pars membranacea was observed. Anteriorly, the trachea appeared to be compressed by a pulsating mass. No abnormal communications between the airways and the digestive tract were found. Given the airway compression, a nocturnal polygraphy with overnight oximetry was carried out and proved the underlying obstructive disorder. In order to define the extrinsic compression and quantify the tracheal collapse, a dynamic chest CT scan with contrast enhancement was carried out and revealed a 4.0 cm wide mediastinal mass closely adherent to the anterior profiles of the first five thoracic vertebra, both compressing and dislocating the trachea and esophagus to the front and to the right, respectively (**Figures 2A,B**). Integration with ultrasound imaging directed at the jugulum confirmed the presence of a thin walled anechoic cyst. The patient underwent median sternotomy followed by opening of the pericardium and lateralization of the great vessels; total thymectomy was also made necessary to access the mass. On lowering the right pulmonary artery, the voluminous mass was appreciated, tightly adherent to the pars membranacea of the trachea and easily detachable from the esophagus. The cyst, filled with clear liquid and not communicating with the foregut, was therefore punched to reduce its size and facilitate dissection. Histopathological analysis later identified a cystic formation covered by respiratory epithelium and without smooth muscle in the walls, namely a bronchogenic cyst. The postoperative endoscopy revealed complete resolution of the tracheal compression at the T2-T3

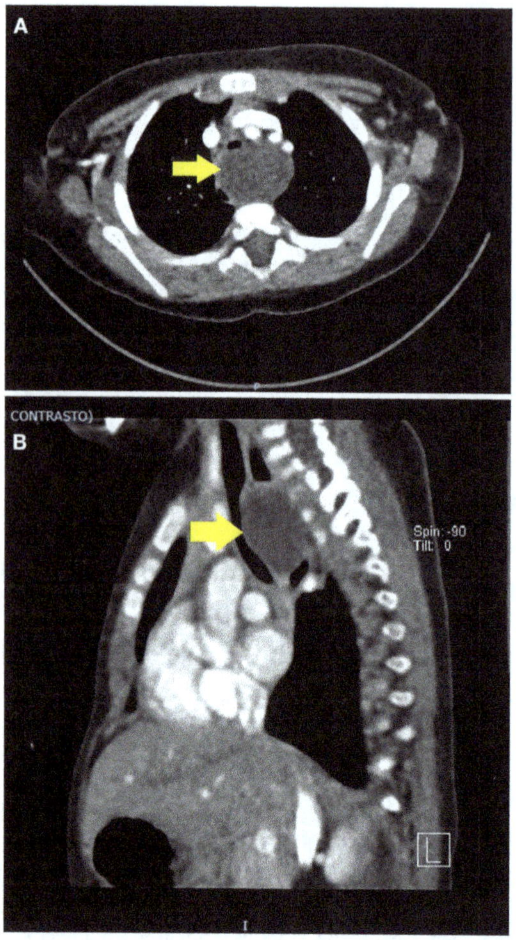

FIGURE 2 | (A,B) Contrast-enhanced chest CT scan. A thin-walled round mass (antero-posterior to lateral diameter, size 30 × 25 × 40 mm) can be seen at the level of the first five dorsal vertebral somas (from D1 to D5). The mass (yellow arrow) occupies the upper and middle mediastinum, displacing the esophagus posteriorly and the trachea anteriorly. In dynamic acquisitions a marked reduction in the size of the trachea to the middle third is documented. The epiaortic vessels appear to be slightly displaced anteriorly without reduction in size.

level. Unfortunately, the patient had a severe respiratory distress with low oxygen saturation, requiring non-invasive ventilation in the intensive care unit (ICU) on the third postoperative day. Both wet and dry crackles could be heard at the right lower lobe. The chest X-ray confirmed the presence of a shaded consolidation at the right lower lobe, consistent with the expected postoperative dysventilation. An urgent endoscopy was required and proved the absence of any fistulous communication between airways and esophagus. Nevertheless, a paralysis of the left vocal cord was detected. Molecular analysis of the sputum later identified an infection by Rhinovirus. The patient respiratory function and imaging gradually improved until she was weaned from ventilatory support. She was discharged 3 weeks after surgery, with only residual expiratory sounds and dysphonia due to the left vocal cord paralysis. One month later, the patient's wheezing completely resolved, and the dysphonia also improved. We obtained informed written consent from the patient's parent authorizing publication of the clinical case and radiologic images. Her anonymity has been preserved.

DISCUSSION

About 20% of mediastinal masses are primary cysts arising in the absence of other underlying pathology (5). Unless they are of unspecified nature, primary cysts can originate from thymus, pericardium, digestive tract and airway system, with the latter being the most frequent type (6). Bronchogenic cysts arise from the precursor of the tracheobronchial tree, the respiratory diverticulum, as proven by their usual location proximal to the trachea or bronchi, either within the lung parenchyma or the mediastinum. In infants, they account for 10% of mediastinal masses and are more common in males (7). The cysts are usually identified by contrast-enhanced chest CT scan as well-defined homogeneous masses adjacent to the lower airways. Two thirds of bronchogenic cysts are asymptomatic, but surgical excision is always necessary as to confirm the diagnosis and rule out malignancies (6). Cyst resection is mandatory in children, even when asymptomatic, as they have a high risk of developing acute respiratory failure later in life, due to compression either of the trachea or bronchi (5). Furthermore, some cases show that half of the patients with bronchogenic cysts may develop complications, such as compression of adjacent structures, infection through a bronchial communication, and rupture into the trachea, the pericardial cavity, or the pleural cavity (8). Other complications of bronchogenic cysts are pneumothorax and pleuritis (9). In our case a common viral infection complicated a difficult postoperative course, given the age of the patient and the size of the cyst that had been removed. The kind of surgery that had been performed also had an intrinsic risk of causing iatrogenic tracheoesophageal fistula (10), thus making frequent endoscopic controls mandatory.

Despite the usual location of bronchogenic cysts within the mediastinum, the given one was well above the carina, compressing both the trachea and esophagus and leading to wheezing without feeding problems. On the basis of cyst's dimension, the symptoms were expected to appear earlier in life, but in our case no respiratory distress was noted at birth or immediately after. Treatment of mediastinal masses, such as the cyst we encountered, is hazardous and should always be managed by a multidisciplinary team. Along with bronchogenic cysts, there are a variety of causes of extrinsic compression of the trachea that may cause wheezing and mimic an asthmatic bronchitis in children, ranging from the more common mediastinal neoplasms to the less frequent vascular rings (11). Therefore, other causes than pre-school asthma have to be taken into account in younger children with wheezing poorly responsive to medical treatment. That is, not all pre-school wheezing means airway reactivity!

ETHICS STATEMENT

We obtained informed written consent from the patient's parent authorizing publication of clinical case and radiologic imagings.

AUTHOR CONTRIBUTIONS

MR made data analysis, wrote the paper and approved the final manuscript. FP contributed to the writing of the paper, revised and approved the final manuscript. PF analyzed the bioptical specimen and made the final diagnosis, revised the paper and approved the final manuscript. AC performed the surgical removal of the cyst, revised the paper and approved the final manuscript. RC contributed to design, revised and approved the final manuscript.

REFERENCES

1. Forgacs P. The functional basis of pulmonary sounds. *Chest.* (1978) 73:399–405. doi: 10.1378/chest.73.3.399
2. Chang AB, Robertson CF, Van Asperen PP, Glasgow NJ, Mellis CM, Masters IB, et al. A multicenter study on chronic cough in children: burden and etiologies based on a standardized management pathway. *Chest.* (2012) 142:943–50. doi: 10.1378/chest.11-2725
3. Brand PLP, Baraldi E, Bisgaard H, Boner AL, Castro-Rodriguez JA, Custovic A, et al. Definition, assessment and treatment of wheezing disorders in preschool children: an evidence-based approach. *Eur Respir J.* (2008) 32:1096–110. doi: 10.1183/09031936.00002108
4. McLaren CA, Elliott MJ, Roebuck DJ. Vascular compression of the airway in children. *Paediatr Respir Rev.* (2008) 9:85–94. doi: 10.1016/j.prrv.2007.12.008
5. Donahue JM, Nichols FC. Primary mediastinal tumors and cysts and diagnostic investigation of mediastinal masses. In: Shields TW, LoCicero J III, Reed CE, editors. *General Thoracic Surgery.* Philadelphia, PA: Lippincott Williams & Wilkins (2009). p. 2195–9.
6. Putnam JB Jr. Lung, chest wall, pleura, and mediastinum. In: Townsend C, Daniel Beauchamp R, Mark Evers B, Mattox K, editors. *Sabiston Textbook of Surgery: The Biological Basis of Modern Surgical Practice.* Elsevier (2017). p. 1580–610.
7. Goswamy J, de Kruijf S, Humphrey G, Rothera MP, Bruce IA. Brochogenic cysts as a cause of infantile stridor: case report and literature review. *J Laryngol Otol.* (2011) 125:1094–97. doi: 10.1017/S0022215111001502
8. Sarper A, Ayten A, Golbasi I, Demircan A, Isin E. Bronchogenic cyst. *Tex Heart Inst J.* (2003) 30:105–8.
9. Aktogu S, Yuncu G, Halilcolar H, Ermete S, Buduneli T. Bronchogenic cysts: clinicopathological presentation and treatment. *Eur Respir J.* (1996) 9:2017–21. doi: 10.1183/09031936.96.09102017
10. Suen HC, Mathisen DJ, Grillo HC, LeBlanc J, McLoud TC, Moncure AC, et al. Surgical management and radiological characteristics of bronchogenic cysts. *Ann Thorac Surg.* (1993) 55:476–81. doi: 10.1016/0003-4975(93)91022-F
11. Backer CL, Mongé MC, Popescu AR, Eltayeb OM, Rastatter JC, Rigsby CK. Vascular rings. *Semin Pediatr Surg.* (2016) 25:165–175. doi: 10.1053/j.sempedsurg.2016.02.009

24

From the Ground Up: Esophageal Atresia Types, Disease Severity Stratification and Survival Rates at a Single Institution

Devon Michael Evanovich [1,2], *Jue Teresa Wang* [1,3], *Benjamin Zendejas* [3,4,5], *Russell William Jennings* [3,4,5] *and Dusica Bajic* [1,3*]

[1] *Department of Anesthesiology, Critical Care and Pain Medicine, Boston Children's Hospital, Boston, MA, United States,* [2] *Tufts School of Medicine, Tufts University, Boston, MA, United States,* [3] *Harvard Medical School, Harvard University, Boston, MA, United States,* [4] *Department of Surgery, Boston Children's Hospital, Boston, MA, United States,* [5] *Esophageal and Airway Treatment Center, Boston Children's Hospital, Boston, MA, United States*

Correspondence:
Dusica Bajic
dusica.bajic@childrens.harvard.edu

Esophageal atresia (EA), although a rare congenital anomaly, represents one of the most common gastrointestinal birth defects. There is a gap in our knowledge regarding the impact of perioperative critical care in infants born with EA. This study addresses EA types, disease severity stratification, and mortality in a retrospective cohort at a single institution. Institutional Review Board approved our retrospective cross-sectional study of term-born (n = 53) and premature infants (28–37 weeks of gestation; n = 31) that underwent primary surgical repair of EA at a single institution from 2009–2020. Demographic and clinical data were obtained from the electronic medical record, Powerchart (Cerner, London, UK). Patients were categorized by (i) sex, (ii) gestational age at birth, (iii) types of EA (in relation to respiratory tract anomalies), (iv) co-occurring congenital anomalies, (v) severity of disease (viz. American Society of Anesthesiologists (ASA) and Pediatric Risk Assessment (PRAm) scores), (vi) type of surgical repair for EA (primary anastomosis vs. Foker process), and (vii) survival rate classification using Spitz and Waterston scores. Data were presented as numerical sums and percentages. The frequency of anatomical types of EA in our cohort parallels that of the literature: 9.5% (8/84) type A, 9.5% (8/84) type B, 80% (67/84) type C, and 1% (1/84) type D. *Long-gap* EA accounts for 88% (7/8) type A, 75% (6/8) type B, and 13% (9/67) type C in the cohort studied. Our novel results show a nearly equal distribution of sex per each EA type, and gestational age (term-born vs. premature) by anatomical EA type. PRAm scoring showed a wider range of disease severity (3–9) than ASA scores (III and IV). The survival rate in our EA cohort dramatically increased in comparison to the literature in previous decades. This retrospective analysis at a single institution shows incidence of EA per sex and gestational status for anatomical types (EA type A-D) and by surgical approach (primary anastomosis vs. Foker process for *short-gap* vs. *long-gap* EA, respectively). Despite its wider range, PRAm score was not more useful in predicting disease severity in comparison to ASA score. Increased survival rates over the last decade suggest a potential need to assess unique operative and perioperative risks in this unique population of patients. Presented findings also represent a foundation for future clinical studies of outcomes in infants born with EA.

Keywords: ASA, EA, LGEA, mortality, term, term-born infant, PRAm, premature

INTRODUCTION

Esophageal atresia (EA), although a rare congenital anomaly with a stable world-wide prevalence (1) represents one of the most common gastrointestinal birth defects with reported incidence of 1 in 3,000 to 1 in 4,500 live births (2). If esophageal lumen interruption is left unrepaired, infants are prone to inadequate nutrition and growth, as well as infections such as pneumonia (3). EA is classified into 4 types (type A, B, C, and D) based on the anatomical description in relation to the airway structures (4) (**Figure 1**), that does not take into account the complexity of underlying disease.

In addition to associated malformation, the EA gap length dictates the complexity of perioperative care. If the gap of the esophagus is too large to be repaired by direct anastomosis (>3 cm or >2 vertebral bodies in length), EA is defined as *long-gap* EA, which is more commonly found in anatomical types A and B of EA (9). At our institution, the latter cases undergo a unique type of EA repair, the Foker process (5–8). Compared to *short-gap* esophageal atresia, *long-gap* EA is also more likely to be an isolated defect and associated with trisomy 21 (9). In contrast, *short-gap* EA is more commonly found with VACTERL anomalies (vertebral, anorectal, cardiac, tracheo-esophageal fistula and/or esophageal atresia, renal, and limb defects/ malformations) relative to *long-gap* EA (9). Last but not least, CHARGE syndrome (coloboma, heart defects, choanal atresia, growth retardation, genital abnormalities, and ear abnormalities) (10) can further complicate the care of infants born with EA.

The complexity of underlying disease with and without other congenital anomalies in the case of EA is undeniable. Although *short-gap* EA is repaired with direct anastomosis and requires shorter pain management, infants are vulnerable to post-operative feeding challenges (11) in addition to the impact of associated anomalies. In cases of *long-gap* EA, the revolutionary Foker process (5–8) encourages the natural growth and lengthening of infant's existing esophageal pouches, but it requires at least two separate thoracotomies/thoracoscopies with a subsequent prolonged postoperative intubation (12, 13) associated with development of physical dependence to drugs of sedation (13–15). The primary goal of this study addresses the severity of EA disease as a blueprint for a subsequent myriad of caregiving conditions that might impose challenges to developing infants born with EA. Specifically, we conducted a retrospective analysis at a single institution to analyze incidence of EA by severity of disease using American Society of Anesthesiologists (ASA) (16) and Pediatric Risk Assessment (PRAm) (17–19) scores in the context of (i) sex, (ii) gestational age (term-born and premature), (iii) anatomical classification of EA types, and (iv) the type of surgical repair (viz. direct anastomosis vs. Foker process with prolonged sedation). Our secondary clinical end-point measures looked into mortality risk in the context of other co-morbidities according to Spitz et al. (20) and Waterson et al. (21) classifications that take into account co-existing pneumonia and cardiac disease, respectively. This study was, in part, previously published as thesis (22).

METHODS

Study Design and Subjects Equations

Institutional Review Board at Boston Children's Hospital approved this retrospective cross-sectional research study (IRB-P000007855) of infants born with esophageal atresia (EA) that underwent primary surgical repair at a single institution. The study conformed to the standards set by the Declaration of Helsinki and Good Clinical Practice guidelines. The patient information was obtained from a prospectively maintained clinical database, *The Esophageal and Airway Treatment Center* REDCap database, established in 2009. Considering our institution is not a birthing center, all infants cared for at our institution are considered outborn. Eligibility criteria included: (1) term-born (defined as birth between 37 and 42 weeks of gestation) and premature infants (28–37 weeks of gestation) born with EA of any type, and (2) patients that received their primary surgical repair at Boston Children's Hospital. Cohort patients underwent surgery in the first month of life with exception of two patients that were born outside of the State and underwent primary surgical repair at our institution at 2 and 3 months of age. Exclusion criteria included: (1) extreme prematurity (<28 weeks of gestation), and (2) any surgical repair at other institutions (including but not limited to EA repair). Our retrospective study included a total of 84 patients ($n = 53$ term-born; $n = 31$ premature) over the period of 11 years (2009–2020).

Chart Review

Electronic medical record, Powerchart (Cerner, London, UK) was used to collect demographic data (viz. date of birth; gestational age at birth (weeks); birth weight (kg)) and clinical data. The latter included several end-point measures.

Esophageal Atresia Types

In addition to classification of EA into 4 anatomical types (type A, B, C, and D) based on the anatomical description in relation to the airway structures (4) – in particular to co-existence with tracheo-esophageal fistula (TEF), we also classified EA cases based on the length of EA gap into: *short-gap* (that was repaired by primary anastomosis) and *long-gap* that underwent repair by Foker process (5–8). Some of the patients with *long-gap* EA were managed with our newer minimally invasive Foker process which entails an internal adjustable traction system that is adjusted every 5–7 days via a thoracoscopy. As such, it leads to less postoperative muscle paralysis and sedation in comparison to the external traction Foker process via thoracotomy (8, 23, 24). For the purpose of this study, we identify *short-gap* EA with direct anastomosis repair, and *long-gap* EA with the Foker

Abbreviations: ASA, American Society of Anesthesiologist; **EA**, Esophageal atresia; **CHARGE**, Coloboma, Heart defects, choanal Atresia, growth Retardation, Genital abnormalities, and Ear abnormalities; **PRAm**, Pediatric Risk Assessment; **TEF**, Tracheo-esophageal fistula; **VACTERL**, Vertebral, Anorectal, Cardiac, Tracheo-esophageal fistula and/or Esophageal atresia, Renal, and Limb defects/malformations.

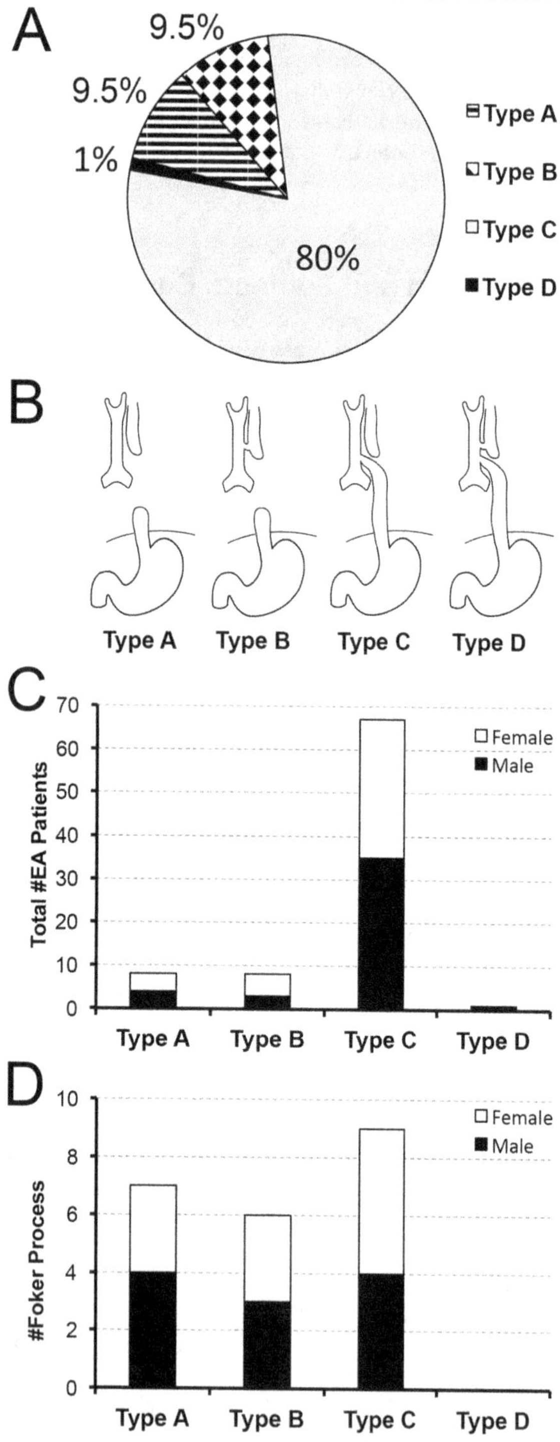

FIGURE 1 | Retrospective Analysis of Incidence of Primary Esophageal Atresia Repair at a Single Institution. Data was retrospectively collected from 2009–2020 ($n = 84$). Pie chart in **(A)** summarizes the percent (%) incidence of esophageal atresia (EA) by anatomical classification that is schematically illustrated in **(B)**. According to our retrospective data analysis, anatomical *type C* of EA is the most frequently encountered. Graph in **(C)** also illustrates nearly equal sex distribution per anatomical type with females found in 50% in *type A*, 62.5% in *type B*, and 48% in *type C*. Graph in **(D)** summarizes the incidence of *long-gap* EA patients ($n = 22$) that underwent Foker process (5–8). Incidence of *long-gap* EA follows the trend per anatomical type and sex, similar to the cohort as a whole (see Results for more detail).

process repair - as these are the two main surgical approaches at our Institution.

Medical/Surgical Comorbidities

As EA often presents with other congenital anomalies and/or co-morbidities, we collected clinical data regarding any other genetic or chromosomal anomalies (e.g., Trisomy 18, 21 etc.), and any other associated congenital anomalies (e.g., vertebral, cardiac, anal anomalies etc.), some of which are a part of the complex congenital syndromes associated with EA such as VACTERL (25) or CHARGE syndrome (26). Co-existing cardiac anomalies were classified as minor (not requiring surgical intervention such as patent foramen ovale, patent ductus arteriosus, atrial septal defect, ventricular septal defect, dextrocardia), or complex (requiring surgical correction such as large ventricular septal defect, large atrial septal defect, coarctation of the aorta, large patent ductus arteriosus, and Tetralogy of Fallow). We quantified the incidence of other associated co-morbidities such as: (i) pneumonia treatment, and (ii) cardiac surgeries, which both served as a basis for mortality risk evaluation (see below). Due to the retrospective study design, characterization of associated co-morbidities was obtained from the medical records as part of the clinical diagnostics and treatment.

Disease Severity

Complexity of clinical status in the context of other comorbidities was assessed using two scoring systems: American Society of Anesthesiologists (ASA) (16) and Pediatric Risk Assessment (PRAm) (17–19) scores at the time of EA repair surgery. Assigning an ASA Physical Status classification level is a clinical decision based on several factors (16) and represents the most commonly used assessment of system level disease severity by anesthesiologists (**Figure 3A**–*Table*). ASA scores are based on several factors and range from ASA I (normal healthy patient) to ASA VI (a declared brain dead patient) (16). In contrast, PRAm scoring is a relatively novel measure introduced in 2017 (17–19) that involves 5 scoring points: urgency of surgical procedure (+1), presence of at least one comorbidity (+2), presence of at least one indication of critical illness (+3), age <12 months at surgery (+3), and co-existing malignancy (+4) for a range of scores from 0 to 13. PRAm scoring has been designed as a less subjective assessment of disease severity for the use specifically in pediatric populations (scores 0 – 13; **Figure 3B**–*Table*).

Mortality Risk Assessment

Considering our retrospective data collection spans period of last 11 years (2009-2020), it was used for comparison to previously published survival rates in infants born with EA as per two different scoring systems: (i) Waterston et al. (21), and (ii) Spitz et al. (20). As originally described by Waterston et al. (21), this scoring system takes into account weight of the patient, co-existence of other congenital anomalies, and pneumonia. Scoring is described as low risk (**group A:** birth weight >2.5 kg with no or co-existing congenital anomaly or pneumonia), moderate risk (**group B:** birth weight 1.8–2.5 kg with co-existing mild pneumonia and mild congenital anomaly), or high risk (**group C:** birth weight 1.8–2.5 kg with co-existing severe pneumonia and severe congenital anomaly).

To improve clarity and transparency with scoring definitions, we modified the original scoring by Waterson et al. (21) for moderate and high risk groups. In this report, the moderate mortality risk group (group B) included infants with co-existing *moderate* pneumonia (defined as receiving antibiotics), and/or a *moderate* congenital anomaly (viz. limb anomalies, cleft lip or palate, atrial-septal defect or small patent ductus arteriosus). High mortality risk (group C) in this study referred to infants with *severe* pneumonia (defined as requiring mechanical ventilation) and/or a *severe* congenital anomaly (viz. defined as making survival difficult or impossible without surgical repair). The second scoring system, described by Spitz et al. (20), takes into account weight and co-existence of a severe cardiac congenital anomaly. The risk is described as low **(I)**, moderate **(II)**, and high **(III)** risk of mortality with major cardiac anomalies defined as one that required medical or surgical treatment.

Statistical Analysis

Data was presented as numerical sums and percentages for (i) sex and anatomical classification of EA, (ii) gestational age at birth, (iii) distribution of *long-gap* EA patients for sex and gestational age, (iv) distribution of congenital anomalies, (v) disease severity scores, and (vi) survival rate. PRAm scores were also presented as numerical sums and as boxplot distributions indicating median scores, first and third quartile ranges, and absolute values for minimum and maximum values.

RESULTS

The retrospective chart review included infants that underwent EA repair at a single institution over a period of 11 years (2009–2020; $n = 84$): 53 term-born, and 31 premature (born between 28 and 37 weeks of gestation).

Demographic Information and Incidence of Esophageal Atresia Types

Anatomical Types

Figures 1A,B illustrate incidence of EA patients according to the anatomical types of EA (4): type A (isolated EA; 8/84, 9.5%), type B (TEF at the upper esophageal pouch; 8/84; 9.5%), type C (the most common type of EA with TEF at the lower esophageal pouch; 67/84; 80%), type D (the rarest type of EA with TEF at each esophageal pouch; 1/84; 1%). Our novel data implicate equal distribution of sex for infants born with EA (**Figure 1C**) with 49% (41/84) female and 51% (43/84) male patients of nearly equal distribution per anatomical types of EA: 50% (4/8) female with type A, 62.5% (5/8) female with type B, and 48% (32/67) female with type C.

Esophageal Gap: Short-Gap vs. Long-Gap

We also distinguished between *short-gap* and *long-gap* EA (see Method's section). The latter is equated to Foker process repair (5–8), that represented 26% of the cohort (22/84). Unlike the cohort as a whole (**Figure 1C**), the incidence of *long-gap* EA cases showed nearly equal distribution by anatomical types (**Figure 1D**): type C (9/22; 41%), type A (7/22; 32%), and type B (6/22; 27%). However, *long-gap* EA accounted for 88% (7/8) of patients in type A, 75% (6/8) in type B, and 13% (9/67) in type C (not graphically shown). Importantly, infants born with *long-gap* EA showed exactly equal distribution of sex (50%; 11/22 female) with nearly equal distribution per anatomical types of EA (**Figure 1D**): 42% (3/7) female with type A, 50% (3/6) female with type B, and 56% (5/9 female) with type C.

Gestational Age

Taking into account exclusion of extreme prematurity, this retrospective cohort shows slightly higher frequency of term-born (53/84, 63%) than premature patients (31/84; 37%) with similar trend per anatomical classification of EA types: 75% (6/8) term-born with type A, 50% (4/8) term-born with type B, and 63% (42/67) term-born with type C (**Figures 2A,B**). There was only one term-born patient with type D EA. Similarly, infants that underwent Foker process for *long-gap* EA repair (**Figure 2C**) had a similar frequency of term-born and premature patients (11/22; 50%). However, term-born patients with *long-gap* EA were predominantly noted in type A (6/7; 86%) while premature infants with *long-gap* EA represented majority in type B (4/6; 67%) and type C (6/9; 67%) as illustrated in **Figure 2C**.

Incidence of Co-existing Congenital Anomalies

Syndromes Associated With Esophageal Atresia

Table 1 summarizes the incidence of other co-existing anomalies with EA. About 42% (35/84) of the cohort patients had complex EA disease as part of a syndrome or known chromosomal abnormality (**Table 1A**). Of those, the most frequent was VACTERL syndrome (31/35, 89%), although we also report cases of CHARGE syndrome (2/35, 6%), trisomy 21 (Down's syndrome; 1/35) and trisomy 18 (Edwards syndrome; 1/35). We also report a similar incidence of VACTERL syndrome in those that underwent primary repair (viz. *short-gap* EA; 24/62; 39%) compared to infants that underwent the Foker process for the repair of *long-gap* EA (7/22; 32%).

Esophageal Atresia in the Absence of Syndrome

For infants born with EA without associated syndrome (49/84; 58%), the majority had either 2 (17/49; 35%) or more than 2 (16/49; 33%) co-occurring congenital anomalies. Only a minority of patients had no co-existing congenital anomalies (6/49, 12%; **Table 1B**). Interestingly, a majority of patients – apart from syndromic patients (49/84; 58%) - had a cardiac anomaly (38/49; 78%) and no patients had a documented anorectal anomaly occurring outside of a syndrome (**Table 1C**).

Cardiac Co-anomalies

Of all the infants born with EA that had co-existing cardiac anomalies (72/84; 86%), only 18% (15/84) had congenital heart disease severe enough to require surgical repair (**Table 2A**). Of those that underwent cardiac surgery, 93% (14/15) had type C EA, and only one patient had type B EA. We report a similar pattern of co-existing congenital cardiac anomalies in

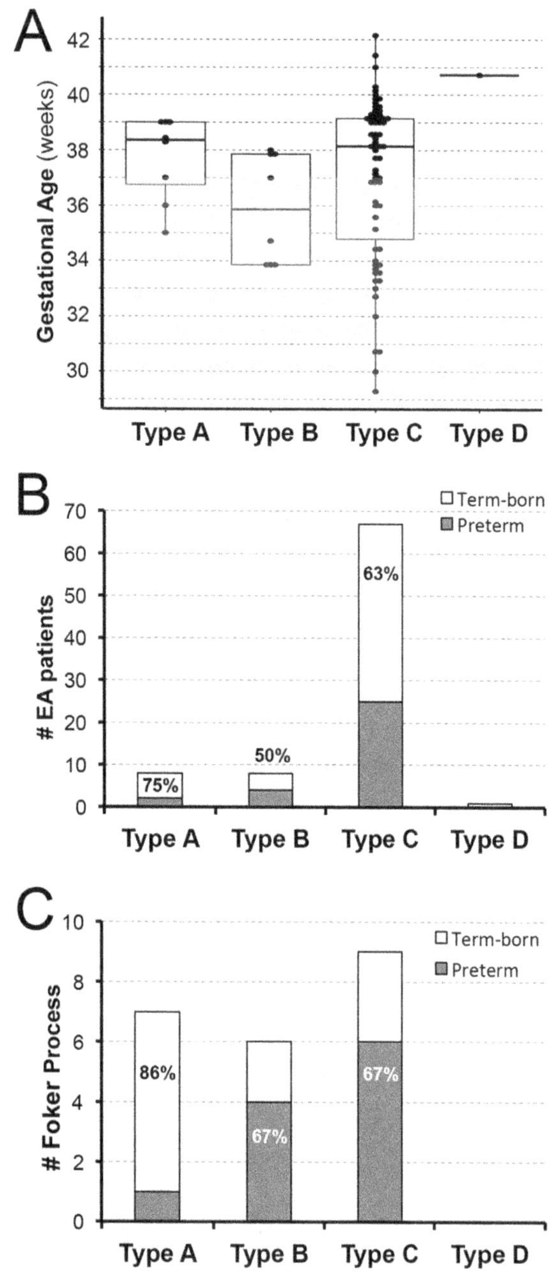

FIGURE 2 | Retrospective Analysis of Esophageal Atresia Classification by Gestational Age at Birth. Retrospective data of infants born with esophageal atresia (EA) was collected from 2009–2020 ($n = 84$) and included infants born ≥28 weeks of gestation that were classified as term-born (37–42 weeks gestation) or premature (28–37 weeks of gestation). **(A)** Illustrates individual distribution of gestational age at birth per EA type (dots), while gray area schematically marks prematurity (<37 weeks of gestation). **(B)** Summarizes percent (%) incidence of EA per anatomical type and gestational age groups with either equal (type B) or predominant incidence of term-born patients (type A and C). In this cohort of infants with primary surgical repair of EA at our institution, we report only one term-born infant with *type D* EA. For illustration of anatomical EA types, please see **Figure 1B**. **(C)** Summarizes incidence of infants that underwent Foker process (5–8) for *long-gap* EA repair. We report equal incidence of term-born and preterm patients. However, term-born patients with *long-gap* EA were predominantly noted in *type A* (6/7; 86%) while premature infants with long-gap EA represented majority in *type B* (4/6; 67%) and *type C* (6/9; 67%) anatomical EA type.

TABLE 1 | Incidence of esophageal atresia in the context of other congenital anomalies.

	Number	Percentage (%)
A. EA as part of complex congenital syndrome (cohort $n = 84$)		
VACTERL	31	37%
CHARGE	2	2%
Other	2	2%
None	49	58%
B. EA with other co-anomalies apart from syndrome ($n = 49$)		
None	6	12%
Isolated anomaly	10	20%
2 anomalies	17	35%
More than 2 anomalies	16	33%
C. Distribution of co-anomalies apart from syndrome ($n = 49$)		
Anorectal	0	0%
Vertebral	10	20%
Cardiac	38	78%
Laryngeal cleft	9	18%
Tracheo(broncho)malacia	23	47%
Limb	2	4%
Renal or Kidney	13	27%

Incidence of esophageal atresia with or without other congenital anomalies. (A) *shows that 42% (35/84) of EA was a part of complex syndrome: VACTERL syndrome (31/35, 89%); CHARGE syndrome (2/35, 6%); Trisomy 21 (Down's syndrome; 1/35); and Trisomy 18 (Edwards syndrome; 1/35). As illustrated in* ***(B)****, of those esophageal atresia (EA) infants with no complex congenital diagnosis (49/84; 58%), a majority had either 2 (17/49; 35%) or > 2 (16/49; 33%) co-occurring congenital anomalies not associated with the syndrome. Incidence of specific co-existing anomalies is listed in* ***(C)****. Interestingly, a majority of patients had a cardiac anomaly (38/49; 78%) and no patients had a documented anorectal anomaly occurring outside of a syndrome. Acronyms: CHARGE, Coloboma, Heart defects, choanal Atresia, growth Retardation, Genital abnormalities, and Ear abnormalities; VACTERL, Vertebral, Anorectal, Cardiac, Tracheo-esophageal fistula and/ or Esophageal atresia, Renal, and Limb defects/ malformations.*

infants with *long-gap* EA that underwent the Foker process repair (**Table 2B**): 86% (19/22) had co-existing cardiac anomalies, but only 14% (3/22) required cardiac surgery and were diagnosed with either type C EA (2/3) or type B EA (1/3). **Table 2** summarizes severity of cardiac findings in this cohort.

Severity Stratification of Underlying Disease

Figure 3 illustrates 2 different disease severity scores by anatomical EA types (types A-D; **Figure 1B**) and gestational age (term-born vs. premature).

American Society of Anesthesiologists Physical Status Classification

Half of the patients of this cohort were rated either ASA Physical Status III (49% (41/84) with severe systemic disease; 76% (31/41) term-born; 24% (10/41) premature), or ASA Physical Status IV (51% (43/84) with severe systemic disease that is a constant threat to life; 51% (22/43) term-born; 49% (21/43) premature). **Figure 3A** shows ASA Physical Status classification of the cohort infants per anatomical types of EA. For the most common type of EA – type C, the majority of term-born patients received ASA

TABLE 2 | Incidence of co-existing congenital cardiac anomalies.

EA type	Total number	Minor (no cardiac surgery)	Major (cardiac surgery)
A. Cohort (*n* = 84)	**72/84 (86%)**	**57/72 (79%)**	**15/72 (21%)**
Type A	6/8 (75%)	6/6 (100%)	0/6 (0%)
Type B	5/8 (63%)	4/5 (80%)	1/5 (20%)
Type C	60/67 (90%)	46/60 (77%)	14/60 (23%)
Type D	1/1 (100%)	1/1 (100%)	0/1 (0%)
B. Foker Process (*n* = 22)	**19/22 (86%)**	**16/19 (84%)**	**3/19 (16%)**
Type A	5/7 (71%)	5/5 (100%)	0/5 (0%)
Type B	5/6 (83%)	4/5 (80%)	1/5 (20%)
Type C	9/9 (100%)	7/9 (78%)	2/9 (22%)
Type D	none	N/A	N/A

Incidence of Congenital Cardiac Anomalies by Esophageal Atresia Types. *Table summarizes incidence of co-existing cardiac anomalies in infants born with esophageal atresia (EA) stratified by anatomical type in relation to the tracheo-esophageal fistula (See also* ***Figure 1****) for the entire cohort* ***(A)****, and in a subset of long-gap EA patients that underwent Foker process repair* ***(B)****. Incidence of cardiac anomalies is shown as total number (left column; n = 84). Of those that underwent cardiac surgery (n = 72), we summarize percent (%) of those with minor cardiac anomaly (not requiring surgery; central column; n = 57), and those that underwent cardiac repair (major anomaly; right column; n = 15).*

III status (27/42; 64%), while the majority of premature infants received ASA IV status (19/25; 76%).

Pediatric Risk Assessment Scores

Considering all patients in this retrospective cohort underwent surgical repair in infancy, and none had any associated malignancy, the PRAm score ranged from 3 to 9 across all anatomical types and gestational age groups (**Figure 3B**). For the cohort as a whole, we report Median PRAm score of 5 for both term-born (interquartile range of 4–6) and premature infants (interquartile range of 5–8). When classified according to anatomical EA types, premature infants had a higher median score for type B EA (Median 7; interquartile range of 4.75–9), but a lower median score for most frequent type C (Median 5; interquartile range 5–8) in comparison to term-born infants (Median 4; interquartile range of 3–5 for type B; Median 5; interquartile range of 4–6 for type C). While type B shows higher PRAm scores for premature infants, there is a limited number of patients in this group (*n* = 8) compared to type C (*n* = 67). Furthermore, we report a wide PRAm score classification (**Figure 4A**) for term-born patients with propensity for lower PRAm scores (25% (13/53) PRAm 3; 9% (5/53) PRAm 9), and premature infants with propensity for higher PRAm scores (10% (3/31) PRAm 3; 23% (7/31) PRAm 9).

Relationship Between ASA Physical Status and PRAm Scores

To better gauge individual relationship of two different scores, **Figure 4B** illustrates relationship between ASA physical status and PRAm scores. Despite wide distribution of PRAm scores irrespective of the gestational age (**Figure 4A**), patients with assigned ASA IV classification had about equal distribution per gestational age groups: premature (21/43; 49%) and term-born patients (22/43; 51%). However, we do not show that premature infants with ASA IV physical classification (*n* = 21/43) align with higher PRAm score distribution (**Figure 4B**).

Disease Severity With Respect to Type of EA Surgical Repair

We also report a wide distribution of PRAm scores (scores 3-9) irrespective of the type of surgical repair (**Figure 5A**). However, infants born with *short-gap* EA undergoing direct anastomosis repair (*n* = 62) have a propensity for lower PRAm scores in term-born patients (62.5% (10/16) PRAm 3; 42% (5/12) PRAm 9) and higher PRAm scores in premature patients (12.5% (2/16) PRAm 3; 17% (2/12) PRAm 9) as illustrated in **Figure 5B**. Similarly, infants born with *long-gap* EA undergoing Foker process repair (*n* = 22) have a propensity for lower PRAm scores in term-born patients (19% (3/16) PRAm 3; 0% (0/12) PRAm 9) and higher PRAm scores in premature patients (6% (1/16) PRAm 3; 42% (5/12) PRAm 9) as illustrated in **Figure 5B**. Considering more premature patients with EA have ASA IV classification status (**Figure 3A**), prematurity should be considered a confounding factor for increased underlying disease severity. As such, other important aspects of prematurity, such as intra-uterine growth retardation and prematurity associated sequelae (e.g., respiratory distress syndrome) should be considered as potential indirect markers of prematurity in assessing outcomes following EA repair. Finally, when PRAm scores (with score range from 3–9) are graphed in relation to ASA physical status (**Figure 5C**), more infants with *long-gap* EA are scored as ASA IV classification (73%; 16/22) compared to *short-gap* EA patients (44%; 27/62). Future goals should include unique scoring system design that would include other potential confounders unique for EA repair, such as length of post-operative mechanical ventilation and antibiotic treatment as indirect markers of postoperative sedation and infections, respectively.

Mortality Risk Assessment of Infants Born With Esophageal Atresia

Mortality Risk Assessment I

Table 3 summarizes the mortality risk assessment as originally described by Waterston et al. (21) in EA patients according to the (i) birth weight, (ii) co-existing congenital anomalies (**Tables 1 and 2**), and (iii) co-morbidity with pneumonia into: low (group A), moderate (group B), and high mortality risk (group C). Indeed, our retrospective study is of similar population size of EA patients (*n* = 84) as in the original report (*n* = 113) (21). However, our cohort had smaller numbers of infants in low risk group and much higher number of infants in high mortality group, group C (**Table 4**). With that in mind, we also show striking survival rates especially in the moderate risk (group B; 100% (42/42) vs. 68% (29/43 in the Waterson's study) and high risk group [group C; 95% (38/40) vs. 6% (2/32) in the original study (21)].

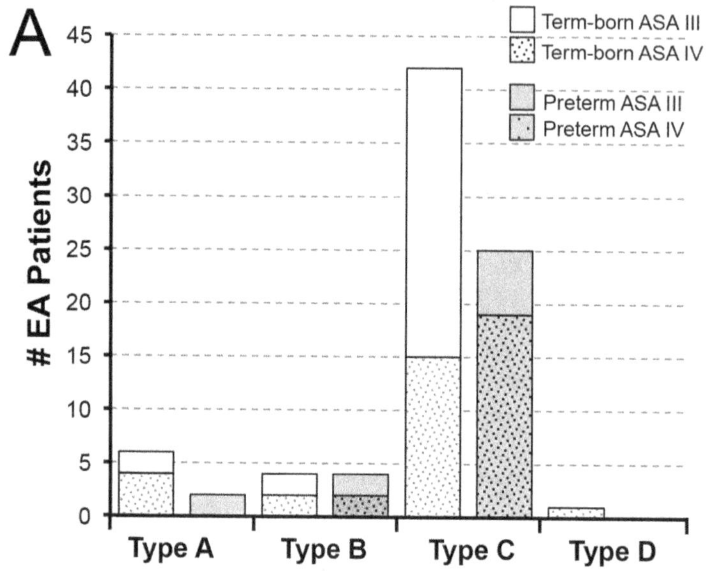

Score	Definition
ASA I	Healthy
ASA II	Mild systemic disease
ASA III	**Severe systemic disease**
ASA IV	**Disease - a threat to life**
ASA V	Moribund patient

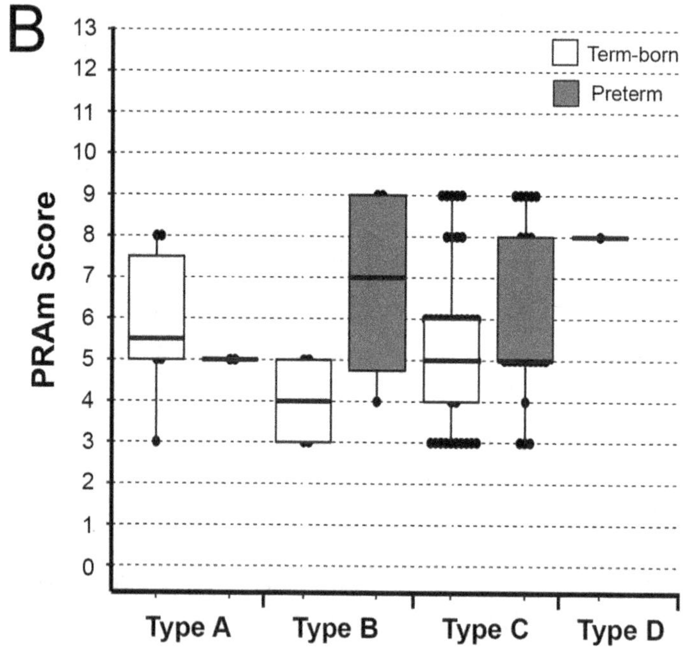

Value	Definition
+1	Urgent Surgical Procedure
+2	At least 1 comorbidity
+3	≥ 1 indication of critical illness
+3	<12 months age at time of surgery
+4	Surgical procedure with neoplasm or preoperative chemotherapy
* Values are added and scored 0-13.	

FIGURE 3 | Underlying Disease Severity Stratification in Esophageal Atresia Cohort. Graphs illustrate incidence of American Society of Anesthesiologists (ASA) Physical Status classification **(A)** and Pediatric Risk Assessment (PRAm) severity scores **(B)** in infants born with esophageal atresia (EA) that underwent primary repair at a single institution from 2009-2020 ($n = 84$). Definition of scoring is shown in summary tables on the right for both the ASA Physical Status (16) and PRAm scoring (17–19). Graphs show stratification by anatomical types of EA (type A-D) and gestational age (term-born and premature; see Methods section). Specifically, all patients in this study were rated as either ASA Physical Status III or IV **(A)**. For the most common *type C* EA, the majority of term-born patients had ASA III status (27/42; 64%), while the majority of premature infants were assigned ASA IV status (19/25; 76%) implicating premature infants were more critically ill in the most common type of EA, *type C*. Graph in **(B)** illustrates distribution of PRAm scores per anatomical type and gestational age. Considering all infants had surgery when <12 months of age, the minimal score was 3. Since none of the infants had co-existing malignancy, the highest score was 9. From the graph in **(B)**, one can infer that premature infants had higher median score for type B EA, but lower median score for type C (thick horizontal line). Individual values are represented as dots, boxes span the interquartile range (IQR) (first and third quartile), and whiskers represent maximum and minimum values.

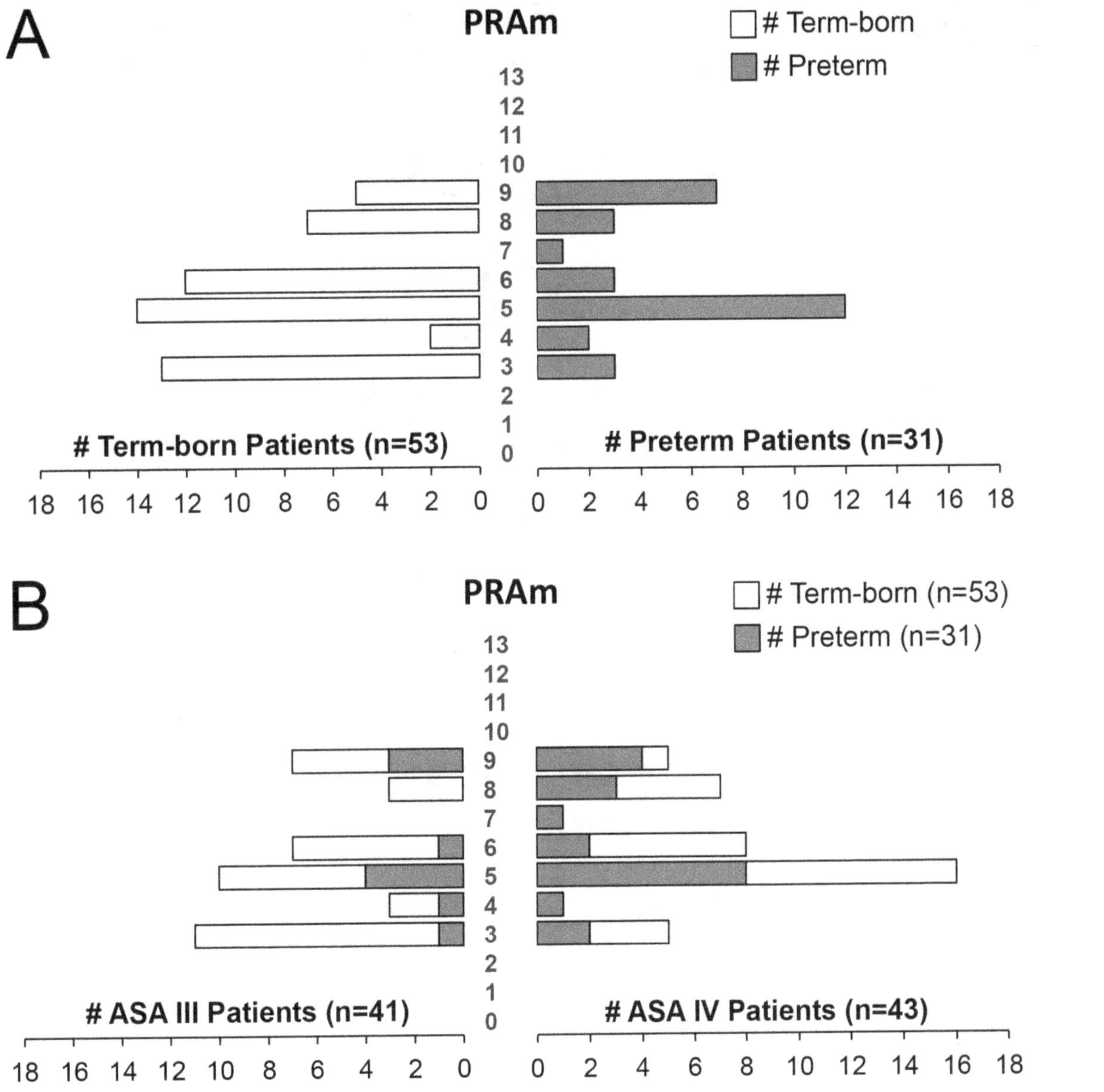

FIGURE 4 | Pediatric Risk Assessment (PRAm) Scores in a Retrospective Cohort of Infants Born with Esophageal Atresia. **(A)** Shows PRAm scores of term-born (left) and preterm patients (right) illustrating a wide range of PRAm score across gestational age of infants born with esophageal atresia (EA; $n = 84$). Note a subtle tendency of term-born patients for lower, and premature patients for higher PRAm scores. **(B)** Plots PRAm scores in relation to American Society of Anesthesiologists (ASA) Physical Status Classification. Despite more premature infants having had higher ASA IV classification (21/31; 68%) in comparison to term-born (22/53; 41%; see also **Figure 3A**), PRAm score shows wide distribution of scores between 3 and 9. Such outlining is in support of ASA and not PRAm scoring in assessing disease severity when gestational age is the primary factor.

Mortality Risk Assessment II

The second scoring system by Spitz et al. (20) takes into account (i) birth weight and (ii) co-existence and (iii) severity of cardiac congenital anomalies. The risk is described as low (I), moderate (II), and high (III) risk of mortality. Although our retrospective cohort has lower power ($n = 84$) in comparison to previous decades' reports: 1980–1992 ($n = 372$) (20) and 1993–2004 ($n = 188$) (27), we report improved survival rates (**Table 4**), especially for low risk group (I; 100%; 62/62) and moderate risk group (II) of 90% (19/21). This data are in stark contrast to moderate risk group (II) survival rates of 59% (41/70) during 1980s (1980–1992) (20) and 82% (41/50) survival rate in the following decade (1993–2004) (27). Since our cohort only had only one patient that met criteria for group III - in part due to the exclusion criteria of extremely premature patients (<28 weeks), future clinical studies are needed to evaluate group III survival rates at our institution.

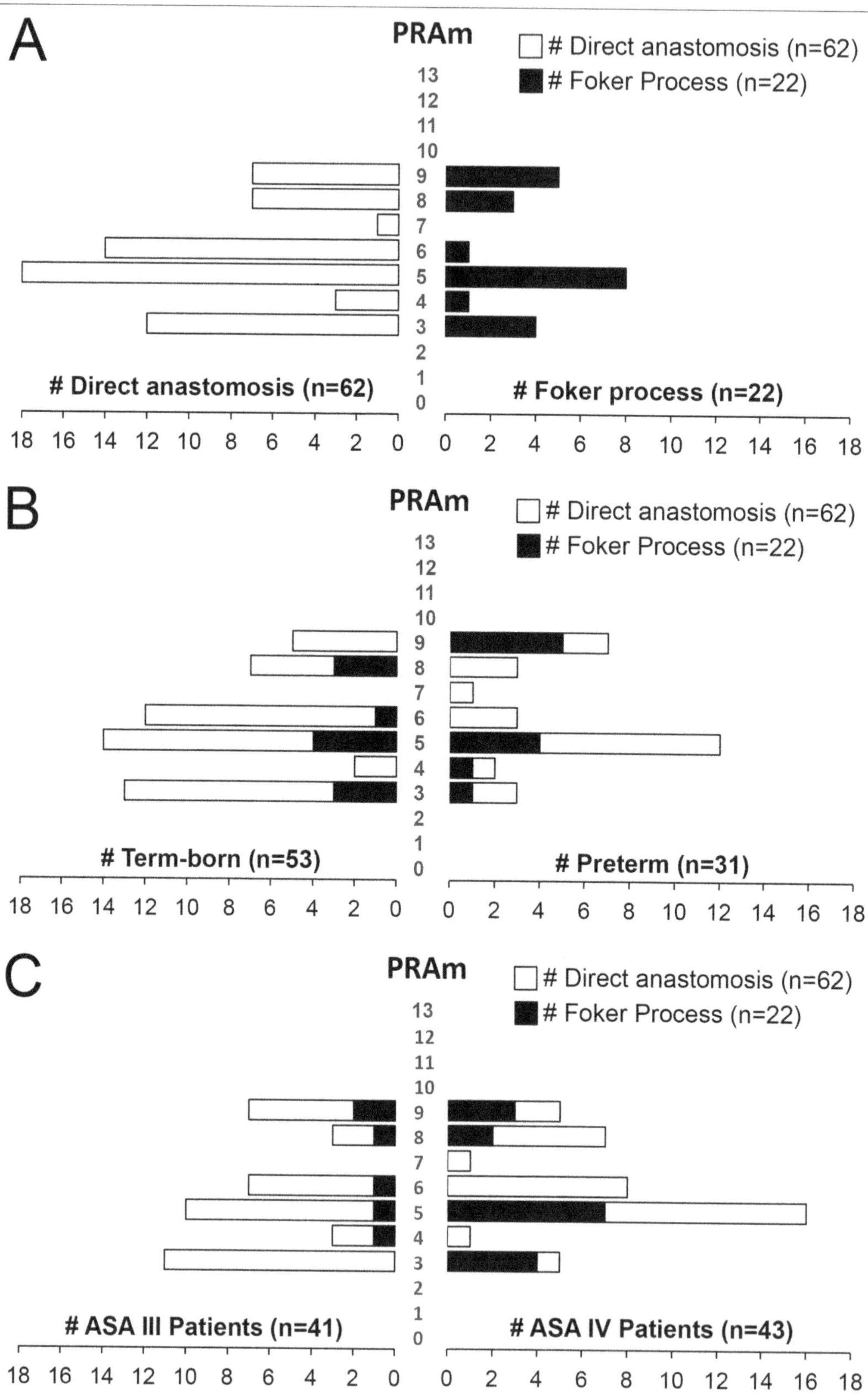

FIGURE 5 | Disease Severity Stratification of Infants Born with Esophageal Atresia by Type of Surgical Repair. **(A)** Illustrates wide distribution of Pediatric Risk Assessment (PRAm) scores (from scores 3–9) by the type of surgical repair: (i) direct anastomosis for *short-gap* esophageal atresia (EA) repair (left), and (ii) Foker process (5–8) for *long-gap* EA repair (right). **(B)** Summarizes severity of disease per type of surgical repair in relation to the gestation age at birth. Similar to data in **Figure 4A**, note the subtle tendency of term-born patients having had lower, and premature patients higher PRAm scores. When PRAm scores are graphed in relation to American Society of Anesthesiologists (ASA) physical status **(C)**, we report more infants with *long-gap* EA with an ASA IV classification (73%; 16/22).

TABLE 3 | Mortality risk assessment I.

Group	Definition	1951–1959 (21) (n = 113)	2009–2020 (n = 84)
A	Birth weight >2.5 kg	36/38 (95%)	2/2 (100%)
B	1.8 kg <Birth weight <2.5 kg or >2.5 kg with moderate congenital anomaly and/or pneumonia	29/43 (68%)	42/42 (100%)
C	Birth weight <1.8 kg or >2.5 kg with a severe congenital anomaly and/or pneumonia	2/32 (6%)	38/40 (95%)

Survival rates of infants born with esophageal atresia according to scores by Waterson et al. *Using a modified Waterston et al. protocol (21), patients born with esophageal atresia (EA) were stratified into 3 categories* ***(A–C)*** *of mortality risk based on birth weight, co-existing anomalies, and presence or absence of pneumonia. The risk is described as low* ***(A)****, moderate* ***(B)****, and high* ***(C)*** *risk of mortality. Previously reported incidence of survival rates for EA patients (1951–1959) (21) is shown along with the current cohort's survival rates (2009–2020). Our results demonstrate increased survival, especially for group with moderate and higher mortality risk, groups B and C, respectively.*

TABLE 4 | Mortality risk assessment II.

Group	Definition	1980–1992 (20) (n = 372)	1993–2004 (27) (n = 188)	2009–2020 (n = 84)
I	Birth weight >1.5 kg and no major cardiac anomaly	283/293 (97%)	130/132 (98.5%)	62/62 (100%)
II	Birth weight <1.5 kg or major cardiac anomaly	41/70 (59%)	41/50 (82%)	19/21 (90%)
III	Birth weight <1.5 kg and major cardiac anomaly	2/9 (22%)	3/6 (50%)	1/1 (100%)

Survival Rates Assessment of Infants Born with Esophageal Atresia According to Scores by Spitz et al. *Using the Spitz et al. protocol (20), patients born with esophageal atresia (EA) were stratified into three categories of mortality risk based on birth weight, and the presence and severity of cardiac anomaly. Major cardiac anomalies were defined as one that required medical or surgical treatment. The risk is described as low* ***(I)****, moderate* ***(II)****, and high* ***(III)*** *risk of mortality. Spitz's original incidence of survival rates of EA patients for two separate decades, (1980–1992) (20) and (1993–2004) (27), are shown along with the current cohort's survival rates (2009–2020). Our results demonstrate increased survival, especially for low and moderate mortality risk groups.*

DICUSSION

Our novel results using retrospective approach from a single institution show near equal distribution of sex and gestational age (term-born vs. premature) by anatomical type of EA (types A–D) and by type of surgical repair (direct anastomosis vs. Foker process). We also share the incidence of co-occurring congenital anomalies with EA, with special emphasis on cardiac anomalies that have been shown to be a major mortality risk factor for infants born with EA (20). Although PRAm score showed a wider range of disease severity (3–9), ASA scores (III and IV) are more useful in predicting disease severity. We also report increased survival rate in our EA cohort in comparison to the literature in previous decades.

Limitations of the Retrospective Chart Review

In keeping with the retrospective study design (28), data collected were originally intended for reasons other than research (29, 30). Due to the dependence of patient information stored for clinical practice, retrospective analysis may represent incomplete or missing documentation, poorly recorded or absent chart information, as well as difficult identification of desired patient data [e.g., attainment of PRAm scores (17) for cases of EA repair prior to 2017].

Study Size

Despite the exclusion of cases with extreme prematurity, and surgical repair at an outside institution, this study retained a moderate sample size with enough power to evaluate EA disease characteristics. The main challenges imposed with the exclusion criteria are that of generalizability since our institution represents a highly specialized level of care.

High-Risk Mortality Scores

Mortality risk assessment scores were quantified according to the scores previously described in the literature by Waterston et al. (21), and Spitz et al. (20). For both types of scoring, the high-risk groups used very low birth weights as surrogates for extreme prematurity. For this study, we defined Waterston risk assessment for the highest risk group (group C) as either (i) a low birth weight (associated with prematurity) or (ii) a standard birthweight with severe congenital anomaly or severe pneumonia. Therefore, analysis of Waterston et al. (21) group C was likely not significantly impacted by the exclusion of extreme prematurity. In contrast, the Spitz risk assessment required a birth weight <1.5 kg for the highest risk group (group III) for which only one patient from our retrospective cohort met criteria. Therefore, risk assessment of group III of the Spitz et al. (20) classification is not powered in our retrospective study.

Characteristics of Esophageal Atresia Cohort

Anatomical Types of Esophageal Atresia

We report similar distribution of EA patients according to the anatomical classification (**Figure 1A**) compared to the literature (4, 31, 32) although one should keep in mind that definition of long-gap EA might differ. Our slightly increased incidence for type A and type B EA could be explained by the fact that data was obtained from a single institution, which pioneered the Foker process (5–8) for repair of *long-gap* EA (9) and receives patients locally, nationally and internationally. Indeed, we report higher incidence of *long-gap* EA in more rare types of EA: types A and type B, despite type C having the highest number of *long-gap* EA patients in this cohort (**Figure 1D**). The definitions for *long-gap* EA have not been agreed upon and can confound the comparison of data within the literature. Currently, a common method of classification is to simply define types A and B as *long-gap EA* and all others as *short-gap* EA (33, 34). The presence of long-gap EA patients with type C EA (**Figure 1D**) is in direct contrast to those studies that classify *long-gap* EA by purely anatomical classification. However, Ure et al. in 1995 (35) reported a total of 9 long-gap EA patients and a majority of them having type C EA. Study by Donoso et al. in 2016 (34) reported that a single patient with type

C EA underwent *long-gap* EA repair despite being classified as *short-gap* in their study. Due to the inconsistency in the literature, we defined *long-gap* EA by surgical procedure [viz. Foker process (5–8)] implicating complex perioperative critical care instead of anatomical definitions based on the location of the EA gap.

Sex Distribution

We report nearly equal sex distribution for the entire cohort ($n = 84$), which is consistent with previous large retrospective reports (36–39). Since sex distribution for EA patients was only reported for the entire cohort (34, 39–41), we indicate - for the first time - that there is nearly equal sex distribution in EA patients by anatomical types (**Figure 1C**). We also report equal sex distribution for *long-gap* EA patients, which is in accordance with previous report in a larger cohort (9). Findings of equal sex distribution indicate that there is possibly no sex preference in infants born with EA - the subject of interest that continues to be investigated.

Distribution as Per Gestational Age

Our study found a slightly higher incidence of term-born patients in comparison to premature infants (28–37 weeks of gestation) with EA (**Figures 2A,B**). This finding stands in contrast to a large national cohort study of EA that included all gestational ages and found a higher prevalence of EA in premature patients (39). This discrepancy could be explained, in part, by our exclusion criteria that eliminated extremely premature patients from the cohort. However, our findings of higher incidence of term-born patients are consistent with the national studies in France (41) and Italy (40) reporting similar results. While the incidence of gestational age in *long-gap* EA patients are reported in the literature (6, 42), our novel results outline incidence of *long-gap* EA by anatomical types (**Figure 1B**). Discrepancy among gestational age within EA studies and novel findings of gestational age distribution in *long-gap* EA patients (with exclusion of extreme prematurity) suggests the need for future analysis to discern demographics of prematurity, as it represents an important risk factor in hospital mortality (43).

Incidence of Associated Congenital Anomalies and Comorbidities With Esophageal Atresia

Congenital co-anomalies with EA can present as a wide spectrum across multiple organ systems (26), and can pose a challenge for care of infants with EA with increased risk of mortality and morbidity (44).

VACTERL Syndrome

The incidence of VACTERL association in this cohort was high at 37% compared to the literature report at around 10% (44) (**Table 1A**). Higher incidences of VACTERL syndrome in our report has previously been recognized in other studies (9) and is likely due to recognized differences in VACTERL diagnostics (45). Our cohort was comprised of sicker infants due to the very low incidence of isolated EA at 12% (**Table 1B**) compared to very large cross-hospital findings of isolated EA at 45% (36), 57.3% (37), and 38.7% (38) at other institutions. Findings of increased incidence of VACTERL and other comorbidities in this study possibly reflects institutional reputation as a national and international referral center for infants born with EA. Our report of higher incidence of VACTERL patients in *short-gap* EA are in accordance with previous report from our institution (9). This is in contrast to the study from Tabriz Children's Hospital and Tehran Mofid Hospital in Iran that reported no difference in incidence of VACTERL spectrum defects irrespective of the type of surgical repair required (42). The analysis of etiology of VACTERL syndrome is outside the scope of this study but is described well in the literature (25, 45, 46) and continues to be investigated.

Congenital Cardiac Anomalies

It is well known that co-occurring cardiac anomalies can impact the length and complexity of care for EA patients (41). We identified that most EA patients had co-existing cardiac anomalies: 86% for the entire cohort (**Table 2A**) and 79% in the non-syndromic cases (**Table 1C**). This is consistent with literature report from the Children's Hospital of Chongqing Medical University, China (71.2%) (47) and a large multicenter study of EA patients across 43 hospitals (70%) (43). We and others (48) report that a great majority of co-existing cardiac anomalies were defined as simple. We also report, for the first time, that only about a fifth of EA patients with co-existing cardiac anomalies had undergone cardiac repair - of which majority were type C EA cases (**Table 2A**). Our novel data in infants with *long-gap* EA show having nearly equal incidence of cardiac co-anomalies compared to the entire cohort with a similar incidence of patients requiring cardiac surgery (**Table 2B**). Our results confirm that (i) non-syndromic patients with EA may present with additional and potentially life-threatening congenital anomalies and that (ii) infants with non-syndromic *long-gap* EA can have cardiac anomalies imposing additional risk to their care (20, 41).

Perioperative Risk Assessment

Underlying Disease Severity

Despite wider PRAm score variability (score 3-9; **Figure 4A**) and the same PRAm median score of 5 irrespective of the gestational age (**Figure 3B**), ASA Physical Status classification remains a golden standard in assessing underlying disease severity. We only noted a trend in term-born patients toward propensity for lower PRAm scores irrespective of the surgical type, while premature patients with *long-gap* EA showed propensity for higher PRAm scores (**Figure 5B**). Latter trends are in alignment with the seminal report in literature of a large cohort of infants undergoing non-cardiac surgery, validating PRAm scoring in predicting perioperative risk (17). Future work should also analyze unique risk factors related to surgical type of EA repair (viz. direct anastomosis vs. Foker process; open vs. laparoscopic approach) to expand on previous risk stratification of patients born with EA (49, 50). Morbidity risk assessment should also possibly include assessment of the neurological findings as our recent pilot study of infants with *long-gap* EA reported incidental brain findings for not only premature but term-born infants following Foker process repair ($n = 13$/group) (12, 15, 51, 52).

Mortality Risk Assessment

We report increased survival rates in this cohort as per two different mortality risk assessment scores. Despite our modification to the scoring schema by Waterston et al. (21), we report the total survival rates have vastly improved in the last decade for each of the described Waterston risk groups (**Table 3**). In addition, Spitz et al. (20) extended Waterston's mortality risk score in 1994 by including co-existing cardiac anomalies with EA. Indeed, the latter mortality risk score represents the most widely used mortality risk stratification that continues to be used for assessing risk in EA patients (27, 34). According to the most recent study of mortality predictors, major congenital heart disease was a significant predictor, while birth weight <1.5 kg was not (53). Indeed, we report increased survival rates in the most recent decade (2009–2020; **Table 4**) when compared to 1980s (20) and 1990s (27, 34) as previously published by Spitz et al. (20, 27). Such data are in support of great improvements in perioperative critical care of EA patients and treatment of their comorbidities, which may account for our reporting of improved survival. As per literature recommendation, the preferred clinical management of infants born with EA should be aided by highly specialized multidisciplinary team at expert centers (54) to help increase survival and decrease the incidence of morbidities (55). Therefore, improved outcomes in this report may be explained – in part, by the highly specialized nature of *The Esophageal and Airway Treatment Center* at our institution. Increased survival rates over the last decade suggest a potential need to assess unique operative and perioperative risks in this unique population of patients, as well as non-survival metrics such as functional status and quality of life.

Last, but not least, previous reports also suggests that extremely low birth weight infants with EA patients are at a higher risk of mortality (56), while a recent study showed potentially improved outcomes for extremely low birth-weight infants that underwent a staged repair for EA (57). Analysis of survival rates of extremely low birth weight infants with EA, especially those that underwent the Foker process for *long-gap* EA repair is needed to validate and potentially expand on these and our findings.

CONCLUSIONS

We present a comprehensive analysis of EA patient classification by anatomical types (type A-D) and by surgical repair type (direct anastomosis vs. Foker process for *short-gap* vs. *long-gap* EA, respectively). Despite a wider PRAm score distribution in infants born with EA, ASA scores remain the gold standard in assessing underlying disease severity stratification. With increase in survival rates over the last decade, future studies should be directed toward assessing unique aspects of EA group in the context of (i) severity of underlying disease with and without comorbidities, (ii) unique complexities of perioperative critical care (with and without prolonged sedation, repeated procedures, and infection/sepsis assessment), and (iii) survival metrics such as functional status (e.g., neurobehavioral outcomes and quality of life). It is our hope that this retrospective study will be of service to research community when designing future clinical studies of risks and outcomes in this uniquely vulnerable population of infant patients.

AUTHOR CONTRIBUTIONS

Authorship credit was based on substantial contribution to (1) the conception and manuscript design (DE, JW, and DB), (2) acquisition (DE, JW, RJ, and DB), analysis (DE and DB), or interpretation of data (all authors), drafting the article (DE and DB) or critical revision for important intellectual content (all authors), (3) final approval of the version to be published (all authors), and (4) are accountable for all aspects of the work in ensuring that questions related to the accuracy or integrity of any part of the work are appropriately investigated and resolved (all authors).

FUNDING

The Boston Children's Hospital 2019 OFD/BTREC/CTREC Faculty Career Development Fellowship, and 2017 Trailblazer Award from the Department of Anesthesiology, Critical Care and Pain Medicine, Boston Children's Hospital supported this work (DB). The content of this article is solely the responsibility of the authors and does not necessarily represent the official views of the funders.

ACKNOWLEDGMENTS

The authors gratefully acknowledge (1) Quality Improvement Consultants, John J. Bennett, BS, MHA, and Heather B. Riley, MS, for their help with accessing *The Esophageal and Airway Treatment Center* REDCap data base; (2) Mark Breibart, Director of Anesthesia Information Technology from Department of Anesthesiology, Critical Care and Pain Medicine, Boston Children's Hospital for his help in obtaining PRAm scores; (3) Mackenzie S. Kagan, BS for help with graphs editing.

REFERENCES

1. Sfeir R, Michaud L, Salleron J, Gottrand F. Epidemiology of esophageal atresia. *Dis Esophagus.* (2013) 26:354–5. doi: 10.1111/dote.12051
2. Moore, KL, Persaud, TVN, Torchia, MG. Alimentary System. In Moore KL, Persaud TVN, Torchia MG, editors. *The Developing Human: Clinically Oriented Embryology.* London: Elsevier India (2012), p. 193–221. Available online at: https://www.elsevier.com/books/the-developing-human-clinically-oriented-embryology-9e/moore/978-81-312-3505-8
3. Pinheiro PF. Simões e Silva AC, Pereira RM. Current knowledge on esophageal atresia. *World J Gastroenterol.* (2012) 18:3662–72. doi: 10.3748/wjg.v18.i28.3662

4. Gross RE. *The Surgery of Infancy and Childhood: its principles and techniques.* Philadelphia, London: WB Saunders (1953).
5. Foker JE, Linden BC, Boyle EM Jr. Marquardt C. Development of a true primary repair for the full spectrum of esophageal atresia. *Ann Surg.* (1997) 226:533–41; discussion 41-3. doi: 10.1097/00000658-199710000-00014
6. Bairdain S, Hamilton TE, Smithers CJ, Manfredi M, Ngo P, Gallagher D, et al. Foker process for the correction of long gap esophageal atresia: primary treatment versus secondary treatment after prior esophageal surgery. *J Pediatr Surg.* (2015) 50:933–7. doi: 10.1016/j.jpedsurg.2015.03.010
7. Kunisaki SM, Foker JE. Surgical advances in the fetus and neonate: esophageal atresia. *Clin Perinatol.* (2012) 39:349–61. doi: 10.1016/j.clp.2012.04.007
8. Foker JE, Kendall Krosch TC, Catton K, Munro F, Khan KM. Long-gap esophageal atresia treated by growth induction: the biological potential and early follow-up results. *Semin Pediatr Surg.* (2009) 18:23–9. doi: 10.1053/j.sempedsurg.2008.10.005
9. Bairdain S, Zurakowski D, Vargas SO, Stenquist N, McDonald M, Towne MC, et al. Long-gap esophageal atresia is a unique entity within the esophageal atresia defect spectrum. *Neonatology.* (2017) 111:140–4. doi: 10.1159/000449241
10. Holland AJ, Fitzgerald DA. Oesophageal atresia and tracheo-oesophageal fistula: current management strategies and complications. *Paediatr Respir Rev.* (2010) 11:100–6; quiz 6–7. doi: 10.1016/j.prrv.2010.01.007
11. Harrington AW, Riebold J, Hernandez K, Staffa SJ, Svetanoff WJ, Zurakowski D, et al. Nutrition delivery and growth outcomes in infants with long-gap esophageal atresia who undergo the Foker process. *J Pediatr Surg.* (2021) 56:2133–39. doi: 10.1016/j.jpedsurg.2021.07.014
12. Mongerson CRL, Wilcox SL, Goins SM, Pier DB, Zurakowski D, Jennings RW, et al. Infant Brain Structural MRI Analysis in the Context of Thoracic Non-cardiac Surgery and Critical Care. *Front Pediatrics.* (2019) 7:315. doi: 10.3389/fped.2019.00315
13. Hodkinson DJ, Mongerson CRL, Jennings RW, Bajic D. Neonatal functional brain maturation in the context of perioperative critical care and pain management: a case report. *Heliyon.* (2019) 5:e02350-e. doi: 10.1016/j.heliyon.2019.e02350
14. Solodiuk JC, Jennings RW, Bajic D. Evaluation of postnatal sedation in full-term infants. *Brain Sci.* (2019) 9:114. doi: 10.3390/brainsci9050114
15. Rudisill SS, Wang JT, Jaimes C, Mongerson CRL, Hansen AR, Jennings RW, et al. Neurologic injury and brain growth in the setting of long-gap esophageal atresia perioperative critical care: a pilot study. *Brain Sci.* (2019) 9:383. doi: 10.3390/brainsci9120383
16. Abouleish AE, Leib ML, Cohen NH. ASA Provides Examples to Each ASA Physical Status Class. *ASA Newsl.* (2015) 79:38–49. Available online at: https://www.asahq.org/standards-and-guidelines/asa-physical-status-classification-system
17. Nasr VG, DiNardo JA, Faraoni D. Development of a pediatric risk assessment score to predict perioperative mortality in children undergoing noncardiac surgery. *Anesth Analg.* (2017) 124:1514–9. doi: 10.1213/ANE.0000000000001541
18. Valencia E, Staffa SJ, Faraoni D, DiNardo JA, Nasr VG. Prospective external validation of the pediatric risk assessment score in predicting perioperative mortality in children undergoing noncardiac surgery. *Anesth Analg.* (2019) 129:1014–20. doi: 10.1213/ANE.0000000000004197
19. Nasr VG, Valencia E, Staffa SJ, Faraoni D, DiNardo JA, Berry JG, et al. Comprehensive risk assessment of morbidity in pediatric patients undergoing noncardiac surgery: an institutional experience. *Anesth Analg.* (2020) 131:1607–15. doi: 10.1213/ANE.0000000000005157
20. Spitz L, Kiely EM, Morecroft JA, Drake DP. Oesophageal atresia: at-risk groups for the 1990s. *J Pediatr Surg.* (1994) 29:723–5. doi: 10.1016/0022-3468(94)90354-9
21. Waterston DJ, Carter RE, Aberdeen E. Oesophageal atresia: tracheo-oesophageal fistula. A study of survival in 218 infants. *Lancet.* (1962) 1:819–22. doi: 10.1016/S0140-6736(62)91837-8
22. Evanovich DM. Retrospective *Analysis of Disease Severity Stratification in Infants Born with Esophageal Atresia at a Single Institution: [Masters in Biomedical Science Thesis].* Boston (MA): Tufts University School of Medicine (2021).
23. Till H, Muensterer OJ, Rolle U, Foker J. Staged esophageal lengthening with internal and subsequent external traction sutures leads to primary repair of an ultralong gap esophageal atresia with upper pouch tracheoesophagel fistula. *J Pediatr Surg.* (2008) 43:E33–5. doi: 10.1016/j.jpedsurg.2008.02.009
24. Svetanoff WJ, Zendejas B, Hernandez K, Davidson K, Ngo P, Manfredi M, et al. Contemporary outcomes of the Foker process and evolution of treatment algorithms for long-gap Esophageal Atresia. *J Pediatr Surg.* (2021) 56:2180–91. doi: 10.1016/j.jpedsurg.2021.02.054
25. Shaw-Smith C. Oesophageal atresia, tracheo-oesophageal fistula, and the VACTERL association: review of genetics and epidemiology. *J Med Genet.* (2006) 43:545–54. doi: 10.1136/jmg.2005.038158
26. Brown AK, Roddam AW, Spitz L, Ward SJ. Oesophageal atresia, related malformations, and medical problems: a family study. *Am J Med Genet.* (1999) 85:31–7. doi: 10.1002/(sici)1096-8628(19990702)85:1<31::aid-ajmg7>3.0.co;2-d
27. Lopez PJ, Keys C, Pierro A, Drake DP, Kiely EM, Curry JI, et al. Oesophageal atresia: improved outcome in high-risk groups? *J Pediatr Surg.* (2006) 41:331–4. doi: 10.1016/j.jpedsurg.2005.11.009
28. Gearing RE, Mian IA, Barber J, Ickowicz A. A methodology for conducting retrospective chart review research in child and adolescent psychiatry. *J Can Acad Child Adolesc Psychiatry.* (2006) 15:126–34.
29. Hess DR. Retrospective studies and chart reviews. *Respir Care.* (2004) 49:1171–4.
30. Jansen AC, van Aalst-Cohen ES, Hutten BA, Büller HR, Kastelein JJ, Prins MH. Guidelines were developed for data collection from medical records for use in retrospective analyses. *J Clin Epidemiol.* (2005) 58:269–74. doi: 10.1016/j.jclinepi.2004.07.006
31. Spitz L. Oesophageal atresia. *Orphanet J Rare Dis.* (2007) 2:24. doi: 10.1186/1750-1172-2-24
32. Vogt EC. Congenital esophageal atresia. *Am J Roentgenol.* (1929) 22:463–5.
33. Deurloo JA, Ekkelkamp S, Hartman EE, Sprangers MA, Aronson DC. Quality of life in adult survivors of correction of esophageal atresia. *Arch Surg.* (2005) 140:976–80. doi: 10.1001/archsurg.140.10.976
34. Donoso F, Kassa AM, Gustafson E, Meurling S, Lilja HE. Outcome and management in infants with esophageal atresia - a single centre observational study. *J Pediatr Surg.* (2016) 51:1421–5. doi: 10.1016/j.jpedsurg.2016.03.010
35. Ure BM, Slany E, Eypasch EP, Gharib M, Holschneider AM, Troidl H. Long-term functional results and quality of life after colon interposition for long-gap oesophageal atresia. *Eur J Pediatr Surg.* (1995) 5:206–10. doi: 10.1055/s-2008-1066206
36. Depaepe A, Dolk H, Lechat MF. The epidemiology of tracheo-oesophageal fistula and oesophageal atresia in Europe. EUROCAT Working Group. *Arch Dis Child.* (1993) 68:743–8. doi: 10.1136/adc.68.6.743
37. Robert E, Mutchinick O, Mastroiacovo P, Knudsen LB, Kjersti Daltveit A, Castilla EE, et al. An international collaborative study of the epidemiology of esophageal atresia or stenosis. *Reproduct Toxicol.* (1993) 7:405–21. doi: 10.1016/0890-6238(93)90085-L
38. Torfs CP, Curry CJ, Bateson TF. Population-based study of tracheoesophageal fistula and esophageal atresia. *Teratology.* (1995) 52:220–32. doi: 10.1002/tera.1420520408
39. Wang B, Tashiro J, Allan BJ, Sola JE, Parikh PP, Hogan AR, et al. A nationwide analysis of clinical outcomes among newborns with esophageal atresia and tracheoesophageal fistulas in the United States. *J Surg Res.* (2014) 190:604–12. doi: 10.1016/j.jss.2014.04.033
40. Cassina M, Ruol M, Pertile R, Midrio P, Piffer S, Vicenzi V, et al. Prevalence, characteristics, and survival of children with esophageal atresia: a 32-year population-based study including 1,417,724 consecutive newborns. *Birth Defects Res A Clin Mol Teratol.* (2016) 106:542–8. doi: 10.1002/bdra.23493
41. Sfeir R, Bonnard A, Khen-Dunlop N, Auber F, Gelas T, Michaud L, et al. Esophageal atresia: data from a national cohort. *J Pediatr Surg.* (2013) 48:1664–9. doi: 10.1016/j.jpedsurg.2013.03.075
42. Aslanabadi S, Ghabili K, Rouzrokh M, Hosseini MB, Jamshidi M, Adl FH, et al. Associated congenital anomalies between neonates with short-gap and long-gap esophageal atresia: a comparative study. *Int J Gen Med.* (2011) 4:487–91. doi: 10.2147/IJGM.S19301
43. Sulkowski JP, Cooper JN, Lopez JJ, Jadcherla Y, Cuenot A, Mattei P, et al. Morbidity and mortality in patients with esophageal atresia. *Surgery.* (2014) 156:483–91. doi: 10.1016/j.surg.2014.03.016
44. Stoll C, Alembik Y, Dott B, Roth MP. Associated malformations in

patients with esophageal atresia. *Eur J Med Genet.* (2009) 52:287–90. doi: 10.1016/j.ejmg.2009.04.004

45. Brosens E, Ploeg M, van Bever Y, Koopmans AE, Ijsselstijn H, Rottier RJ, et al. Clinical and etiological heterogeneity in patients with tracheo-esophageal malformations and associated anomalies. *Eur J Med Gene.* (2014) 57:440–52. doi: 10.1016/j.ejmg.2014.05.009
46. Shaw-Smith C. Genetic factors in esophageal atresia. tracheo-esophageal fistula and the VACTERL association: roles for FOXF1 and the 16q241 FOX transcription factor gene cluster, and review of the literature. *Eur J Med Gene.* (2010) 53:6–13. doi: 10.1016/j.ejmg.2009.10.001
47. Li XW, Jiang YJ, Wang XQ, Yu JL, Li LQ. A scoring system to predict mortality in infants with esophageal atresia: a case-control study. *Medicine (Baltimore).* (2017) 96:e7755. doi: 10.1097/MD.0000000000007755
48. Rokitansky A, Kolankaya A, Bichler B, Mayr J, Menardi G. Analysis of 309 cases of esophageal atresia for associated congenital malformations. *Am J Perinatol.* (1994) 11:123–8. doi: 10.1055/s-2007-994571
49. Faraoni D, Zou X, DiNardo JA, Nasr VG. Integration of the intrinsic surgical risk with patient comorbidities and severity of congenital cardiac disease does not improve risk stratification in children undergoing noncardiac surgery. *Anesth Analg.* (2020) 131:1083–9. doi: 10.1213/ANE.0000000000004906
50. Nasr VG, Staffa SJ, Zurakowski D, DiNardo JA, Faraoni D. Pediatric risk stratification is improved by integrating both patient comorbidities and intrinsic surgical risk. *Anesthesiology.* (2019) 130:971–80. doi: 10.1097/ALN.0000000000002659
51. Mongerson CRL, Jaimes C, Zurakowski D, Jennings RW, Bajic D. Infant corpus callosum size after surgery and critical care for long-gap esophageal atresia: qualitative and quantitative MRI. *Sci Rep.* (2020) 10:6408. doi: 10.1038/s41598-020-63212-3
52. Bajic D, Rudisill SS, Jennings RW. Head circumference in infants undergoing Foker process for long-gap esophageal atresia repair: Call for attention. *J Pediatr Surg.* (2021) 56:1564–9. doi: 10.1016/j.jpedsurg.2021.01.030
53. Lazow SP, Ben-Ishay O, Aribindi VK, Staffa SJ, Pluchinotta FR, Schecter SC, et al. Predictors of index admission mortality and morbidity in contemporary esophageal atresia patients. *J Pediatr Surg.* (2020) 55:2322–8. doi: 10.1016/j.jpedsurg.2020.02.005
54. van der Zee DC, Tytgat SHA, van Herwaarden MYA. Esophageal atresia and tracheo-esophageal fistula. *Semin Pediatr Surg.* (2017) 26:67–71. doi: 10.1053/j.sempedsurg.2017.02.004
55. van der Zee DC, van Herwaarden MYA, Hulsker CCC, Witvliet MJ, Tytgat SHA. Esophageal atresia and upper airway pathology. *Clin Perinatol.* (2017) 44:753–62. doi: 10.1016/j.clp.2017.08.002
56. Petrosyan M, Estrada J, Hunter C, Woo R, Stein J, Ford HR, et al. Esophageal atresia/tracheoesophageal fistula in very low-birth-weight neonates: improved outcomes with staged repair. *J Pediatr Surg.* (2009) 44:2278–81. doi: 10.1016/j.jpedsurg.2009.07.047
57. Oztan MO, Soyer T, Oztorun CI, Firinci B, Durakbaşa Ç U, Dokumcu Z, et al. Outcome of very low and low birth weight infants with esophageal atresia: results of the turkish esophageal atresia registry. *Eur J Pediatr Surg.* (2020) 31:226–35. doi: 10.1055/s-0040-1713663

25

Robotic-Assisted Bladder Neck Procedures for Incontinence in Pediatric Patients

Patricio C. Gargollo [1*] *and Lindsay A. White* [2]

[1] *Division of Pediatric Urology, The Mayo Clinic and Mayo Medical School, Rochester, MN, United States,* [2] *The University of Washington School of Medicine, Seattle, WA, United States*

***Correspondence:**
Patricio C. Gargollo
gargollo.patricio@mayo.edu*

Purpose: To review the current status of bladder neck procedures for incontinence in pediatric patients, focusing on the increasing role of robotic-assisted laparoscopic surgical techniques.

Methods: A comprehensive review of the literature on open and robotic-assisted bladder neck procedures was conducted, with a focus on articles published in the last 20 years. This data was subsequently compared with published results from robotic-assisted bladder neck reconstruction series completed at our institution.

Results: The principal bladder neck procedures for incontinence in pediatric patients include: Artificial Urinary Sphincter, Bladder Neck Sling, Bladder Neck Closure and Bladder Neck Reconstruction. Continence rates range from 60 to 100% with a lack of expert consensus on the preferred procedure (or combination of procedures). Robotic-assisted approaches are associated with longer operative times, especially early in the surgical experience, but demonstrate equivalent continence rates with potential benefits including: low intraoperative blood loss, improved cosmesis, and decreased intra-abdominal adhesion formation.

Conclusions: Robotic-assisted procedures of the bladder neck are safe, feasible, follow the same steps and principles as those of open surgery and produce equivalent continence rates. Robotic-assisted techniques can be adapted to a variety of bladder neck procedures and safely expanded to selected patients with previous open abdominal surgery.

Keywords: robotic surgery, urinary incontinence, bladder neck reconstruction, appendicovesicostomy, artificial urinary sphincter, bladder neck sling, bladder neck closure

INTRODUCTION

Minimally invasive techniques are at the forefront of urologic surgery. As advances in laparoscopic instrumentation and robotic technology continue, the use of these techniques in the pediatric population has expanded. Robotic-assisted procedures in the pediatric population are well established for nephrectomy, pyeloplasty, ureteral reimplantation, and bladder surgery, but the use of this technology remains limited in more complex reconstructive cases. Longer operative times are often cited as a barrier to the use of minimally invasive techniques in complex reconstruction, but it has been demonstrated that much of the difference in operative time can be mitigated with increased surgeon experience (1, 2). Even with longer operative times, advantages over open surgery may include lower intraoperative blood loss, decreased post-operative narcotic use, and superior cosmesis (3, 4). These benefits have the potential to be accentuated in the pediatric population due to the relatively confined working spaces and a heightened awareness of cosmesis. In addition, the potential for decreased intra-abdominal adhesion formation in laparoscopic and robotic procedures, as compared to open, cannot be discounted. In patient populations that are at high risk of undergoing multiple lifetime abdominal surgeries, the benefits of decreased adhesions could have significant implications in reducing both technical difficulty and operative time in re-operation (5, 6).

Furthermore, as the use of minimally invasive surgical techniques increases, so too does the pool of patients considered to be candidates for this approach. While previous open abdominal surgery (PAS) was traditionally considered a relative contraindication to a laparoscopic or robotic-assisted approach, emerging studies indicate safety and efficacy of complex robotic reconstructions in these populations (1). In this review, we will discuss the surgical interventions available for pediatric incontinence, the increasing role of robotic-assisted techniques, complex reconstruction of the bladder neck, and our cumulative experience and approach to treating these patients.

SURGICAL INTERVENTION FOR URINARY INCONTINENCE

Urine leakage in the absence of a detrusor contraction, regardless of the primary cause (exstrophy/epispadias, cloacal anomalies, or neurogenic bladder secondary to spinal cord injury or dysraphisms) is the definition of an incompetent urinary sphincter mechanism (7). The basic goal behind surgical procedures to address this incompetent sphincter mechanism is to tighten the bladder outlet. This can be achieved in many ways including: placement of an artificial urinary sphincter (AUS), placement of a bladder neck sling (BNS), bladder neck reconstruction (BNR), and bladder neck closure (BNC). We will review the current status of each of these surgical interventions for incontinence, and more specifically, how these procedures are being adapted for robotic-assisted laparoscopic surgery (RALS). Whether or not a concomitant bladder augmentation procedure should be performed with the procedures listed above is a highly contested topic and beyond the scope of this review, and thus will not be covered here.

ARTIFICIAL URINARY SPHINCTER

The AUS has been used for surgical intervention in pediatric incontinence for decades. The historical benefits of AUS placement include the ability to maintain the potential for spontaneous voiding, decreasing the percentage of patients required to complete obligatory clean intermittent catheterization (CIC), and the potential to delay, or avoid, fixed resistance procedures such as BNS, BNR, or BNC. Continence rates following AUS placement in the pediatric population have remained similar across decades with Simeoni et al. reporting overall success rates of 77% in 1996 (8) and Catti et al. demonstrating similar results with 73% of patients achieving continence in 2008 (9). Despite good continence, both studies also demonstrated relatively high complication rates, with device removal required in 19 and 20% of patients, respectively (8, 9). In addition, post-operative changes in detrusor dynamics following AUS placement are concerning as they have been shown to lead to renal failure in 16% of patients and the need for augmentation cystoplasty in 31% of patients (10).

In patients with previous surgery of the bladder neck or proximal urethra success rates of AUS placement become extremely variable. Castera et al. evaluated AUS placement in 49 patients with 67% of all patients achieving continence, but further comparison demonstrated that of patients with no previous surgery ($n = 25$), 86% achieved urinary continence, whereas only 37.5% of patients who had undergone prior bladder neck surgical procedures ($n = 8$) achieved continence (11). Ruiz et al. followed this study with examination of AUS placement in 23 patients without spina bifida, but with previous surgery of the bladder neck or proximal urethra and achieved continence in 87% of the 19 sphincters that remained in place (86.3% survival rate) (12). Levesque et al. looked beyond efficacy to evaluate long-term survival of the AUS in the pediatric population and found that the mean survival time of the prostheses was 12.5 years (95% CI, 10.3–14.6), and was independent of patient sex or incontinence etiology (13). In addition, Bauer conducted a meta-analysis encompassing 585 pediatric patients from reported series of AUS placement between 1996 and 2006 and found that 32% of patients voided spontaneously to completion without the aid of CIC, demonstrating that AUS may provide large advantages over other bladder outlet procedures for patients in which spontaneous voiding is a priority (10).

Recently, Moscardi et al. reported the first described case of robotic-assisted laparoscopic (RAL)-AUS placement in the pediatric population. The procedure was safely accomplished, and the patient remained continent between volitional voids at

Abbreviations: APV, Appendicovesicostomy; AUS, Artificial Urinary Sphincter; BNC, Bladder Neck Closure; BNR, Bladder Neck Reconstruction; BNS, Bladder Neck Sling; CIC, Clean Intermittent Catheterization; LM, Leadbetter/Mitchell; PAS, Previous open abdominal surgery; RAL-AUS, Robotic-assisted laparoscopic artificial urinary sphincter; RALS, Robotic-assisted laparoscopic surgery.

3-month follow-up (14). This report demonstrates that RAL-AUS placement is feasible in the pediatric population, which may be advantageous in facilitating concomitant intra-abdominal procedures, but further experience will be required to compare the safety, efficacy, and long-term outcomes, as it remains unclear if robotic-assistance will affect previously reported continence or complication rates.

BLADDER NECK SLING

Comparison of published data regarding the effectiveness of BNS for pediatric incontinence is challenging because most published series include patients with previous or concurrent procedures. In a review article from 2000, Kryger et al. reported overall continence for fascial sling placement varying from 40 to 100%, but with very limited follow-up (15). Snodgrass and colleagues completed BNS placement with appendicovesicostomy (APV) in 30 children with satisfactory continence (defined as 2 or fewer damp pads daily) achieved in 83% of patients (16). In addition, Snodgrass and Barber compared success rates of 34 consecutive patients with neurogenic incontinence receiving BNS alone and 37 patients receiving BNS plus Leadbetter-Mitchell (LM) BNR. They found that 46% of BNS alone cases did not require pads post-operatively whereas 82% of BNS plus LM BNR did not require pads (17). In addition, 6-month follow-up demonstrated that no patients had hydronephrosis and only 2 patients (BNS plus LM BNR) had transient low-grade reflux (grade I or II) on postoperative urodynamics, which resolved on subsequent studies 2 and 4 months later (17). It was initially believed that this may represent BNS superiority for preservation of the upper tracts, but this idea was later called into question by Grimsby et al. when they found that upon long-term assessment, 30% of these patients had postoperative vesicoureteral reflux (VUR)/hydronephrosis and 17% required ureteral reimplantation or subureteral injection of bulking agent (18). This further demonstrates the effects of limited clinical series and limited follow-up when comparing the success and long-term safety of BNS placement to alternative bladder outlet procedures.

These same confounders and limitations exist when comparing open vs. robotic-assisted BNS placement. Rare reports of BNS placement without concurrent BNR or APV exist, again making it difficult to compare to the open series described above. This author has extensive experience with RAL-BNS placement, but as this procedure is performed concurrently with BNR and APV, results will be discussed in subsequent sections. Finally, due to the superior continence rates now being achieved with BNS placement plus concurrent procedures, it is unlikely that the success of BNS alone will be able to be evaluated without these confounding factors.

BLADDER NECK CLOSURE

Closure of the bladder neck is perhaps the most radical option for achieving continence, as it is irreversible and requires compliance with obligatory CIC of a cutaneous stoma. Bergman et al. showed an 88% dry rate in a retrospective review of patients with mixed etiology incontinence who failed medical therapy and underwent bladder neck closure as their primary surgery (19). This is similar to findings by Liard et al. who evaluated 21 patients with BNC as primary surgical therapy and showed an 80% dry rate (20). Another retrospective study by Hoebeke et al. evaluated 17 children undergoing BNC and demonstrated a dry rate of 100% but difficulty with catheterization in 47% of patients (21). Kavanagh et al. more recently reviewed 28 consecutive patients undergoing BNC and found an initial success rate in 96.4% (27 of 28) of patients. Importantly, 68% of these patients had undergone previous unsuccessful bladder neck procedures, demonstrating safety and efficacy of BNC as a secondary surgical intervention, though a relatively high total surgical re-intervention rate of 39.3% (11 of 28) should be noted (22).

Robotic BNC has been reported in the literature (23), but all current reports include BNC as a concomitant procedure performed as part of a larger study. Murthy et al. preformed 4 RAL-BNC in conjunction with RAL-augmentation ileocystoplasty and APV with good short-term results, but updated interim results revealed that 3 of 4 RAL-BNC required further surgical intervention due to dehiscence (23). The feasibility of RAL-BNC is expected given the excellent exposure to the pelvis and bladder provided by a robotic-assisted approach, but to date published literature on RALS-BNC in the pediatric population is too limited to confirm safety, provide continence rates or compare to open series.

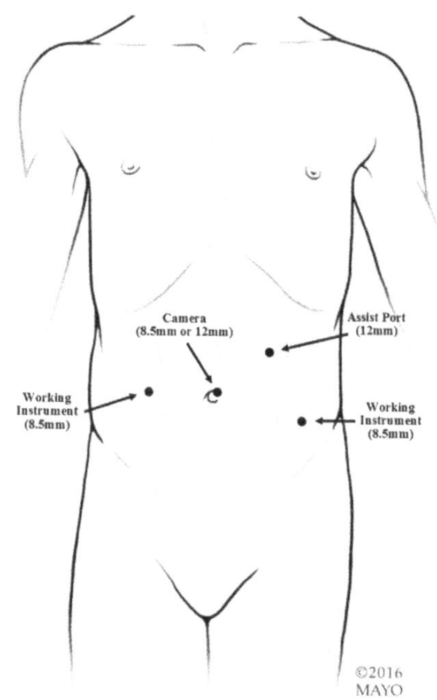

FIGURE 1 | Port placement. We use an 8.5-mm or 12-mm camera and two 8.5-mm working ports. If any bowel work is going to be performed or if a sling is going to be used, we suggest a 12-mm assist in the left upper quadrant. If just an APV is going to be performed, a 5-mm assist port can be used.

BLADDER NECK RECONSTRUCTION

Various reconstructive procedures and operative techniques are available to increase the resistance at the bladder outlet, including the Young-Dees Leadbetter (YDL), the Pippi-Salle, the Kropp repair, and the modified LM repair. To date, no single technique has demonstrated consistently superior outcomes, in large part due to multiple limitations of the published literature including: retrospective studies with significant confounders (various primary diagnoses, previous or concurrent procedures, use of augmentation cystoplasty), non-standardized protocols, and multiple definitions of what constitutes urinary continence. Cole et al. compared these techniques in a retrospective review of 49 continence procedures for patients with varying etiologies of incontinence and found continence rates of 79% for YDL and 75% for Kropp and Pippi-Salle repairs (24). Another retrospective review of 18 children with neurogenic incontinence showed a dry rate (4 h or more between catheterizations) of 61% following Pippi-Salle reconstruction (25). As previously described, Snodgrass and Barber were able to achieve 82% continence rate with LM BNR plus BNS with a mean follow-up of 13 months, with 60% still dry at maximum follow-up of 55 months (17). Despite the limitations in evaluation, these open BNR series demonstrate continence rates ranging from 50 to 85% (2).

Grimsby and colleagues reviewed the perioperative and short-term outcomes between 26 open and 19 RAL-BNRs. They found that while operative time was significantly longer in the robotic group (8.2 vs. 4.5 h, $p < 0.001$), there was no difference in length of stay (median 4 days), acute complications or continence outcomes (26). Re-operation rates were slightly less in the robotic group with 56% (14 patients) in the open group undergoing a total of 23 subsequent surgeries, compared to 42% (8 patients) in the robotic group undergoing 12 additional procedures ($p = 0.5$), although follow-up was longer in the open group (26). Operative time at re-operation was not reported in this study, but a previous report by the same authors comparing 28 open APVs and 39 RAL-APVs, found that while there was no difference in number of complications ($p = 0.788$) or number of re-operations ($p = 0.791$), the first re-operation had a significantly shorter operative time in the robotic group (6).

At our institution, the procedure of choice for management of neurogenic bladder with persistent urinary incontinence (despite CIC and anticholinergic therapy) includes creation of a RAL-APV (or Monti channel when the appendix is inadequate) and LM BNR along with BNS placement. This combination of procedures and the specific technique to complete them robotically was first described by this author in "Robotic-assisted bladder neck repair: feasibility and outcomes" in 2015, with relatively few adjustments made to the procedure since this date (2). Our RAL approach to BNR allows for minimal incisions, limited to an inverted "V"-shaped incision in the umbilicus, an assist port in the left upper quadrant and two 8.5-mm working ports, as represented in **Figure 1**. In addition, this technique

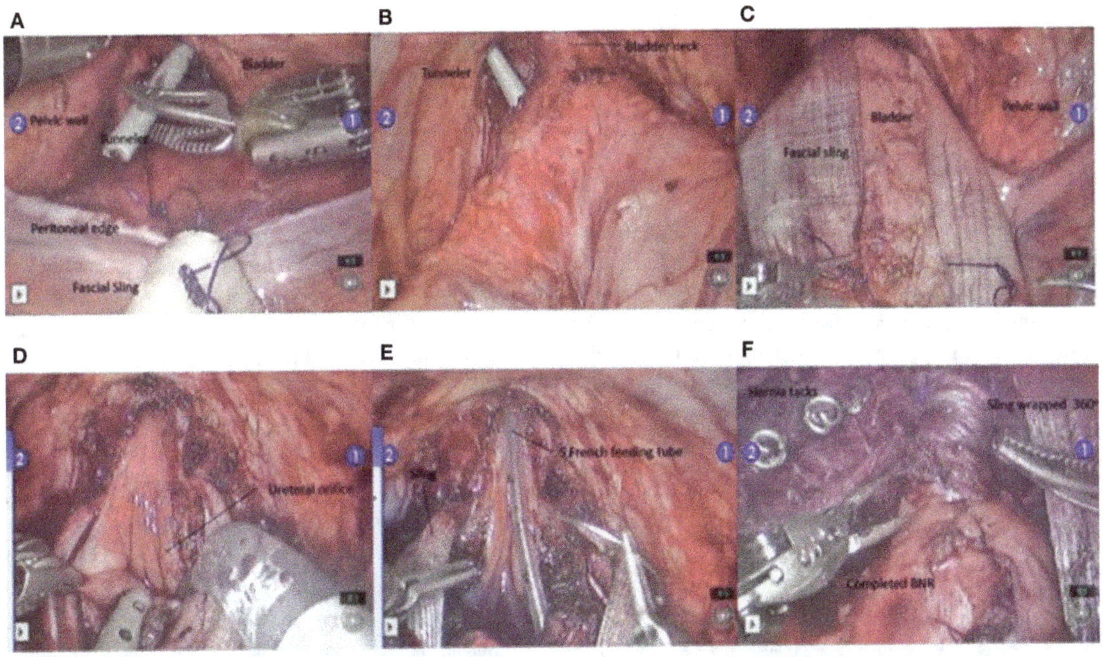

FIGURE 2 | Steps in the BNR. The tunnelers are passed ventrally from the posterior bladder dissection into the developed space of Retzius **(A,B)**. Once the sling is passed from posterior to anterior **(C)**, the urethra is unroofed up through the bladder neck to the level of the interureteric ridge **(D)**. At this point, the Foley catheter is exchanged for a 5-F feeding tube, and the urethra is retubularized in 2 layers with a running simple suture of 4-0 Vicryl followed by 3-0 Vicryl **(E)**. After the LM repair is completed, the sling is tightly wrapped 360° and attached to the pubic bone using 6 screws from a hernia tacker **(F)**. Permission for use of this figure has been obtained from Elsevier Publishing Company. The originally published form can be found at Gargollo (2).

facilitates dissection, creating excellent exposure to the pelvis and the bladder, and providing the ability to accommodate any type of bladder neck repair (e.g., LM, Pippi-Salle, Kropp and YDL). As previously described, our institution utilizes retrovesicular placement of the sling, LM BNR, retubularization of the urethra around a 5-Fr feeding tube and 360 degree sling wrapping, as shown in **Figure 2**. We then hitch the bladder to the anterior abdominal wall prior to creation of the APV.

Using this technique in 38 patients, 82% ($n = 31$) became completely dry during the day on CIC every 3 h and of the 7 patients who were wet, 4 were non-compliant with CIC (2). This is consistent with the 85.2% initial continence rate reported by Gundeti et al. in a multi-institutional review of 88 patients undergoing RAL-APV and various concomitant bladder neck procedures (including BNR in 21, BNS in 17, and BNC in 4) (27).

Our mean operative time for this reconstruction is 5.8 h (3.6–12.25 h), with longer operative times being significantly higher in the first 10 vs. the last 28 cases ($P = 0.0001$), demonstrating the ability to mitigate some of the increase in operative time with increased surgeon experience (2). In follow-up, 5.3% ($n = 2$) required augmentation cystoplasty due to the post-operative development of decreased bladder compliance, 10.5% ($n = 4$) developed *de novo* reflux (grades 2 and 3), and 5.3% ($n = 2$) developed bladder stones (2). These complications are consistent with those seen in the bladder outlet procedures described previously, but to date, have occurred at a relatively lower rate, though direct comparison is challenged by multiple confounders.

Finally, the majority of the BNR procedures described above have occurred as primary surgical intervention in patients with neurogenic bladder, but the techniques utilized in this repair have already been expanded to include a broader patient population. Last year, our institution presented the first RAL-BNR in a patient with classic bladder exstrophy at the American Urologic Association Annual Meeting (Gargollo et al., under review). This year, our institution published the first study demonstrating the feasibility and safety of RAL-BNR in patients with PAS. In 36 patients with PAS, the mean operative time was 8.2 h, with the first 18 cases taking significantly longer than the last 18 cases (mean 9.1 h vs. mean 7.5 h, $p = 0.002$), again demonstrating a learning curve for this procedure. Throughout this study, there were 5 cases that were converted to open due to failure to progress. All conversions were secondary to intra-abdominal adhesions and all occurred in patients with multiple previous ventriculoperitoneal (VP) shunt revisions. At a mean follow-up of 2 years (range 2–36 months), 5.5% ($n = 2$) of patients who had previously undergone a BNR required a BNC for persistent incontinence and 8% ($n = 3$) underwent surgery for bladder calculi. While further studies comparing open and robotic approaches to BNR are needed in patients with PAS to determine equivalency or superiority of one approach over the other, our initial reports to date of RAL-BNR appear promising.

CONCLUSION

RAL surgical techniques have immense potential in the surgical treatment of pediatric incontinence. Our review demonstrates that RAL techniques can be adapted to a variety of procedure types with equivalent continence rates. In addition, the added benefits of improved cosmesis, less intraoperative blood loss, less post-operative pain and decreased adhesion formation make a robotic approach the preference at our institution. Longer operative times can be expected, especially early in the surgical experience, but over time, operative times become significantly shorter and more similar to the duration expected for traditional open surgery for these procedures. Our data also support the feasibility and safety of expanding the range of RAL surgical candidates to include selected patients with PAS. Overall, while there is still a lack of expert consensus on the preferred reconstructive procedure (or combination of procedures) for the treatment of pediatric incontinence, it appears that RAL surgical techniques will continue to push the frontier.

AUTHOR CONTRIBUTIONS

PG conceived of the presented idea, developed the surgical technique described, participated in drafting of the manuscript and critically revised the manuscript for important intellectual content. LW completed the comprehensive literature review, participated in drafting of the manuscript and formatted the manuscript for submission, under supervision of PG. All authors reviewed and approved the final manuscript.

REFERENCES

1. Gargollo PC, Granberg C, Gong E, Tu D, Whittam B, Dajusta D. Complex robotic lower urinary tract surgeries in patients with previous open surgery. *J Urol.* (2018) 1:162–168. doi: 10.1016/j.juro.2018.06.017
2. Gargollo PC. Robotic-assisted bladder neck repair: feasibility and outcomes. *Urol Clin.* (2015) 42:111–20. doi: 10.1016/j.ucl.2014.09.013
3. Bagrodia A, Gargollo P. Robot-assisted bladder neck reconstruction, bladder neck sling, and appendicovesicostomy in children: description of technique and initial results. *J Endourol.* (2011) 25:1299–305. doi: 10.1089/end.2011.0031
4. Freilich DA, Penna FJ, Nelson CP, Retik AB, Nguyen HT. Parental satisfaction after open versus robot assisted laparoscopic pyeloplasty: results from modified Glasgow Children's benefit inventory survey. *J Urol.* (2010) 183:704–8. doi: 10.1016/j.juro.2009.10.040
5. Pattaras JG, Moore RG, Landman J, Clayman RV, Janetschek G, McDougall EM, et al. Incidence of postoperative adhesion formation after transperitoneal genitourinary laparoscopic surgery. *Urology.* (2002). 59:37–41. doi: 10.1016/S0090-4295(01)01474-1
6. Grimsby GM, Jacobs MA, Gargollo PC. Comparison of complications of robot-assisted laparoscopic and open appendicovesicostomy in children. *J Urol.* (2015) 194:772–6. doi: 10.1016/j.juro.2015.02.2942
7. Abrams P. The standardization of terminology of lower urinary tract function: report from the standardization sub-committee of the international continence society. *Neurourol Urodyn.* (2002) 21:167–78.
8. Simeoni J, Guys JM, Mollard P, Buzelin JM, Moscovici J, Bondonny JM, et al. Artificial urinary sphincter implantation for neurogenic bladder: a multi-institutional study in 107 children. *Br J Urol.* (1996) 78:287–93.

9. Catti M, Lortat-Jacob S, Morineau M, Lottmann H. Artificial urinary sphincter in children—voiding or emptying? An evaluation of functional results in 44 patients. *J Urol.* (2008) 180:690–3. doi: 10.1016/j.juro.2008.04.039
10. Bauer SB. Long-term efficacy of artificial urinary sphincters in children. *J Urol.* (2008) 180:441. doi: 10.1016/j.juro.2008.05.082
11. Castera R, Podestá ML, Ruarte A, Herrera M, Medel R. 10-year experience with artificial urinary sphincter in children and adolescents. *J Urol.* (2001) 165:2373–6. doi: 10.1016/S0022-5347(05)66207-6
12. Ruiz E, Puigdevall J, Moldes J, Lobos P, Boer M, Ithurralde J, et al. 14 years of experience with the artificial urinary sphincter in children and adolescents without spina bifida. *J Urol.* (2006) 176:1821–5. doi: 10.1016/j.juro.2006.05.024
13. Levesque PE, Bauer SB, Atala A, Zurakowski D, Colodny A, Peters C. Ten-year experience with the artificial urinary sphincter in children. *J Urol.* (1996) 156:625–8.
14. Moscardi PRM, Ballesteros N, Abd-El-Barr AE, Salvitti M, Castellan M. Robotic-assisted laparoscopic artificial urinary sphincter and MACE procedure on a pediatric patient. *J Pediatr Urol.* (2017) 13:527–8. doi: 10.1016/j.jpurol.2017.06.011
15. Kryger JV, Gonzalez R, Barthold JS. Surgical management of urinary incontinence in children with neurogenic sphincteric incompetence. *J Urol.* (2000) 163:256–63. doi: 10.1016/S0022-5347(05)68031-7
16. Snodgrass WT, Elmore J, Adams R. Bladder neck sling and appendicovesicostomy without augmentation for neurogenic incontinence in children. *J Urol.* (2007) 177:1510–5. doi: 10.1016/j.juro.2006.11.080
17. Snodgrass W, Barber T. Comparison of bladder outlet procedures without augmentation in children with neurogenic incontinence. *J Urol.* (2010) 184:1775–80. doi: 10.1016/j.juro.2010.04.017
18. Grimsby GM, Menon V, Schlomer BJ, Baker LA, Adams R, Gargollo PC, et al. Long-term outcomes of bladder neck reconstruction without augmentation cystoplasty in children. *J Urol.* (2016) 195:155–61. doi: 10.1016/j.juro.2015.06.103
19. Bergman J, Lerman SE, Kristo B, Chen A, Boechat MI, Churchill BM. Outcomes of bladder neck closure for intractable urinary incontinence in patients with neurogenic bladders. *J Pediatr Urol.* (2006) 2:528–33. doi: 10.1016/j.jpurol.2005.12.001
20. Liard A. The Mitrofanoff procedure: 20 years later. *J Urol.* (2001) 165(6 Pt 2):2394–8. doi: 10.1016/S0022-5347(05)66213-1
21. Hoebeke P, De Kuyper P, Goeminne H, Van Laecke E, Everaert K. Bladder neck closure for treating pediatric incontinence. *Eur Urol.* (2000) 38:453–6. doi: 10.1159/000020323
22. Kavanagh A, Afshar K, Scott H, MacNeily AE. Bladder neck closure in conjunction with enterocystoplasty and Mitrofanoff diversion for complex incontinence: closing the door for good. *J Urol.* (2012) 188:1561–6. doi: 10.1016/j.juro.2012.02.027
23. Murthy P, Cohn JA, Selig RB, Gundeti MS. Robot-assisted laparoscopic augmentation ileocystoplasty and Mitrofanoff appendicovesicostomy in children: updated interim results. *Eur Urol.* (2015) 68:1069–75. doi: 10.1016/j.eururo.2015.05.047
24. Cole EE, Adams MC, Brock JW 3rd, Pope JC 4th. Outcome of continence procedures in the pediatric patient: a single institutional experience. *J Urol.* (2003) 170(2 Pt 1):560–3 (discussion: 563). doi: 10.1097/01.ju.0000078015.55801.52
25. Jawaheer G, Rangecroft L. The Pippi Salle procedure for neurogenic urinary incontinence in childhood: a three-year experience. *Eur J Pediatr Surg.* (1999) 9(Suppl. 1):9–11.
26. Grimsby GM, Jacobs MA, Menon V, Schlomer BJ, Gargollo PC. Perioperative and short-term outcomes of robotic vs open bladder neck procedures for neurogenic incontinence. *J Urol.* (2016) 195:1088–92. doi: 10.1016/j.juro.2015.11.043
27. Gundeti MS, Petravick ME, Pariser JJ, Pearce SM, Anderson BB, Grimsby GM, et al. A multi-institutional study of perioperative and functional outcomes for pediatric robotic-assisted laparoscopic Mitrofanoff appendicovesicostomy. *J Pediatr Urol.* (2016) 12:386.e1–5. doi: 10.1016/j.jpurol.2016.05.031

Congenital Bronchobiliary Fistula: A Case Report and Literature Review

Zhen Bing†, Rui Chen†, Pengchao Xing†, Yueyi Ren† and Kefeng Hou†*

Heart Center, Qingdao Women and Children's Hospital, Qingdao, China

***Correspondence:**
Kefeng Hou
xhxf1221@163.com

Congenital bronchobiliary fistula (CBBF) is a rare disease. Children with CBBF mostly have atypical clinical manifestations that can be easily missed. We report a case of a child with CBBF who was diagnosed with fistulography with the help of an endobronchial blocker and a fiberoptic bronchoscope. The CBBF was successfully removed by thoracoscopic surgery.

Keywords: congenital bronchobiliary fistula, bronchoscope, endobronchial blocker, fistulography, thoracoscopic surgery

INTRODUCTION

Congenital bronchobiliary fistula (CBBF) is a rare disease, which was first reported by Neuhauser et al. (1). It is a rare developmental anomaly, i.e., fistula between the respiratory and biliary tract. Its clinical manifestations are recurrent and persistent refractory pulmonary inflammation. We reported a 2-year-old boy with CBBF, who was successfully diagnosed with fistulography and treated by thoracoscopic surgery.

CASE PRESENTATION

A 2-year-old boy was hospitalized in our center for recurrent pneumonia. He was hospitalized three times for pneumonia in the past 6 months. The main symptom was cough. The child is too young to cough sputum out. There was no typical yellow-greenish sputum in the period of pneumonia. There was also no cyanosis, respiratory distress, or jaundice. Chest x-ray showed chronic inflammatory changes on the right side at the beginning of the disease. Application of antibiotics and drug-aerosol inhalation can relieve cough symptoms. Chest CT showed multiple patchy hyperdense shadows in both lungs. The 3D-CT reconstruction showed that the wall of the right main bronchus has a conical cleft-like protrusion with the end pointing downward last time (**Figure 1A**).

In the catheter room, fiberoptic bronchoscopy and bronchography were performed at the same time. Under general anesthesia, a standard 5.5-mm-inner diameter (ID) endotracheal tube (ETT) without cuffed was successfully inserted into the trachea. A multiport airway adapter (Tappa, Common type, EBT0105) was used to connect endotracheal intubation (**Figure 2**) (2). An electronic fiberoptic bronchoscope was inserted into the trachea through the multiport airway adapter, whose outside diameter is 2.8 mm. We can see yellow secretions attached to the glottis and trachea through the fiberoptic bronchoscope. An abnormal opening was found at the level of the tracheal carina, and yellow secretions could be seen at the opening (**Figure 3A**). The pediatric endobronchial blocker (5-Fr) was inserted into the tube through the multiport airway adapter. Different models of endobronchial blockers have clear matching endotracheal intubation diameter and fiberoptic bronchoscope specification (**Table 1**). With the assistance of an electronic fiber bronchoscope, the endobronchial blocker was inserted into the fistula (**Figures 3B–D**). Two milliliters of gas was injected into the endobronchial blocker through the end lateral hole, and

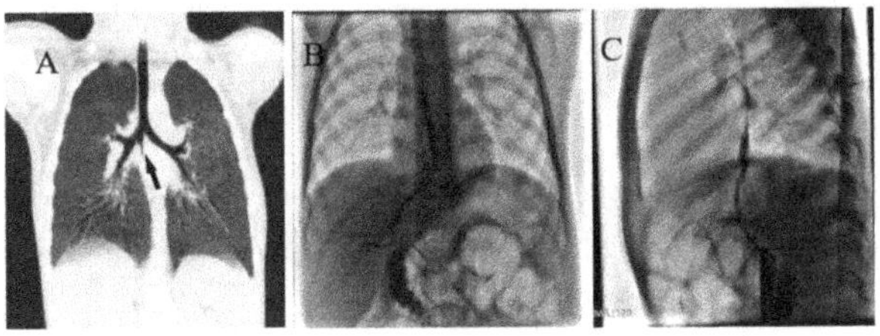

FIGURE 1 | (A) Right main bronchus wall with conical cleft-like protrusion (black arrow). **(B)** Anteroposterior angiography of BBF. **(C)** Lateral angiography of BBF.

the cuff of the endobronchial blocker was filled to close the fistula. Iodixanol was used as the contrast agent. A 20-ml syringe was used to connect the exhaust pipe of the endobronchial blocker to inject the fistula, and DSA was performed at the same time. It can be seen that the contrast medium is connected to the left hepatic duct through the esophageal hiatus, and the contrast medium sequentially fills the left intrahepatic bile duct, the right intrahepatic bile duct, the common hepatic duct, the common bile duct, the gallbladder, and the duodenum (**Figures 1B,C**). No other biliary malformation was found. Ultrasound examination of the liver and gallbladder showed no abnormality. The examination of hydatidosis and other parasites was normal. By way of aspiration of intratracheal lavage fluid examination, the total bile acid was found to be 306.20 μmol/L. Esophagotracheal fistula was not found by upper gastrointestinal angiography.

We discussed the diagnosis and treatment of CBBF with the guardian of the child and signed the informed consent for the operation. The CBBF was cut off and sutured by video-assisted minimally invasive thoracoscopic surgery. Two endobronchial blockers were used. For one-lung ventilation, one endobronchial blocker was inserted into the right main bronchus under bronchoscope guidance before intubation. After that, a standard 5.5-mm ETT without cuff was inserted into the trachea and connected to the multiport airway adapter. Under bronchoscope guidance, the second endobronchial blocker was inserted into the CBBF through the multiport airway adapter and ETT. The right posterior axillary line in the sixth intercostal space was used as the observation hole, and a 30° 5-mm thoracoscope was inserted. The fourth intercostal space in the right anterior axillary line and the seventh intercostal space in the middle axillary line were the operation holes. A 6-mm-diameter fistula was found at the beginning of the right main bronchus below the tracheal carina (**Figure 4A**). The fistula runs down the right side of the spine and passes through the diaphragm. By shaking the endobronchial blocker in the fistula, the BBF shaking can be seen under the thoracoscope. The fistula was fully exposed and the whole course of the fistula was free intrathoracic (**Figure 4B**). After double ligation with No. 10 mousse thread at both ends (**Figure 4C**), the fistula was double clamped with a hemolock clamp, and the fistula was removed with an ultrasonic knife (**Figure 4D**). Lastly, the thoracic drainage tube was placed through the seventh intercostal operation hole. The operation lasted 105 min. Tracheal intubation was removed 1 h after the operation. The excised fistula was sent for pathological examination. Microscopically, the specimen presented as a tubular structure of cartilage and muscle, lined with squamous and pseudostratified ciliated columnar epithelial mucosa and submucosal glands. It was considered as tracheal malformation. The lung shadow disappeared, which was demonstrated by chest CT after 6 months of the operation.

DISCUSSION

CBBF is associated with abnormal embryonic development. Its symptoms can occur from newborn to adult (3, 4). The severity of CBBF is different, which is related to the diameter of the fistula and whether combined with bile tract malformation. The earlier the symptoms appear, the more severe the condition is. This patient began to cough repeatedly at 2 years old but did not expectorate typical yellow-greenish sputum. Typical yellow-greenish sputum is rarely seen in infants. Infants also cannot describe whether the sputum is bitter or not. Therefore, it is easy to miss a diagnosis in infancy. If infants show recurrent pneumonia, yellow-greenish sputum can be seen during sputum suction, and cone-shaped fissure-like protrusion can be seen on chest 3D-CT reconstruction. In this situation, CBBF should be suspected, and relevant examinations should be further improved to make a definite diagnosis.

There are various diagnostic methods for CBBF. The increase of total bile acids in sputum or intratracheal lavage fluid is helpful for the diagnosis of CBBF. Chest CT scan and 3D-CT reconstruction can show the abnormal branches of the trachea. It is difficult to directly show the whole shape of the fistula, but it can evaluate the severity of pulmonary inflammation and guide whether the lobectomy should be performed at the same time. Abdominal CT examination can diagnose primary diseases such as liver abscess and bile duct stones. In addition, some patients can see a gas shadow in the bile duct. Abnormal branches of the trachea and gas shadow in the bile duct are important indirect signs of BBF. In this case, the abnormal branch of the trachea was found in the previous chest CT examination. It was ignored and diagnosis was missed. Percutaneous transhepatic cholangiography (PTC) and endoscopic retrograde cholangiopancreatography (ERCP) can show the origin and course of the fistula. In addition, it can also confirm whether there are other bile duct malformations. At present, PTC and ERCP are the main methods for the diagnosis of acquired bronchobiliary fistula (ABBF) in adults (5). Because the PTC and ERCP are complex and traumatic, it is not widely carried out in children (6, 7). Contrast-enhanced magnetic resonance cholangiography can show the anatomy of the biliary tract and provide physiological or pathological bile flow function information. Compared with conventional magnetic resonance cholangiopancreatography (MRCP), contrast-enhanced magnetic resonance cholangiopancreatography has more obvious diagnostic advantages. However, it needs longer operation time and higher technical requirements (8). Bronchoscopy is the first choice for the diagnosis of CBBF.

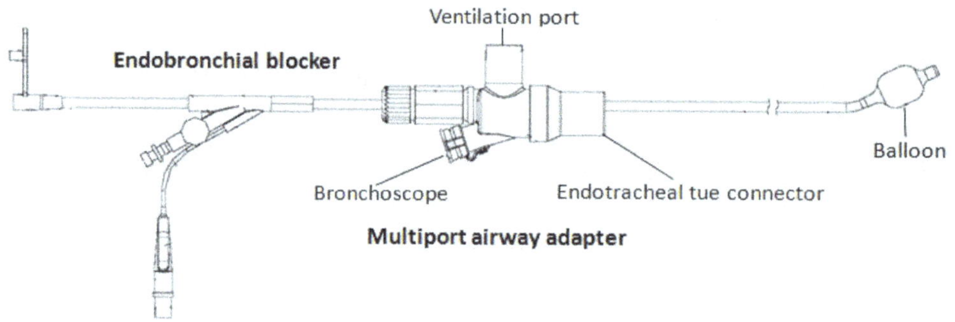

FIGURE 2 | The pediatric endobronchial blocker system.

Through the bronchoscope, we can see the yellow-green liquid overflowing from the fistula, and it will still overflow again after lavage. The bile acid test of lavage fluid is positive, which has an important diagnostic value. The bronchoscopy cannot show the whole course of the fistula. Bronchography can show the course of CBBF. Traditional bronchography involves the catheter being inserted into the trachea through the biopsy hole of the bronchoscope and a contrast agent is injected (9, 10). Li et al. (9) retrospectively analyzed 44 cases of CBBF. It showed that the orifice of CBBF was near the tracheal carina, with 45.4% opening in the right main bronchus, 43.2% opening in the tracheal carina, and 11.4% opening in the left main bronchus. Because the position of the fistula is very high, the contrast medium fistulography is easy to flow to the lower bronchi and alveoli. If the fistula is thin, the fistula is often not displayed, let alone the bile duct. We used the endobronchial blocker to block the orifice of CBBF. The whole shape and course of the BBF could be displayed by injecting contrast agents under x-ray fluoroscopy. There are three advantages to increase the injection pressure of the contrast agents and prolong fluoroscopy time. First of all, in addition to clearly showing the fistula, the left intrahepatic bile duct, the right intrahepatic bile duct, the common hepatic duct, the common bile duct, the gallbladder, and the duodenum can also be displayed in sequence. To determine whether there is a biliary malformation, ERCP cholangiography is not necessary. It can provide an important reference for the choice of surgical methods. Secondly, CBBF can be located by anteroposterior and lateral fluoroscopy. It can help to select the position of the observation hole and the operation hole for the thoracoscopic surgery. Finally, the CBBF tracheal fistula was occluded for angiography, which can avoid contrast media reflux to the bronchus and alveoli.

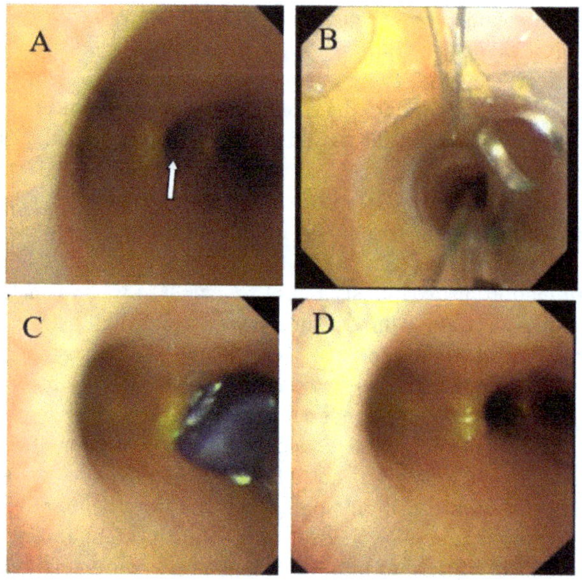

FIGURE 3 | **(A)** Abnormal opening of the tracheal carina (white arrow). **(B)** Endobronchial blocker enter into the trachea. **(C)** Endobronchial blocker enter into the fistula. **(D)** The endobronchial blocker was inflated and fixed after entering the fistula.

The main treatment method of CBBF is operation, which depends on the location of the fistula and whether it is combined with other liver and biliary diseases. It includes fistulectomy and plugging under bronchoscopic guidance. In case of CBBF with bile duct malformation, absence of common bile duct, abnormal bile intestinal drainage, and so on, fistula jejunum Roux-en-Y anastomosis, hilar jejunum anastomosis, and gallbladder jejunum anastomosis, among others, are feasible to fully drain bile and avoid fistula recurrence (11–13). The plugging of the fistula under bronchoscope guidance has the advantages of less trauma and quick recovery. At present, it is mainly used in adult ABBF, and there are few reports in children (14–19). Video-assisted thoracoscopic surgery in the treatment of CBBF can provide an unparalleled surgical vision compared to thoracotomy. In addition, it has less trauma and faster postoperative recovery. However, it is rarely reported in children (20–22). The CBBF-ectomy of this case is through mini-incision by video-assisted thoracoscopy surgery. One-lung ventilation was performed by an endobronchial blocker. The BBF was cut off and sutured. At present, the commonly used single lung ventilation technology includes double-lumen bronchial catheter ventilation and endobronchial blocker blocking one

TABLE 1 | Different models of endobronchial blocker have clear matching endotracheal intubation diameter and fiberoptic bronchoscope specification.

Endobronchial blocker (Fr)		5			7			9	
Endotracheal intubation (mm)	4.5	5.0	5.5	6.0	6.5	7.0	7.5	8.0	8.5
Bronchoscope (mm)	2.2		2.8		3.5			4.0	

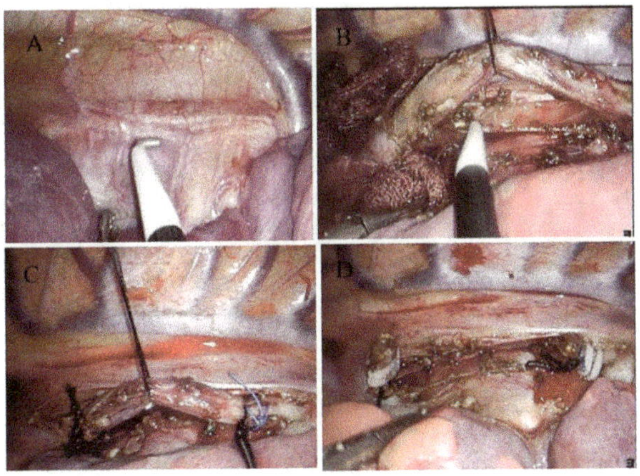

FIGURE 4 | Video-assisted thoracoscopic surgery to cut and suture the fistula. **(A)** CBBF was detected. **(B)** Free CBBF. **(C)** Ligation of CBBF. **(D)** CBBF was cut and sutured.

side of the main bronchus (23, 24). The smallest double-lumen bronchus tube is 26F. For children under 8 years old, one-lung ventilation with a double-lumen bronchus tube is impossible. The peripheral diameter of an endobronchial blocker is significantly smaller than a double-lumen endobronchial tube. The applicable age range of the endobronchial blocker is wider than the double-lumen endobronchial tube (2, 25, 26). The bronchial orifice of the CBBF was occluded by an endobronchial blocker. It can prevent bile acid from reflux into the trachea when squeezing the fistula during operation. Then, it can avoid asphyxia and chemical inflammatory injury of the lung. The course of the BBF should be confirmed before resection. We can confirm the target fistula along the abnormal branch of the trachea. Besides, the fistula can be seen by shaking the endobronchial blocker.

In conclusion, if the patient has recurrent cough and refractory pneumonia, we should be alert to CBBF. The airway reconstruction can show abnormal tracheal branches and abdominal CT can find a gas shadow in the liver. Bronchography can make a definite diagnosis of CBBF with the help of the bronchoscope and endobronchial blocker. The application of a double endobronchial blocker during operation can not only effectively implement one-lung ventilation for children but also help to determine the course of BBF and prevent bile acid reflux to the lung. It is a simple, feasible, accurate, and reliable diagnostic and treatment method to block the fistula with an endobronchial blocker. Video-assisted thoracoscopic surgery is a safe (with minimal trauma) and effective way to cut off the fistula.

AUTHOR CONTRIBUTIONS

ZB was responsible for data interpretation, drafting of the manuscript, and approval of the final version to be published. RC, PX, YR, and KH were responsible for the study concept, data collection and interpretation, revision of the manuscript, and approval of the final version to be published. All authors read and approved the final manuscript.

REFERENCES

1. Neuhauser EB, Elkin M, Landing B. Congenital direct communication between the biliary system and respiratory tract. *AMA Am J Dis Child.* (1952) 83:654–9. doi: 10.1001/archpedi.1952.02040090100012
2. Wu C, Liang X, Liu B. Selective pulmonary lobe isolation with Arndt pediatric endobronchial blocker for an infant: a case report. *Medicine.* (2019) 98:e18262. doi: 10.1097/MD.0000000000018262
3. Carvalho CD, Barbas CS, Guarnieri RM, Campos JD, Filomeno LT, Saldiva PH, et al. Congenital bronchobiliary fistula: first case in an adult. *Thorax.* (1988) 43:792–3. doi: 10.1136/thx.43.10.792
4. Pathak S, Jethi S, Saoji R. Isolated congenital tracheobiliary fistula. *Indian Pediatr.* (2018) 55:995–6. doi: 10.1007/s13312-018-1426-x
5. Yin H, Zhao G, Du Y, Zhao P. Anesthesia management in neonatal congenital bronchobiliary fistula: a case report and literature review. *BMC Anesthesiol.* (2020) 20:1–7. doi: 10.1186/s12871-020-01052-4
6. Lou Q, Sun J, Zhang X, Shen H. Successful therapeutic ERCP in a 99-day-old child with common bile duct stones: a case report and discussions on the particularities of the ERCP in children. *Front Pediatr.* (2020) 8:435. doi: 10.3389/fped.2020.00435
7. Deng Z, Zeng J, Lv C, Jiang L, Ji J, Li X, et al. Prevalence and factors associated with post-endoscopic retrograde cholangiopancreatography pancreatitis in children. *Digest Dis Sci.* (2020) 66:224–30. doi: 10.1007/s10620-020-06179-5
8. Karabulut N, Cakmak V. Kiter G. Confident diagnosis of bronchobiliary fistula using contrast-enhanced magnetic resonance cholangiography. *Korean J Radiol.* (2010) 11:493–6. doi: 10.3348/kjr.2010.11.4.493
9. Li TY. Zhang ZB. Congenital bronchobiliary fistula: a case report and review of the literature. *World J Clin Cases.* (2019) 7:881–90. doi: 10.12998/wjcc.v7.i7.881
10. JohnWagget M, Stool S, Bishop HC, Kurtz MB. Congenital bronchobiliary fistula. *J Pediatr Surg.* (1970) 5:566–9. doi: 10.1016/0022-3468(70)90012-6
11. Günlemez A, Tugay M, Elemen L, Türker M, Gürcan NI, Demir H, et al. Surgical experience in a baby with congenital broncho-biliary fistula. *Ann Thorac Surg.* (2009) 87:318–20. doi: 10.1016/j.athoracsur.2008.06.028
12. Chan YT, Ng WD, Mak WP, Kwong ML, Chow CB. Congenital bronchobiliary fistula associated with biliary atresia. *Br J Surg.* (2010) 71:240–1. doi: 10.1002/bjs.1800710329
13. Salzedas Netto AA, Silva PCM, Vicentine FPP, Takamatsu FY, Gonzalez AM, Succi JE, et al. Congenital tracheo-biliary fistula: staged surgical

treatment. *J Pediatr Surg Case Rep.* (2017) 32:11–3. doi: 10.1016/j.epsc.2017.12.019

14. Kim JH, Man DK, Lee YK, Hwang SG, Ji HL, Kim EK, et al. Bronchobiliary fistula treated with histoacryl embolization under bronchoscopic guidance: a case report. *Respirat Med CME.* (2008) 1:164–8. doi: 10.1016/j.rmedc.2008.04.002
15. Goldman SY, Greben CR, Setton A, Mckinley MJ, Axelrod DJ, Charles HW, et al. Bronchobiliary fistula successfully treated with n-butyl cyanoacrylate *via* a bronchial approach. *J Vasc Interv Radiol.* (2007) 18:151–5. doi: 10.1016/j.jvir.2006.10.012
16. Shang Y, Bai C, Yao XP, Huang Y, Zhao LJ, Li Q. Transnasal flexible bronchoscopic implantation of a nickel-titanium (NiTi) bronchial occlusive device for a bronchobiliary fistula. *Endoscopy.* (2010) 42:225–6. doi: 10.1055/s-0029-1244059
17. Prieto-Nieto MI, Pérez-Robledo JP, lvarez-Luque A, Suz JIA, Torres JN. Cutaneous bronchobiliary fistula treated with Tissucolsealant. *Cardiovasc Intervent Radiol.* (2011) 34(Suppl.2):232–5. doi: 10.1007/s00270-010-9807-0
18. Mukkada RJ, Antony R, Francis JV, Chettupuzha AP, Augustine P, Venugopal B, et al. Bronchobiliary fistula treated successfully with endoscopic microcoils and glue. *Ann Thorac Surg.* (2014) 98:e33–4. doi: 10.1016/j.athoracsur.2014.04.052
19. Kostopanagiotou K, George RS, Kefaloyannis E, Papagiannopoulos K. Novel technique in managing bronchobiliary fistula in adults: endobronchial embolization using silicone spigots in 2 cases. *Ann Thoracic Med.* (2015) 10:67–8. doi: 10.4103/1817-1737.146889
20. Kuo Y-S, Lee S-C, Chang H, Hsieh C-B, Huang T-W. Thoracoscopic surgery for bronchobiliary fistula: a case report. *J Cardiothorac Surg.* (2014) 9:139. doi: 10.1186/s13019-014-0139-z
21. Na KJ, Jung JC, Hwang Y, Lee HJ, Park IK, Kang CH, et al. Minimally invasive surgical repair for congenital bronchobiliary fistula in an adult. *Ann Thoracic Surg.* (2016) 101:1584–7. doi: 10.1016/j.athoracsur.2015.05.126
22. Wang Z, Chen Y, Huang J, Peng C, Cao Z. Minimally invasive thorascopic surgery in treating congenital bronchobiliary fistula: a case report and a brief review of the literature. *J Pediatr Surg Case Rep.* (2020) 57:101445. doi: 10.1016/j.epsc.2020.101445
23. Zhang ZJ, Zheng ML, Nie Y, Niu ZQ. Comparison of Arndt-endobronchial blocker plus laryngeal mask airway with left-sided double-lumen endobronchial tube in one-lung ventilation in thoracic surgery in the morbidly obese. *Brazil J Med Biol Res.* (2018) 51:e6825. doi: 10.1590/1414-431x20176825
24. Zhang C, Yue J, Li M, Jiang W, Pan Z. Bronchial blocker versus double-lumen endobronchial tube in minimally invasive cardiac surgery. *BMC Pulmonary Med.* (2019) 19:956. doi: 10.1186/s12890-019-0956-x
25. Yoo JY, Chae YJ, Park SY, Haam S, Kim M, Kim DH. Time to tracheal intubation over a fibreoptic bronchoscope using a silicone left double-lumen endobronchial tube versus polyvinyl chloride single-lumen tube with bronchial blocker: a randomized controlled non-inferiority trial. *J Thorac Dis.* (2019) 11:901–8. doi: 10.21037/jtd.2019.01.108
26. Guo X, Song X, Chen X, Liu W, Wang H, Xia H, et al. novel technique for endobronchial blocker placement for one-lung ventilation in children under 2 years. *Acta Anaesthesiol Scand.* (2018) 62:765–72. doi: 10.1111/aas.13099

27

Mentoring in Pediatric Thoracoscopy: From Theory to Practice

Francesco Macchini [1], Ernesto Leva [1,2], Valerio Gentilino [3], Anna Morandi [1] and Steven Scot Rothenberg [4]*

[1] Department of Pediatric Surgery, Fondazione IRCCS Ca' Granda Ospedale Maggiore Policlinico, Milan, Italy, [2] Department of Clinical Sciences and Community Health, University of Milan, Milan, Italy, [3] Department of Pediatric Surgery, Ospedale Filippo Del Ponte, Azienda Socio Sanitaria Territoriale Sette Laghi, Varese, Italy, [4] Rocky Mountain Hospital for Children, Denver, CO, United States

***Correspondence:**
Francesco Macchini
francesco.macchini@policlinico.mi.it

Introduction: Thoracoscopy represents the most challenging area of pediatric minimally invasive surgery due to its technical difficulty. A standardized training program would be advisable. The aim of this study is to evaluate the results of our surgical training.

Materials and Methods: A retrospective, single-center, cohort study was performed. The following four-step program was tested: (1) theoretical part; (2) experimental training; (3) training in centers of reference; (4) personal operative experience. Particular attention was focused on the choice of mentor. Times and modality of adherence to the program were evaluated. The effectiveness and safety of the training were evaluated according to the surgical results of esophageal atresia (EA/TEF) repair and resection of congenital lung malformations (CLM). The study was conducted from January 2014 to May 2020. Attending surgeons with previous experience in neonatal and pediatric laparoscopy were selected for the training program after being evaluated by the head of Department.

Results: The training program was fully completed in 2 years. Twenty-four lobectomies, 9 sequestrectomies, 2 bronchogenic cyst resections and 20 EA/TEF repair were performed. Thoracoscopy was always feasible and effective, with no conversion. The operative times progressively decreased. Only three minor complications were recorded, all treated conservatively.

Conclusions: A standardized training program is highly desirable to learn how to safely perform advanced pediatric thoracoscopy. The 4-steps design seems a valid educational option. The choice of the mentor is crucial. An experience-based profile for pediatric surgeons who may teach thoracoscopy is advisable.

Keywords: thoracoscopy, training, mentoring, teacher education, congenital lung malformation, esophageal atresia

INTRODUCTION

After the extensive diffusion of minimally invasive surgery (MIS) in the adult population, this surgical approach gradually involved the more challenging pediatric world (1).

In the last two decades MIS extended to an ever-growing number of indications in pediatric surgery and became the gold standard for certain diseases (2).

Among different applications of MIS in childhood, thoracoscopy is the most challenging as the thorax was the last area to be approached by MIS pediatric surgeons. Thoracoscopy is currently regarded by many pediatric surgeons as the last step in MIS training (1). In fact, it is technically more difficult than open surgery and requires a stepwise learning curve (LC). In particular, two factors are currently implicated to achieve competence: first case volume, but frequencies are typically low in pediatric surgery, so that a significantly longer time is required to reach a plateau of competence. Secondly, a standardized pediatric thoracoscopic training program does not exist yet (2, 3). As a consequence, only a limited number of pediatric surgeons are currently experts on this topic.

The recent development of instruments that are suitable for children has been crucial to making thoracoscopy feasible also in neonates and infants, so that even difficult procedures, such as esophageal atresia/tracheo-esophageal fistula (EA/TEF) repair and resection of congenital lung malformation (CLM), can be safely performed thoracoscopically (4).

In 2015, the European Society of Pediatric Endoscopic Surgeons (ESPES) published the guidelines for training program in pediatric minimally invasive surgery, recommending a four-steps training program (2).

The aim of our study is to evaluate the results of the surgical training in pediatric thoracoscopy in our Center, since the establishment of a new thoracoscopic program.

MATERIALS AND METHODS

We conducted a retrospective, single-center, cohort study at the Pediatric Surgery Department, Fondazione IRCCS Ca' Granda Ospedale Maggiore Policlinico in Milan, Italy. Parents gave written informed consent for surgical procedures and for the publication of this series in accordance with the Declaration of Helsinki. In 2012 we started a thoracoscopic training program.

The adherence of our training program to the ESPES guidelines for training program in pediatric minimally invasive surgery was evaluated, with the focus to verify the completion of all of the steps and the collection of the number of required procedures. In addition the surgical outcomes of our procedures were analyzed and also compared to the results of open surgery in our Center.

According to ESPES guidelines, a valid MIS training curriculum is represented by the "Peyton's Four-Step Approach" consisting in (5):

1. Theoretical part: attendance of at least 1 theoretical course in thoracoscopy;
2. Experimental training (MIS trainer, animal models, 3-D *ex vivo* models): spending at least 10–20 h of training on a pelvic trainer and at least 10 h of training on an animal model;
3. Training in a center of reference for pediatric MIS: attendance of 1–3 months of training in a center with high volume of MIS activity;
4. Personal operative experience: performing at least 30 procedures as assistant controlling the camera and more than 50 basic procedures as primary surgeon helped by a tutor (2).

Training Curriculum

Only attending surgeons with previous experience in neonatal and pediatric laparoscopy were selected for the training program after being evaluated by the head of department. The training process started with the delivery of educational material and attendance to national and international courses (6). High-fidelity simulation sessions were performed according to two different modalities. The "dry lab" was performed with the use of traditional and high-fidelity MIS trainers (7, 8). Next hands-on training was delivered through "wet labs," animal-based simulation sessions (9). An observership program at an international high volume referral center for pediatric thoracoscopy was the subsequent step (7). Professor S.S. Rothenberg from the Department of Pediatric Surgery of the Rocky Mountain Hospital for Children, Denver, Colorado (USA) was chosen as reference surgical mentor in view of his universally recognized experience in pediatric thoracoscopy (10, 11). Department directed by Prof. S.S. Rothenberg is a high-volume training center (>200 MIS procedures per year) (2) and trains pediatric surgeons from all over the world during the whole year. The first cases and the wider series of EA repairs and CLM resections come from this center, that published some of the most recent and updated papers (10, 11).

The next step consisted of performing a series of selected cases at our Hospital with the mentoring of Rothenberg (11). The first cases were performed by him with the training surgeons acting as first assistant. The following cases were managed by the local surgeons under his assistance and guidance. The last step was for the local team to manage the cases independently. For complex cases, pre-operative advice from the mentor was always required, by sharing through internet/web the history and images of patients. Patient's data were treated according to Data Protection Act.

The second end point of our study was the evaluation of the effectiveness and safety of our training according to our surgical results. This target was achieved focusing on two of the most difficult thoracoscopic procedures in pediatric surgery: EA/TEF repair in newborns and CLM resection during infancy (4). No modifications were made to the standard of care for newborns and infants requiring thoracoscopy for the studied diseases. Regarding EA/TEF, criteria for the thoracoscopic approach were: suspected standard type C EA/TEF, birth weight $\geq$2,000 g, absence of major associated malformations, and cardio-respiratory stability (no medical cardiac support and no mechanical ventilation). Reasons for conversion from thoracoscopy to open thoracotomy were any intraoperative adverse event or lack of progress for more than 15 min (12–14). According to the last step of our training program, the techniques recommended by Prof. Rothenberg in his last publications were selected as procedures of choice (10, 11).

Two additional aspects of our general approach deserve to be mentioned.

First, all cases are preoperatively evaluated by a multidisciplinary dedicated team, consisting of neonatologist, radiologist, pneumonologist, surgeon, anaesthesiologist.

Images are collectively evaluated, with 3D reconstructions when possible (15).

Secondly, the surgical team, including anesthetists and scrub nurses, always performs a preoperative meeting and a post-operative critical analysis of the procedures. During the first one, the surgical anatomy and the technical steps are revised in details, with the support of internal schemes and videos, e-learning (www.websurg.com; www.globalcastmd.com), and videos from the mentor. In the post-operative meetings, one soon after surgery and one a month later, an evaluation of the entire procedure and of the related criticisms and complications are carried out. Surgical criticisms are also evaluated on the basis of the analysis of video recordings of the procedures.

Surgical Outcome

To evaluate the impact of the surgical expertise on pediatric thoracoscopy, we retrospectively analyzed our case-series from the beginning of our surgical activity (January 2014) to present (May 2020). Only patients operated independently from the tutor were analyzed. We retrieved the following data: indications to thoracoscopy and demographic data; number of procedures performed with success; number of procedures needing conversion and reasons; length of surgery; perioperative, and postoperative complications.

A further comparison between the results of the thoracoscopic approach and the "open" traditional one was performed too, focusing on length of surgery and perioperative and postoperative complications. The population operated with the open technique was chosen among patients with characteristics similar to the thoracoscopic group, in terms of patients' age, indications for surgery and study period. It deserves to be specified that the open interventions were performed by a larger group of trained surgeons, including the surgeons selected for the thoracoscopic training.

The severity of every complication was assessed according to the Clavien-Dindo Classification of Surgical Complications (**Table 1**). It is a morbidity scale based on the therapeutic consequences of complications, that constitutes a simple, objective, and reproducible approach for comprehensive surgical outcome assessment (16).

The analysis of the results in terms of operative times and complications was limited to procedures with the higher number of patients and with the relatively lower variables, i.e., lobectomies, sequestrectomies and EA/TEF repairs.

Variables were expressed as mean ± standard deviation (SD) for demographic and baseline variables, and as median and range for length of follow-up. The learning curves were analyzed using linear regression.

Parametric variables were compared with the Student's *t*-test. Categorical variables were evaluated by Fisher exact test. Statistical analysis was performed using SigmaStat® (Systat Software Inc., San Jose, CA, USA). A $p < 0.05$ was considered significant.

RESULTS

Training Curriculum

Two surgeons previously trained in neonatal and pediatric laparoscopy and with experience in basic thoracoscopic procedures were selected. As regards laparoscopy, Nissen fundoplication, extra-mucosal pyloromyotomy, appendectomy, cholecystectomy, and surgery for Hirschsprung disease, were the most common and well-known performed procedures. Regarding previous thoracoscopic experience, neonatal removal of thoraco-amniotic shunts dislodged in thorax, treatment of pleural empyema and lung biopsies have been performed in a satisfactory number of patients. In particular, selected surgeons had a previous personal experience in more than 500 neonatal and pediatric minimally invasive procedures. The four-step training program was fully completed in 2 years (June 2012–2014).

Here following the details of every single step are reported.

- Theoretical knowledge: 4 theoretical national and 2 theoretical international courses were attended by the selected surgeons. All courses were focused on minimally invasive thoracic surgery and were organized under the sponsorship of national, European and international societies.
- Practice-based learning and improvement in experimental setting: 1 national and 1 international "dry lab" courses were attended, using both traditional and high-fidelity MIS trainers. Simulations were performed systematically even after treating the first patients in order to maintain a high level of technical ability. One national and 1 international "wet lab" courses were attended, both using young anesthetized piglets. During dry and wet labs, thoracoscopic lobectomies and esophageal anastomosis were performed. These steps were further developed by attending the post-graduate Master program in Pediatric Minimally Invasive Surgery at Alma Mater Studiorum—Università di Bologna—Italy.
- Stages in centers of reference: as previously described, a 15 day observer-ship was completed at the Department of Pediatric Surgery of the Rocky Mountain Hospital for Children, Denver, Colorado (USA), under the mentoring of Professor S.S. Rothenberg. During this period many thoracoscopic procedures were observed, such as pulmonary lobectomies, sequestrectomies, closures of patent ductus arteriosus, bronchogenic and pleural cysts resections, corrections of pectus excavatum.
- personal operative experience: within 6 months after the observership in USA, the first 10 cases of CLM were operated on as assistant with Professor S.S. Rothenberg working as main surgeon. In particular, trainees operated 5 pulmonary lobectomies, 1 bronchogenic cysts and 1 extra-lobar pulmonary sequestration as first assistant. The series included also 1 closure of patent ductus arteriosus and 1 esophageal duplication. Then, 2 pulmonary lobectomies and a resection of bronchogenic cyst were operated as first surgeon helped by the mentor. Finally the thoracoscopic procedures were approached without the presence of the tutor. In cases with challenging malformations, images, and advices were

TABLE 1 | Classification of surgical complications grades definition (modified from Clavien-Dindo Classification).

Grade I	Any deviation from the normal postoperative course without the need for pharmacological treatment or surgical, endoscopic, and radiological interventions. Acceptable therapeutic regimens are: drugs as antiemetics, antipyretics, analgesics, diuretics, and electrolytes and physiotherapy. This grade also includes wound infections opened at the bedside
Grade II	Requiring pharmacological treatment with drugs other than such allowed for Grade I complications. Blood transfusions and total parenteral nutrition are also included
Grade III	Requiring surgical, endoscopic, or radiological intervention Grade III-a: intervention not under general anesthesia
Grade III-b	Intervention under general anesthesia
Grade IV	Life-threatening complication (including CNS complications)‡ requiring IC/ICU-management
Grade IV-a	Single organ dysfunction (including dialysis)
Grade IV-b	Multi-organ dysfunction
Grade V	Death of a patient

‡*Brain hemorrhage, ischemic stroke, subarachnoidal bleeding, but excluding transient ischemic attacks (TIA); CNS, Central Nervous System; IC, Intermediate care; ICU, Intensive care unit.*

shared by web the days before. The first neonatal thoracoscopy for EA/TEF correction was performed after almost 1 year since the first thoracoscopic CLM resection. Due to the urgent need for surgery, typical of this malformation, the procedure was done without the mentor. Also in this case images and videos were shared before surgery. As for the personal experience, dedicated surgeons were selected among those highly trained in neonatal and pediatric surgery and with previous high experience in minimally invasive pediatric surgery. At the end of the training period, more than 30 thoracoscopic procedures were performed as cameraman and more than 80 as primary surgeon.

Surgical Outcome

As regards the 2 thoracoscopic procedures selected for the present study, 35 CLM resections and 20 EA/TEF repairs were performed as main surgeons in the study period in Fondazione IRCCS Ca' Granda Ospedale Maggiore Policlinico in Milan, Italy.

The CLM population received the following operations: 24 lobectomies, 9 sequestrectomies, and 2 bronchogenic cyst resections. Mean age at surgery was 7.6 ± 3.3 months, 19 patients were males. Thoracoscopy was feasible and effective in all cases, no conversion was observed. No major anatomical variants were detected in patients where a 3D CT scan reconstruction was possible. This data was consistent with the intraoperative findings. Mean operative time was 167 ± 65 min for lobectomies and 84 ± 27 min for sequestrectomies. As regards lobectomies, a significant reduction in operative times (p = 0.0001) was observed while increasing the surgical experience (**Figure 1**). Also operative times of sequestrectomies progressively reduced, though not reaching statistical significance probably due to the small number of patients (p = 0.21).

Regarding the comparison between traditional and MIS surgery, in the same study period 34 lobectomies, 2 sequestrectomies, and 2 bronchogenic cyst resections were performed in our Center with a thoracotomic approach. Mean operative time was 163 ± 45 min for lobectomies (p = 0.83). The mean surgery length was 110 min for sequestrectomies and 100 min for bronchogenic cyst resections but the limited numbers of both populations don't allow a statistical analysis.

The EA/TEF population consisted of 20 patients (13 males). Eleven newborns (55%) had a distal TEF (type C according to Gross classification), 5 (25%) an isolated TEF (type E), 3 (15%) had no fistulas and were classified as long gap (type A), and 1 (5%) proximal and distal fistulas (type D). The satisfactory results obtained with the first 5 EA/TEF cases prompted us to treat long gap forms too.

For EA with distal TEF (type C), mean gestational age at surgery was 38 ± 1.6 weeks, mean age was 1.7 ± 1 days and mean weight 2.763 ± 466,6 g.

Thoracoscopy was feasible and effective in all cases. No need for conversion was observed. Mean operative time was 134 25 min. The operative times rapidly decreased after the first case, though not reaching statistical significance (p = 0.67) probably due to the small number of patients, and remained stable for the subsequent procedures.

In the study period 18 type C EA were traditionally approached. Mean operative length was 126 ± 34 min (p = 0.07).

A total of 3 patients with a long gap malformation were operated on thoracoscopically. MIS was effective in performing a direct esophageal anastomosis in all cases and no conversion was recorded.

Regarding the MIS post-operative period, only 1 CLM patient (3%) developed an early complication. One male with an extralobar sequestration, that was prenatally ablated, had a post-operative bleeding that resolved after tranexanic acid iv therapy, probably as a consequence of the extensive blunt adhesiolysis between the lung and the ES (Grade II according to Clavien-Dindo Classification).

Two damages to the middle lobe requiring additional resections (Grade III b) occurred in the thoracotomic group.

Within C-type EA repair, 2 minor leakages were observed in both groups (MIS 18% vs. Open 11%; p = 1). Patients were treated conservatively with i.v. antibiotics and fasting, and presented a spontaneous resolution of the leakage. These complications were classified as Grade II according to Clavien-Dindo Classification. Six (50%) MIS vs. 9 (50%) open patients developed an anastomotic stricture (p = 1) requiring dilations (mean ± DS number of dilations: MIS 0.83 ± 1.0 vs. Open 0.94 ± 1.2; p = 0.4). These complications were classified as Grade IIIb according to Clavien-Dindo Classification. No significant

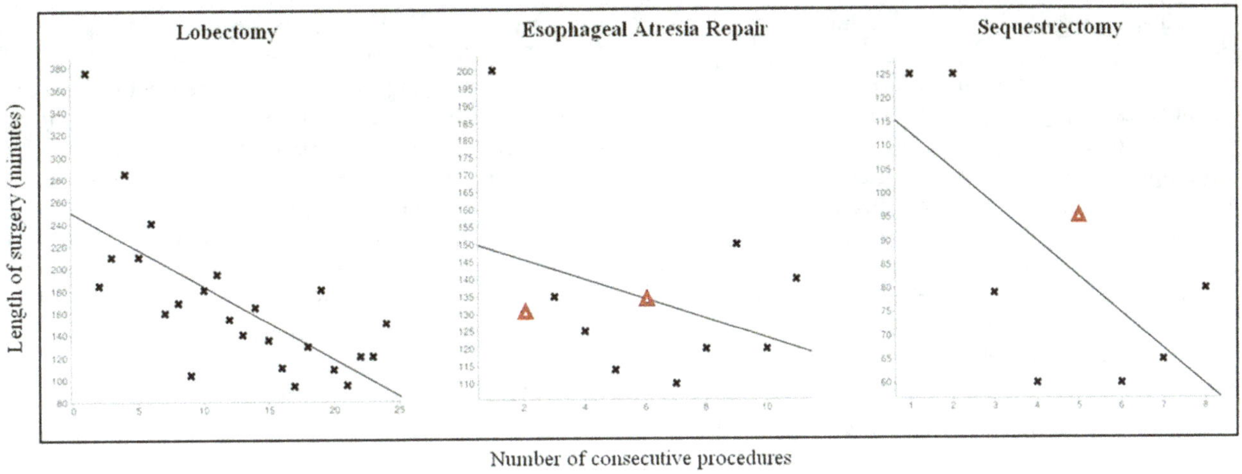

FIGURE 1 | Personal learning curve for different pediatric thoracoscopic procedures. **Δ**: Patients with Grade II complication according to Clavien-Dindo Classification.

differences in the prevalence of gastro-esophageal reflux disease was observed between the two studied groups (MIS 3/12–25% vs. Open 7/18–39%; $p = 0.69$).

As previously reported, all procedures were analyzed during the multidisciplinary post-operative meeting, where an evaluation of the entire procedure and of the related criticisms was done, and the follow-up was revised during the monthly meeting.

The mid-term follow-up was uneventful too. At follow-up (median time 24 months, range 1–46) children with CLM resection are clinically and radiologically healthy. Children with EA/TEF repair at a median follow-up time of 30 months (range 3–39) are clinically in good health. From an endoscopic point of view, 5 children (45%) developed a post-anastomotic stenosis that was successfully treated in the first 6 months of life with a mean of 1.8 ± 0.8 pneumatic dilations. In our series, the incidence of esophageal post-anastomotic stenosis is similar to the population operated with an open technique and to experiences from other centers (12, 17).

DISCUSSION

In the last few decades, MIS has significantly developed, extending to infancy and childhood. This progress was also due to the introduction of advanced techniques and specific devices for the management of little spaces and little anatomical structures.

However, among the different applications of MIS in childhood, thoracoscopy represented the last area to be reached. Although thoracoscopy represents a well-established approach for infants and children, reducing pain and morbidity and avoiding the long-term consequences of a thoracotomy (11), it is not still widely adopted, due to the fact that it is technically more difficult under different aspects. Main difficulties are due to anatomical features in children: pleural and mediastinal areas are minimal; intercostal spaces are limited, especially in neonates, not allowing the use of instruments >5 mm; the anatomy may be distorted by the original malformation; manipulated structures are thin and eventual complications may be fatal (1).

Technical aspects are involved in the delay in pediatric thoracoscopy too: the discrepancy between limited operative spaces and the large size of the available instruments, with a length and thickness of the jaws often disproportionate to the operative space of the infant (4). In addition, case volume and frequency are typically low in pediatric surgery, and a significantly longer time is required to reach competence. Finally, capnothorax is not always well-tolerated by neonates and infants, further reducing the number of procedures (18).

The final difficulties concern training. In many regions worldwide the training in pediatric surgery does not include a fellowship in adult cardio-thoracic surgery. Moreover, a standardized pediatric thoracoscopic training program does not exist yet (3).

Recently, the European Society of Pediatric Endoscopic Surgeons (ESPES) proposed guidelines for an European MIS training program for pediatric surgeons, with the aim to construct a curriculum that provides a safe, uniform, efficient and procedure-specific training program to gain experience, while maintaining patient safety. ESPES hoped that European countries would adopt this program so as to secure a standardized technical qualification in MIS for all future pediatric surgeons (2).

We tried to reproduce the suggestions by ESPES in our training program in pediatric thoracoscopy. The four-steps training program was fully completed in 2 years.

All steps reached high levels of satisfaction from the participants.

The basic knowledge of MIS procedures by the training surgeons was an important starting point, thanks to the acquired knowledge in handling thin structures and operating in limited spaces as in neonatal and infant thoracoscopic and laparoscopic procedures, as well as in doing intracorporeal knots. This condition allowed to overcome the mentioned limits of pediatric MIS training, especially due to low volume and frequency of cases.

In our personal experience, the theoretical step represented a significant occasion to go deep into the topic.

According to the participants, the practice-based learning appeared more similar to reality and crucial from a surgical point of view to develop adequate technical skills.

Previous steps reached a high level of interest and utility, but we think that a special notice has to be given to the choice of the mentor that has to be highly accurate. In fact it represents not only the step immediately before the starting of surgery, but also the on-going support when the trained surgeons begin to operate independently.

We think that some points about this step need to be critically analyzed.

The first point is how to choose the mentor. At the moment there are a lot of training centers for MIS, but standardized essential requirement to certify them still does not exist. As suggested by ESPES guidelines, a training center should be able to offer a complete MIS training, with structured "dry" and "wet" laboratories. Trainees should participate in complex surgery and undergo structured training in all aspects of the procedure and then perform a designated number of cases under supervision (2).

In our experience some points of mentoring revealed crucial: to study the tutor's technique, reading his papers and watching the videos of his operations; to see and help him as assistant, trying to learn his tips and tricks; to operate with him as primary surgeon, following his live suggestions; to keep in strict connection even after the period of training. As regards tips and tricks, our mentor recommended us to introduce the use of miniaturized instruments, especially designed for neonates and infants. In our experience, these new instruments facilitated the thoracoscopic procedure and helped us to reduce the length of surgery (4).

As a general consideration, our experience shows that the surgical approaches suggested by Prof. S.S. Rothenberg are safe and reproducible, after an appropriate training. Results similar to other international centers (12) are achievable in a relatively short time frame.

Another important contribution to this last aspect may come from tele-mentoring: to overcome the lacking continuity in oversight by instructors, a remote teacher–student interaction is established through the web in different ways. Instructors use the connection to assess video recorded training sessions of students at distant locations and guide them through the MIS procedures with specific and personalized feedback. Tele-mentoring may be as effective as in-person instruction in teaching advanced MIS surgical skills, providing an effective method of teaching remotely and allowing expansion of robust simulation training curricula (19). We never adopted this tool but we think it may be very useful and will develop significantly in a near future.

According to all these considerations, we think that a step should be added to the training course, specifically dedicated to the choice and modalities of mentoring.

The results of our training program seem promising. Considerable numbers of thoracoscopic CLM resections and EA/TEF repairs were effectively performed in a relatively short period. Despite being still in training, the length of surgery did not significantly differ from the open group, thus not increasing the surgical and anesthesiological patient's exposure.

As regards the patients' safety, no major intra- and early post-operative complications, such as complications requiring surgical, endoscopic or radiologic intervention, life-threatening complications or death (16), were recorded. Focusing on CLM resection, the open group presented two major complications requiring additional surgery. One possible explanation of these results may be related to the magnification provided by the thoracoscopic approach that helps in a better anatomical vision. As regards EA/TEF repairs, no significant differences were recorded between the two groups, both in early and in late complication rate.

Pediatric thoracoscopy represents a fascinating and innovative technique, encountering in our experience a high level of satisfaction both for families and for the whole team.

The traditional "Master–Apprentice Model" revealed useful in the first part of our training, allowing us to reach the basic knowledge and technical competences to perform thoracoscopy in children. In this model, the apprentice first learns to perform a procedure by observing the master or surgeon how it needs to be done; then the trainee has to assist the surgeon several times; finally he will gradually be allowed to perform parts of the operation under the master's supervision until the apprentice can eventually perform it by himself (2, 20). The collaboration with the mentor in our experience also led to research projects and the organization of international workshops on pediatric thoracic surgery in 2017 and 2019.

In summary, in our experience a multistep training program as previously described seems effective to start pediatric thoracoscopy safely. A support to this consideration also comes from results we obtained following the same steps in other surgical areas, such as the fetoscopic correction of myelomeningocele (21) and the setting of a neonatal ECMO team (22).

We think that some further points of our method concurred to provide adequate surgical skills for an effective execution of thoracoscopy, especially in neonates and infants. A dedicated team including anesthetists, neonatologist, radiologist, pneumologist, and nurses, should be selected at the beginning of the training program and all steps should be shared with all the team. A multidisciplinary approach ensures a detailed preoperative assessment; a specific neonatal stabilization and study of the child; an appropriate intra-operative management; and a right post-operative and long-term follow-up.

A preoperative meeting and a post-operative critical analysis of the procedures are valuable. During the first one, the surgical anatomy and the technical steps are revised, and the intervention is planned in details. In our experience, an important help in deepening the anatomy and any anatomical variants of the lungs is guaranteed by the CT-scan images and, when possible, by the use of 3D reconstructions. In fact, as reported by previous studies (23), variations in lung anatomy are frequent and the benefits of a precise pre-operative evaluation are currently stressed by many authors. In the post-operative meeting, the evaluation of the entire procedure and of the related criticisms and complications are always an opportunity to make steps forward. A significant help to this came in our experience from the systematic recording of the procedures, that were subsequently always reviewed and analyzed. This last step revealed useful also in our hospital to organize local and international meetings on this specific topic.

A last issue may be of some help in reducing the problem of low case volume and frequency and the subsequent slowness of the LC. Whenever possible, the opportunity to attend the operatory rooms of adult thoracic surgery may be useful for a constant revision of anatomy. Although the approaches in adult surgery are different from the pediatric ones, a significant improve may come from their experience and high volume activity. In addition, a centralization of the studied malformations in high level centers should be advisable. CLM and EA are considered rare diseases and need a dedicated training with high skill levels to provide the best management and outcome. Centralizing these patients would ensure higher volumes and accordingly better expertise.

After the completion of the described process, since 2018 the same training program involving other surgeons and trainees has started, being mentored by the already skilled local surgeons.

We think that the main limitation of the present study is represented by being a single center observational study. Despite this aspect provides uniformity of the studied population, we strongly advocate further multicentric studies to verify the reproducibility and safety of our training program.

CONCLUSIONS

Pediatric thoracoscopy represents the most challenging area of MIS. A standardized and certified training program is advisable. The 4-steps training seems a valuable educational proposal. The choice of the mentor is crucial.

AUTHOR CONTRIBUTIONS

FM contributed conception and design of the study. FM and VG collected and analyzed the data retrospectively. FM, AM, EL, and SR wrote the first draft of the manuscript. All authors contributed to manuscript critical revision, read, and approved the submitted version.

ACKNOWLEDGMENTS

The authors would like to thank nurses and neonatologists of the NICU, surgeons of the Department of Pediatric Surgery, anesthesiologists of the Pediatric Anesthesiology and Intensive Care Unit, nurses of the operating room and Pediatric Surgery Department, and the administrative staff of Fondazione IRCCS Ca' Granda Ospedale Maggiore Policlinico.

REFERENCES

1. Lau C-T, Wong KKY. Pediatric minimal invasive surgery - thoracoscopic lobectomy. *Ann Laparosc Endosc Surg.* (2018) 3:94. doi: 10.21037/ales.2018.11.09
2. Esposito C, Escolino M, Saxena A, Montupet P, Chiarenza F, De Agustin J, et al. European Society of Pediatric Endoscopic Surgeons (ESPES) guidelines for training program in pediatric minimally invasive surgery. *Pediatr Surg Int.* (2015) 31:367–73. doi: 10.1007/s00383-015-3672-5
3. Macdonald AL, Haddad M, Clarke SA. Learning curves in pediatric minimally invasive surgery: a systematic review of the literature and a framework for reporting. *J Laparoendosc Adv Surg Tech A.* (2016) 26:652–9. doi: 10.1089/lap.2016.0193
4. Macchini F, Zanini A, Morandi A, Ichino M, Leva E. Thoracoscopic surgery for congenital lung malformation using miniaturized 3 mm vessel sealing and 5-mm stapling devices: single-center experience. *J Laparoendosc Adv Surg Tech A.* (2020) 30:444–7. doi: 10.1089/lap.2019.0589
5. Romero P, Günther P, Kowalewski KF, Friedrich M, Schmidt MW, Trent SM, et al. Halsted's "See One, Do One, and Teach One" versus Peyton's four-step approach: a randomized trial for training of laparoscopic suturing and knot tying. *J Surg Educ.* (2018) 75:510–5. doi: 10.1016/j.jsurg.2017.07.025
6. Iwanaka T, Morikawa Y, Yamataka A, Nio M, Segawa O, Kawashima H, et al. Skill qualifications in pediatric minimally invasive surgery. *Pediatr Surg Int.* (2011) 27:727–31. doi: 10.1007/s00383-011-2871-y
7. Teixeira DF, Carvalho TS, Alcântara MC, Ribeiro ACB, Antunes AG, Gadelha AAB, et al. Simulation in pediatric video surgery: training with simple and reproducible exercises elaborated by residents. *J Laparoendosc Adv Surg Tech A.* (2019) 29:1362–7. doi: 10.1089/lap.2019.0207
8. Reino-Pires P, Lopez M. Validation of a low-cost do-it-yourself model for neonatal thoracoscopic congenital diaphragmatic hernia repair. *J Surg Educ.* (2018) 75:1658–63. doi: 10.1016/j.jsurg.2018.04.005
9. Bidarkar SS, Deshpande A, Kaur M, Cohen RC. Porcine models for pediatric minimally invasive surgical training–a template for the future. *J Laparoendosc Adv Surg Tech A.* (2012) 22:117–22. doi: 10.1089/lap.2011.0057
10. Rothenberg SS. Thoracoscopic repair of esophageal atresia and tracheoesophageal fistula in neonates, first decade's experience. *Dis Esophagus.* (2013) 26:359–64. doi: 10.1111/dote.12054
11. Rothenberg SS, Middlesworth W, Kadennhe-Chiweshe A, Aspelund G, Kuenzler K, Cowles R, et al. Two decades of experience with thoracoscopic lobectomy in infants and children: standardizing techniques for advanced thoracoscopic surgery. *J Laparoendosc Adv Surg Tech A.* (2015) 25:423–8. doi: 10.1089/lap.2014.0350
12. Dingemann C, Zoeller C, Ure B. Thoracoscopic repair of oesophageal atresia: results of a selective approach. *Eur J Pediatr Surg.* (2013) 23:14–8. doi: 10.1055/s-0032-1326953
13. Zobel M, Gologorsky R, Lee H, Vu L. Congenital lung lesions. *Semin Pediatr Surg.* (2019) 28:1–9. doi: 10.1053/j.sempedsurg.2019.07.004
14. Downard CD, Calkins CM, Williams RF, Renaud EJ, Jancelewicz T, Grabowski J, et al. Treatment of congenital pulmonary airway malformations: a systematic review from the APSA outcomes and evidence based practice committee. *Pediatr Surg Int.* (2017) 33:939–53. doi: 10.1007/s00383-017-4098-z
15. Macchini F, Borzani I, Cavalli S, Morandi A, D'Angelo ID, Zanini A, et al. Thoracoscopic resection of congenital lung malformation: looking for the right preoperative assessment. *Eur J Pediatr Surg.* (2019) 6:452–8. doi: 10.1055/s-0039-1696669
16. Dindo D, Demartines N, Clavien P-A. Classification of surgical complications: a new proposal with evaluation in a cohort of 6,336 patients and results of a survey. *Ann Surg.* (2004) 240:205–13. doi: 10.1097/01.sla.0000133083.54934.ae
17. van der Zee DC, Bax KN. Thoracoscopic treatment of esophageal atresia with distal fistula and of tracheomalacia. *Semin Pediatr Surg.* (2007) 16:224–30. doi: 10.1053/j.sempedsurg.2007.06.003

18. Bishay M, Giacomello L, Retrosi G, Thyoka M, Garriboli M, Brierley J, et al. Hypercapnia and acidosis during open and thoracoscopic repair of congenital diaphragmatic hernia and esophageal atresia: results of a pilot randomized controlled trial. *Ann Surg.* (2013) 258:895–900. doi: 10.1097/SLA.0b013e31828fab55
19. Quezada J, Achurra P, Jarry C, Asbun D, Tejos R, Inzunza M, et al. Minimally invasive tele-mentoring opportunity-the Mito project. *Surg Endosc.* (2020) 34:2585–92. doi: 10.1007/s00464-019-07024-1
20. Bethlehem MS, Kramp KH, van Det MJ, ten Cate Hoedemaker HO, Veeger NJ, Pierie JP. Development of a standardized training course for laparoscopic procedures using Delphi methodology. *J Surg Educ.* (2014) 71:810–6. doi: 10.1016/j.jsurg.2014.04.009
21. Carrabba G, Macchini F, Fabietti I, Schisano L, Meccariello G, Campanella R, et al. Minimally invasive fetal surgery for myelomeningocele: preliminary report from a single center. *Neurosurg Focus.* (2019) 47:E12. doi: 10.3171/2019.8.FOCUS19438
22. Raffaeli G, Ghirardello S, Vanzati M, Baracetti C, Canesi F, Conigliaro F, et al. Start a neonatal extracorporeal membrane oxygenation program: a multistep team training. *Front Pediatr.* (2018) 6:151. doi: 10.3389/fped.2018.00151
23. Gossot D, Seguin-Givelet A. Anatomical variations and pitfalls to know during thoracoscopic segmentectomies. *J Thorac Dis.* (2018) 10:S1134–44. doi: 10.21037/jtd.2017.11.87

28

Robotic Management of Urolithiasis in the Pediatric Population

Natalia Ballesteros [1], Zachary A. Snow [2], Paulo R. M. Moscardi [3], George A. Ransford [1], Pablo Gomez [4] and Miguel Castellan [1,3,5]*

[1] Division of Pediatric Urology, Nicklaus Children's Hospital, Miami, FL, United States, [2] Dr. Kiran C. Patel College of Osteopathic Medicine, Nova Southeastern University, Fort Lauderdale, FL, United States, [3] Division of Pediatric Urology, Jackson Memorial Hospital, Miami, FL, United States, [4] Division of Pediatric Urology, Florida Hospital for Children, Orlando, FL, United States, [5] Division of Pediatric Urology, Joe DiMaggio Children's Hospital, Hollywood, FL, United States

***Correspondence:**
Natalia Ballesteros
natabal4@gmail.com

A variety of surgical techniques exist for the management of urolithiasis. Minimally invasive techniques have replaced open surgery in the last few decades. For complex stone management, robotic-assisted laparoscopic surgery (RALS) has emerged as a safe and feasible alternative in adults. The literature for RALS for urolithiasis (RALS-UL) in the pediatric population is scarce. Herein, we present a review of the literature in both adult and pediatric patients as well as our experience using RALS-UL at our institutions. Special attention is given to the synchronous management of urolithiasis when surgery is performed for other conditions such as ureteropelvic junction obstruction (UPJO), and a supplemental video is provided.

Keywords: robotic, pyelolithotomy, nephrolithotomy, urolithiasis, renal stones, ureteropelvic junction obstruction, pediatric

INTRODUCTION

Urolithiasis is a very common condition affecting both men and women of all age groups. When surgical management is indicated, there are a variety of minimally invasive techniques that have gradually replaced open surgery as the preferred approach (1). Although most patients with kidney or ureteric stones are treated via ureteroscopy (URS) and retrograde intrarenal surgery (RIRS), percutaneous nephrolithotomy (PCNL) or extracorporeal shock wave lithotripsy (ESWL); the use of laparoscopic surgery in stone disease has increased over the last two decades (2), and open surgical interventions such as anatrophic nephrolithotomy and ureterolithotomy are now rarely done. Besides the significant laparoscopic skills needed, drawbacks to laparoscopic stone surgery include challenges with ureteral stenting and suturing, limited dissection and intracorporal reconstruction, as well as increased risk of urinary leak (3–6). The use of the robotic platform allows for improved ergonomics and visualization (magnified, three-dimensional) as well as ease of instrument dexterity that most closely imitates the open technique maintaining the advantages associated with minimally invasive surgery. Robotic assisted laparoscopic surgery for urolithiasis (RALS-UL) overcomes most of the issues associated with open or laparoscopic urolithiasis surgery and the training curve, like most skills, is attainable. Robot-assisted pyelolithotomy, robot-assisted ureterolithotomy and robot-assisted flexible URS are now part of the urologist's arsenal for the treatment of large volume stones and become particularly useful in conditions requiring simultaneous reconstruction (1, 7). In the pediatric population the incidence of urolithiasis appears to be increasing globally (8). The standard procedures to treat stone disease in children have been similar as those used in the adult population (9). However, there is very limited data regarding the use of robotic-assisted surgery in the management of pediatric urolithiasis.

Lee et al. (10) demonstrated safe and effective use of robotic-assisted pyelolithotomy in 5 adolescent patients with large stone burdens. To our knowledge, this is the only study dedicated to the surgical management of stone disease robotically within the pediatric population. In this literature review, we will highlight the current advances in the field of robotics for stone disease among the general population.

MATERIALS AND METHODS

We performed a review of the major studies in adult and pediatric robotic-assisted laparoscopic surgery for urolithiasis (RALS-UL) from 2005 to 2018. Search words included, but were not limited to: robotic, laparoscopic, urolithiasis, stone, pyelolithotomy, nephrolithotomy, and pediatric.

RESULTS

Since 2005, 22 articles for RALS-UL have been published in the adult population for management of various conditions: concomitant management of UPJO and nephrolithiasis (4), concomitant management of caliceal diverticuli with stones (2), pyelolithotomy (2), pyelolithotomy with nephrolithotomy (1), extended pyelolithotomy (4), ureterolithotomy (1 proximal, 1 distal), anatrophic nephrolithotomy (3), and management of stones when ectopic and other renal anomalies are present (2 pelvic kidney, 1 horseshoe kidney, 1 cross-fused ectopic kidney). Of note, many of these studies did not include detailed information regarding the initial patient stone burden. Additionally, the video section of one journal in 2012 reported a case of anatrophic nephrolithotomy. This video was not available for viewing.

In the pediatric population, an article from 2007 is the only one that describes RALS-UL: 4 pyelolithotomies and 1 concomitant management of UPJO and nephrolithiasis. Furthermore, the video section of one journal in 2014 depicted a technique using intraoperative ultrasound probing during RALS-UL in children. This video and further details of the study were not available for reviewing.

DISCUSSION

According to the American Urological Association (AUA) and Endourological Society guidelines on adult urolithiasis, when surgical intervention is necessary, URS/RIRS and ESWL are considered to be first-line treatment for kidney stones < 2 cm, whereas for > 2 cm, PCNL is the therapy of choice (11). This is also the case for pediatric patients, with the addition that ESWL can be implemented as well when stones are >2 cm (12). Although these guidelines do not include RALS as a standard of treatment for routine patients, they do include open, laparoscopic, or robotic interventions as an option for patients with rare anatomic anomalies and complex stone disease or for those requiring concomitant reconstruction (12). This is further supported by the European Association of Urology (EAU) guideline for the management of urinary stone disease in children which states that open or laparoscopic alternatives may be inevitable in such situations (13). Ample literature has shown that laparoscopic and robotic-assisted approaches to stone disease are both viable options for patients with large stones, abnormal collecting system anatomy, and complex stone burden (14). The earliest report of laparoscopy for the management of stone disease was published in the 1979, when Wickham first documented his results of laparoscopic ureterolithotomy via a retroperitoneal approach (15). Then, over a decade later, clinical trials investigating this minimally-invasive method began to expand largely due to the creation of new laparoscopic technologies and the widespread adoption of laparoscopic surgical skills (2). In 1994, Gaur et al. (16) demonstrated the safe and effective use of retroperitoneal laparoscopic pyelolithotomy in 5 patients with medium-sized pelvic stones not amenable to ESWL or PCNL. Since then, multiple studies have been performed showing that laparoscopic pyelolithotomy is comparable to PCNL for kidney stones > 2 cm in the renal pelvis, with certain advantages such as less blood loss and less post-operative analgesia requirement (14, 17). As for laparoscopic ureterolithotomy, clinical trials comparing this approach to traditional flexible ureteroscopy for large upper tract stones (> 2 cm) show comparable to higher stone-free rates, less need for any additional procedures and lower complication rates (18). The success of conventional laparoscopic techniques in the management of large volume stones in combination with the development of the da Vinci® Surgical System by Intuitive Surgical Inc. eventually gave way to the use of robotic-assisted surgery in the treatment of urolithiasis. The use of RALS-UL was first reported by Atug et al. (19). Since then, RALS-UL has become a great tool in the urologist armamentarium for managing diverse complex and challenging cases of urolithiasis where other known modalities may not be feasible or when multiple prior procedures have been attempted.

General Considerations

Preoperative Urine Culture and Antibiotics

The importance of documented urine sterilization prior to urologic surgical intervention cannot be overstated, especially in the setting of intraperitoneal and/or retroperitoneal urine spillage during robotic cases (20). Likewise, perioperative antibiotic prophylaxis should be used based on urologic guidelines and preoperative culture sensitivity.

Ureteral Stents

In general, placement of ureteral double J (JJ) stents is performed depending on the case and at the surgeon's discretion. They can be conducted antegrade during the procedure in similar fashion as when placed in open cases. In other instances, stents may have been already placed preoperatively to relieve obstruction. For other cases, such as in anatrophic nephrolithotomies, routine ureteral stent placement is not done (20). At one of our institutions, we prefer to perform a retrograde pyelogram (RPG) and JJ stent placement prior to all RAL pyeloplasties; therefore, it is done in this manner for concurrent management of renal stones. At another institution (FHC), retrograde pyelogram is not routinely performed and urinary drainage (JJ stenting or nephrostomy tube) is avoided in the majority of RAL pyeloplasties. Indications for JJ stenting at this institution include massive reduction of the renal pelvis, solitary kidney and age < 6 months. Additionally, for isolated pyelolithotomies, we do not leave a ureteral stent when the ureteropelvic junction (UPJ) is not compromised. On infants, we place 3.7 Fr stents, and in older children we use either 3.7 or 4.8 Fr stents.

Nephroscopy and Stone Retrieval

Regardless of stone location in the upper collecting system, the use of the flexible or rigid ureteroscope is a great addition to the surgical intervention. The scope is deployed through an assistant port, when available, or through a robotic trocar after one of the arms is undocked. A ureteral access sheath can be telescoped through the trocar if multiple stones are found or if a large stone burden warrants it. This maneuver decreases surgical time. At our institutions we prefer the use of a flexible ureteroscope for nephroscopy when multiple stones are present to maximize stone clearance (**Figure 1**). The stones can be retrieved with the ProGrasp forceps (Intuitive Surgical INC, Sunnyvale, CA, USA), when easily visible, or using endoscopic graspers or baskets. Laser lithotripsy can be employed as necessary to break large stones into smaller fragments that are easier to retrieve (21). Furthermore, for removing stones from the abdominal cavity, simultaneous removal through the trocar or the use of a commercially available or homemade bag is possible. One article mentioned the use of the fingers of a sterile glove as retrieval bags (21). Interestingly, the use of a flexible cystoscope has also been described to ease intraperitoneal stone removal after pyelolithotomy is closed (22).

Intraoperative Ultrasonography

The use of the laparoscopic ultrasound probe is an additional tool that can aid in localizing calculi before or after nephroscopy and can also be used to identify hilar vessels when needed, for example in anatrophic nephrolithotomy cases (20, 23, 24).

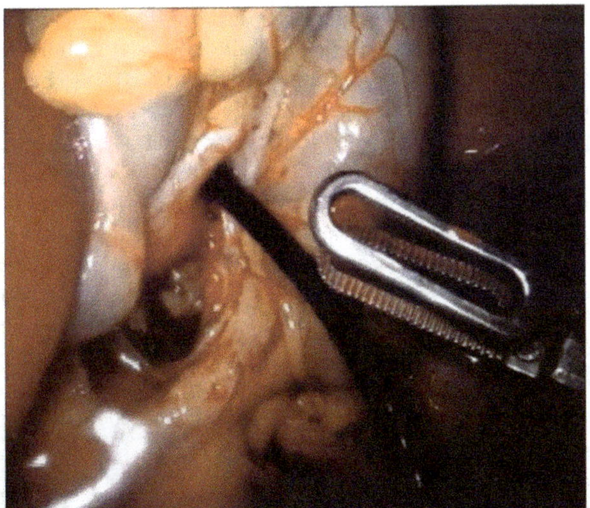

FIGURE 1 | Nephroscopy using a standard digital flexible ureteroscope.

Type of Suture

The collecting system is closed with interrupted or continuous absorbable suture depending on surgeon's preference. In cases of nephrolithotomy, the renal parenchyma can be closed with braided or barbed absorbable suture.

Drain Placement

In many cases, a JP or similar suction drain has been left intraperitoneally for 1–2 days (24–26). At our institutions, for robotic pyeloplasties and other pediatric surgeries, we do not traditionally leave such drain and instead we leave a Foley catheter for 1–2 days. If a JJ stent is left, it is removed 4–6 weeks later. For cases of RALS-UL, we have not had urinary leaks or other complications in this manner.

Urolithiasis and Concomitant UPJO

When presented with cases of UPJO and renal stone disease, options for surgical management are limited. The European Association of Urology guidelines currently recommend that robotic-assisted pyeloplasty (RALP) and surgical intervention for stones be performed in separate procedures (27). However, due to the potential risks of general anesthetics on the brain development of children undergoing multiple and lengthy procedures (28, 29), one should consider as an alternative to perform both surgeries concurrently. Laparoscopic pyeloplasty with pyelolithotomy with or without flexible URS to completely clear stone burden has been widely described in the adult literature. Concomitant RALP and pyelolithotomy (RALP +P) in these patients was first reported by Atug et al. (19). After pyelotomy, flexible renoscopy with stone removal was achieved on 8 patients with 100% stone clearance confirmed on imaging. Since then, 3 more studies looking specifically at RALP + P have emerged supporting the safety and feasibility of the procedure along with high stone-free rates (27, 30, 31). Of these, Zheng et al. (27) reported their experience removing renal calculi with a rigid ureteroscope in 9 patients. The stone-fee rate was 89% with one patient requiring one ESWL session for complete stone clearance. Most recently, in 2017 Jensen et al. (30) demonstrated that although the median operative time for concomitant RALP and RALS-UL was 31 min more than RALP alone, no statistical difference in the blood loss or length of stay were observed.

In the pediatric population, only one case has been described of concomitant RALP and pyelolithotomy on an adolescent. Further details regarding the stone burden was not reported but the patient was rendered stone free with a single procedure (10). At our institutions, over the last 5 years we have performed concomitant RALP + P on 10 patients from 5 to 26 years of age (supplementary video: https://doi.org/10.6084/m9.figshare.8799269.v1). All cases had preoperatively been diagnosed with UPJO and ipsilateral nephrolithiasis. As above mentioned, after pyelotomy, nephroscopy and stone removal was performed (**Figure 2**). Length of stay was 1 day in 7 cases. The extra day spent by the remaining patients was for pain control or for observation. Nine of 10 patients were rendered stone free with robotic intervention. In 2 patients, no stone was found. One of them had a punctate stone recognized on preoperative computed tomography (CT) and was believed to have been flushed out

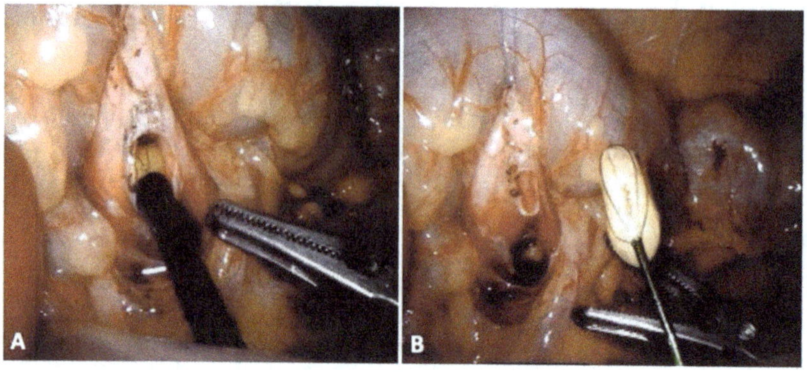

FIGURE 2 | Patient with UPJO and nephrolithiasis undergoing pyeloplasty and concomitant nephrolithotomy. Through the flexible ureteroscope **(A)**, a standard basket device is used for stone extraction **(B)**.

with irrigation as it was not visualized later on postoperative imaging. The other patient had a history of a small lower pole calculus. This was missed during nephroscopy and shortly after the pyeloplasty he passed the stone spontaneously. Of note, this patient later underwent other interventions for recurrent urolithiasis, including on the contralateral kidney.

Pyelolithotomy, Extended Pyelolithotomy, and Nephrolithotomy

With the above-mentioned success of concurrent RALP + P, robotic pyelolithotomy has become the most common approach in the RALS-UL literature and further applications have been explored to include nephrolithotomy and extended pyelolithotomy procedures. Pyelolithotomy involves incision of the renal pelvis with subsequent stone extraction. Further involvement of the calyceal system calls for an extended approach. Nephrotomy and nephrolithotomy is performed to allow stone extraction when there is a narrow infundibulum or part of the calculus is attached to the parenchyma. In 2006, Badani et al. (32) reported their experience with robotic extended pyelolithotomy (REP). The patient is positioned in modified lateral decubitus with minimal to no flexion and without kidney rest elevation. After adequate exposure of the renal pelvis, a pyelotomy is performed away from the UPJ. The authors demonstrated complete stone removal and minimal blood loss in 12 patients with partial staghorn calculi. Of note, a 13th patient with complete staghorn stones was unsuccessfully cleared, leading to the conclusion that REP is not a suitable technique for full staghorn calculi. Other authors have described REP with similar experiences (33–35), with the latest one being a case report of a 31-year-old non-diabetic woman with emphysematous pyelonephritis caused by on a 6.5 cm gas-containing calculus (35). In 2015, Rajiv et al. (25) described a case of bilateral large stone disease managed with simultaneous bilateral robot-assisted pyelolithotomy, showing minimal morbidity, a short hospital course and the avoidance of adjuvant procedures. A multi-center evaluation of robotic pyelolithotomy and robotic nephrolithotomy in 27 patients between 2008 and 2014 concluded that both techniques are safe (minimal bleeding and low risk of sepsis) and effective (maximum stone free clearance and infrequent retreatment rates) for patients with large renal pelvis and calyceal stones (36). Cystine stones account for 1–2% and 6–8% of urolithiasis in the adult and pediatric population, respectively (21). Although cystinuria is best treated medically for stone prevention, the surgical management of large stones can be quite a challenge and may require multiple endourologic procedures. On the other hand, robotic pyelolithotomy is a feasible alternative. In 2017, Megiatto et al. (21) reported a case of a 20-year-old woman who was poorly compliant with medical treatment and had undergone several procedures through the years for her disease. On one side, there was a single stone that required both URS and ESWL to clear. For her large, multiple stone burden contralaterally (36 stones), she underwent robotic pyelolithotomy with concomitant renoscopy and laser lithotripsy. In the only published report of RALS-UL in the pediatric population, 4 patients, between the ages of 10 and 23, underwent robotic-assisted laparoscopic lithotomy for the treatment of large cystine stones 2–7 cm in size (10). These stones had been refractory to previous PCNL and ESWL. Additionally, one patient required open conversion due to an intrarenal pelvis and inability to remove the stone. This patient required 3 additional procedures (ESWL and 2 URS) to become stone free. In 2014, Ghani et al. (23) published a video that depicts a technique for using intraoperative ultrasound probing during RALS-UL in 4 children to aid in stone localization. This video was not available for viewing but is worth mentioning as an additional tool that can be applied to RALS-UL. At one of our institutions, we performed metachronous bilateral pyelolithotomies in a 15-year-old girl with bilateral staghorn calculi and a new diagnosis of cystinuria (**Figure 3**). In both cases, no ureteral stents were left indwelling as the UPJs were not compromised. She had a 1-night hospitalization per each surgery. There were no overall complications and she was 100% stone free following the procedures.

Calyceal Diverticular Calculi

Another example of approaching urolithiasis concomitantly with the management of another condition is in the treatment of

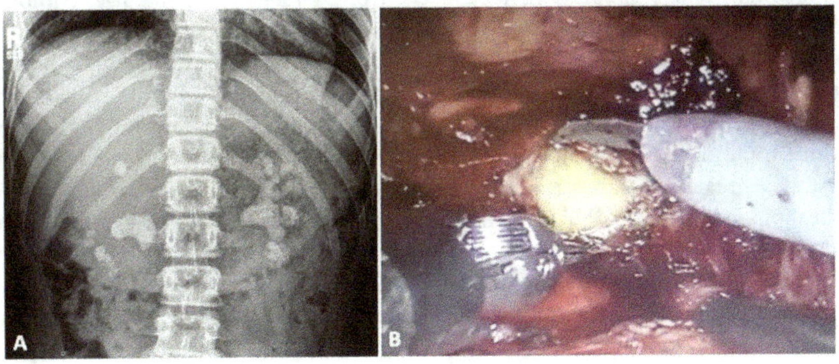

FIGURE 3 | Patient with bilateral staghorn calculi and cystinuria **(A)** undergoes metachronous bilateral pyelolithotomies **(B)**.

calyceal diverticular calculi. The incidence of stones within a calyceal diverticulum ranges from 1 to 10% (37). Although these are managed primarily with ESWL, RIRS and PCNL; laparoscopic and robotic assisted interventions are feasible alternatives. Furthermore, laparoscopic intervention has been proposed to be the approach for management of anteriorly-located calyceal diverticuli that have failed prior endourologic attempts or for anteriorly-located stones > 3 cm (38). In 2014, Torricelli et al. (37) reported the first case managed robotically in a 33-year old obese woman with a symptomatic 2 cm, anterior mid polar calyceal diverticular calculus. She had undergone two prior failed URS attempts: one with diverticular laser incision but inability to remove stone fragments after lithotripsy and the second had found the diverticular neck to be obliterated. After RALS-UL, the diverticulum was managed with fulguration. The patient was in a 45-degree lateral decubitus position with the table flexed, and the ports were placed in similar fashion as for robotic-assisted laparoscopic partial nephrectomy (RALPN). As in RALPN, the renal vasculature was clamped for warm ischemia. Likewise, an intraperitoneal drain was left in place for 2 days. More recently, Verbrugghe et al. (39) described their similar experience with an anterior calyceal diverticulum with stone burden in the lower pole of a 55-year old woman with an additional history of pyelonephritis. In the first case, the use of a robotic ultrasound probe was used for identification of the diverticulum while in the second case a CT-guided puncture of the calyx was done with a harpoon left in place for localization.

Congenital Renal Anomalies

Ectopic pelvic and horseshoe kidneys are a surgical challenge in the management of ureterolithiasis. They are located in close proximity to the bony pelvis and are surrounded by important visceral organs. In addition to abnormal vasculature, they have intrinsic anatomical anomalies such as malrotation, anteriorly displaced renal pelves, and high ureteral insertions. These often lead to partial or complete urinary obstruction and hydronephrosis. UPJO is found in 70% of ectopic kidneys with hydronephrosis (5). Concomitant urolithiasis poses a challenge for endourological interventions, including PCNL requiring modified renal access. RALS-UL is an alternative that has been demonstrated in the literature to be safely feasible. Pyeloplasty with concomitant pyelolithotomy on an ectopic pelvic kidney with UPJO and nephrolithiasis was first described in 2010 by Zheng et al. (27). The patient was a 55-year old man who presented with abdominal pain, a serum creatinine (Cr) of 2.3 mg/dL, and the aforementioned renal anomalies. Six months after surgical intervention, the patient was doing well, Cr had significantly improved, and renal function had increased from 19 to 24%. In the management of isolated large-burden urolithiasis in these anomalous kidneys, the traditional surgical modalities have been employed in the past such as RIRS, ESWL, and PCNL. However, due to the above-mentioned anatomic challenges, these surgeries are often difficult and unsuccessful for complete stone clearance (24). In these cases, endopyelotomy with subsequent pyelolithotomy can be accomplished. Examples described in the literature include an ectopic pancake, or fused lumped kidney, with a 2.5 cm stone in one of the moieties (40) and a horseshoe kidney with multiple pelvicalyceal calculi (25). In most cases, patient positioning and robotic port placement were done in a prostatectomy-like configuration. In the pediatric population, this would be comparable to positioning and port placement for bilateral vesicoureteral reimplantations. A transmesenteric approach was utilized for endopyelotomy and subsequent pyelolithotomy thus avoiding mobilization of the colon and its increased operative time and potential risk for injury (22, 25).

Ureterolithiasis

RALS-UL is also helpful in the setting of complex ureteral calculi and prior surgical interventions. It's use in the upper urinary tract with good outcomes has been previously reported (41). In 2015 Olvera-Posada et al. (3) reported the case of a 66-year-old female with a history of recurrent ureterolithiasis, recurrent urinary tract infections (UTIs), two large obstructing right proximal ureteral calculi, and a right split renal function of 37%. Despite a remote successful ureteroscopy in the past on that same kidney, the patient underwent failed attempts at antegrade or retrograde access to the stone in this instance; partially due to ureteral tortuosity and significant inflammatory changes. She underwent robotic assisted ureteropyelostomy for the stone removal followed by pyeloplasty for closure. At 1-year follow up renogram the right renal function was 42% and there was good drainage. Likewise, RALS-UL has been performed successfully in the lower ureters. In 2013 Dogra et al. (4) published outcomes on 16 patients (mean age 27) treated with robotic-assisted distal ureterolithotomies for impacted stones over 2 cm in size. Their mean operative time was 45.3 min with a mean console time of 20.3 min, which was significantly shorter when compared with a traditional endoscopic approach. Additionally, they demonstrated greater clearance rates and a lower incidence of complications compared to URS. Of note, all patients underwent urethral catheterization, intraperitoneal ureteral stenting, and placement of intraperitoneal drain. The drain was removed on postoperative day (POD) 1 and the Foley on POD 2, with the ureteral stents removed around 4 weeks later.

Robotic Anthropic Nephrolithotomy

Open anatrophic nephrolithotomy is done now rarely despite its high rate of stone clearance due to the morbidity of the procedure. In the majority, the laparoscopic method has been performed with warm ischemia, due to the difficulties achieving renal icing intraperitoneally (24). This modality is not ideal for preservation of renal function. Sotelo (42) was the first to report a case of robotic-assisted anatrophic nephrolithotomy (RANL). This was done via video submission and it was not available for viewing at this time. They reported implementation of vascular control with early unclamping and controlled hypotension. Like in the laparoscopic approach, warm ischemia was replicated with a time of 26 min. The patient required intraoperative blood transfusion, a residual 1 cm stone was later identified, and furosemide renogram showed 10% renal function loss at 1 month of follow up. In 2013, using their practice with cold ischemia for partial nephrectomies, Ghani et al. (24) then reported their experience performing RANL on three patients. They described their technique which includes initial cystoscopic placement of a JJ ureteral stent and the patient is then placed in a traditional flank position. Port placement includes a gel port placed in the midline, with a camera and assistant port through it, two more robotic arm ports and an additional assistant port. Renal hypothermia was achieved with ice slush which was introduced through the gel port. Following this, Mannitol was administered, and the hilum was clamped. The incision was made through the avascular plane and after nephrolithotomy, the collecting system was closed with monofilament suture and running barbed suture was used for the renal parenchyma. The mean cold ischemia time was 57 min. The authors achieved a stone-free rate of 33%, with intraoperative knowledge that 2 of the 3 patients had incomplete stone clearance, despite having used intraoperative ultrasonography. These 2 patients required PCNL to remove the residual calculi. One patient had a drain placed as a nephrostomy tube for drainage of pyonephrosis at the time of stone removal. There were no complications including no need for blood transfusion. Renal function preservation was corroborated upon follow up based on creatinine clearance. Another study of RANL in 2014 was performed by King et al. (26) on 7 patients, 5 with complete staghorn calculi. The mean warm ischemia time was 35 min. They demonstrated a 29% stone-free rate with minimal hospital length of stay and few post-operative complications, including a blood transfusion and continuous bladder irrigation in one patient for hematuria. Although these studies failed to demonstrate significant stone-free rates as compared to the open technique, both studies highlight the successful debulking of large staghorn stones in a traditionally difficult to manage population and with improved morbidity. Also, further research needs to be done to determine if there is a significant long-term difference in renal function with regards to the use of cold vs. warm ischemia. Another advantage of performing this surgery robotically, is the application of intraoperative near infrared fluorescence (NIRF) with indocyanine green (ICG) dye. Although not performed in humans, NIRF has been assessed in porcine models to detect the avascular renal plane for proper demarcation of the site of nephrolithotomy (43). Madi et al. (20) described their use of NIRF intraoperative to assess if there is any residual renal perfusion after vascular clamping perhaps from an accessory or unclamped vessel. They do not mention if a dose of ICG was given before obtaining vascular control for use on the kidney to identify the avascular plane.

CONCLUSION

Minimally invasive management of stones in general has evolved in the last few decades.

Although URS, RIRS, ESWL, and PCNL are still first line treatment in the management of pediatric and adult urolithiasis, RALS-UL has been demonstrated to be safe, effective, and with high stone-free rates in some specific cases. Although all authors stated encouraging results, no study compared the robotic approach to first-line minimally-invasive surgery. RALS-UL is a viable option for patients in whom the above minimally invasive techniques are not applicable or in circumstances where their use is hampered: complex urinary tract calculi, failed prior procedures, or abnormal genitourinary anatomy. Furthermore, concomitant RALS-UL can be performed when other reconstructive interventions are planned. For example, RALP + P should constitute the first choice of treatment for concomitant renal stones and UPJO. The use of flexible URS aids in localizing and extracting stone burden. We have successfully performed RALS-UL at our institution and though the pediatric literature is scarce, this area continues to be one that needs further research.

AUTHOR CONTRIBUTIONS

NB and ZS contributed to the conception and design of the study. NB, GR, and PG contributed to database acquisition and analysis. NB and ZS co-wrote the first drafts of the manuscript. PM, PG, and MC wrote sections of the manuscript. All authors contributed to manuscript revision, read and approved the submitted version, and agree to be accountable for all aspects of the work.

ACKNOWLEDGMENTS

We are grateful to all the personnel that was involved in the medical and surgical treatment of these patients.

REFERENCES

1. Müller PF, Schlager D, Hein S, Bach C, Miernik A, Schoeb DS. Robotic stone surgery—Current state and future prospects: a systematic review. *Arab J Urol.* (2018) 16:357–64. doi: 10.1016/j.aju.2017.09.004
2. Humphreys MR. The emerging role of robotics and laparoscopy in stone disease. *Urol Clin North Am.* (2013) 40:115–28. doi: 10.1016/j.ucl.2012.09.005
3. Olvera-Posada D, Dion M, Alenezi H, Razvi H, Pautler SE. Robotic proximal ureteropyelostomy after unsuccessful endourologic management of complicated proximal ureteral stone disease. *J Endourol Case Rep.* (2015) 1:30–2. doi: 10.1089/cren.2015.29012.dop
4. Dogra PN, Regmi SK, Singh P, Saini AK, Nayak B. Lower ureteral stonesrevisited: expanding the horizons of robotics. *Urology.* (2013) 82:95–9. doi: 10.1016/j.urology.2013.02.059
5. Nayyar R, Singh P, Gupta NP. Robot-assisted laparoscopic pyeloplasty withstone removal in an ectopic pelvic kidney. *JSLS.* (2010) 14:130–2. doi: 10.4293/108680810X12674612015102
6. Gaur DD, Trivedi S, Prabhudesai MR, Madhusudhana HR, Gopichand M. Laparoscopicureterolithotomy: technical considerations and long-term follow-up. *BJU Int.* (2002) 89:339–43. doi: 10.1046/j.1464-4096.2001.01562.x
7. Siddiqui KM, Albala DM. Robotic-assisted surgery and treatment of urolithiasis. *Int J Surg.* (2016) 36 (Pt D):673–5. doi: 10.1016/j.ijsu.2016.11.031
8. Hwang K, Mason MD, Peters CA. Clinical practice: surgical approaches to urolithiasis in children. *Eur J Pediatrics.* (2011) 170:681–8. doi: 10.1007/s00431-010-1373-6
9. Aydogdu O, Karakose A, Celik O, Atesci YZ. Recent management of urinary stone disease in a pediatric population. *World J Clin Pediatrics.* (2014) 3:1–5. doi: 10.5409/wjcp.v3.i1.1
10. Lee RS, Passerotti CC, Cendron M, Estrada CR, Borer JG, Peters CA. Early results of robot assisted laparoscopic lithotomy in adolescents. *J Urol.* (2007) 177:2306–9; discussion 2309–10. doi: 10.1016/j.juro.2007.01.178
11. Assimos D, Krambeck A, Miller NL, Monga M, Murad MH, Nelson CP, et al. Surgical management of stones: American Urological Association/Endourological Society Guideline, Part I. *J Urol.* (2016) 196:1153–60. doi: 10.1016/j.juro.2016.05.090
12. Assimos D, Krambeck A, Miller NL, Monga M, Murad MH, Nelson CP, et al. Surgical management of stones: American Urological Association/Endourological Society Guideline, Part II. *J Urol.* (2016) 196:1161–9. doi: 10.1016/j.juro.2016.05.091
13. Radmayr C, Bogaert G, Dogan HS, Kocvara R, Nijman JM, Stein R, Tekgul S, et al. *European Association of Urology Guidelines on Paediatric Urology: Urinary Stone Disease.* (2018). Available online at: https://uroweb.org/guideline/paediatric-urology/#3_14 (accessed April 8, 2019).
14. Pedro RN, Buchholz N. Laparoscopic and robotic surgery for stone disease. *Urolithiasis.* (2018) 46:125–7. doi: 10.1007/s00240-017-1014-x
15. Wickham JE. The surgical treatment of renal lithiasis. In: Wickham JE, editor. *Urinary Calculous Disease.* Edinburg: Churchill Livingstone (1979).
16. Gaur DD, Agarwal DK, Purohit KC, Darshane AS. Retroperitoneal laparoscopic pyelolithotomy. *J Urol.* (1994) 151:927–9. doi: 10.1016/S0022-5347(17)35124-8
17. Singh V, Sinha RJ, Gupta DK, Pandey M. Prospective randomized comparison of retroperitoneoscopic pyelolithotomy versus percutaneous nephrolithotomy for solitary large pelvic kidney stones. *Urol Int.* (2014) 92:392–5. doi: 10.1159/000353973
18. Kumar A, Vasudeva P, Nanda B, Kumar N, Jha SK, Singh H. A prospective randomized comparison between laparoscopic ureterolithotomy and semirigid ureteroscopy for upper ureteral stones >2 cm: a single-center experience. *J Endourol.* (2015) 29:1248–52. doi: 10.1089/end.2013.0791
19. Atug F, Castle EP, Burgess SV, Thomas R. Concomitant management of renalcalculi and pelvi-ureteric junction obstruction with robotic laparoscopicsurgery. *BJU Int.* (2005) 96:1365–8. doi: 10.1111/j.1464-410X.2005.05819.x
20. Madi R, Hemal A. Robotic pyelolithotomy, extended pyelolithotomy,nephrolithotomy, and anatrophic nephrolithotomy. *J Endourol.* (2018) 32:S73–81. doi: 10.1089/end.2017.0718
21. Meggiato L, Cattaneo F, Zattoni F, Dal Moro F, Beltrami P, Zattoni F. Complex cystine kidney stones treated with combined robot-assisted laparoscopicpyelolithotomy and intraoperative renoscopy. *Urologia.* (2018) 85:76–8. doi: 10.5301/uro.5000215
22. Al-Yousef R, Almarzouq A, Aldousari S. Robotic pyelolithotomy in a congenital pelvic kidney: side docking and robotic prostatectomy port - site approach. *Int Braz J Urol.* (2017) 43:374. doi: 10.1590/s1677-5538.ibju.2016.0059
23. Ghani KR, Trinh QD, Jeong W, Friedman A, Lakshmanan Y, Omenon M, et al. Robotic nephrolithotomy and pyelolithotomy with utilization of the roboticultrasound probe. *Int Braz J Urol.* (2014) 40:125–6; discussion 126. doi: 10.1590/S1677-5538.IBJU.2014.01.19
24. Ghani KR, Rogers CG, Sood A, Kumar R, Ehlert M, Jeong W, et al. Robot-assisted anatrophic nephrolithotomy with renal hypothermia for managing staghorn calculi. *J Endourol.* (2013) 27:1393–8. doi: 10.1089/end.2013.0266
25. Rajiv Y, Kumar A, Poonam Y. Bilateral simultaneous robot-assistedpyelolithotomy for large (>6 cm) kidney stones: technique and review ofliterature. *J Robot Surg.* (2015) 9:263–6. doi: 10.1007/s11701-015-0524-1
26. King SA, Klaassen Z, Madi R. Robot-assisted anatrophic nephrolithotomy: description of technique and early results. *J Endourol.* (2014) 28:325–9. doi: 10.1089/end.2013.0597
27. Zheng J, Yan J, Zhou Z, Chen Z, Li X, Pan J, et al. Concomitant treatment ofureteropelvic junction obstruction and renal calculi with robotic laparoscopicsurgery and rigid nephroscopy. *Urology.* (2014) 83:237–42. doi: 10.1016/j.urology.2013.08.008
28. FDA. *FDA Drug Safety Communication: FDA Review Results in New Warnings about Using General Anesthetics and Sedation Drugs in Young Children and Pregnant Women.* Available online at: https://Www.Fda.Gov/Drugs/Drugsafety/Ucm532356.Htm (accessed April 8, 2019).
29. FDA. *FDA Drug Safety Communication: FDA Approves Label Changes for Use of General Anesthetic and Sedation Drugs in Young Children.* https://www.fda.gov/Drugs/DrugSafety/ucm554634.htm (accessed April 8, 2019).
30. Jensen PH, Berg KD, Azawi NH. Robot-assisted pyeloplasty and pyelolithotomy inpatients with ureteropelvic junction stenosis. *Scand J Urol.* (2017) 51:323–8. doi: 10.1080/21681805.2017.1300188
31. Mufarrij PW, Woods M, Shah OD, Palese MA, Berger AD, Thomas R, et al. Robotic dismembered pyeloplasty: a 6-year, multi-institutional experience. *J Urol.* (2008) 180:1391–6. doi: 10.1016/j.juro.2008.06.024
32. Badani KK, Hemal AK, Fumo M, Kaul S, Shrivastava A, Rajendram AK, et al. Robotic extended pyelolithotomy for treatment of renal calculi: a feasibility study. *World J Urol.* (2006) 24:198–201. doi: 10.1007/s00345-006-0099-6
33. Nayyar R, Wadhwa P, Hemal AK. Pure robotic extended pyelolithotomy: cosmeticreplica of open surgery. *J Robot Surg.* (2007) 1:207–11. doi: 10.1007/s11701-007-0039-5
34. Sotelo R, Astigueta JC, Giedelman C, de Andrade R, Carmona O, Ramirez D, et al. Robotic extended pyelolithotomy for complete staghorn calculus. *J Robot Surg.* (2010) 4:99–102. doi: 10.1007/s11701-010-0192-0
35. Manny TB, Manny JS, Hemal AK. Transmesocolic robotic extended pyelolithotomyof a large gas-containing renal stone: case report and review of the literature. *Urol Ann.* (2013) 5:126–8. doi: 10.4103/0974-7796.110015
36. Swearingen R, Sood A, Madi R, Klaassen Z, Badani K, Elder JS, et al. Zero-fragment nephrolithotomy: a multi-center evaluation of robotic pyelolithotomy and nephrolithotomy for treating renal stones. *Eur Urol.* (2017) 72:1014–21. doi: 10.1016/j.eururo.2016.10.021
37. Torricelli FC, Batista LT, Colombo JR Jr, Coelho RF. Robotic-assistedlaparoscopic management of a caliceal diverticular calculus. *BMJ Case Rep.* (2014) 2014:bcr2014205437. doi: 10.1136/bcr-2014-205437
38. Koopman SG, Fuchs G. Management of stones associated with intrarenal stenosis: infundibular stenosis and caliceal diverticulum. *J Endourol.* (2013) 27: 1546–50. doi: 10.1089/end.2013.0186
39. Verbrugghe A, Gaillandre L, Mouton D, Deschildre F, Koenig P, Ballereau C, et al. Robot-assisted laparoscopic management of caliceal diverticular calculi. *Urol Case Rep.* (2017) 13:133–6. doi: 10.1016/j.eucr.2017.04.004

40. Kumar S, Bishnoi K, Panwar VK, Kumar A, Sharma MK. Stone in ectopic pelvicpancake kidney: a surgical challenge overcome by robotic surgery. *J Robot Surg.* (2018) 12:181–3. doi: 10.1007/s11701-017-0704-2
41. Hemal AK, Nayyar R, Gupta NP, Dorairajan LN. Experience with robotic assisted laparoscopic surgery in upper tract urolithiasis. *Can J Urol.* (2010) 17:5299–305.
42. Sotelo R. Robotic assisted laparoscopic anatrophic nephrolithotomy: first case report. J Endourol (2012) 26:P1–572. doi: 10.1016/S1569-9056(13)61621-8
43. Sood A, Hemal AK, Assimos DG, Peabody JO, Menon M, Ghani KR. Robotic anatrophic nephrolithotomy utilizing near-infrared fluorescence image-guidance: idea, development, exploration, assessment, and long-term monitoring (IDEAL) stage 0 animal model study. *Urology.* (2016) 94:117–22. doi: 10.1016/j.urology.2016.04.051

29

Ongoing Laryngeal Stenosis: Conservative Management and Alternatives to Tracheostomy

Cláudia Schweiger [1,2] and Denise Manica [1]*

[1] Otolaryngology Department, Hospital de Clínicas de Porto Alegre, Porto Alegre, Brazil, [2] Programa de Pós-Graduação em Saúde da Criança e do Adolescente, Universidade Federal do Rio Grande do Sul, Porto Alegre, Brazil

***Correspondence:**
Cláudia Schweiger
causch@hotmail.com

Background: Following tracheal intubation, some children may develop stridor, which is an indication of an obstructive lesion in the airway, such as an ongoing laryngeal stenosis (LS). This review focuses on evaluation of stridor and possible endoscopic predictors of progression to LS and, once post-intubation acute lesions are established, therapeutic choices to manage this disorder in avoidance of tracheostomy. Tracheostomy, due to its inherent increased morbidity, mortality and influence on social stigma, should be viewed only as a last resort. In this article, available conservative and alternative therapies for ongoing LS are thoroughly reviewed.

Methods: A systematic review concerning randomized clinical trials and prospective studies on treatment modalities for LS was performed. A search strategy was developed for MEDLINE comprising terms related to disease, intervention and population. Title and abstract from captured references were peer-reviewed for eligibility. Selected studies full-texts were peer-reviewed and the results were compiled in a structured and narrative review. Stridor evaluation and post-extubation acute lesion classification were studied. Treatments such as balloon dilation, rigid dilation, corticosteroid-coated small tube intubation, and corticosteroid nebulization were described and evidence supporting their usage was discussed.

Keywords: airway stenosis, larynx, acute lesions, intubation, laryngoplasty

INTRODUCTION

Laryngeal stenosis occurs mainly as a consequence of endotracheal intubation. Endotracheal tube induced mucosal injury is a well-recognized etiopathogenic factor leading to stenosis but contributing factors are still a matter of debate. Among these, sedation level (1) and length of intubation (2) have already been demonstrated as definite risk factors.

Definition of acute lesions comprises those identified in <30 days since extubation (3, 4). Moderate to severe lesions pose the highest probability of progressing to chronic stenosis. Recently a classification for acute lesions was proposed with high sensitivity and specificity for the development of laryngeal stenosis. This classification is showed in **Table 1** (5).

Endoscopic treatment of acute lesions may avoid eventual tracheostomy and need for open surgery; or result in a less obstructive lesion that may present a better probability of success for a following intervention.

A range of different endoscopic approaches can be used, both isolated or combined. The use of endoscopic treatment is resurging and this can be attributed to the availability of new and

TABLE 1 | Classification of acute laryngeal Injuries (CALI) as mild, moderate, or severe, according to anatomical location and type of injury.

	Group 1	Group 2	
	Mild	**Moderate**	**Severe**
Supraglottis	■ Edema ■ Hyperemia		
Glottis	■ Edema ■ Hyperemia	■ Uni- or bilateral ulceration ■ Arytenoid GT	■ Inter-arytenoid ulceration ■ Inter-arytenoid GT ■ Immobility
Subglottis	■ Edema ■ Hyperemia	■ Partial ulceration (<360°)	■ Complete ulceration (3,600) ■ GT

GT, granulation tissue.

TABLE 2 | Search strategy for MEDLINE (accessed: 07/07/2019).

Search term	Number of entries
#1: ("Laryngostenosis"[Mesh] OR "laryngeal stenosis"[tw] OR "subglottic stenosis"[tw] OR "laryngeal stenosis"[All fields] OR "subglottic stenosis" [All fields]) OR ("stridor" AND "intubation" [All fields]) OR ("acute laryngeal stenosis" [All fields])	4,192
#2: (Infant[MeSH] OR Infant* OR infancy OR Newborn* OR Baby* OR Babies OR Neonat* OR Preterm* OR Prematur* OR Postmatur* OR Child[MeSH] OR Child* OR Schoolchild* OR School age* OR Preschool* OR Kid or kids OR Toddler* OR Adolescent[MeSH] OR Adoles* OR Teen* OR Boy* OR Girl* OR Minors[MeSH] OR Minors* OR Puberty[MeSH] OR Pubert* OR Pubescen* OR Prepubescen* OR Pediatrics[MeSH] OR Pediatric* OR Pediatric* OR Peadiatric* OR Schools[MeSH] OR Nursery school* OR Kindergar* OR Primary school* OR Secondary school* OR Elementary school* OR High school* OR Highschool*)	4,582,304
#3: (corticosteroid[tw] OR steroid[tw] OR balloon*[tw] OR dilat*[tw] OR rigid*[tw] OR "Mitomycin"[Mesh] OR "1a-docosahexaenoyl mitomycin C" [Supplementary Concept] OR "mitomycin C-N (2)-deoxyguanosine adduct" [Supplementary Concept] OR "mitomycin C-DNA adduct" [Supplementary Concept] OR "mitomycin C-immunoglobulin M antibody conjugate" [Supplementary Concept] OR "mitomycin C-dextran" [Supplementary Concept] OR "mitomycin C-anti-alpha-fetoprotein antibody conjugate" [Supplementary Concept] OR mitomycin[tw] OR "cricoid split"[tw])	543,280
#1 AND **#2** AND **#3**	428

more sophisticated endoscopic instrumentation and the adjunctive use of new pharmaceuticals (6). Besides, endoscopic treatment results in a shorter operative time, decreased length of hospitalization, avoidance of external incisions, and less emotional and financial burden on the family.

Despite important advances in the management of subglottic stenosis over the last decades, its treatment remains complex and challenging. The aim of this systematic review is to identify current available endoscopic approaches for this disease and evaluate their success rates.

METHODS

Information Sources and Search Strategy

We have performed a comprehensive systematic review in order to identify all reports concerning ongoing laryngeal stenosis and therapeutic strategies. Search strategy was developed for MEDLINE and comprised terms defining laryngeal stenosis and related disorders, and available therapies. Annals from major international meetings in otolaryngology and pediatric airway surgery were also consulted. We have also hand searched references from all retrieved publications and prior systematic reviews. The search strategy for MEDLINE is available in **Table 2**. Further search strategies followed the same structure.

Duplicates were excluded before proceeding to study selection. All titles and abstracts retrieved were screened independently by two researchers. Full-text articles also had its eligibility evaluated by two independent researchers. The last date of the search was July 7th, 2019. We have followed Preferred Reporting Items for Systematic Reviews and Meta-Analyses (PRISMA) statement for conducting this study and reporting our results (7, 8).

Eligibility Criteria

Inclusion Criteria

We have included all references concerning randomized clinical trials (RCT), phase I and II prospective studies, case series and case reports, involving neonatal (0–28 days old) and pediatric (29 days to 18 years) patients, and reporting results on pharmacologic and endoscopic treatments as primary approaches for ongoing laryngeal stenosis. Only reports in English, Portuguese, Spanish, Italian and German were eligible.

Exclusion Criteria

We have not included other types of publications such as reviews, editorials, letters to the editor, guidelines, study protocols or position papers. All open surgical approaches (even if endoscopic procedures were performed as adjunctive treatment) were excluded. Also, studies pertaining to population samples concerning adult patients (both exclusively or alongside pediatric patients) were excluded. Congenital stenosis or those acquired by other causes not associated with endotracheal intubation were excluded because they do not share the same pathologic mechanisms.

Study Selection and Review

Two reviewers participated in the screening and full-text evaluation. All abstracts screened and articles selected were reviewed by the same two reviewers, while a third reviewer would intervene if there was any discordance over eligibility. Reports were classified based on their main focus, whether diagnosis, prognosis, treatment and complications. All reviews were proceeded independently, and final drafts from both reviewers were eventually compiled into one final review article.

RESULTS

Search Results

The initial search resulted in 432 references. After excluding duplicates and articles not concerning study's population and/or intervention, 106 were eventually assessed as full text. Finally, 22 articles fulfilled eligibility criteria and were included in qualitative synthesis. No quantitative meta-analysis of data was possible due to heterogeneity of interventions and scarcity of comparative trials. Studies content was summarized below. PRISMA flow diagram is depicted in **Figure 1**.

Elective Endotracheal Intubation

Hoeve et al. described 23 patients with a mean age of 37 days who presented extubation failure due to acute laryngeal lesion. They were re-intubated with a "loose fit" tube (inferior in diameter to what would be recommended concerning patient age, permitting leakage of air at the end of an insufflation) for a period of 17 days. Only one of these patients progressed to tracheostomy. When the airway finding was edema or superficial lesions, mean time for intubation was only 8 days and more than half of these patients were extubated within 3 days. When ulceration and edema was found, the mean intubation time was 13 days. However, when granulation was present, intubation longed for weeks afterwards (9).

Graham reported 10 newborn patients undergoing a protocol of 2 weeks of intubation after extubation failure due to acute lesion. Six patients were successfully extubated; two were tracheostomized and decannulated afterwards, with no need for further surgical procedures; one underwent tracheal reconstruction; and the other tracheostomized patient died due to other causes (10).

Monnier recommends that, when dealing with soft-tissue stenosis without mucosal necrosis, a re-intubation should be performed with a one-size smaller endotracheal tube with topical application of an endolaryngeal plug of gentamycin-corticosteroid ointment. Most of these patients can be extubated after a mean re-intubation period of 2–4 days (11).

Endoscopic Balloon Dilation (EBD)

Balloon dilation was first described in 1984 as a method to treat tracheal and bronchial stenosis (12) Subsequently, other case reports were published (13–15). All of them, however, applied balloon dilation for patients with chronic stenoses. The analysis of balloon dilation results for chronic and acute stenoses as separate diseases was only recently attempted.

Compared to previous methods of dilation such as bougies and endotracheal tubes, this new technique has the theoretical advantage of exerting radial pressure on the airway, which projects the stenosis away from the center of the airway, reducing the incidence of shear-related trauma of the epithelium that may occur with rigid dilation (16). Balloon dilation has been studied in several case series since 1991, but its indications, safety and efficacy were still under debate.

The literature search identified 24 abstracts about balloon dilation. After review of the full-length articles, 14 were excluded, due to its use for chronic stenoses (15, 17–20), due to its lack of differentiation between acute or chronic stenosis (16, 19, 21–27), and/or because the paper did not differentiate between rigid or balloon dilations (27, 28). The 10 remaining papers were selected for this review (3, 29–37).

Technique

Balloon dilation is performed under general anesthesia in all articles, using a high pressure, non-compliant balloon catheter. The technique has a slight variability in the studies.

Some authors used the INSPIRA AIRTM balloon (Acclarent Inc., CA, U.S.A.) (33, 37). Other authors do not mention the brands of their balloons and/or use many different brands (3, 29–32, 34–36). The balloon size was selected according to the ideal subglottic diameter for the patient's age (3, 29, 32–34, 36, 37). An inflation/deflation handle mounted with a syringe and gauge assembly designed to monitor and maintain the pressure was used by all authors (29–38). The balloon was inflated to rated burst pressure by some authors (33, 36, 37). Other authors specifically mentioned pressures between 2 and 15 atm, (3) 2 atm, (29, 31, 34), 4 atm, (32), 7 atm (30). The balloon was maintained inflated for 30–60 s or until the patient's oxygen saturation level dropped below 90–92% (3, 29–37). Some authors repeated the procedure 2–3 times during each session (31–37).

Outcomes of Balloon Dilation

The 10 case reports and series (nine retrospectives, one prospective), published between 2007 and 2017, included 109 pediatric patients who underwent 1–6 dilations each, with an average 1.8 dilations per patient. Follow-up ranged from 5 days to 7 years (3, 29–37). Included studies are summarized on **Table 3**.

Success was defined as an improvement of symptoms, decrease in Myer-Cotton level of stenosis, decannulation of previous tracheostomy, or avoidance of reconstructive surgeries and tracheostomy in all studies. Success rate ranged from 66 to 100%, with a total of 97 of the 109 patients (88.99%) reaching a successful outcome.

None of the studies described complications of the procedure. Avelino et al. described that four patients presented dysphagia in the post-operative period, but they do not specify whether these patients had previous acute or chronic SGS (3).

Balloon Adjunctive Treatments

Mitomycin-C

Mitomycin-C is an antibiotic produced by *Strepnomyces caespitosus* exhibiting antiproliferative and antineoplastic properties. It inhibits fibroblast proliferation and synthesis of extracellular matrix proteins, and thereby modulates wound healing and scarring.

Ortiz et al. described 16 children presenting SGS managed with balloon dilation and topical application of mitomycin solution 1 mg/mL in the dilated area for 1 min, reporting a 100% success rate. Authors describe that laryngoscopy was performed as soon as symptoms appeared, but do not specify the time interval between extubation and examination. Mean number of dilation procedures was 2.5, and the number of sessions was proportional to the grade of stenosis (39).

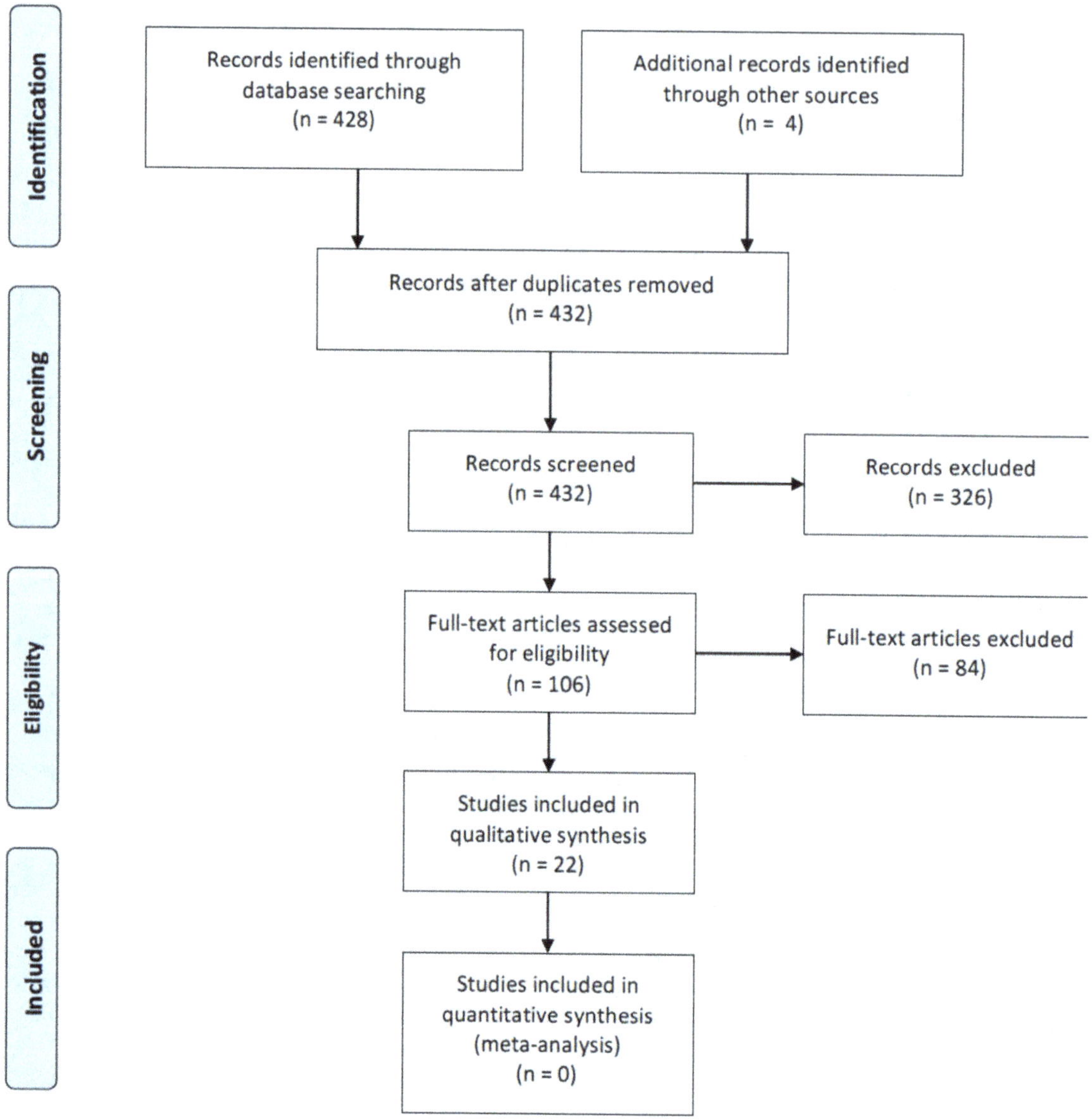

FIGURE 1 | PRISMA flow diagram.

Endoscopic Anterior Cricoid Split (EACS)

Open surgical approach was first described by Cotton as an alternative to performing tracheotomy in premature infants with prolonged intubation. As the aim of the present review is conservative treatments, only EACS is reviewed.

Mirabile et al. (40) described for the first time EBD-associated EACS. They reported five acquired stenosis patients without tracheostomy in whom a 100% success rate was attained. After this first study, Chen et al. (36) described three children presenting acute SGS undergoing EBD + EACS with a success rate of 66.7%. Similarly, Horn et al. (41) described success with the technique in two out of three children presenting extubation failure. Carr et al. (42) described a 100% success rate in five intubated children with extubation failure, using this same approach.

Rigid Dilation

The literature search identified 14 abstracts about rigid dilation. After review of the full-length articles, only one of those studies clearly separated acute and chronic lesion groups, which was eventually included (4).

Dilations were performed with increasing diameter endotracheal tubes, depending on the patient's age. Dilation was started with Silastic (a portmanteau of "silicone"and "plastic") bougies when stenosis prevented the introduction of a 2.5 mm endotracheal tubes. In 12 patients, adjuvant treatment was administered locally, but authors did not separate groups (acute or chronic) for this intervention. Success rate was 96.4% (27/28) and researchers determined that acute stenosis was a predictor of success, while chronic stenosis showed a success rate of 57.1%.

TABLE 3 | Balloon dilation: case reports and case series (n = 109).

Author, year. Retrospective X prospective	Number of patients. Age	Description of the type of SGS. Grade of SGS	Number of dilations. Mean number of dilations per patient	Adjuvant treatment	Success rate. Follow-up length
Durden and Sobol (29). Retrospective case series	Four patients. 3–7 mo	Soft. Grades 2–3	1–2 dilations per patient. Mean: 1.2	Topical steroid applied + intubation for 24–48h + systemic steroid	75% success.[a] Mean of 3.5 months of follow-up
Rossetti et al. (30). Retrospective case report	One patient. 10 mo	Acute. Grade 3	1 dilation.	None	100% success. 5 days of follow-up
Schweiger et al. (31). Prospective case series	Eight patients. 2–14 mo	Acute (<60 days after intubation, with GT). Grades 1–3	1–2 dilations per patient. Mean: 1.37 dilations per patient	Systemic steroids	100% success. 6 months of follow-up
Collins et al. (32). Retrospective case series	Two patients.[b] 1 mo (both)	Thin, circumferential SGS. Grade 3	2 dilations. Mean: 1	Topical Mitomycin (1 patient) and topical triamcinolone (1 patient)	100% success. 1–23 months of follow-up
Whigham et al. (33). Retrospective case series	Nine patients.[c] 1–31 mo (mean = 10.8 mo)	Soft. Grade 2–3	14 dilations. Mean: 1.55 per patient	None	66% success. 12–24 months of follow-up
Filiz and Ulualp (34). Retrospective case series	Three patients. 14 weeks-1 yo	Acute (5 days to 6 weeks after extubation). Grades 2–3	3–4 dilations per patient. Mean: 3.33 per patient	Systemic steroids	100% success. 14–21 months of follow-up
Avelino et al. (3). Retrospective	17 patients.[d] Mean: 4.2 mo	Acute (<30 days after extubation). Grades 1–3	Mean: 2 dilations per patient.	Oral prednisolone + steroid nebulization	100% success. 3–15 months of follow-up (mean 7.8 months)
Ozturk et al. (35). Retrospective case report	One patient. 23 days-old	Acute. Grade 3	2 dilations.		100% success. 8 months of follow-up
Alshammari et al. (37). Retrospective	45 patients.[e] 1 mo–15 yo	40 soft, 5 mature. Grades 1–3	1–6 dilations per patient. Mean: 2	1–2 ml Kenalog	82.3% success. 1 year of follow-up
Chen et al. (36). Retrospective	19 patients.[f] 0.3–144 mo (mean = 4 mo)	Acute. Grades 2–4.	1–8 dilations per patient. Mean: 2.6 per patient		100% success. 0.5–7 years of follow-up

mo, months-old; yo, years-old; SGS, subglottic stenosis; GT, granulation tissue.

[a] *One patient in the study needed a tracheostomy.*

[b] *Only patients number two and four were included in this analysis (not clearly described in the paper if the other three patients presented acute or chronic lesions).*

[c] *Only nine patients with soft stenosis and primary balloon dilation (excluded those who underwent adjuvant balloon dilation and those who had firm lesions).*

[d] *Only patients with acute lesions were included in this analysis.*

[e] *Authors described 40 patients with acute lesions and five with chronic ones. They do not separate outcomes of acute and chronic lesions, but since chronic ones accounted for only 12.5% of their patients, it was decided to include all their patients in this analysis.*

[f] *Only patients with acute SGS and who underwent balloon dilation were included in the analysis. Of the 22 patients with acute lesions, three were excluded because they were submitted to balloon dilation + endoscopic anterior cricoid split.*

CO_2 Laser and Coblation

Studies concerning different laser and coblation techniques in laryngeal stenosis deal mainly with chronic stenosis (43–46). Regarding acute lesions, a study by Koufman et al. (47) was found describing five non-tracheostomized patients undergoing stenosis treatment with carbon dioxide (CO_2) surgical laser. Two of them needed tracheostomy, but eventually were decannulated. Dilation and steroid injection were adjunctive measures. Bollig and Gov-Ari (48) described a 9-months-old girl successfully managed with bipolar radiofrequency plasma ablation (coblation) after prior multiple endoscopic balloon dilations.

Microdebrider

Rees et al. (49) described one case of subglottic granulation treated with microdebrider. This was the sole publication reporting the use of this technique in acute lesions.

DISCUSSION

In 1984, Cotton stated that endoscopic techniques were effective in the early phases of wound healing, when the scar tissue is soft and pliable (50). Since then, many techniques have been described, with variable rates of success. Recent technological advances have facilitated endoscopic approaches that promise fewer wound complications, decreased postoperative pain, shortened hospital stays, and no external scarring (40). The success of endoscopic techniques for acute stenosis is defined by the long-term resolution of stenosis and the avoidance of open surgery such as laryngotracheal reconstruction.

Rigid dilations have been used for a long time, with highly variable and essentially disappointing results (51, 52). Rigid dilation studies found in this review do not report clear inclusion criteria especially concerning mature or in evolution stenosis status. Also, miscellaneous etiologies and different age groups were enrolled. Furthermore, reported dilatation techniques and

TABLE 4 | Comparison of therapeutic approaches success rates.

Therapeutic option in acute laryngeal lesions	Success rates*
Elective endotracheal intubation	60 (10)–95.6%(9)
EBD	66 (33)–100% (36)
EBD + mitomycin-C	100% (39)
EBD + EACS	66.7 (36)–100% (40)
Rigid dilation	96.4% (4)
CO_2 laser	60% (47)
Coblation	1 successful case (48)
Microdebrider	1 successful case (49)

EBD, Endoscopic Balloon Dilation; EACS, Endoscopic Anterior Cricoid Split.
**Included studies did not report on complications rates from therapeutic approaches.*

ancillary treatments are heterogeneous. It is known that although this technique is effective, significant sheer forces are generated across the area of stenosis, and ongoing serial dilatations are often required. Studies on rigid dilation showed the need of a high number of repeated dilations but again did not segregate chronic from acute lesions. The only one found stratifying this information reported a mean number of procedures of two and a success rate of 96.4%.

Balloon dilation emerged as a promising alternative to those dilations with bougies, bronchoscopes and endotracheal tubes. It was initially designed for endovascular interventions and later adapted for use in tracheobronchial stenoses by interventional radiologists and pediatric surgeons (12, 13). The absence of shearing forces minimizes subglottic trauma, both at the mucosal level and in deeper planes, thereby decreasing the tendency to re-stenosis. As with conventional dilation techniques, balloon dilation is more likely to succeed in the presence of immature scar tissue (15).

While the number of reports on balloon dilation is still currently small, encouraging reports of this simple technique suggest that balloon dilation is probably the single most promising treatment for acute subglottic stenosis.

There is very little information available in the literature to guide balloon sizing, inflation pressure and length of inflation time. Currently, surgeons often use their own breadth of experience to guide the parameters used in the procedure. Excessively high inflation pressures or big balloon sizes can damage or rupture the airway, and inadequately low pressures or small balloon sizes can reduce the effectiveness of procedures and result in the requirement for even more procedures.

Lee et al. (28) was excluded of the balloon dilation analysis, but interestingly its results showed that, independently of the kind of therapy (bougination, incision using cold knife or laser, and balloon dilation), the success rate for acute SGS (within 30 days after extubation) is 88.8%, compared to 9.09% for chronic stenosis (more than 30 days after extubation). Their success rate sharply equals the success rate of this systematic review (88.99%). In the discussion, authors mention that the success rate is probably related to the SGS grade and nature of the scar tissue, since fine membranous scars and acute membranous type of SGS (immature scar tissue) can be expanded more easily than total cartilaginous fibrosis (mature scar tissue).

However, since the outcome of the dilation was not 100% in many studies, adjuvant therapies, such as steroid local injection, systemic steroids have been added to the therapeutic options in some cases. As we could notice in this systematic review, evidences about these adjuvant therapies are scarce. Also concerning other approaches such as CO_2 laser, coblation and microdebridor, further studies are necessary in acute lesions to settle debate over those specific treatments.

The establishment of endoscopic management protocols is complex due to technique variability and multiplicity among different institutions and patient's individual characteristics. Success of endoscopic treatment is probably also significantly influenced by the skill and ability of the collaborative staff, especially anesthesiologists and neonatal/pediatric critical care specialists. **Table 4** summarizes success rates from therapeutic approaches discussed in this review.

As far as authors are concerned, if the acute lesion is restricted to subglottis, EBD is the best option. In the postoperative period, steroid nebulization and proton pump inhibitor use has become a promising adjuvant treatment. Review laryngoscopy around the seventh postoperative day should always be performed, or even earlier if symptoms become noticeable. Procedure may be repeated many times, as long as the subglottic lumen is improving with each dilation. If the lumen is still not good enough after the second dilation, adjuvant treatment as topic steroids are advisable. Authors do not recommend more than 4 dilations–if the patient would require more than 4 dilations, it seems reasonable to change the therapeutic approach. When there is an associated glottic lesion or widespread airway edema or granulation tissue, reintubation with a one-or two-size smaller endotracheal tube with topical application of a steroid ointment for 48–72 h seems to be an attractive approach. Soon after extubation, we also recommend the use of inhaled corticosteroid and proton pump inhibitor.

Future studies should examine the effects of different balloon diameters and pressures, the role of adjuvant therapies such as steroid local injections and systemic steroids, and also the difference between rigid and balloon dilation. There are currently no evidence-based guidelines for the treatment of post-intubation acute laryngeal lesions, and the clinical experience of each team often guides the therapeutic approach.

AUTHOR CONTRIBUTIONS

CS and DM participated in study design, search strategy elaboration, peer-review, narrative review, manuscript writing, and final revision.

REFERENCES

1. Schweiger C, Manica D, Pereira DRR, Carvalho PRA, Piva JP, Kuhl G, et al. Undersedation is a risk factor for the development of subglottic stenosis in intubated children. *J Pediatr.* (2017) 93:351–5. doi: 10.1016/j.jped.2016.10.006
2. Manica D, Schweiger C, Marostica PJ, Kuhl G, Carvalho PR. Association between length of intubation and subglottic stenosis in children. *Laryngoscope.* (2013) 123:1049–54. doi: 10.1002/lary.23771
3. Avelino M, Maunsell R, Jube Wastowski I. Predicting outcomes of balloon laryngoplasty in children with subglottic stenosis. *Int J Pediatr Otorhinolaryngol.* (2015) 79:532–6. doi: 10.1016/j.ijporl.2015.01.022
4. Cuestas G, Rodriguez V, Doormann F, Bellia Munzon P, Bellia Munzon G. Endoscopic treatment of acquired subglottic stenosis in children: predictors of success. *Arch Argent Pediatr.* (2018) 116:418–25. doi: 10.5546/aap.2018.eng.422
5. Schweiger C, Manica D, Kuhl G, Sekine L, Marostica PJ. Post-intubation acute laryngeal injuries in infants and children: a new classification system. *Int J Pediatr Otorhinolaryngol.* (2016) 86:177–82. doi: 10.1016/j.ijporl.2016.04.032
6. Rutter MJ, Cohen AP, De Alarcon A. Endoscopic airway management in children. *Curr Opin Otolaryngol Head Neck Surg.* (2008) 16:525–9. doi: 10.1097/MOO.0b013e3283184479
7. Hutton B, Salanti G, Caldwell DM, Chaimani A, Schmid CH, Cameron C, et al. The PRISMA extension statement for reporting of systematic reviews incorporating network meta-analyses of health care interventions: checklist and explanations. *Ann Intern Med.* (2015) 162:777–84. doi: 10.7326/M14-2385
8. Shamseer L, Moher D, Clarke M, Ghersi D, Liberati A, Petticrew M, et al. Preferred reporting items for systematic review and meta-analysis protocols (PRISMA-P) 2015: elaboration and explanation. *BMJ.* (2015) 349:g7647. doi: 10.1136/bmj.g7647
9. Hoeve LJ, Eskici O, Verwoerd CD. Therapeutic reintubation for post-intubation laryngotracheal injury in preterm infants. *Int J Pediatr Otorhinolaryngol.* (1995) 31:7–13. doi: 10.1016/0165-5876(94)01061-2
10. Graham JM. Formal reintubation for incipient neonatal subglottic stenosis. *J Laryngol Otol.* (1994) 108:474–8. doi: 10.1017/S0022215100127148
11. Monnier P, Bernath MA, Chollet-Rivier M, Cotting J, George M, Perez MH. *Pediatric Airway Surgery: Management of Laryngotracheal Stenosis in Infants and Children* Lausanne: Springer.
12. Cohen MD, Weber TR, Rao CC. Balloon dilatation of tracheal and bronchial stenosis. *AJR Am J Roentgenol.* (1984) 142:477–8. doi: 10.2214/ajr.142.3.477
13. Hebra A, Powell DD, Smith CD, Othersen HBJr. Balloon tracheoplasty in children: results of a 15-year experience. *J Pediatr Surg.* (1991) 26:957–61. doi: 10.1016/0022-3468(91)90843-I
14. Elkerbout SC, Van Lingen RA, Gerritsen J, Roorda RJ. Endoscopic balloon dilatation of acquired airway stenosis in newborn infants: a promising treatment. *Arch Dis Child.* (1993) 68:37–40. doi: 10.1136/adc.68.1_Spec_No.37
15. Axon PR, Hartley C, Rothera MP. Endoscopic balloon dilatation of subglottic stenosis. *J Laryngol Otol.* (1995) 109:876–9. doi: 10.1017/S0022215100131561
16. Wentzel JL, Ahmad SM, Discolo CM, Gillespie MB, Dobbie AM, White DR. Balloon laryngoplasty for pediatric laryngeal stenosis: case series and systematic review. *Laryngoscope.* (2014) 124:1707–12. doi: 10.1002/lary.24524
17. Gungor A. Balloon dilation of the pediatric airway: potential for disaster. *Am J Otolaryngol.* (2012) 33:147–9. doi: 10.1016/j.amjoto.2011.05.004
18. Guarisco JL, Yang CJ. Balloon dilation in the management of severe airway stenosis in children and adolescents. *J Pediatr Surg.* (2013) 48:1676–81. doi: 10.1016/j.jpedsurg.2012.12.035
19. Gunaydin RO, Suslu N, Bajin MD, Kuscu O, Yilmaz T, Unal OF, et al. Endolaryngeal dilatation versus laryngotracheal reconstruction in the primary management of subglottic stenosis. *Int J Pediatr Otorhinolaryngol.* (2014) 78:1332–6. doi: 10.1016/j.ijporl.2014.05.022
20. Lisy J, Groh D, Chovanec M, Markova M, Suchanek V, Polaskova P, et al. Balloon dilatation of pediatric subglottic laryngeal stenosis during the artificial apneic pause: experience in 5 children. *Biomed Res Int.* (2014) 2014:397295. doi: 10.1155/2014/397295
21. Bent JP, Shah MB, Nord R, Parikh SR. Balloon dilation for recurrent stenosis after pediatric laryngotracheoplasty. *Ann Otol Rhinol Laryngol.* (2010) 119:619–27. doi: 10.1177/000348941011900909
22. Hautefort C, Teissier N, Viala P, Van Den Abbeele T. Balloon dilation laryngoplasty for subglottic stenosis in children: 8 years' experience. *Arch Otolaryngol Head Neck Surg.* (2012) 138:235–40. doi: 10.1001/archoto.2011.1439
23. Maturo SC, Hartnick CJ. Pediatric airway balloon dilation. *Adv Otorhinolaryngol.* (2012) 73:112–5. doi: 10.1159/000334461
24. Chueng K, Chadha NK. Primary dilatation as a treatment for pediatric laryngotracheal stenosis: a systematic review. *Int J Pediatr Otorhinolaryngol.* (2013) 77:623–8. doi: 10.1016/j.ijporl.2013.02.003
25. Maresh A, Preciado DA, O'connell AP, Zalzal GH. A comparative analysis of open surgery vs endoscopic balloon dilation for pediatric subglottic stenosis. *JAMA Otolaryngol Head Neck Surg.* (2014) 140:901–5. doi: 10.1001/jamaoto.2014.1742
26. Talwar R, Virk JS, Bajaj Y. Paediatric subglottic stenosis–have things changed? Our experience from a developing tertiary referral centre. *Int J Pediatr Otorhinolaryngol.* (2015) 79:2020–2. doi: 10.1016/j.ijporl.2015.08.031
27. Bavishi A, Boss E, Shah RK, Lavin J. Outcomes after endoscopic dilation of laryngotracheal stenosis: an analysis of ACS-NSQIP. *J Clin Outcomes Manag.* (2018) 25:111−6.
28. Lee JC, Kim MS, Kim DJ, Park DH, Lee IW, Roh HJ, et al. Subglottic stenosis in children: our experience at a pediatric tertiary center for 8 years in South Korea. *Int J Pediatr Otorhinolaryngol.* (2019) 121:64–7. doi: 10.1016/j.ijporl.2019.02.044
29. Durden F, Sobol SE. Balloon laryngoplasty as a primary treatment for subglottic stenosis. *Arch Otolaryngol Head Neck Surg.* (2007) 133:772–5. doi: 10.1001/archotol.133.8.772
30. Rossetti E, Germani A, Onofri A, Bottero S. Non-invasive ventilation with balloon dilatation of severe subglottic stenosis in a 10-months infant. *Intensive Care Med.* (2011) 37:364–5. doi: 10.1007/s00134-010-2069-0
31. Schweiger C, Smith MM, Kuhl G, Manica D, Marostica PJ. Balloon laryngoplasty in children with acute subglottic stenosis: experience of a tertiary-care hospital. *Braz J Otorhinolaryngol.* (2011) 77:711–5. doi: 10.1590/S1808-86942011000600006
32. Collins WO, Kalantar N, Rohrs HB, Silva RC. The effects of balloon dilation laryngoplasty in children with congenital heart disease. *Arch Otolaryngol Head Neck Surg.* (2012) 138:1136–40. doi: 10.1001/jamaoto.2013.676
33. Whigham AS, Howell R, Choi S, Pena M, Zalzal G, Preciado D. Outcomes of balloon dilation in pediatric subglottic stenosis. *Ann Otol Rhinol Laryngol.* (2012) 121:442–8. doi: 10.1177/000348941212100704
34. Filiz A, Ulualp SO. Long-term outcomes of balloon dilation for acquired subglottic stenosis in children. *Case Rep Otolaryngol.* (2014) 2014:304593. doi: 10.1155/2014/304593
35. Ozturk K, Erdur O, Sofiyev F, Onal IO, Annagur A. Non-invasive treatment of acquired subglottic stenosis. *J Craniofac Surg.* (2016) 27:e492–3. doi: 10.1097/SCS.0000000000002809
36. Chen C, Ni WH, Tian TL, Xu ZM. The outcomes of endoscopic management in young children with subglottic stenosis. *Int J Pediatr Otorhinolaryngol.* (2017) 99:141–5. doi: 10.1016/j.ijporl.2017.06.012
37. Alshammari J, Alkhunaizi AA, Arafat AS. Tertiary center experience with primary endoscopic laryngoplasty in pediatric acquired subglottic stenosis and literature review. *Int J Pediatr Adolesc Med.* (2017) 4:33–7. doi: 10.1016/j.ijpam.2016.11.001
38. Avelino MG, Fernandes EJ. Balloon laryngoplasty for subglottic stenosis caused by orotracheal intubation at a tertiary care pediatric hospital. *Int Arch Otorhinolaryngol.* (2014) 18:39–42. doi: 10.1055/s-0033-1358577
39. Ortiz R, Dominguez E, De La Torre C, Hernandez F, Encinas JL, Lopez-Fernandez S, et al. Early endoscopic dilation and mitomycin application in the treatment of acquired tracheal stenosis. *Eur J Pediatr Surg.* (2014) 24:39–45. doi: 10.1055/s-0033-1357754
40. Mirabile L, Serio PP, Baggi RR, Couloigner VV. Endoscopic anterior cricoid split and balloon dilation in pediatric subglottic stenosis. *Int J Pediatr Otorhinolaryngol.* (2010) 74:1409–14. doi: 10.1016/j.ijporl.2010.09.020
41. Horn DL, Maguire RC, Simons JP, Mehta DK. Endoscopic anterior cricoid split with balloon dilation in infants with failed extubation. *Laryngoscope.* (2012) 122:216–9. doi: 10.1002/lary.22155
42. Carr S, Dritsoula A, Thevasagayam R. Endoscopic cricoid split in a tertiary referral paediatric centre. *J Laryngol Otol.* (2018) 132:753–6. doi: 10.1017/S0022215118001226

43. Duncavage JA, Ossoff RH, Toohill RJ. Carbon dioxide laser management of laryngeal stenosis. *Ann Otol Rhinol Laryngol.* (1985) 94:565–9. doi: 10.1177/000348948509400608
44. Zawadzka-Glos L, Chmielik M, Gabryszewska A. The endoscopic treatment of postintubation laryngeal stenosis in children, using argon plasma coagulation. *Int J Pediatr Otorhinolaryngol.* (2003) 67:609–12. doi: 10.1016/S0165-5876(03)00064-8
45. Monnier P, George M, Monod ML, Lang F. The role of the CO2 laser in the management of laryngotracheal stenosis: a survey of 100 cases. *Eur Arch Otorhinolaryngol.* (2005) 262:602–8. doi: 10.1007/s00405-005-0948-8
46. Fastenberg JH, Roy S, Smith LP. Coblation-assisted management of pediatric airway stenosis. *Int J Pediatr Otorhinolaryngol.* (2016) 87:213–8. doi: 10.1016/j.ijporl.2016.06.035
47. Koufman JA, Thompson JN, Kohut RI. Endoscopic management of subglottic stenosis with the CO_2 surgical laser. *Otolaryngol Head Neck Surg.* (1981) 89:215–20. doi: 10.1177/019459988108900214
48. Bollig CA, Gov-Ari E. A novel use of coblation in the treatment of subglottic stenosis. *Int J Pediatr Otorhinolaryngol.* (2018) 111:108–10. doi: 10.1016/j.ijporl.2018.05.023
49. Rees CJ, Tridico TI, Kirse DJ. Expanding applications for the microdebrider in pediatric endoscopic airway surgery. *Otolaryngol Head Neck Surg.* (2005) 133:509–13. doi: 10.1016/j.otohns.2005.06.029
50. Cotton RT, Myer CM 3rd. Contemporary surgical management of laryngeal stenosis in children. *Am J Otolaryngol.* (1984) 5:360–8. doi: 10.1016/S0196-0709(84)80006-X
51. Grahne B. Operative treatment of severe chronic traumatic laryngeal stenosis in infants up to 3 years old. *Acta Otolaryngol.* (1971) 72:134–7. doi: 10.3109/00016487109122465
52. Louhimo I, Grahne B, Pasila M, Suutarinen T. Acquired laryngotracheal stenosis in children. *J Pediatr Surg.* (1971) 6:730–7. doi: 10.1016/0022-3468(71)90853-0

30

Congenital Pulmonary Airway Malformation in Children: Advantages of an Additional Trocar in the Lower Thorax for Pulmonary Lobectomy

Hiroyuki Koga [1], Takanori Ochi [1], Shunki Hirayama [2], Yukio Watanabe [2], Hiroyasu Ueno [2], Kota Imashimizu [2], Kazuhiro Suzuki [3], Ryohei Kuwatsuru [3], Kinya Nishimura [4], Geoffrey J. Lane [1], Kenji Suzuki [2] and Atsuyuki Yamataka [1]*

[1] *Department of Pediatric General and Urogenital Surgery, Juntendo University School of Medicine, Tokyo, Japan,* [2] *Department of General Thoracic Surgery, Juntendo University School of Medicine, Tokyo, Japan,* [3] *Department of Radiology, Juntendo University School of Medicine, Tokyo, Japan,* [4] *Department of Anesthesiology and Pain Medicine, Juntendo University School of Medicine, Tokyo, Japan*

Correspondence:
Hiroyuki Koga
h-koga@juntendo.ac.jp

Aim: To present the use of an additional trocar (AT) in the lower thorax during thoracoscopic pulmonary lobectomy (TPL) in children with congenital pulmonary airway malformation.

Methods: For a lower lobe TPL (LL), an AT is inserted in the 10th intercostal space (IS) in the posterior axillary line after trocars for a 5-mm 30° scope, and the surgeon's left and right hands are inserted conventionally in the 6th, 4th, and 8th IS in the anterior axillary line, respectively. For an upper lobe TPL (UL), the AT is inserted in the 9th IS, and trocars are inserted in the 5th, 3rd, and 7th IS, respectively. By switching between trocars (6th⟷8th for the scope, 4th⟷6th for the left hand, and 8th⟷10th for the right hand during LL and 5th⟷7th, 3rd⟷5th, and 7th⟷9th during UL, respectively), vital anatomic landmarks (pulmonary veins, bronchi, and feeding arteries) can be viewed posteriorly. The value of AT was assessed from blood loss, operative time, duration of chest tube insertion, requirement for post-operative analgesia, and incidence of perioperative complications.

Results: On comparing AT+ ($n = 28$) and AT– ($n = 27$), mean intraoperative blood loss (5.6 vs. 13.0 ml), operative time (3.9 vs. 5.1 h), and duration of chest tube insertion (2.2 vs. 3.4 days) were significantly decreased with AT ($p < 0.05$, respectively). Differences in post-operative analgesia were not significant. There were three complications requiring conversion to open/mini-thoracotomy: AT– ($n = 2$; bleeding), AT+: ($n = 1$; erroneous stapling).

Conclusions: An AT and switching facilitated posterior dissection during TPL in children with congenital pulmonary airway malformation enhancing safety and efficiency.

Keywords: thoracoscopic surgery, pulmonary lobectomy, congenital pulmonary airway malformation, child, anterior approach, posterior approach

INTRODUCTION

Thoracoscopic pulmonary lobectomy (TPL) is now an accepted, well-described procedure for treating congenital cystic lung disease. Reports of TPL being used for congenital pulmonary airway malformation (CPAM) are increasing, because of improvements in prenatal diagnosis and better understanding of its prognosis. In infants and children, TPL has the advantages of better cosmetic outcome, less musculoskeletal chest wall sequelae, better shoulder motility, and unimpaired future breast development compared with conventional open thoracotomy (1–3).

Being minimally invasive, TPL is associated with less post-operative pain, shorter hospitalization, and decreased long-term morbidity (4, 5); the general consensus is that while it is a safe, efficient procedure, it can be technically challenging in children because everything is physically smaller, the anatomy is often anomalous, and the working space is limited. In particular, in neonates, the distance a trocar can be inserted is limited which compromises maneuverability and the visual field. In other words, the ability to correctly identify vital structures (both normal and anomalous), assess what can be preserved or not, then safely secure the large pulmonary vessels can be so daunting, that even well-experienced pediatric surgeons with expertise have opted to wait until patients are larger if possible, rather than operate during the neonatal period.

In order to address these limitations, the concept of adding an additional trocar (AT) in the lower thorax to allow instruments and hands to be switched between trocars as required for comfort and effectiveness during a task was trialed during TPL. Here, a comparison of TPL performed with and without an AT was used to assess the impact of using an AT.

MATERIALS AND METHODS

The medical records of 55 consecutive CPAM cases treated by TPL at a single institution between June 2009 and November 2019 were reviewed retrospectively. All procedures were performed by one of two senior board-certified pediatric surgeons (AY or HK) under the direct supervision of one of five thoracic surgeons with extensive experience of TPL (KeS, YW, KI, HU, and SH).

Conventional TPL performed with an AT (AT+; five trocars) was compared with TPL performed without an AT (AT–; four trocars) for prenatal diagnosis, incidence of pre-operative infections, age and weight at surgery, blood loss, operative time, duration of chest tube insertion, requirement for post-operative analgesia, and incidence of perioperative complications.

Thoracoscopic Pulmonary Lobectomy

Essentially, TPL involves the same principles as open lobectomy, namely, isolation and division of the pulmonary artery, vein, and bronchus to the affected lobe, with separation of lung parenchyma using a combination of sharp and blunt dissection and electrocautery to define and isolate the pathologic lesion. All subjects were treated using the same equipment and devices. Details of the TPL performed in this series are described elsewhere (6–8). Briefly, after induction of general anesthesia and tracheal intubation, the patient is placed in the lateral decubitus position to allow access to the hilum both anteriorly and posteriorly. For thoracoscopy, the surgeon and assistant stand facing the patient while viewing a monitor positioned behind the patient (**Figure 1**). A closed technique is used to place the initial 5 mm optical trocar 1 cm below the inferior angle of the scapula to prevent leakage around the trocar site when an artificial pneumothorax is established to complete collapse of the lung. The initial trocar is used to define the position and status of the fissure and evaluate the general condition of the lung parenchyma and later for lung retraction. Carbon dioxide insufflated at low flow (0.5–1.0 L/min) and under low pressure (4–6 mmHg) is used to collapse the lung. A Fogarty catheter is used for single-lung ventilation. A chest tube is placed under direct vision in all cases.

Lower Lobe TPL

The initial trocar is used to retract the lung. For a left lower lobe TPL (LL), 5-mm trocars for a 5-mm 30° scope, the surgeon's left hand, and the surgeon's right hand are placed in the 6th, 4th, and 8th intercostal spaces (IS) in the anterior axillary line, respectively. The AT is placed in the 10th IS in the posterior axillary line to dissect or view vital structures, such as the pulmonary veins, bronchus, and feeding artery from a posterior perspective as well as observe the entire pulmonary artery, aortic arch, and course of the vagus nerve by switching the scope between the 6th and 8th IS trocars, the left hand between the 4th and 6th IS trocars, and the right hand between the 8th and 10th IS trocars (**Figure 2**). For a right LL, the procedure is the same, but the left and right hand trocars are reversed.

Upper Lobe TPL

For upper lobe TPL (UL), trocar positions on either side are one IS higher than for LL; i.e., 5th IS for the scope, 3rd IS for the left hand, 7th IS for the right hand, and 9th IS for the AT (**Figure 3**). The scope is switched between the 5th and 7th IS, the left hand between the 3rd and 5th IS trocars, and the right hand between the 7th and 9th IS trocars.

Middle Lobe TPL

Trocars for the scope, left hand, and right hand are placed in the 5th, 4th, and 7th IS in the anterior axillary line, respectively. To create more space between the scope trocar and the right-hand trocar, the scope trocar can be placed slightly more anteriorly than the right-hand trocar, which will prevent the scope and right-hand instruments from colliding.

Statistics/Ethics

Data were expressed as mean ± standard deviation. The Student's t-test and chi-square test were used for statistical analysis. A p-value <0.05 was considered to be statistically significant. This study was approved by the Juntendo University School of Medicine Institutional Review Board (IRB number: 17-209) and complies with the Helsinki Declaration of 1975 (revised1983).

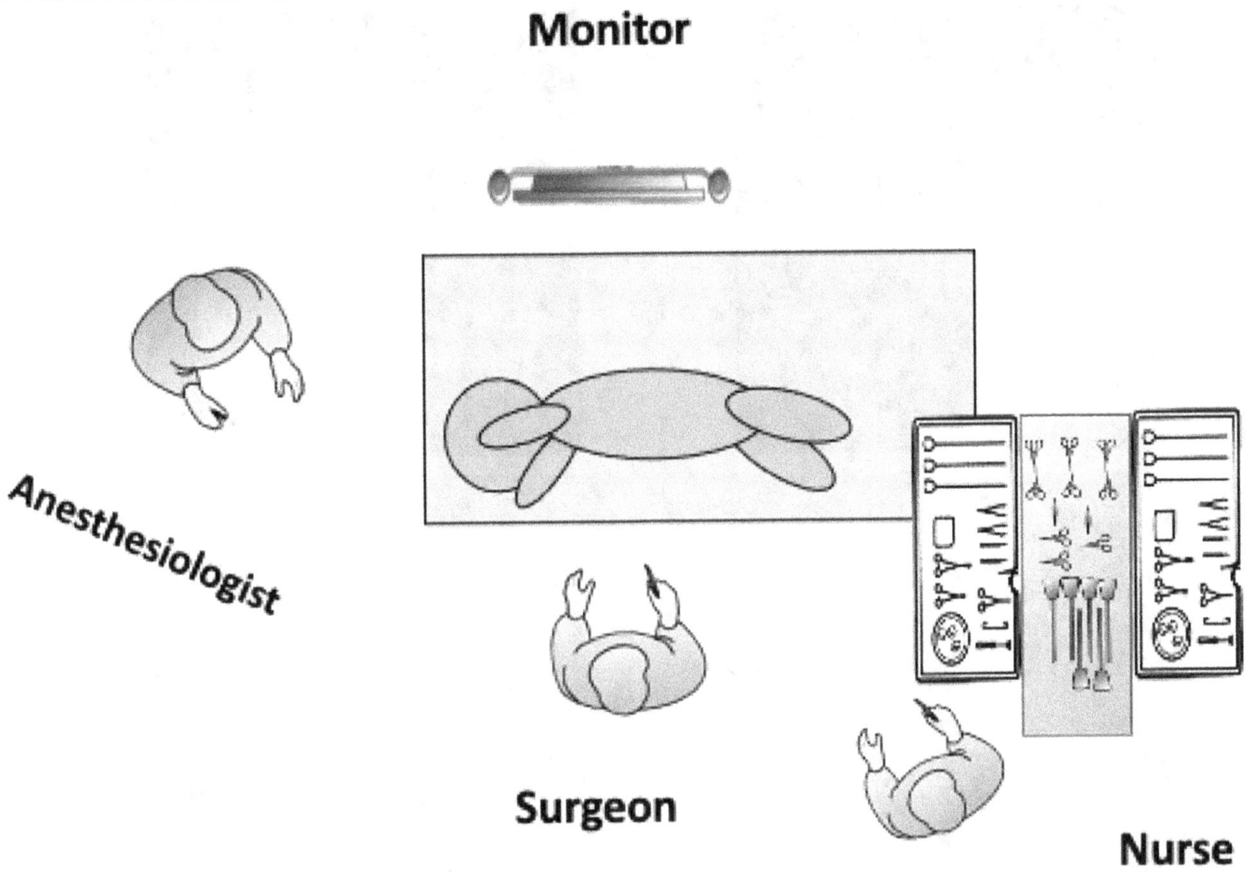

FIGURE 1 | Operating room layout and patient positioning for a left TPL. The patient is placed in the lateral decubitus position and should be placed toward the edge of the operating table in front of the operating surgeon to enhance maneuverability and prevent instruments from hitting the table. The operating surgeon stands facing the patient while viewing a monitor positioned behind the patient.

RESULTS

All 55 CPAM cases were Japanese. Groups were AT+ ($n = 28$) and AT− ($n = 27$). Both AT+ and AT− were similar for patient demographics and location of pathology. Prenatal diagnosis and incidence of pre-operative infections were not significantly different: 20 cases (71%) in AT+ vs. 20 cases (74%) in AT− for prenatal diagnosis ($p = 0.87$) and 7 cases (25%) in AT+ vs. 7 cases (28%) in AT− for pre-operative infections ($p = 0.93$), respectively. Mean ages and mean weights at TPL for AT+ and AT− were not significantly different (2.9 ± 2.3 vs. 2.6 ± 1.6 years old, $p = 0.57$, and 12.8 ± 5.1 vs. 12.0 ± 3.7 kg, $p = 0.80$, respectively). Pulmonary fissures were absent or incomplete in 13/28 (46%) cases in AT+ and 11/27 (41%) cases in AT−; these differences were not statistically significant ($p = 0.67$).

Types of TPL performed were the following: for AT+: left UL ($n = 4$), left LL ($n = 7$), right UL/right middle lobe TPL (ML) ($n = 1$), right ML/right LL ($n = 1$), right ML ($n = 2$), and right LL ($n = 13$); and for AT−: left UL ($n = 5$), left LL ($n = 10$), right UL ($n = 1$), right UL/right ML ($n = 1$), right ML ($n = 3$), and right LL ($n = 7$). There was no significant difference between AT+ and AT− for duration of post-operative analgesia (2.1 ± 1.1 vs. 2.6 ± 1.0 days; $p = 0.08$). However, differences for mean blood loss and mean operative time were significantly different between AT+ and AT− (5.6 ± 3.8 vs. 13.0 ± 5.6 ml, $p < 0.0001$ and 3.9 ± 1.5 vs. 5.1 ± 1.4 h, $p = 0.003$), respectively.

There were three intraoperative complications: bleeding from a bronchial artery during anterior-to-posterior dissection of a bronchus in AT− ($n = 2$) and accidental stapling of the Fogarty catheter used for single-lung ventilation in AT+ ($n = 1$). All three cases required conversion to open/mini-thoracotomy. Chest tubes were removed significantly earlier in AT+ than in AT− (2.2 ± 1.4 vs. 3.4 ± 2.0 days; $p = 0.01$). One case in AT− actually required a chest tube for 14 days post-operatively because of a persistent air leak from a sealed fissure.

DISCUSSION

To the best of our knowledge, this is the first report detailing the benefits of an AT in the lower thorax during TPL in children with CPAM. However, CPAM is rare (9–11), and the learning curve for TPL in children is steep. As with any surgical procedure, confidence comes from experience, and obtaining

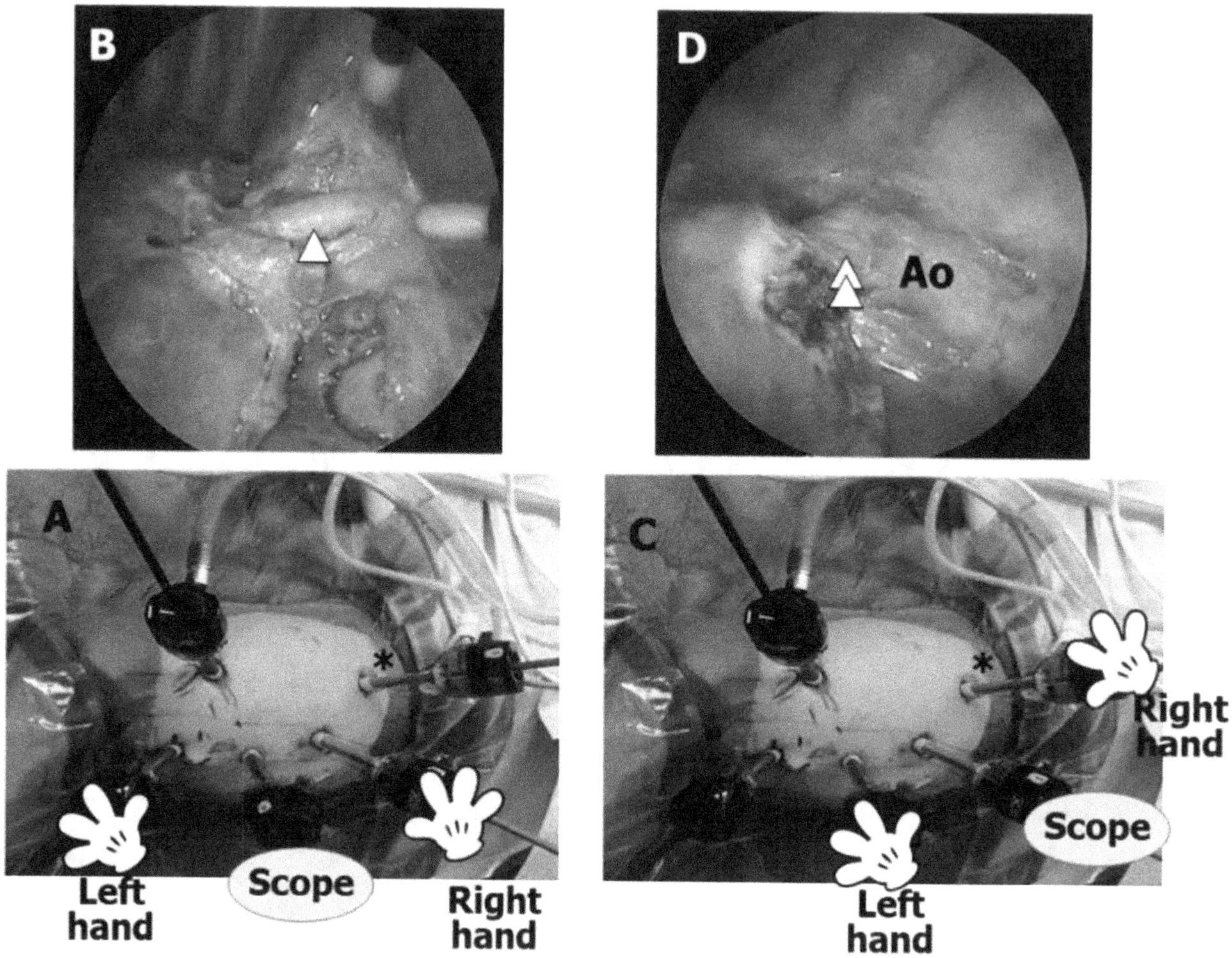

FIGURE 2 | Trocar positions for a left lower lobectomy TPL (left LL). **(A)** Most surgeons perform a LL with the scope in the 6th IS for the entire procedure without using an additional trocar (AT). **(B)** Anterior view using conventional trocar placement is adequate for dissecting the interlobar arteries, such as A8–10 (arrowhead), but dissection can only be viewed progressing in the anterior/posterior plane without viewing the posterior aspects of the bronchus and pulmonary vein and posterior mediastinum. By inserting an AT (asterisk) in the 10th IS, the same dissection can be observed from a different angle. **(C)** Asterisk shows the AT in the 10th IS. **(D)** Posterior view through the AT. The AT facilitates safe dissection of a feeding artery (double arrowhead) originating from the aorta (Ao) and visualization of the posterior aspects of the inferior pulmonary vein and left bronchus as well as the pulmonary artery, aortic arch, and course of the vagus nerve.

enough experience to perform TPL safely and efficiently is difficult. The literature reflects this, with most reports about TPL being from single specialist centers or, if they are from larger referral centers, involving few subjects. Despite improvements in technology and availability, TPL is generally considered too technically demanding for most pediatric surgeons to offer as a routine procedure. With this in mind, an AT in the lower thorax with switching between trocars as required was trialed during TPL in this series.

Conventional wisdom would dictate an anterior approach for TPL, particularly in children and especially in neonates because there is more space from the chest wall to the mediastinum where the pulmonary vessels arise. An anterior approach would also seem more logical because the visual field is easier to secure and allows hilar vascular structures to be viewed safely for orientation; dissection of bronchi and branches of pulmonary arteries could also be facilitated. However, an anterior approach is inadequate for viewing and understanding anatomic relationships in the mediastinum completely because the posterior aspects of bronchi and pulmonary veins, as well as the posterior mediastinum, cannot be viewed readily. AT trialed in this series expanded the visual field posteriorly to enable vital structures, such as the pulmonary veins, bronchi, and feeding vessels, to be inspected from a posterior perspective as well as allow the entire pulmonary artery, the aortic arch, and the vagus nerve to be viewed. Thus, by switching trocars using AT, the surgeon has access to the surgical field from all sides and can inspect and check progress from various angles, enhancing safety and reliability, especially during dissection of a feeding artery originating from the aorta and dissection of the posterior wall of the inferior pulmonary vein and bronchus during LL. During UL, A1+2, A3, and A6 branches located postero-lateral to the interlobar pulmonary artery can be

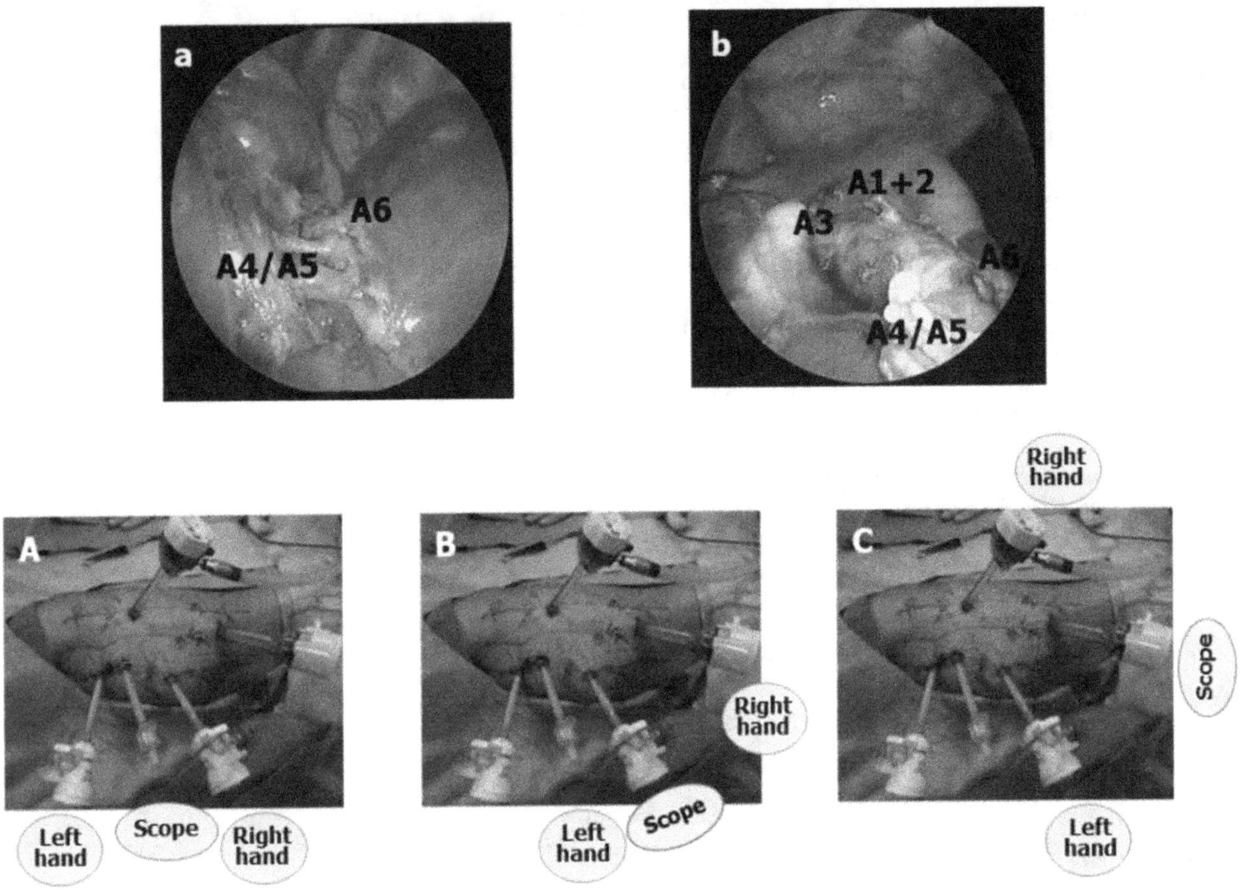

FIGURE 3 | Trocar positions for a left upper lobectomy TPL (left UL). **(A)** All trocar positions are one IS higher than for LL. By switching the scope from the 5th IS trocar to a trocar in the 7th or 9th IS, the entire course of the interlobar pulmonary artery can be visualized as well as the pulmonary hilum from the posterior mediastinum. **(B,C)** When the scope is switched from the trocar in the 5th IS to either one of the trocars in the 7th or 9th IS, interlobar pulmonary artery branches A1+2 and A3 can be observed more easily, enhancing the safety of TPL.

seen readily, ensuring added safety during TPL. In other words, without AT, the pulmonary hilum cannot be viewed from the posterior aspect throughout an entire TPL, with the result that a TPL can only be performed in the anterior–posterior plane which is stressful even for an experienced surgeon, because of the blind aspects, and further complicated if fissures are anomalous.

From experience, fissure cases can be handled with confidence by using an AT to switch instruments to view the same structures from a slightly different angle. In general, during TPL in infants and children, the view through the scope is from front to back and limited by the small size of the thorax, so treating an incomplete fissure located anteriorly, such as an incomplete fissure between S4+5 and S8 in the left lung, between the right UL and ML, or between the right ML and LL, is more difficult than treating an incomplete fissure located posteriorly, such as an incomplete fissure between S1+2 and S6 in the left lung or between the right UL and LL. Thus, by switching between trocars, there is less risk for injury because both anterior and posterior views are possible. As shown in this series, blood loss and operative time for AT+ were lower, although there were no significant differences in location or incidence of incomplete fissures between the two groups (AT+ and AT–). An AT with switching was crucial for preventing accidental injury to the pulmonary arterial wall during TPL with normal fissures but even more so when fissures were incomplete or absent.

Operator disorientation may also arise because of patient positioning during TPL. In conventional open thoracotomy, the surgeon and assistant usually stand behind the patient (5), but in TPL, they stand in front of the patient because the patient is in the lateral decubitus position. A thorough grasp of the anatomic relationships of each lobe cannot be overemphasized because intraoperatively, the three-dimensional relationships of vessels and bronchi to each lobe must be readily imaginable because the field of view through a scope is two-dimensional and everything may not be visible, so an operating surgeons must be completely comfortable with the anatomy of the lungs. In other words, anatomic relationships both normal and anomalous must be second nature, so the operating surgeon is always prepared and aware of the potential for the unexpected, especially important when no landmarks are present, for example, in cases of absent or incomplete fissure. In such patients, incising lung parenchyma that otherwise lacks superficial landmarks can cause air leakage which is one of the commonest complications of lung surgery and can require chest tube insertion if prolonged. Chest tube insertion extends hospitalization resulting in higher costs and greater risks for pleural infections. While an AT alone will not prevent air leakage absolutely, having a better grasp of the operative field from additional perspectives will provide more information about anatomic relationships (or lack thereof) and allow operating surgeons to make decisions with greater confidence.

In this series, there were three intraoperative complications. Of these, two were bleeding from bronchial arteries that occurred in AT– cases and have not occurred again since AT use became routine. The third, accidental stapling of the Fogarty catheter used for single-lung ventilation, was due to operator carelessness. Although subject numbers are limited, AT should be considered as improving safety of TPL in children.

Although there are limitations to this study because of its retrospective nature and the small number of cases, the results obtained attest to the value of using an AT, and as a result, TPL in children should really be considered a five-trocar procedure henceforth. While the concept of an AT may seem somewhat unconventional because skilled experienced surgeons can perform TPL with just three trocars, an AT with switching is a simple technique that effectively enhances safety by facilitating visualization and as shown in this series improves TPL in children with CPAM.

In conclusion, AT could be applied to any minimally invasive procedure that is challenging technically, anatomically, or logistically.

AUTHOR CONTRIBUTIONS

HK and AY designed the study. HK, TO, SH, YW, HU, KI, KaS, RK, KN, KeS, and AY were involved in clinical treatment. HK and TO collected and analyzed the data. HK and GL prepared and revised the manuscript. All authors contributed to the article and approved the submitted version.

ACKNOWLEDGMENTS

The authors would like to thank the nurses and surgeons from the Department of Pediatric General and Urogenital Surgery and Department of General Thoracic Surgery, anesthesiologists from the Department of Anesthesiology and Pain Medicine, radiologists from the Department of Radiology, operating room nursing staff, and Juntendo University Hospital administrative staff for their support and encouragement.

REFERENCES

1. Diamond IR, Herrera P, Langer JC, Kim PC. Thoracoscopic versus open resection of congenital lung lesions: a case-matched study. *J Pediatr Surg.* (2007) 42:1057–61. doi: 10.1016/j.jpedsurg.2007.01.043
2. Rothenberg SS. First decade's experience with thoracoscopic lobectomy in infants and children. *J Pediatr Surg.* (2008) 43:40–4. doi: 10.1016/j.jpedsurg.2007.09.015
3. Vu LT, Farmer DL, Nobuhara KK, Miniati D, Lee H. Thoracoscopic versus open resection for congenital cystic adenomatoid malformations of the lung. *J Pediatr Surg.* (2008) 43:35–9. doi: 10.1016/j.jpedsurg.2007.09.012
4. Lawal TA, Gosemann JH, Kuebler JF, Gluer S, Ure BM. Thoracoscopy versus thoracotomy improves midterm musculoskeletal status and cosmesis in infants and children. *Ann Thorac Surg.* (2009) 87:224–28. doi: 10.1016/j.athoracsur.2008.08.069
5. Rothenberg SS, Middlesworth W, Kadennhe-Chiweshe A, Aspelund G, Kuenzler K, Cowles R, et al. Two decades of experience with thoracoscopic lobectomy in infants and children: standardizing techniques for advanced thoracoscopic surgery. *J Laparoendosc Adv Surg Tech A.* (2015) 25:423–28. doi: 10.1089/lap.2014.0350
6. Koga H, Suzuki K, Nishimura K, Okazaki T, Lane GJ, Inada E, et al. Traction sutures allow endoscopic staples to be used safely during thoracoscopic pulmonary lobectomy in children weighing less than 15 kg. *J Laparoendosc Adv Surg Tech A.* (2013) 23:81–3. doi: 10.1089/lap.2012.0063
7. Sueyoshi R, Koga H, Suzuki K, Miyano G, Okawada M, Doi T, et al. Surgical intervention for congenital pulmonary airway malformation (CPAM) patients with preoperative pneumonia and abscess formation: "open versus thoracoscopic lobectomy". *Pediatr Surg Int.* (2016) 32:347–51. doi: 10.1007/s00383-015-3848-z
8. Yamataka A, Koga H, Ochi T, Imashimizu K, Suzuki K, Kuwatsuru R, et al. Pulmonary lobectomy techniques in infants and children. *Pediatr Surg Int.* (2017) 33:483–95. doi: 10.1007/s00383-016-4052-5
9. Duncombe GJ, Dickinson JE, Kikiros CS. Prenatal diagnosis and management of congenital cystic adenomatoid malformation of the lung. *Am J Obstet Gynecol.* (2002) 187:950–54. doi: 10.1067/mob.2002.127460
10. Laberge JM, Flageole H, Pugash D, Khalife S, Blair G, Filiatrault D, et al. Outcome of the prenatally diagnosed congenital cystic adenomatoid lung malformation: a Canadian experience. *Fetal Diagn Ther.* (2001) 16:178–86. doi: 10.1159/000053905
11. Park S, Kim ER, Hwang Y, Lee HJ, Park IK, Kim YT, et al. Serial improvement of quality metrics in pediatric thoracoscopic lobectomy for congenital lung malformation: an analysis of learning curve. *Surg Endosc.* (2017) 31:3932–38. doi: 10.1007/s00464-017-5425-0

Permissions

All chapters in this book were first published by Frontiers; hereby published with permission under the Creative Commons Attribution License or equivalent. Every chapter published in this book has been scrutinized by our experts. Their significance has been extensively debated. The topics covered herein carry significant findings which will fuel the growth of the discipline. They may even be implemented as practical applications or may be referred to as a beginning point for another development.

The contributors of this book come from diverse backgrounds, making this book a truly international effort. This book will bring forth new frontiers with its revolutionizing research information and detailed analysis of the nascent developments around the world.

We would like to thank all the contributing authors for lending their expertise to make the book truly unique. They have played a crucial role in the development of this book. Without their invaluable contributions this book wouldn't have been possible. They have made vital efforts to compile up to date information on the varied aspects of this subject to make this book a valuable addition to the collection of many professionals and students.

This book was conceptualized with the vision of imparting up-to-date information and advanced data in this field. To ensure the same, a matchless editorial board was set up. Every individual on the board went through rigorous rounds of assessment to prove their worth. After which they invested a large part of their time researching and compiling the most relevant data for our readers.

The editorial board has been involved in producing this book since its inception. They have spent rigorous hours researching and exploring the diverse topics which have resulted in the successful publishing of this book. They have passed on their knowledge of decades through this book. To expedite this challenging task, the publisher supported the team at every step. A small team of assistant editors was also appointed to further simplify the editing procedure and attain best results for the readers.

Apart from the editorial board, the designing team has also invested a significant amount of their time in understanding the subject and creating the most relevant covers. They scrutinized every image to scout for the most suitable representation of the subject and create an appropriate cover for the book.

The publishing team has been an ardent support to the editorial, designing and production team. Their endless efforts to recruit the best for this project, has resulted in the accomplishment of this book. They are a veteran in the field of academics and their pool of knowledge is as vast as their experience in printing. Their expertise and guidance has proved useful at every step. Their uncompromising quality standards have made this book an exceptional effort. Their encouragement from time to time has been an inspiration for everyone.

The publisher and the editorial board hope that this book will prove to be a valuable piece of knowledge for researchers, students, practitioners and scholars across the globe.

List of Contributors

Catherine J. Chen and Craig A. Peters
Pediatric Urology, Children's Health System Texas, University of Texas Southwestern, Dallas, TX, United States

Mohammad Ashkan Moslehi
Pediatric Interventional Pulmonology Division, Department of Pediatrics, School of Medicine, Shiraz University of Medical Sciences, Shiraz, Iran

E. Sofie van Tuyll van Serooskerken
Department of Pediatric Surgery, Pediatric Wilhelmina Children's Hospital, University Medical Center Utrecht, Utrecht, Netherlands

Stefaan H. A. J. Tytgat, Johannes W. Verweij, David C. van der Zee and Maud Y. A. Lindeboom
Department of Pediatric Surgery, Pediatric Wilhelmina Children's Hospital, University Medical Center Utrecht, Utrecht, Netherlands
Congenital Esophageal and Airway Team Utrecht, Pediatric Wilhelmina Children's Hospital, University Medical Center Utrecht, Utrecht, Netherlands

Arnold J. N. Bittermann and Saskia Coenraad
Congenital Esophageal and Airway Team Utrecht, Pediatric Wilhelmina Children's Hospital, University Medical Center Utrecht, Utrecht, Netherlands
Department of Pediatric Otorhinolaryngology, Pediatric Wilhelmina Children's Hospital, University Medical Center Utrecht, Utrecht, Netherlands

Hubertus G. M. Arets
Congenital Esophageal and Airway Team Utrecht, Pediatric Wilhelmina Children's Hospital, University Medical Center Utrecht, Utrecht, Netherlands
Department of Pediatric Pulmonology, Pediatric Wilhelmina Children's Hospital, University Medical Center Utrecht, Utrecht, Netherlands

Mario Navarrete Arellano
Hospital Central Militar, SEDENA, Mexico City, Mexico

Francisco Garibay González
Department of Pediatrics, Hospital Militar de Especialidades de la Mujer y Neonatología, SEDENA, Mexico City, Mexico

Ali Kamran and Russell W. Jennings
Department of General Surgery, Harvard Medical School, Boston Children's Hospital, Boston, MA, United States

Chenyu Liu, Kaisheng Cheng, Dengke Luo, Miao Yuan, Taozhen He and Chang Xu
Department of Pediatric Surgery, West China Hospital of Sichuan University, Chengdu, China

Xuejiao Yu
Department of Clinical Pathology, West China Hospital of Sichuan University, Chengdu, China

Ramphis A. Morales-López, Marcos Pérez-Marchán and Marcos Pérez Brayfield
Division of Urology, Department of Surgery, University of Puerto Rico School of Medicine, San Juan, PR, United States
HIMA-San Pablo Group, Caguas, PR, United States

Xiling Wu
Department of Pulmonology, The Children's Hospital, Zhejiang University School of Medicine, National Clinical Research Center for Child Health, Hangzhou, China

Alireza Basharkhah, Christoph Castellani, Michael Höllwarth, Georg Singer and Holger Till
Department of Pediatric and Adolescent Surgery, Medical University of Graz, Graz, Austria

Herwig Lackner, Anna Karastaneva, Martin Benesch and Christian Urban
Division of Pediatric Hematology-Oncology, Department of Pediatrics and Adolescent Medicine, Medical University of Graz, Graz, Austria

Marko Bergovec
Department of Orthopedics and Trauma, Medical University of Graz, Graz, Austria

Stephan Spendel
Division of Plastic, Aesthetic and Reconstructive Surgery, Department of Surgery, Medical University of Graz, Graz, Austria

Erich Sorantin
Division of Pediatric Radiology, Department of Radiology, Medical University of Graz, Graz, Austria

Bernadette Liegl-Atzwanger
Diagnostic and Research Center of Pathology, Medical University of Graz, Graz, Austria

Freyja-Maria Smolle-Jüttner
Division of Thoracic and Hyperbaric Surgery, Department of Surgery, Medical University of Graz, Graz, Austria

Ramnath Subramaniam
Consultant Paediatric Urologist, Leeds Teaching Hospitals NHS Trust, Leeds, United Kingdom
Department of Paediatric Urology, University of Leeds, Leeds, United Kingdom
Department of Paediatric Urology, University of Ghent, Ghent, Belgium

Michael Rutter
Division of Pediatric Otolaryngology, Aerodigestive and Esophageal Center, Cincinnati Children's Hospital Medical Center, Cincinnati, OH, United States

I-Chun Kuo
Division of Pediatric Otolaryngology, Aerodigestive and Esophageal Center, Cincinnati Children's Hospital Medical Center, Cincinnati, OH, United States
Department of Otolaryngology-Head and Neck Surgery, Chang Gung Memorial Hospital, Taoyuan, Taiwan

Giovanna Riccipetitoni, Mirko Bertozzi, Marta Gazzaneo, Alessandro Raffaele and Fabrizio Vatta
Department of Pediatric Surgery, Fondazione Istituti di Ricovero e Cura a Carattere Scientifico (IRCCS) Policlinico San Matteo, University of Pavia, Pavia, Italy

Walid A. Farhat
Division of Urology, Hospital for SickKids, University of Toronto, Toronto, ON, Canada

Nicolas Fernandez
Division of Urology, Hospital for SickKids, University of Toronto, Toronto, ON, Canada
Department of Urology, Fundación Santa Fe de Bogota, Bogota, Colombia
Division of Urology, Hospital Universitario San Ignacio, Pontificia Universidad Javeriana, Bogota, Colombia

Shuxian Li and Zhimin Chen
Department of Pulmonology, The Children's Hospital, Zhejiang University School of Medicine, National Clinical Research Center for Child Health, Hangzhou, China

Lei Wu
Department of Pulmonology, The Children's Hospital, Zhejiang University School of Medicine, National Clinical Research Center for Child Health, Hangzhou, China
Department of Endoscopy Center, The Children's Hospital, Zhejiang University School of Medicine, National Clinical Research Center for Child Health, Hangzhou, China

Wei Chen
Department of Endoscopy Center, The Children's Hospital, Zhejiang University School of Medicine, National Clinical Research Center for Child Health, Hangzhou, China
Department of Pediatrics, The First Affiliated Hospital of USTC, Division of Life Sciences and Medicine, University of Science and Technology of China, Hefei, China

PengCheng Li
Department of Endoscopy Center, The Children's Hospital, Zhejiang University School of Medicine, National Clinical Research Center for Child Health, Hangzhou, China
Department of Pediatrics, Affiliated Hospital of Nantong University, Nantong, China

Aylin N. Bilgutay
Department of Pediatric Urology, Children's Healthcare of Atlanta, Atlanta, GA, United States

Andrew J. Kirsch
Department of Pediatric Urology, Children's Healthcare of Atlanta, Atlanta, GA, United States
Department of Urology, Emory University School of Medicine, Atlanta, GA, United States

Marilena Trozzi, Duino Meucci, Antonio Salvati, Maria Luisa Tropiano and Sergio Bottero
Airway Surgery Unit, Pediatric Surgery Department, Bambino Gesù Children's Hospital, Rome, Italy

Farahnaz Sadegh Beigee and Kambiz Sheikhy
Department of Thoracic Surgery, Lung Transplantation Research Center, National Research Institute of Tuberculosis and Lung Diseases, Masih Daneshvari Hospital, Shahid Beheshti University of Medical Sciences, Tehran, Iran

Ali Sheikhy
Research Department, Tehran Heart Center, Tehran University of Medical Sciences, Tehran, Iran
Non-communicable Disease Research Center, Endocrinology and Metabolism Population Sciences Institute, Tehran University of Medical Sciences, Tehran, Iran

Ardavan Akhavan
Institute for Pediatric Urology, Komansky Children's Hospital, New York Presbyterian-Weill Cornell, New York, United States

John S. Barlog
SUNY Downstate Medical Center, Brooklyn, NY, United States

Marta Filauro, Francesco Mazzola, Frank Rikki Canevari and Giorgio Peretti
IRCCS Ospedale Policlinico San Martino, Genoa, Italy
Unit of Otorhinolaryngology—Head and Neck Surgery, University of Genoa, Genoa, Italy

Francesco Missale
IRCCS Ospedale Policlinico San Martino, Genoa, Italy
Unit of Otorhinolaryngology—Head and Neck Surgery, University of Genoa, Genoa, Italy
Department of Molecular and Translational Medicine, University of Brescia, Brescia, Italy

Martin Riis Ladefoged
Copenhagen Trial Unit, Department 7812, Centre for Clinical Intervention Research, Copenhagen University Hospital Rigshospitalet, Copenhagen, Denmark
Department of Clinical Medicine, University of Copenhagen, Copenhagen, Denmark

Steven Kwasi Korang
Copenhagen Trial Unit, Department 7812, Centre for Clinical Intervention Research, Copenhagen University Hospital Rigshospitalet, Copenhagen, Denmark
Department of Anesthesiology Critical Care Medicine, Childrens Hospital Los Angeles, Los Angeles, CA, United States

Simone Engmann Hildorf and Jacob Oehlenschlæger
Department of Paediatric Surgery, Copenhagen University Hospital Rigshospitalet, Copenhagen, Denmark

Susanne Poulsen and Ulrik Lausten-Thomsen
Department of Neonatology, Copenhagen University Hospital Rigshospitalet, Copenhagen, Denmark

Magdalena Fossum
Department of Clinical Medicine, University of Copenhagen, Copenhagen, Denmark
Department of Paediatric Surgery, Copenhagen University Hospital Rigshospitalet, Copenhagen, Denmark
Department of Women's and Children's Health, Karolinska Institutet, Stockholm, Sweden

Ravindra Sahadev, Katelyn Spencer, Arun K. Srinivasan, Christopher J. Long and Aseem Ravindra Shukla
Division of Pediatric Urology, Children's Hospital of Philadelphia, Philadelphia, PA, United States

Marco Roversi
Academic Department, University of Rome Tor Vergata, Rome, Italy

Federica Porcaro and Renato Cutrera
Paediatric Pulmonology and Respiratory Intermediate Care Unit, Sleep and Long-Term Ventilation Unit, Academic Department of Paediatrics, Research Institute, Bambino Gesù Children's Hospital, Rome, Italy

Paola Francalanci
Department of Pathology, Research Institute, Bambino Gesù Children's Hospital, Rome, Italy

Adriano Carotti
Unit of Pediatric Cardiac Surgery, Research Institute, Bambino Gesù Children's Hospital, Rome, Italy

Devon Michael Evanovich
Department of Anesthesiology, Critical Care and Pain Medicine, Boston Children's Hospital, Boston, MA, United States
Tufts School of Medicine, Tufts University, Boston, MA, United States

Jue Teresa Wang and Dusica Bajic
Department of Anesthesiology, Critical Care and Pain Medicine, Boston Children's Hospital, Boston, MA, United States
Harvard Medical School, Harvard University, Boston, MA, United States

Benjamin Zendejas and Russell William Jennings
Harvard Medical School, Harvard University, Boston, MA, United States
Department of Surgery, Boston Children's Hospital, Boston, MA, United States
Esophageal and Airway Treatment Center, Boston Children's Hospital, Boston, MA, United States

Patricio C. Gargollo
Division of Pediatric Urology, The Mayo Clinic and Mayo Medical School, Rochester, MN, United States

Lindsay A. White
The University of Washington School of Medicine, Seattle, WA, United States

Zhen Bing, Rui Chen, Pengchao Xing, Yueyi Ren and Kefeng Hou
Heart Center, Qingdao Women and Children's Hospital, Qingdao, China

Anna Morandi and Francesco Macchini
Department of Pediatric Surgery, Fondazione IRCCS Ca' Granda Ospedale Maggiore Policlinico, Milan, Italy

Ernesto Leva
Department of Pediatric Surgery, Fondazione IRCCS Ca' Granda Ospedale Maggiore Policlinico, Milan, Italy
Department of Clinical Sciences and Community Health, University of Milan, Milan, Italy

Valerio Gentilino
Department of Pediatric Surgery, Ospedale Filippo Del Ponte, Azienda Socio Sanitaria Territoriale Sette Laghi, Varese, Italy

Steven Scot Rothenberg
Rocky Mountain Hospital for Children, Denver, CO, United States

Natalia Ballesteros and George A. Ransford
Division of Pediatric Urology, Nicklaus Children's Hospital, Miami, FL, United States

Zachary A. Snow
Dr. Kiran C. Patel College of Osteopathic Medicine, Nova Southeastern University, Fort Lauderdale, FL, United States

Paulo R. M. Moscardi
Division of Pediatric Urology, Jackson Memorial Hospital, Miami, FL, United States

Pablo Gomez
Division of Pediatric Urology, Florida Hospital for Children, Orlando, FL, United States

Miguel Castellan
Division of Pediatric Urology, Nicklaus Children's Hospital, Miami, FL, United States
Division of Pediatric Urology, Jackson Memorial Hospital, Miami, FL, United States
Division of Pediatric Urology, Joe DiMaggio Children's Hospital, Hollywood, FL, United States

Denise Manica
Otolaryngology Department, Hospital de Clínicas de Porto Alegre, Porto Alegre, Brazil

Cláudia Schweiger
Otolaryngology Department, Hospital de Clínicas de Porto Alegre, Porto Alegre, Brazil
Programa de Pós-Graduação em Saúde da Criança e do Adolescente, Universidade Federal do Rio Grande do Sul, Porto Alegre, Brazil

Hiroyuki Koga, Takanori Ochi Geoffrey J. Lane and Atsuyuki Yamataka
Department of Pediatric General and Urogenital Surgery, Juntendo University School of Medicine, Tokyo, Japan

Shunki Hirayama, Yukio Watanabe, Hiroyasu Ueno, Kota Imashimizu and Kenji Suzuki
Department of General Thoracic Surgery, Juntendo University School of Medicine, Tokyo, Japan

Kazuhiro Suzuki and Ryohei Kuwatsuru
Department of Radiology, Juntendo University School of Medicine, Tokyo, Japan

Kinya Nishimura
Department of Anesthesiology and Pain Medicine, Juntendo University School of Medicine, Tokyo, Japan

Index

www.ingramcontent.com/pod-product-compliance
Lightning Source LLC
LaVergne TN
LVHW060057220926
848484LV00008BA/2124